Register Now for O[n] to Your Boo[k]

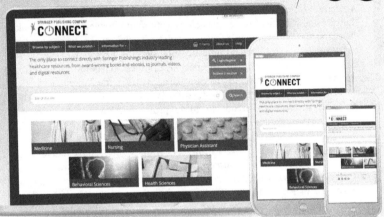

Your print purchase of *Public Health Nutrition* **includes online access to the contents of your book**—increasing accessibility, portability, and searchability!

Access today at:

http://connect.springerpub.com/content/book/978-0-8261-4685-4 or scan the QR code at the right with your smartphone and enter the access code below.

WJNRVAP2

Scan here for quick access.

SPRINGER PUBLISHING COMPANY
View all our products at springerpub.com

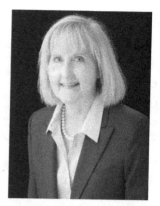

M. Margaret Barth, PhD, MPH, serves as Professor and Chair of Nutrition and Health Care Management at Appalachian State University. Dr. Barth received her PhD in Nutrition and Food Science from University of Illinois, Urbana–Champaign; MPH from University of Illinois, Chicago; MBA from The Kellogg School of Management, Northwestern University; and BS in Nutrition and Medical Dietetics from University of Illinois, Chicago. Dr. Barth has served in leadership roles in academia and food organizations in areas of nutrition, food systems, and sustainability and developed research and service learning projects in the United States, Mexico, South America, Philippines, and China. Publications include authorship of more than 50 scientific research papers along with invited review articles, book chapters, and government references on nutritional quality, public health nutrition, food safety, and community food systems. Recipient of the highest alumni award from the University of Illinois, College of Agriculture, Consumer and Environmental Sciences in 2014. In addition to professional activities in the American Public Health Association (APHA), World Public Health Nutrition Association (WPHNA), and Association of State Public Health Nutritionists (ASPHN), she serves as an advisor to nonprofit organizations.

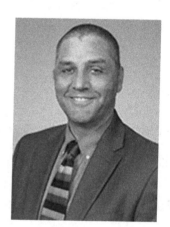

Ronny A. Bell, PhD, MS, is Professor (with Tenure) and Chair of the Department of Public Health in the Brody School of Medicine at East Carolina University (ECU). Prior to his appointment at ECU, Dr. Bell was Professor of Public Health Sciences and Director of the Maya Angelou Center for Health Equity at Wake Forest Baptist Medical Center. Dr. Bell received his undergraduate degree in Public Health Nutrition from the University of North Carolina at Chapel Hill and his master's and doctorate in Foods and Nutrition at the University of North Carolina at Greensboro. He completed a postdoctoral fellowship in Gerontology and a master's degree in Epidemiology at the Wake Forest School of Medicine. Dr. Bell's research focuses on chronic disease epidemiology and prevention in racial and ethnic minority populations with a focus on American Indian populations. He currently chairs the North Carolina Diabetes Advisory Council and the North Carolina American Indian Health Board and co-chairs the Healthy North Carolina 2030 Task Force. Nationally, he currently serves on the American Diabetes Association Health Disparities Committee.

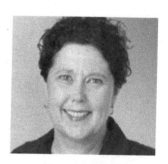

Karen Grimmer, PhD, MMedSci, CertHlthEc, is a Senior Researcher in Clinical Education and Training in the College of Nursing and Health Sciences at Flinders University in Adelaide, South Australia and Professor Extraordinaire at Stellenbosch University in Cape Town, South Africa. She served there as the scientific lead on Project SAGE (South African Guidelines Excellence), a Flagship grant from the South African Medical Research Council designing and testing new ways of producing and translating evidence effectively into primary care settings in South Africa. Dr. Grimmer is the former inaugural director of the International Centre for Allied Health Evidence (iCAHE), UniSA. She has been publishing peer-reviewed scientific articles since 1989 and has authored and co-authored more than 350 papers to date. Her scholarly work reflects public health and interprofessional health quality and service delivery issues; evidence-based practice theory, practice, and implementation; discharge planning quality and aging in place; and adolescent spinal health. Dr. Grimmer has published eight invited book chapters, conceptualized and edited two niche textbooks on evidence-based practice and clinical guidelines, and presented hundreds of conference presentations. She has established long-term, valued, and formal linkages with research institutions in South Africa, Tokyo, Manila, Hong Kong, California, and North Carolina. She was awarded the Lifetime Achievement Award in Allied Health in 2014 at the 10th Allied Health Conference in Malaysia. This award was conferred by the International Chief Allied Health Professionals Organisation. She has established The Sihlalo Outreach mission to create advantage out of disadvantage for young people through personal, societal, and professional training opportunities in Cape Town, South Africa.

PUBLIC HEALTH NUTRITION

Rural, Urban, and Global Community-Based Practice

M. Margaret Barth, PhD, MPH
Ronny A. Bell, PhD, MS
Karen Grimmer, PhD, MMedSci, CertHlthEc
Editors

Kyle L. Thompson, DCN, RDN, LDN
Adam Hege, PhD, MPA, CHES
Associate Editors

SPRINGER PUBLISHING COMPANY

No part of this publication may be reproduced, stored in a retrieval system, or transmitted in any form or by any means, electronic, mechanical, photocopying, recording, or otherwise, without the prior permission of Springer Publishing Company, LLC, or authorization through payment of the appropriate fees to the Copyright Clearance Center, Inc., 222 Rosewood Drive, Danvers, MA 01923, 978-750-8400, fax 978-646-8600, info@copyright.com or on the Web at www.copyright.com.

Springer Publishing Company, LLC
11 West 42nd Street, New York, NY 10036
www.springerpub.com
connect.springerpub.com

Acquisitions Editor: David D'Addona
Compositor: Exeter Premedia Services Private Ltd.

ISBN: 978-0-8261-4684-7
ebook ISBN: 978-0-8261-4685-4
DOI: 10.1891/9780826146854

Qualified instructors may request supplements by emailing textbook@springerpub.com
Instructor's Manual: 978-0-8261-4686-1
Test Bank: 978-0-8261-4688-5
Image Bank: 978-0-8261-4687-8
Sample Syllabus: 978-0-8261-4689-2
PowerPoints: 978-0-8261-4687-2

20 21 22 23/ 5 4 3 2 1

The author and the publisher of this Work have made every effort to use sources believed to be reliable to provide information that is accurate and compatible with the standards generally accepted at the time of publication. The author and publisher shall not be liable for any special, consequential, or exemplary damages resulting, in whole or in part, from the readers' use of, or reliance on, the information contained in this book. The publisher has no responsibility for the persistence or accuracy of URLs for external or third-party Internet websites referred to in this publication and does not guarantee that any content on such websites is, or will remain, accurate or appropriate.

Library of Congress Cataloging-in-Publication Data

Names: Barth, M. Margaret, editor. | Bell, Ronny A., editor. |
   Grimmer-Somers, Karen, editor. | Thompson, Kyle L., editor. | Hege,
   Adam, editor.
Title: Public health nutrition : rural, urban, and global community-based
   practice / M. Margaret Barth, Ronny A. Bell, Karen Grimmer, editors;
   Kyle L. Thompson, Adam Hege, associate editors.
Other titles: Public health nutrition (Barth)
Description: New York, NY: Springer Publishing Company, LLC, [2020] |
   Includes bibliographical references and index.
Identifiers: LCCN 2020000603 (print) | LCCN 2020000604 (ebook) | ISBN
   9780826146847 (paperback) | ISBN 9780826146861 (instructor's manual) |
   ISBN 9780826146885 (test bank) | ISBN 9780826146878 (image bank) | ISBN
   9780826146892 (sample syllabus) | ISBN 9780826146854 (ebook) | ISBN
   9780826146872 (PowerPoints)
Subjects: MESH: Diet, Healthy | Public Health | Community Health Services |
   Global Health | Rural Population | Urban Population
Classification: LCC RA427.8 (print) | LCC RA427.8 (ebook) | NLM QT 235 |
   DDC 362.1—dc23
LC record available at https://lccn.loc.gov/2020000603
LC ebook record available at https://lccn.loc.gov/2020000604

Contact us to receive discount rates on bulk purchases.
We can also customize our books to meet your needs.
For more information please contact: sales@springerpub.com

Publisher's Note: **New and used products purchased from third-party sellers are not guaranteed for quality, authenticity, or access to any included digital components.**

Printed in the United States of America.

To the public health nutrition leaders of the future, that their efforts would encourage and bless all those they serve.

CONTENTS

3. **Nutrition Epidemiology Research Methods**   *43*
Erin Bouldin, Karen Grimmer, Jamie Griffin, M. Margaret Barth, and Ronny A. Bell

4. **Behavioral Aspects of Public Health Nutrition**   *69*
Karen Chapman-Novakofski and Kristen N. DiFilippo

PART II: CULTURAL ASPECTS OF PUBLIC HEALTH NUTRITION

PART IV: CURRENT AND FUTURE CHALLENGES IN PUBLIC HEALTH NUTRITION AND SUSTAINABILITY

CONTRIBUTORS

Becky Adams, DrPH, RD, CDE, Director, Partnership and Policy Support/Section Chief, Nutrition and Physical Activity, Association of State Public Health Nutritionists, Little Rock, Arkansas

Alice Ammerman, DrPH, Mildred Kaufman Distinguished Professor, Department of Nutrition, Gillings School of Global Public Health and Director, Center for Health Promotion and Disease Prevention, University of North Carolina at Chapel Hill, Chapel Hill, North Carolina

Olivia Anderson, PhD, RD, Clinical Assistant Professor, Department of Nutritional Sciences, School of Public Health, University of Michigan, Ann Arbor, Michigan

M. Margaret Barth, PhD, MPH, Professor and Chair, Department of Nutrition and Health Care Management, Appalachian State University, Boone, North Carolina

Ronny A. Bell, PhD, MS, Professor and Chair, Department of Public Health, East Carolina University, Greenville, North Carolina

Erin Bouldin, PhD, Assistant Professor, Department of Health and Exercise Science, Appalachian State University, Boone, North Carolina

Hilary A. Campbell, **PharmD, JD,** Research Associate, Margolis Center for Health Policy, Duke University, Durham, North Carolina

Karen Chapman-Novakofski, PhD, RDN, Professor, Department of Food Science and Human Nutrition, College of Agricultural, Consumer and Environmental Sciences, University of Illinois at Urbana–Champaign, Urbana, Illinois

John Coveney, PhD, Professor, Global Food, Culture and Health, Flinders University, Adelaide, South Australia

David N. Cox, PhD, Principal Research Scientist, CSIRO Health and Biosecurity, Adelaide, South Australia

Joanna Cummings, MS, RD, CNSC, Director, OHSU-Lao Nutrition Education and Research Partnership, Instructor, Oregon Health & Science University, Portland, Oregon

Amy Dailey, PhD, MPH, Associate Professor, Department of Health Sciences, Director of Community Based Learning and Research, Gettysburg College, Gettysburg, Pennsylvania

Arelis Moore de Peralta, MD, PhD, MPH, MEd, Assistant Professor of Community Health, Department of Languages, Clemson University, Clemson, South Carolina

Jigna M. Dharod, PhD, Associate Professor, Director of Graduate Studies, Department of Nutrition, University of North Carolina at Greensboro, Greensboro, North Carolina

Kristen N. DiFilippo, PhD, RDN, Teaching Assistant Professor, Department of Kinesiology and Community Health, College of Agricultural, Consumer and Environmental Sciences, University of Illinois at Urbana–Champaign, Champaign, Illinois

Michelle Eichinger, MS, MPA, Doctoral Student, Department of Planning, Design and the Built Environment, Clemson University, Clemson, South Carolina

Alisha Farris, PhD, RD, CSP, Assistant Professor of Nutrition, Department of Nutrition and Health Care Management, Beaver College of Health Sciences, Appalachian State University, Boone, North Carolina

Claude Fischler, PhD, Directeur de recherche CNRS emeritus, IIAC, Ecole des Hautes Etudes en Sciences Sociales, Paris, France

Jamie Griffin, PhD, RD, Assistant Professor, Department of Nutrition, Appalachian State University, Boone, North Carolina

Karen Grimmer, PhD, MMedSci, CertHlthEc, Former Director, Center for Allied Health Evidence, University of Flinders, Adelaide, South Australia; Professor Extraordinaire, Faculty of Medical and Health Science, Stellenbosch University, Cape Town, South Africa; Senior Researcher, College of Nursing and Health Sciences, Flinders University, Adelaide, South Australia; Adjunct Professor, Faculty of Medicine, University of Santo Tomas, Manila, Philippines

Melissa Gutschall, PhD, RD, LDN, Associate Professor and Director, Appalachian State University Graduate Program in Nutrition, Department of Nutrition and Health Care Management, Beaver College of Health Sciences, Appalachian State University, Boone, North Carolina

Carol Anne Hartwick-Pflaum, PhD, Flinders University, Adelaide, South Australia

Nihal Destan Aytekin Hatik, MSc, Knowledge Management Specialist, HarvestPlus, International Food Policy Research Institute (IFPRI), Washington, District of Columbia

Lindsey Haynes-Maslow, PhD, MHA, Assistant Professor and Extension Specialist, Department of Agricultural and Human Sciences, North Carolina State University, Raleigh, North Carolina

Adam Hege, PhD, MPA, CHES, Assistant Professor and Public Health Program Director, Department of Health and Exercise Science, Beaver College of Health Sciences, Appalachian State University, Boone, North Carolina

Amanda S. Hege, MPH, RDN, LD, Sustainable Food Systems Project Manager, Academy of Nutrition and Dietetics Foundation, Chicago, Illinois; Former Director of Community Outreach, University of Kentucky, Lexington, Kentucky

Caitlin Hildebrand, MD, MPH, Graduate Research Assistant, UNC Center for Health Promotion and Disease Prevention and Department of Nutrition, University of North Carolina at Chapel Hill, Chapel Hill, North Carolina

Leslie Hossfeld, PhD, Dean, College of Behavioral, Social and Health Sciences, Clemson University, Clemson, South Carolina

Sonya Jones, PhD, Associate Professor, Department of Health Promotion, Education and Behavior, University of South Carolina, Columbia, South Carolina

Maria Julian, MPA, Director of Community Health Services, Appalachian District Health Department, AppHealthCare, Boone, North Carolina

Dennis Lanigan, Organic Farmer, Hendersonville, North Carolina

Danielle L. Nunnery, PhD, RDN, LDN, Assistant Professor, Department of Nutrition and Health Care Management, Leon Levine Hall of Health Sciences, Appalachian State University, Boone, North Carolina

Kendra Oo, MS, RD, LD, Director of Community Outreach, Department of Dietetics and Human Nutrition, University of Kentucky, Lexington, Kentucky

Stephanie Bell Jilcott Pitts, PhD, Professor, Department of Public Health, East Carolina University, Greenville, North Carolina

Karen L. Probert, MS, RDN, Executive Director, Association of State Public Health Nutritionists, Tucson, Arizona

Dominique M. Rose, PhD, MPH, Program Manager, Department of Population and Quantitative Health Sciences, Mary Ann Swetland Center for Environmental Health, Case Western Reserve University, Cleveland, Ohio

Lauren R. Sastre, PhD, RDN, LDN, Assistant Professor, Department of Nutrition Science, East Carolina University, Health Sciences Building, Greenville, North Carolina

Courtney Schand, MS, RDN, LDN, Owner, Registered Dietitian, CS Nutrition, Nashville, Tennessee

Jessica Soldavini, MPH, RD, LDN, Graduate Research Assistant, UNC Center for Health Promotion and Disease Prevention and Department of Nutrition, University of North Carolina at Chapel Hill, Chapel Hill, North Carolina

Marsha Spence, PhD, MPH, RDN, LDN, Associate Professor of Practice, Director, Public Health Nutrition Graduate Program, University of Tennessee, Knoxville, Tennessee

Gizem Templeton, PhD, Associate in Research, World Food Policy Center, Sanford School of Public Policy, Duke University, Durham, North Carolina

Kyle L. Thompson, DCN, RDN, LDN, Assistant Professor of Nutrition, Coordinator, Appalachian State University Graduate Programs in Public Health Nutrition, Department of Nutrition and Health Care Management, Beaver College of Health Sciences, Appalachian State University, Boone, North Carolina

FOREWORD

Public health nutrition is concerned with promoting and maintaining the nutritional health of populations. While grounded in nutritional science, the practice of public health nutrition must take a public health approach that considers the cultural, political, economic, and environmental influences on how local, national, and global communities access and use food for optimum nutrition. Food security, which is defined by sustainable access to adequate, safe, and nutritious food that meets individual dietary needs and food preferences for an active and healthy life, is a fundamental human right that must underpin the mission of public health nutrition. Today, nearly one in 10 persons globally is food insecure, one in three suffers from at least one form of malnutrition—undernutrition, micronutrient deficiency, overweight or obesity—and diet-related noncommunicable diseases are endemic. The root causes of and factors contributing to food insecurity and malnutrition are complex and multidimensional. To address these, public health nutritionists must work in partnership with those committed to an equitable, evidence-based approach to the prevention of problems at their source. This requires empowerment of those affected and advocacy and action to encourage policy-makers and decision-takers, at all levels from global to local, to create social, economic, and physical environments that support healthy food security.

The public health nutrition workforce brings a critical set of nutrition competencies to the planning and delivery of what is otherwise a public health approach to preventing food insecurity, hunger, diet-related ill health, and disease. The competent public health nutritionist can apply nutrition science, epidemiology, and systems theory to help to identify the nature and determinants of healthy and unhealthy diets and food security. They can identify the interactions of food with biological, cultural, social, and environmental systems, and will advocate for upstream level interventions, recognizing the importance of policies and food systems in shaping access to sustainable healthy foods. They can apply behavioral and implementation sciences skills in the design and implementation of nutrition education strategies, both for community members and other professionals, for prevention and management of undernutrition and diet-related chronic diseases. The public health nutrition workforce can therefore function at many levels, contributing to advocacy and policy decisions in many sectors such as health, agriculture, education, social services, business, and others; capacity development of other professionals in these sectors; education, skills development, and empowerment of community members; and research and evaluation to identify effective actions and best practice. A fully competent workforce working across the dimensions of public health nutrition is essential to improve global food systems and nutrition for better health. Now more than ever the public health nutrition field must embrace the interdisciplinary nature of its mission and work upstream of immediate nutrition problems. Public health nutrition is at the crossroads of food supply, health, and education systems, but it also has social, economic, and political dimensions. Inequity and inequality leading to food insecurity and malnutrition are perpetuated by social, cultural, political, and economic policy decisions.

Zero hunger and good health and well-being are two of the 17 United Nations Sustainable Development Goals for 2030, but 10 others address indicators highly relevant to nutrition. The most pressing of these relate to reducing poverty, inequity, and inequality; increasing access to education, productive work, and health services; improving sanitation and access to clean water and addressing displacement due to changes in land ownership and use, conflict, and natural disasters. Pressures are also growing from new and emerging challenges and trends such as climate change, population growth, urbanization, changing lifestyles, and changing food systems. Much of the work to eliminate hunger and improve health and well-being will need to be done to address determinants defined by goals in other sectors. Public health nutritionists have a leadership role to influence policies and practices impacting nutrition in each sector as well as to motivate and train in nutrition those whose work will impact nutrition. Engagement with communities and individuals affected is also critical. Public health nutritionists must support communities to engage in self-identified and self-selected actions, thus achieving more self-reliance, empowerment, and sustainability. The public health nutrition field needs well-trained and supported nutrition professionals able to advocate at local, national, and international levels to promote our purpose. We need to collaborate and work collectively toward common goals with many different groups and organizations. This work must follow ethical principles, including those of transparency, equity, respect, and unconflicted interest. It must also acknowledge that food security and good health are basic human rights. As its unique contribution, the profession must continue to provide leadership and scholarship to strengthen the evidence base for effective action to improve nutrition-related health, particularly in the worst off and most disadvantaged communities in the world. Reflective practice and commitment to evaluation of our work are needed to learn lessons about what has and has not worked. Armed with this evidence, we must step up and show leadership in advocating for evidence-based policies and actions to improve nutrition. Part of this role is also to develop the capacity of other health professionals, community members, and policy-makers to understand the need for and how to achieve healthy sustainable diets.

As professionals, public health nutritionists need to be trained, mentored, and supported throughout their careers. This begins with an understanding and consensus on the competencies, or combination of knowledge, skills, and attitudes, required to effectively perform public health nutrition work. Curriculum and learning and teaching methods should then be developed based on the competencies. This will ensure relevant workforce preparation and training to perform effectively in the workplace. Curricula for courses need to be revised to match local circumstances, and there is a need for work-based experience and mentoring to help students develop their skills and learn reflective practice. Ongoing structured professional learning is also critical to maintaining competence of the workforce relevant to contemporary issues and needs. To achieve all of this requires high-level support, proper manpower planning, and a strong professional structure to set and help maintain standards. This text recognizes the importance of building and sustaining a professional workforce of public health nutrition leaders. It provides the foundations for building the competencies needed by public health nutritionists to recognize and address contemporary public health nutrition challenges.

It is not a text that dwells on the facts of nutrition sciences but instead explores the means through which such facts can be interpreted, applied, and evaluated for impact at population and community levels. It leads the reader to understand that food supply systems and cultural, social, political, and economic factors are key determinants of sustainable individual and community access to nutritious food. It emphasizes the critical importance of consulting with communities to identify their needs and opportunities for change, while working with them and across sectors to ensure that key determinants at systems levels are also addressed to support sustainable change.

Throughout the text, information, models, processes, examples, and practice activities are provided to help readers develop the understanding and skills needed for effective work in the field. While many of the examples are in the context of the United States, they remain useful in other settings to illustrate key concepts and to provide a focus for comparative discussion.

Margaret Miller
President
World Public Health Nutrition Association

PREFACE

Our team began our work as an exploration to identify an introductory text for the latest in-depth, evidence-based training of future public health nutrition professionals and leaders regionally, nationally, and internationally. In the process, our efforts turned into an incredible journey of working with some of the most outstanding professionals, mentors, and experts in the field of public health nutrition.

The overall goal of this text is to support the missions of various outstanding organizations devoted to the growing field of public health nutrition to promote optimal health and well-being of communities and populations through nutrition-related services, program planning, interventions, and policy, environmental, and systems change. These include the Association of State Public Health Nutritionists (ASPHN), the World Public Health Nutrition Association (WPHNA), the Academy of Nutrition and Dietetics (AND), the Food and Nutrition working group of the American Public Health Association (APHA), the Association of Graduate Programs in Public Health Nutrition (AGPPHN), and the Southeastern University Consortium on Hunger, Poverty and Nutrition, among others.

Some commonalities of the missions of these organizations include the following:

- To provide advanced training in nutrition and public health to develop in-depth knowledge of the latest nutrition-related evidence base, competencies and skills related to the core public health functions, and essential services of public health and public health nutrition

- To strengthen nutrition policy, programs, and environments for all people through the development of culturally competent public health nutrition leaders and collaborative interprofessional advocacy of practitioners nationwide and globally

- To build workforce capacity over the next several decades to meet the desperate need for public health nutrition professionals and practitioners to address the social determinants of health and serve growing population needs in rural, urban, and global settings

The text is organized into four main parts with content highlights as follows:

- *Part I: Foundations of Public Health Nutrition* includes history and principles of public health nutrition, introduction to nutritional epidemiology, behavioral aspects of public health nutrition, and an overview of food policy.

- *Part II: Cultural Aspects of Public Health Nutrition* includes cultural aspects of nutrition, health promotion within communities, and a focus on interprofessional practice in rural, urban, and global public health nutrition settings.

- *Part III: Community Assessment, Planning, Implementing, and Evaluation* includes methods of community nutrition assessment, program planning, and public health nutrition intervention delivery and evaluation.

■ *Part IV: Current and Future Challenges in Public Health Nutrition and Sustainability* includes current nutrition-related health issues, professional development needs and strategies, sustainability concerns, food systems and environmental health trends, and opportunities.

Each chapter provides learning objectives, key concepts, a glossary of terms, and a variety of learning resources including case studies, reflective questions, suggestions for learning activities, and resources for further study.

It is the sincere hope of the editors and authors that this text will be an effective tool for training and inspiring future public health nutrition professionals to engage in transformative practice everywhere in the world to nourish the physical, emotional, and spiritual dimensions of all human beings.

The editors of this text would like to acknowledge each of the authors and the editorial leadership team at Springer Publishing Company. Please accept our sincere thanks and appreciation for your valued contributions.

M. Margaret Barth, PhD, MPH
Ronny A. Bell, PhD, MS
Karen Grimmer, PhD, MMedSci, CertHlthEc

Qualified instructors may obtain access to supplementary material (Instructor's Manual, Test Bank, PowerPoints, Image Bank, and Syllabus) by emailing textbook@springerpub.com.

I

FOUNDATIONS OF PUBLIC HEALTH NUTRITION

INTRODUCTION TO PUBLIC HEALTH NUTRITION

MARSHA SPENCE AND COURTNEY SCHAND

LEARNING OBJECTIVES

1. Provide the definition of public health nutrition (PHN) given by the Academy of Nutrition and Dietetics Public Health Nutrition Task Force in 2012.

2. Explain five key roles of a **public health nutritionist** within a public health agency.

3. Describe the **Social-Ecological Model** and how it can be used by public health nutritionists to understand the multiple levels of influence on nutrition- and other health-related behaviors.

4. Describe the core functions of public health including assessment, assurance, and policy development.

5. List the 10 essential public health services and 16 essential public health nutrition services that support these core functions.

6. Describe essential areas of training for public health nutritionists, including advanced training in nutrition and public health, knowledge of current nutrition-related **evidence-based** skills, and the core functions of public health.

INTRODUCTION

History of PHN in the United States

Mary Egan,[1] a leader in shaping contemporary PHN education and practice in the United States, delineated the history of PHN with major milestones that influenced its development from the mid-1800s to the mid-1990s. During the mid-1800s, which was described as the "great sanitary awakening,"[2] the modern public health system (Figure 1.1)[3] began with a focus on sanitation efforts to decrease the spread of communicable diseases.[4] At this time, PHN was in its infancy with origins in home economics and public health and a focus on food safety and meal preparation on a budget. In the early 1900s, morbidity and mortality rates were high, especially among the working poor, infants, children, and mothers. In 1906, the **Food and Drug Act** was passed by Congress to begin oversight of food production, sales, and labeling.[4] In 1909, under the leadership of President Theodore Roosevelt, the White House held its first conference, the **White House Conference on the Care of Dependent Children**.[5] Because of this conference, the Children's

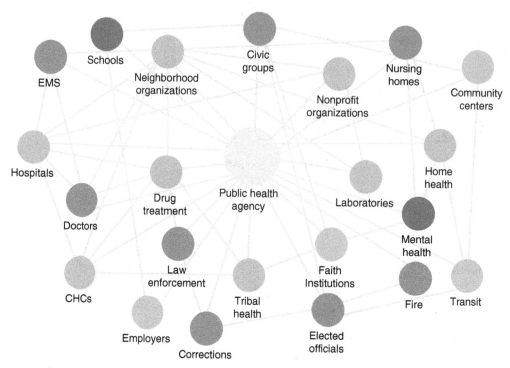

FIGURE 1.1 The modern public health system in the United States.
CHC, community health center; EMS, emergency medical services.
Source: From Centers for Disease Control and Prevention. *The Public Health System.* 2018, June. https://www.cdc
.gov/publichealthgateway/publichealthservices/essentialhealthservices.html

Bureau was created, which in effect launched the field of PHN.[1] The Sheppard–Towner Act in 1921 and the **Social Security Act** in 1935 had profound influences on public health infrastructure and the subsequent growth of PHN. Funds available to state health departments for maternal and child health through Title V of the Social Security Act stimulated rapid growth in the field. Prior to 1935, only three public health nutritionists were employed in three states, but by 1939, 39 public health nutritionists were employed in 24 states. In 1938, public health nutritionists' qualifications were first delineated. The Social Security Act was amended in 1939, and funds were available to train public health nutritionists. In 1942, based in part on nutrition studies conducted by the Public Health Service, nutrition clinics were developed in some state and local public health agencies. By the mid-1940s, 45 of the 48 states employed one or more PHN consultants, and funding to train graduate students in PHN and provide continuing education for practicing PHN professionals was allocated.[1]

During the 1950s, growth of the profession became more organized with the establishment of the Association of Faculties of Graduate Programs in Public Health Nutrition (currently, the **Association of Graduate Programs in Public Health Nutrition**)[6] in 1950 and the Association of State and Territorial Public Health Nutrition Directors (currently, the **Association of State Public Health Nutritionists**) in 1952. In the mid-1960s, legislation passed to reduce poverty in the United States provided funding for projects like the Maternity and Infant Care Program, the Compressive Health Projects for Children and Youth, Head Start, and the Medicare and Medicaid programs. These programs opened many more positions for public health nutritionists as practitioners in the programs or as consultants. The 1969 White House Conference on Food, Nutrition, and Health suggested actions to reduce malnutrition and hunger.[7] One of the recommendations was to provide nutrition services to pregnant women, infants, and young children from impoverished households. In 1972, the **Special Supplemental Nutrition Program for Women, Infants, and Children (WIC)** began as a pilot program, and in 1975, it was funded as a permanent nutrition education and supplemental food program.[8] To assess the nutrition status of the population, the Children's Bureau and the Public Health Service began collecting data in the late 1960s and early 1970s via the *Study of Nutritional Status of Preschool Children in the United States*,[9] the *Ten State Survey, 1968-1970*,[10] and the *National Health and Nutrition Examination Survey, 1971-1975*.[11] These programs and studies expanded positions and the scope of practice of public health nutritionists.[1]

In the 1970s and 1980s, several landmark documents were released that focused on the importance of nutrition in the prevention of chronic diseases and to provide dietary guidance for the U.S. population. First, in 1977, the *Dietary Goals for the United States*[12] were released, followed by *Healthy People: The Surgeon General's Report on Health Promotion and Disease Prevention* in 1979,[13] which outlined the first set of national health goals and objectives that focused on health promotion and disease prevention and highlighted the role of nutrition in these areas. The next year, two important documents were released. First, *Promoting Health/Preventing Disease: Objectives for the Nation* was released[13] and included 226 health-related objectives and action steps for improving population health over the next decade. These documents were the forerunners for the **Healthy People** series of documents,[14] which are science-based health objectives for the U.S. population that are released every 10 years. The second landmark document released that year was *Nutrition and Your Health: Dietary Guidelines for Americans*.[15] This was the first edition of dietary guidance for the U.S. population that focused on healthful dietary patterns based on the most accurate scientific evidence at the time.[16]

During the past two decades of the 1900s, as scientific understanding of chronic diseases and their relationship to nutrition continued to develop, public health nutritionists began working across the life course in the areas of health promotion and disease prevention. The Centers for Disease Control and Prevention (CDC) established the National Center for Chronic Disease Prevention and Health Promotion in 1988 and expanded the roles of public health nutritionists at the federal level working with states and other agencies to decrease chronic disease.[17] Also, in 1988, the Institute of Medicine (IOM) released a groundbreaking document, *The Future of Public Health*.[4,18] This document outlined the three core functions of public health—assessment, policy development, and assurance—and the 10 essential services of public health (Figure 1.2).[19] In 1996, the book, *Moving to the Future: Developing Community-Based Nutrition Services*[20] delineated the essential PHN services, which are still relevant today based on a recent article that defined a similar list of core functions of the PHN workforce in Australia.[21] Table 1.1 delineates the essential PHN services, as outlined by Probert, in relationship to the core functions of public health.

The *Healthy People*[14] series of national health objectives began with *Healthy People 2000*,[22] released September 1990. Since the introduction of these national health objectives, major progress has been made in the reduction of preventable illness and death, including nutrition-related diseases, cardiovascular disease, and cancer, along with risk factors such as hypertension and hyperlipidemia.[23] However, there is much work to be done still. Two nutrition-related leading health indicators, "reduce the proportion of adults who are obese" and "reduce the proportion of children and adolescents aged 2 to 19 years who are considered obese," have not met the 2020 targets and have actually increased from 33.9% to 38.6% and 16.1% to 17.8%, respectively. *Healthy People 2020* objectives related to dietary intake need improvement as well. Although

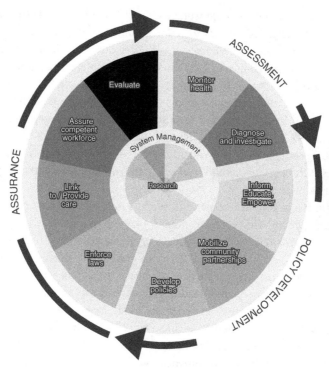

FIGURE 1.2 The 10 essential public health services.
Source: From Centers for Disease Control and Prevention. *The 10 Essential Public Health Services.* 2018, June.
https://www.cdc.gov/publichealthgateway/publichealthservices/essentialhealthservices.html

these objectives have improved from baseline, National Health and Nutrition Examination Survey (NHANES) data show that for the U.S. population, the mean daily intake of vegetables is still below the national objective of 1.6 cup equivalents per 1,000 calories (age-adjusted) and mean percentage of total daily calorie intake from added sugars (age-adjusted) and mean daily sodium intake (age-adjusted) are above the objectives of 9.7% and 2,300 mg, respectively. *Healthy People 2030*,[24] the newest edition of the *Healthy People* series, has seven foundation principles, five overarching goals, and eight action areas (Box 1.1). With a continued focus on prevention of chronic diseases, public health nutritionists will continue to play vital roles in improving population health.

GLOBAL PHN

Global PHN practice and services are much more recent concepts than PHN practice and services in developed nations. Like the United States, developed, transitioning, and developing countries have their own unique histories related to the foundations of public health and, subsequently, the growth of PHN. From the mid-1990s until now, international dietary intake patterns and physical activity levels and sedentary behaviors changed rapidly as a result of greater industrialization, changes in the world food economy, technology, and globalization.[25] Because of these dietary intake and activity changes, there was an ensuing increase in nutrition-related chronic diseases; poorer communities, especially in developing and newly developed countries, experience a disproportionate burden of morbidity and mortality from chronic diseases such

TABLE 1.1 PUBLIC HEALTH CORE FUNCTIONS AND ESSENTIAL PUBLIC HEALTH NUTRITION SERVICES

PUBLIC HEALTH CORE FUNCTION(S)	ESSENTIAL PUBLIC HEALTH NUTRITION SERVICES
Assessment	Assessing the nutritional status of specific populations or geographic areas
	Identifying priority populations that may be at nutritional risk
	Initiating and participating in nutrition data collection
Policy development	Providing leadership in the development of and planning for health and nutrition policies
	Raising awareness among key policy-makers on the potential impact of nutrition and food regulations on budget decisions on the health of the community
	Acting as an advocate for priority populations on food and nutrition issues
Assurance	Planning for nutrition services in conjunction with other health services, based on information obtained from an adequate and ongoing database focused on health outcomes
	Recommending and providing specific training and programs to meet identified nutrition needs
	Identifying or assisting in development of accurate, up-to-date nutrition education materials
	Ensuring the availability of quality nutrition services to priority populations, including nutrition screening, assessment, education, counseling, and referral for food assistance and follow-up
	Providing community health promotion and disease prevention activities that are population-based
	Providing quality assurance guidelines for practitioners dealing with food and nutrition issues
	Facilitating coordination with other providers of health and nutrition services within the community
Assessment/ Assurance/ Policy development	Participating in nutrition research, demonstration, and evaluation projects
	Providing expert nutrition consultation to the community
	Evaluating the impact of the health status of populations who receive public health nutrition services

Sources: From Probert K. *Moving to the Future: Developing Community-Based Nutrition Services.* Washington, DC: Association of State and Territorial Public Health Nutrition Directors; 1996; Institute of Medicine Committee for the Study of the Future of Public Health. *The Future of Public Health.* Washington, DC: National Academies Press; 1988. https://www.ncbi.nlm.nih.gov/books/NBK218224

as diabetes, cardiovascular disease, and cancer.[26] Like most official health agencies, the **World Health Organization (WHO)**, created in 1948 as part of the United Nations, was formed to combat communicable diseases and to improve maternal, infant, and child health and nutrition.[27] Now, WHO is the most prominent health agency in the world and assists public health agencies around the globe in responding to both communicable and noncommunicable diseases.

BOX 1.1

HEALTHY PEOPLE 2030 FOUNDATION PRINCIPLES, OVERARCHING GOALS, AND PLAN OF ACTION

Foundational Principles

- Health and well-being of all people and communities are essential to a thriving, equitable society.
- Promoting health and well-being and preventing disease are linked efforts that encompass physical, mental, and social health dimensions.
- Investing to achieve the full potential for health and well-being for all provides valuable benefits to society.
- Achieving health and well-being requires eliminating health disparities, achieving health equity, and attaining health literacy.
- Healthy physical, social, and economic environments strengthen the potential to achieve health and well-being.
- Promoting and achieving the nation's health and well-being is a shared responsibility that is distributed across the national, state, tribal, and community levels, including the public, private, and not-for-profit sectors.
- Working to attain the full potential for health and well-being of the population is a component of decision-making and policy formulation across all sectors.

Overarching Goals

- Attain healthy, thriving lives and well-being, free of preventable disease, disability, injury, and premature death.
- Eliminate health disparities, achieve health equity, and attain health literacy to improve the health and well-being of all.
- Create social, physical, and economic environments that promote attaining full potential for health and well-being for all.
- Promote healthy development, healthy behaviors, and well-being across all life stages.
- Engage leadership, key constituents, and the public across multiple sectors to take action and design policies that improve the health and well-being of all.

Plan of Action

- Set national goals and measurable objectives to guide evidence-based policies, programs, and other actions to improve health and well-being.
- Provide data that is accurate, timely, accessible, and can drive targeted actions to address regions and populations with poor health or at high risk for poor health in the future.
- Foster impact through public and private efforts to improve health and well-being for people of all ages and the communities in which they live.
- Provide tools for the public, programs, policy-makers, and others to evaluate progress toward improving health and well-being.

(continued)

BOX 1.1

HEALTHY PEOPLE 2030 FOUNDATION PRINCIPLES, OVERARCHING GOALS, AND PLAN OF ACTION (*CONTINUED*)

- Share and support the implementation of evidence-based programs and policies that are replicable, scalable, and sustainable.
- Report biennially on progress throughout the decade from 2020 to 2030.
- Stimulate research and innovation toward meeting *Healthy People 2030* goals and highlight critical research, data, and evaluation needs.
- Facilitate development and availability of affordable means of health promotion, disease prevention, and treatment.

Source: From U.S. Department of Health and Human Services. Office of Disease Prevention and Health Promotion. *Healthy People 2030 Framework.* 2019, November 4. https://www.healthypeople.gov/2020/about-healthy-people/development-healthy-people-2030/framework

PHN: DEFINITIONS

Several organizations have made efforts to define PHN and public health nutritionist for the past several decades.[28-32] PHN professionals and academicians in the United States, the United Kingdom, Australia, and Canada, as well as other countries in the European Union, have worked separately and together to develop working definitions of PHN. One of the first formal definitions of public health nutritionist in the United States was provided by Margaret Kaufmann in *Personnel in Public Health Nutrition in the 1980s* as

> that member of the public health agency staff who is responsible for assessing community nutrition needs and planning, organizing, managing, directing, coordinating, and evaluating the nutrition component of the health agency's services . . . establishes linkages with related community nutrition programs, nutrition education, food assistance, social or welfare services, child care, services to the elderly, other human services, and community-based research.[32]

Hughes,[33] an international PHN workforce development researcher, called for a standard definition of PHN among a working group from nine countries so that that workforce requirements could be assessed internationally. The international work group recommended various key descriptors from various aspects of the profession so that each country could develop its own definition that was best suited to the core functions and services that were unique to each country. The **key descriptors to define PHN** were "solution-oriented, social and cultural aspects, advocacy, disease prevention, and interventions based on systems, communities and organizations."[33]

In the ensuing years, definitions of PHN were formalized by several organizations and authors. Table 1.2 outlines organizations' definitions of PHN since 1998. As seen, there are commonalities among the PHN definitions and for the scope of practice of PHN professionals, for example, advocating for a healthful environment for all; developing policies based on system- and population-level assessments and program evaluations in priority populations; and collaborating with

TABLE 1.2 DEFINITIONS OF PUBLIC HEALTH NUTRITION BY ORGANIZATION AND DATE

ORGANIZATION	DATE	DEFINITION
United Kingdom Nutrition Society	1998	The application of nutrition and physical activity to the promotion of good health, the primary prevention of diet-related illness of groups, communities, and populations (not individuals)[34]
Strategic Intergovernmental Nutrition Alliance (Australia)	2001	Focuses on issues affecting the whole population rather than the specific dietary needs of individuals The impact of food production, distribution, and consumption on the nutritional status and health of particular population groups is taken into account, together with the knowledge, skills, attitudes, and behaviors in the broader community[35]
World Public Health Nutrition Association	2006	The promotion and maintenance of nutrition-related health and well-being of populations through organized efforts and informed choices of society[31]
Dietitians of Canada	2006	Health promotion through awareness raising, education and skill building, supportive environments and policy development, collaborations and partnerships, research and evaluation, and the mentoring and education of future nutrition and health professionals as well as other congruent descriptors[29]
Academy of Nutrition and Dietetics PHN Task Force	2012	The application of nutrition and public health principles to improve or maintain optimal health of populations and targeted groups through enhancements in programs, systems, policies, and environments[28]

Sources: From Uauy R. Understanding public health nutrition. *Lancet.* 2007;370(9584):309–310. doi:10.1016/S0140-6736(07)61145-3; Strategic Intergovernmental Nutrition Alliance. *Eat Well Australia: An Agenda for Action for Public Health Nutrition 2000–2010.* Canberra, Australia: Department Health and Aged Care; 2001; Hughes R. Workforce development: challenges for practice, professionalization and progress. *Public Health Nutr.* 2008;11(8):765–767. doi:10.1017/S1368980008002899; Chenhall C. *Public Health Nutrition Competencies: Summary of Key Informant Interviews.* Toronto, Canada: Dietitians of Canada. 2006, September. https://www.dietitians.ca/Downloads/Public/Public-Health-Nutrition-Competencies--key-informant.aspx; Academy of Nutrition and Dietetics. Public health nutrition: it's every member's business. *HOD Backgrounder.* 2012(Fall):1–22. https://www.eatrightpro.org/-/media/eatrightpro-files/leadership/hod/mega-issues/backgrounders/09-public-health-nutrition-backgrounder.pdf?la=en&hash=06B0F66D994A6BA0C574AB9A27FBA4A155AFD428

key stakeholders to improve programs, services, and policies. Regardless of the definition used for PHN, the similarity of ideas is central to the distinct differentiation between PHN practice and clinical nutrition practice. Thus, these definitions indicate that PHN professionals should have advanced training in nutrition and public health to develop an in-depth knowledge of the most up-to-date nutrition-related evidence base and competencies and skills related to the core public health functions and the essential services of public health and PHN.

PHN: TRAINING AND WORKFORCE

In recent years, PHN has received more attention and greater research funding owing to problems both domestically and globally related to the obesity epidemic, chronic diseases, and food insecurity.[36] As the U.S. population and populations in other developed countries continue to get older and become more diverse, population needs and public health and clinical healthcare, including nutrition, will need to adjust. Longer life spans increase the duration of chronic diseases and rate of comorbidities, which increase the necessity of lifestyle interventions that target culturally appropriate nutrition and physical activity behaviors. Further, because of economic hardships in recent years, food assistance programs, such as the Supplemental Nutrition Assistance Program (SNAP, formerly the Food Stamp Program) and WIC, have had some of the greatest utilization rates in years. Because these programs are often targeted by proposed budget cuts, many Americans, especially low-income and other disenfranchised populations, may be at increased risk for nutrition-related chronic diseases. In the United States and globally, it is essential to have highly trained PHN practitioners who can meet the needs of these populations and advocate for positive nutrition-related health outcomes for vulnerable populations across the life course.[28,36,37] PHN practitioners' knowledge and skills are essential to improving population health; they are essential members of interprofessional public health teams and assist with policy- and system-level decisions for health promotion and disease prevention.[37] Public health nutritionists' competencies are particularly important now; the **Patient Protection and Affordable Care Act**[38] underscores the need for primary prevention as well as screening and treatment of chronic diseases.[39]

The IOM[40] delineated recommendations for training public health professionals, the myriad of health concerns, and the essentiality of multidisciplinary and interdisciplinary/interprofessional approaches in *Who Will Keep the Public Healthy? Educating Public Health Professionals for the 21st Century*. The document asserts that to improve the nation's health, all members of multidisciplinary/interdisciplinary/interprofessional teams must be well trained and use evidence-based guidelines and best practices. It is essential that public health nutritionists have the competencies needed to help curtail obesity epidemic rates and decrease rates of other nutrition-related chronic diseases. Thus, PHN training should include in-depth exposure to the Social-Ecological Model,[41] along with other behavioral theories, and the **social determinants of health** because it is essential for public health nutritionists to understand how behavioral, environmental, biological, societal, and economic factors influence individual health and, subsequently, population health.[37,42] Further, training in PHN should include applied nutrition science; nutrition across the life course; policy development, implementation, and evaluation; biostatistics; epidemiology; public policy related to nutrition and food assistance; community assessment; and program planning, implementation, and evaluation.[43]

PHN: POSITIONS AND CAREER SETTINGS

Position descriptions, classifications, educational requirements, and career settings for PHN practitioners are outlined in *Personnel in Public Health Nutrition for the 2000s*.[44] In this document, PHN professionals are described as "specialized nutrition professionals and paraprofessionals who provide and/or plan nutrition programs through organizations that reach people living in a designated community".[44] PHN professionals may be employed in numerous career settings at state, local, and national agencies and organizations in both the public and private sectors. In addition to local and state public health agencies, other common places that employ or contract with PHN practitioners include federally qualified community health clinics, nonprofit organizations, state departments of education, food assistance programs, hunger-relief agencies, early childhood education settings such as Head Start, and local education agencies, where they are employed as nutrition educators, school health coordinators, or directors of nutrition services. In addition, public health nutritionists work in federally sponsored programs at the local level, such as WIC, SNAP-Ed, and the Expanded Food and Nutrition Education Program, and many federal agencies such as the U.S. Department of Health and Human Services, the U.S. Department of Agriculture, the CDC, Food and Drug Administration, Maternal and Child Health Bureau, and Indian Health Services. Although this list is not all inclusive, it does show the variety of job settings for PHN personnel.

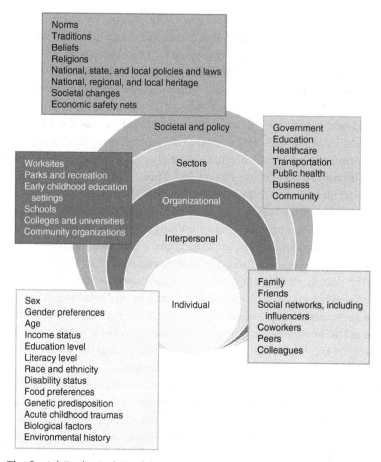

FIGURE 1.3 The Social-Ecological Model.

Source: Data from U.S. Department of Health and Human Services. Office of Disease Prevention and Health Promotion. *The 2015-2020 Dietary Guidelines.* The Social-Ecological Model. 2015. https://health.gov/dietaryguidelines/2015/guidelines/chapter-3/social-ecological-model; Centers for Disease Control and Prevention. *The Social Ecological Model: A Framework for Prevention.* 2019, January. http://www.cdc.gov/violenceprevention/overview/social-ecologicalmodel.html; World Health Organization. Violence Prevention Alliance. *The Ecological Framework.* 2019. https://www.who.int/violenceprevention/approach/ecology/en.; Bronfenbrenner U. Toward an experimental ecology of human development. *Am Psychol.* 1977;32(7):513–531. doi:10.1037/0003-066X.32.7.513

PHN positions can be classified across a continuum of services and functions from direct care services to population and systems focused work.[44] To influence individual and population health, professionals in PHN work across the spheres of influence in the Social-Ecological Model (Figure 1.3).[41,45,46,58] However, most often, these practitioners focus on the outer spheres at the societal and policy levels and within sectors and organizations. Personnel in management positions, which include directors, assistant directors, and supervisors, work predominantly in administrative roles and have little direct contact with their priority populations. Public health nutritionists, consultants, clinical nutritionists, nutritionists, and nutrition educators are classified as professional positions. While public health nutritionists and consultants may have some direct interactions with community members, much of their work is in program planning, implementation, and evaluation. Other professional positions, including clinical nutritionists, nutritionists, and nutrition educators, along with positions classified as technical and support positions, such as nutrition technicians and community nutrition workers, usually have direct contact with the public with a focus on delivery of services. Personnel at the management level and public health nutritionists and consultants at the professional level require advanced training in public health and nutrition so that they are competent in community assessment; are able to plan, implement, and evaluate population- and systems-level programs and services; and have the knowledge and skills required to collaborate and lead interprofessional teams to promote population health.[44]

According to the U.S. Bureau of Labor Statistics,[47] career growth in nutrition and dietetics is projected to increase over the next decade by 11%, which is higher than growth in many other professions. Job growth in PHN may increase even more if the healthcare system continues to shift from a medical treatment model to one of primary prevention.[39] In 2018, the average pay for dietitians/nutritionists was $64,670 annually, with higher paying positions in states on the West Coast and in large metropolitan areas.[47]

PHN: FUTURE TRENDS

In 2006, the World Congress of PHN, an international association of PHN practitioners, academicians, researchers, clinical and public health professionals, policy-makers, and epidemiologists from 79 countries, convened a discussion session to examine the future trends and educational needs of PHN professionals nationally, regionally, and globally.[48] The panel outlined a global need for research, improved technology, and strong collaborations between academia and both private and public sectors to find solutions to malnutrition, both under- and overnutrition, and other nutrition-related health problems. The panel recommended that multiple disciplines from both developed and developing countries should collaborate to find solutions to the global problems, similar to how multinational, multidisciplinary teams have worked to eliminate or dramatically reduce communicable diseases via immunization. Also, the panel recommended that once formed, the collaborations would need to be guided by shared ethical principles, transparency, and open communication. Thus far, such collaborations have been limited, but in May 2008, based on recommendations from the World PHN Congress, the World Association of PHN was incorporated.[49] The purpose of the association is to bring people together to promote and improve PHN and to be the international voice of PHN.

Because current PHN professionals must work to meet the nutrition-related needs of the public to promote population health through nutrition services, interventions, initiatives and policy, systems, and environmental change, it is important that this workforce be trained through graduate coursework and experiential learning and, after entry into the workforce via continuing education, have opportunities for leadership development and other professional development training.[50] Hughes,[31] in an editorial about PHN workforce development, outlined key areas that should be examined to increase the capacity and quality of highly trained PHN professionals, including increased scholarship for the PHN workforce, strong assessment to determine workforce needs, in both developing and developed nations, and funding to conduct such research and train the workforce. Shrimpton et al.[50] noted that development of workforce capacity in PHN should be assessed at each of the following levels: in the PHN workforce, within communities, and at organizational and systems levels.

Currently, PHN workforce development needs are addressed via multiple training avenues, including online certificate training, such as the Academy of Nutrition and Dietetics Center for Lifelong Learning Public Health Nutrition Online Certificate Training;[51] academic graduate certificate programs, such as Appalachian State University Graduate Certificate in Public Health Nutrition Practice;[52] academic coursework in nutrition and public health; graduate programs in PHN and community nutrition;[6] and certification programs, for example, Certification in Public Health[53] and Certified Health Education Specialist.[54] Although an undergraduate degree in nutrition is necessary and advanced education at the graduate level and the registered dietitian/nutritionist credential is preferred, currently there is no specific credential or licensure available to denote a professional's advanced training in PHN. Thus, some public health nutritionists may not have the advanced training and competencies to adequately perform their role. Without advanced training and practice, PHN professionals may be ill-prepared to carry out the core functions of public health and the essential PHN services and work at the system, population, and community levels.[29] Thus, in the future to protect population health, all public health nutritionists should have graduate-level PHN coursework and/or degrees to ensure that the workforce is competent in the areas of community nutrition assessment; program planning, implementation, and evaluation; policy development, implementation, and evaluation; and policy systems and environmental change.[29,37,43]

Another key area of future focus for the PHN workforce is leadership development to ensure organization-, community-, policy-, and systems-level competencies to promote health and prevent nutrition-related diseases for populations.[55] The current workforce in PHN is aging;[56] this will lead to many retirements and the absence of PHN practitioners in leadership roles in the profession.[55,56] Thus, future demands on the PHN workforce must be addressed to help close these gaps. Leadership development is and will continue to be imperative to the PHN profession, as it will allow entry- and midlevel career personnel in PHN to be better equipped to fill vacant leadership positions in public health and PHN and mentor students, trainees, and interns in the field.[57] Because the number of PHN practitioners needed domestically and globally may take several decades to reach the capacity to serve population needs, increased graduate programs in PHN and continuing education for current practitioners are necessary.[50]

Closely aligned with leadership development, developing skilled mentors will also be key to increasing the capacity of the PHN workforce in the future. Palermo et al.,[57] Australian advocates for and researchers on PHN workforce development, recommended the development of PHN mentoring circles, that is, pairing an experienced PHN professional with a group of entry-level PHN practitioners. This could increase each mentor's capacity and effectiveness. Although the effectiveness of these mentoring circles would depend on the commitment, significance, and involvement of everyone in the group, it could be a valid solution to the shortage of experienced PHN practitioners who can assist in the development of new PHN practitioners and leaders.

CONCLUSION

PHN has a rich history of improving population health and a challenging, ambitious, and exciting future in decreasing nutrition-related health disparities, ensuring access to food, and improving the health status of populations across the globe. This text guides readers through three parts related to domestic and global PHN. It presents a comprehensive survey of where the field has been taken due to the work of Mary Egan and other notable leaders in the field, allowing for groundbreaking new opportunities for practitioners, researchers, policy-makers, and other public health professionals.

KEY CONCEPTS

1. Public health nutrition, as defined by the Academy of Nutrition and Dietetics Public Health Nutrition Task Force is, "the application of nutrition and public health principles to improve or maintain optimal health of populations and targeted groups through enhancements in programs, systems, policies, and environments".[28]

2. Public health nutritionist, as defined my Margaret Kaufman, is "that member of the public health agency staff who is responsible for assessing community nutrition needs and planning, organizing, managing, directing, coordinating, and evaluating the nutrition component of the health agency's services . . . establishes linkages with related community nutrition programs, nutrition education, food assistance, social or welfare services, child care, services to the elderly, other human services, and community-based research".[32]

3. The Social-Ecological Model can be used by public health nutritionists to help them understand the multiple levels of influence on nutrition- and other health-related behaviors. The spheres of influence include:

   a. The individual level, which encompasses age, sex, literacy level, race and ethnicity, food preferences, acute childhood traumas, and more

   b. The interpersonal level, which includes families, friends, social networks, coworkers, and peers

   c. The organizational level, which includes worksites, parks and recreation facilities, early childhood education settings, schools, colleges and universities, and community organizations

   d. Sectors, including governmental, educational, healthcare, transportation, public health, community, and business sectors

   e. Societal and policy levels, such as traditions, beliefs, religions, policies and laws, societal changes, and economic safety nets

4. The core functions of public health are assessment, assurance, and policy development. There are 10 essential public health services and 16 essential PHN services that support these core functions.

5. Public health nutritionists should have advanced training in nutrition and public health to develop knowledge of current nutrition-related evidence-based skills related to the core functions of public health and the essential health services of public health and PHN.

CASE STUDY: A PUBLIC HEALTH NUTRITIONIST'S PROCESS FOR INCREASING ACCESS TO HEALTHFUL FOODS IN URBAN AND RURAL COMMUNITIES WITH MOBILE FOOD MARKETS

A public health nutritionist is working with other public health and nutrition professionals on a state coalition to increase access to healthful foods in urban and rural communities. The team begins by assessing the number and types of retail food stores across the state. After finding this information, they then look at the U.S. Department of Agriculture (USDA) Economic Research

Service Food Access Research Atlas (www.ers.usda.gov/Data/FoodDesert). They find that many low-income populations in the state have low access to food stores and low vehicle access. Further, the assessment data show that these areas have the highest rates of child and adult obesity and type 2 diabetes. These findings lead the coalition to seek funds for mobile food markets in collaboration with a local food bank and a local grocery store chain. After writing a successful grant application to the Robert Wood Johnson Foundation (www.rwjf.org) and receiving funding, the coalition begins marketing the mobile food markets in eight of the lowest income counties in the state with the lowest access to healthful foods. To reach the most people, the coalition uses social media, provides infographics at the SNAP office (www.fns.usda.gov/snap/supplemental-nutrition-assistance-program) and at area schools and religious organizations, and runs advertisements about the opening day via radio, television, and billboards.

On the opening day, the mobile markets provide low-cost and no-cost healthful foods and beverages to 2,800 families (over 10,000 individuals). In addition, coalition volunteers help eligible participants enroll in SNAP and survey participants to determine barriers and challenges to preparing the foods that the mobile markets carry. The survey results show that participants would like to learn more about how to prepare healthful foods; thus, coalition members contact extension agents in the area to see if they can do cooking demonstrations at the next mobile market via SNAP-Ed and other USDA programs. In addition, they contact the state department of education to propose high school curricular changes that allow students to take nutrition courses that include healthy food preparation methods. Last, coalition members advocate for improved zoning rules in the priority counties to attract full-service grocery stores to the areas.

Case Study Questions

a. Identify at least 10 essential PHN services described in the case study and categorize them by the associated core functions of public health.

b. Use the Economic Research Service Food Access Research Atlas to find your home county and determine if there are low-income, low-access areas there.

c. In what other areas could the coalition advocate to improve food access for the priority communities?

SUGGESTED LEARNING ACTIVITIES

1. Explore the Association of State Public Health Nutrition website (www.asphn.org) and complete the following:

    i. List the association's mission and vision.

    ii. Describe at least two committees or councils in the association.

    iii. List one way you could become involved in the association.

2. Visit the SNAP website (www.fns.usda.gov/snap/supplemental-nutrition-assistance-program) and find the following:

    i. Based on the website, provide a brief description of SNAP in your own words.

    ii. What are the eligibility requirements for SNAP?

    iii. What can be purchased with SNAP benefits?

REFLECTION QUESTIONS

1. Discuss why it is important for public health nutritionists to have advanced training in both nutrition and public health?

2. This chapter lists several definitions of PHN; compare and contrast these definitions by discussing the commonalities and differences among them.

3. Describe at least five ways that public health nutritionists can work with other public health professionals to improve population health.

4. List and describe at least five historical milestone events and/or legislation that led to expanded roles of public health nutritionists in the United States.

5. Describe the purpose of the World Public Health Nutrition Association.

CONTINUE YOUR LEARNING RESOURCES

American Public Health Association Food and Nutrition Section. https://www.apha.org/apha-communities/member-sections/food-and-nutrition/who-we-are

Association of Graduate Programs in Public Health Nutrition. www.agpphn.org

Centers for Disease Control and Prevention—Nutrition. https://www.cdc.gov/nutrition/index.html

Centers for Disease Control and Prevention National Center for Chronic Disease Prevention and Health. https://www.cdc.gov/chronicdisease/index.htm

Healthy People 2030. https://www.healthypeople.gov/2020/About-Healthy-People/Development-Healthy-People-2030/Framework

The Academy of Nutrition and Dietetics Public Health/Community Nutrition Dietetic Practice Group. https://www.phcnpg.org/page/about

U.S. Department of Agriculture Food and Nutrition Service. https://www.usda.gov/topics/food-and-nutrition

GLOSSARY

Association of Graduate Programs in Public Health Nutrition: One of the first formalized organizations for the profession, created in 1950.

Association of State Public Health Nutritionists: One of the first formalized organizations for the profession, created in 1952.

Evidence-based: Practice that relies on scientific evidence for decision-making and informing practice.

Food and Drug Act: Passed by Congress in 1906 to begin oversight of food production, sales, and labeling.

Global PHN practice: Developed, transitioning, and developing countries have their own unique histories related to the foundations of public health and growth of PHN.

Healthy People: Series of documents that are science-based health objectives for the U.S. population, released every 10 years.

Key descriptors to define PHN: Solution-oriented, social and cultural aspects, advocacy, disease prevention, and interventions based on systems, communities, and organizations.

Mary Egan: Leader in shaping contemporary PHN education and practice in the United States.

Moving to the Future: Developing Community-Based Nutrition Services: Text providing the delineation of the essential PHN services in relationship to the core functions of public health.

Nutrition and Your Health: Dietary Guidelines for Americans: Hallmark document providing dietary guidance for the U.S. population that focused on healthful dietary patterns.

Patient Protection and Affordable Care Act: Legislation that underscores the need for primary prevention as well as screening and treatment of chronic diseases; passed in 2010.

Public health nutritionist: A member of the public health agency staff responsible for assessing community nutrition needs and planning, organizing, managing, directing, coordinating, and evaluating the nutrition component of the health agency's services.

Social determinants of health: Behavioral, environmental, biological, societal, and economic factors that influence individual and population health.

Social-Ecological Model: Key model for application by public health nutritionists to understand how behavioral, societal, and economic factors influence health.

Social Security Act: Legislation that influenced public health infrastructure and subsequent growth of PHN, passed in 1935.

Special Supplemental Nutrition Program for Women, Infants, and Children (WIC): One of the first programs to provide nutrition services to pregnant women, infants, and children, established in 1972.

The Future of Public Health: Groundbreaking document outlining the three core functions of public health—assessment, policy development, and assurance—and the 10 essential services of public health, released by the IOM in 1988.

White House Conference on the Care of Dependent Children: First conference, held in 1909, by the White House related to PHN.

World Health Organization (WHO): Created in 1948 as part of the United Nations, formed to combat communicable diseases and to improve maternal, infant, and child health and nutrition.

World Public Health Nutrition Association: First international organization to promote and improve PHN and to be the international voice of PHN.

REFERENCES

1. Egan M. Public health nutrition: a historical perspective. *J Am Diet Assoc.* 1994;94(3):298–304. doi:10.1016/0002-8223(94)90372-7
2. Winslow CEA. *The Evolution and Significance of the Modern Public Health Campaign.* New Haven, CT: Yale University Press; 1923.
3. Centers for Disease Control and Prevention. *The Public Health System.* 2018, June. https://www.cdc.gov/publichealthgateway/publichealthservices/essentialhealthservices.html
4. Institute of Medicine. *The Future of Public Health.* Washington, DC: National Academies Press; 1988. https://www.ncbi.nlm.nih.gov/books/NBK218224
5. Michael J, Goldstein M. Reviving the White House Conference on Children. *Children's Voice.* 2008;17(1). https://www.cwla.org/reviving-the-white-house-conference-on-children
6. Association of Graduate Programs in Public Health Nutrition. *Directory.* 2019, October. https://agpphn.org/directory
7. White House Conference on Food, Nutrition, and Health, 1970. https://academic.oup.com/nutritionreviews/article/27/9/247/1875780

8. National WIC Association. *WIC Program Overview and History.* https://www.nwica.org/overview-and
   -history
9. Owen GM, Kram KM, Garry PJ, et al. A study of nutritional status of preschool children in the United
   States, 1968-1970. *Pediatrics.* 1974;52(suppl):597–646.
10. Center for Disease Control and Prevention. *Ten-state nutrition survey, 1968-1970.* Atlanta, GA: U.S.
    Department of Health, Education, and Welfare. Publication no. HSM 72-8134; 1972.
11. Centers for Disease Control and Prevention. National Center for Health Statistics (NCHS). National
    Health and Nutrition Examination Survey Data. *History.* 2015, November 6. https://www.cdc.gov/nchs/
    nhanes/history.htm
12. U.S. Senate Select Committee on Nutrition and Human Needs. *Dietary Goals for the United States.* 2nd
    ed. Washington, DC: U.S. Government Printing Office; 1977.
13. Center for Disease Control and Prevention. Year 2000 national health objectives. *MMWR Morb Mortal
    Wkly Rep.* 1989;38(37):629–633.
14. U.S. Department of Health and Human Services. Office of Disease Prevention and Health Promotion.
    Healthy People. 2019, November 4. https://www.healthypeople.gov
15. U.S. Department of Agriculture and U.S. Department of Health and Human Services. Nutrition and
    Your Health: Dietary Guidelines for Americans. *Home and Garden Bulletin No. 232;* 1980. https://pubs
    .nal.usda.gov/sites/pubs.nal.usda.gov/files/hgb.htm#nbr220
16. U.S. Department of Agriculture, Agricultural Research Service, Dietary Guidelines Committee. *Report
    of the Dietary Guidelines Advisory Committee on the Dietary Guidelines for Americans, 1995, to the
    Secretary of Health and Human Services and the Secretary of Agriculture. Appendix I: History of Dietary
    Guidelines for Americans.* 1995. https://health.gov/dietaryguidelines/dga95/12DIETAP.HTM
17. Remington PL, Brownson RC. Fifty years of progress in chronic disease epidemiology and control. *Morb
    Mortal Wkly Rep.* 2011;60(4):70–77.
18. Haughton B, Story M, Keir B. Profile of public health nutrition personnel: challenges for population/
    system-focused roles and state-level monitoring. *J Am Diet Assoc.* 1998;98(6):664–670.
19. Centers for Disease Control and Prevention. *The 10 Essential Public Health Services.* 2018, June. https://
    www.cdc.gov/publichealthgateway/publichealthservices/essentialhealthservices.html
20. Probert K. *Moving to the Future: Developing Community-Based Nutrition Services.* Washington, DC:
    Association of State and Territorial Public Health Nutrition Directors; 1996.
21. Hughes R, Begley A, Yeatman H. Consensus on the core functions of the public health nutrition
    workforce in Australia. *Nutr Diet.* 2016;73(1):103–111.
22. U.S. Department of Health and Human Services. Office of Disease Prevention and Health Promotion.
    History and Development of Healthy People. 2019, November 4. https://www.healthypeople.gov/2020/
    About-Healthy-People/History-Development-Healthy-People-2020
23. U.S. Department of Health and Human Services. Office of Disease Prevention and Health Promotion.
    Healthy People 2020 Leading Health Indicators: Progress Update. 2019, November 4. https://
    www.healthypeople.gov/2020/leading-health-indicators/Healthy-People-2020-Leading-Health-
    Indicators%3A-Progress-Update
24. U.S. Department of Health and Human Services. Office of Disease Prevention and Health Promotion.
    Healthy People 2030 Framework. 2019, November 4. https://www.healthypeople.gov/2020/about
    -healthy-people/development-healthy-people-2030/framework
25. Fielding JE. Public health in the twentieth century: Advances and challenges. *Annu Rev Public Health.*
    1999;20(1):xiii–xxx. doi:10.1146/annurev.publhealth.20.1.0
26. Schmidt H. Chronic disease prevention and health promotion. In: Barrett DH, Ortmann LH, Dawson
    A, et al. eds. *Public Health Ethics: Cases Spanning the Globe.* Cham, Switzerland: Springer; 2016. https://
    www.ncbi.nlm.nih.gov/books/NBK435779
27. World Health Organization. *History of WHO.* 2019. https://www.who.int/about/who-we-are/history.
28. Academy of Nutrition and Dietetics. *Public Health Nutrition: It's Every Member's Business.* HOD
    Backgrounder. 2012. https://www.eatrightpro.org/-/media/eatrightpro-files/leadership/hod/mega
    -issues/backgrounders/09-public-health-nutrition-backgrounder.pdf?la=en&hash=06B0F66D994
    A6BA0C574AB9A27FBA4A155AFD428
29. Chenhall C. *Public Health Nutrition Competencies: Summary of Key Informant Interviews.* Dietitians
    of Canada. 2006, September. https://www.dietitians.ca/Downloads/Public/Public-Health-Nutrition
    -Comptencies--key-informant.aspx

30. Hughes R. Competencies for effective public health nutrition practice: a developing consensus. *Public Health Nutr.* 2004;7(5):683–691.

31. Hughes R. Workforce development: challenges for practice, professionalization and progress. *Public Health Nutr.* 2008;11(8):765–767. doi:10.1017/S1368980008002899

32. Kaufman M, ed. *Personnel in Public Health Nutrition for the 1980's.* McLean, VA: Association of State and Territorial Health Officials Foundation; 1982.

33. Hughes R. Definitions for public health nutrition: a developing consensus. *Public Health Nutr.* 2003;6(6):615–620. doi:10.1079/PHN2003487

34. Uauy R. Understanding public health nutrition. *Lancet.* 2007;370(9584):309–310. doi:10.1016/S0140-6736(07)61145-3

35. Strategic Intergovernmental Nutrition Alliance. *Eat Well Australia: An Agenda for Action for Public Health Nutrition 2000–2010.* Canberra, Australia: Department of Health and Aged Care; 2001.

36. Rhea M, Bettles C. Future changes driving dietetics workforce supply and demand: future scan 2012-2022. *J Acad Nutr Diet.* 2012;112(3):S10–S24. doi:10.1016/j.jand.2011.12.008

37. Haughton B, Stang J. Population risk factors and trends in health care and public policy. *J Acad Nutr Diet.* 2012;112(3):S35–S46. doi:10.1016/j.jand.2011.12.011

38. Patient Protection and Affordable Care Act, 42 USC §18001 (2010).

39. Wells EV, Sarigiannis AN, Boulton ML. Assessing integration of clinical and public health skills in preventive medicine residencies: using competency mapping. *Am J Prev Med.* 2012;42(6):S107–S116. doi:10.1016/j.amepre.2012.04.004

40. Institute of Medicine. *Who Will Keep the Public Healthy? Educating Public Health Professionals for the 21st Century.* Washington, DC: National Academies Press; 2003. doi:10.17226/10542

41. Bronfenbrenner U. Toward and experimental ecology of human development. *Am Psychol.* 1977;32(7):513–531. doi:10.1037/0003-066X.32.7.513

42. Institute of Medicine. *Promoting Health: Intervention Strategies from Social and Behavioral Research.* Washington, DC: National Academy Press; 2000.

43. Spence ML, ed. *Strategies for Success: Curriculum Guide (Didactic and Experiential Learning).* 3rd ed. Association of Graduate Programs in Public Health Nutrition; 2013.

44. Dodds JM. *Personnel in Public Health Nutrition for the 2000s.* Tucson, AZ: Association of State Public Health Nutritionists; 2009. https://www.asphn.org/resource_files/105/105_resource_file1.pdf

45. U.S. Department of Health and Human Services. Office of Disease Prevention and Health Promotion. *The 2015-2020 Dietary Guidelines. The Social-Ecological Model.* 2015. https://health.gov/dietaryguidelines/2015/guidelines/chapter-3/social-ecological-model

46. Centers for Disease Control and Prevention. *The Social Ecological Model: A Framework for Prevention.* 2019, January. http://www.cdc.gov/violenceprevention/overview/social-ecologicalmodel.html

47. Bureau of Labor Statistics, U.S. Department of Labor. *Occupational Outlook Handbook, Dietitians and Nutritionists.* 2019, September 4. https://www.bls.gov/ooh/healthcare/dietitians-and-nutritionists.htm

48. Serra-Majem L. Moving forward in public health nutrition: the I World Congress of Public Health Nutrition. *Nutr Rev.* 2009;67(suppl 1):S2–S6. doi:10.1111/j.1753-4887.2009.00150.x

49. World Public Health Nutrition Association. *Our Work. Our History.* 2018. https://www.wphna.org/about

50. Shrimpton R, Hughes R, Recine E, et al. Nutrition capacity development: a practice framework. *Public Health Nutr.* 2013;7(3):682–688. doi:10.1017/S1368980013001213

51. Academy of Nutrition and Dietetics. *Certificates of Training.* Public Health Nutrition-Modules 1-5. https://www.eatrightstore.org/cpe-opportunities/certificates-of-training?pageSize=20&pageIndex=3&sortBy=namedesc

52. Appalachian State University. *App State Online.* Public Health Nutrition Practice Graduate Certificate. https://online.appstate.edu/programs/id/public-health-nutrition

53. National Board of Public Health Examiners. *Credentialing Public Health Leaders.* 2019. https://www.nbphe.org

54. National Commission for Health Education Credentialing, Inc. *Health Education Credentialing.* https://www.nchec.org/health-education-credentialing

55. Wright K, Rowitz L, Merkle A, et al. Competency development in public health leadership. *Am J Public Health.* 2000;90(8):1202–1207. doi:10.2105/AJPH.90.8.1202

56. Haughton B, George A. The Public Health Nutrition workforce and its future challenges: the US experience. *Public Health Nutr.* 2008;11(8):782–791. doi:10.1017/S1368980008001821

57. Palermo C, Hughes R, McCall L. An evaluation of a public health nutrition workforce development intervention for the nutrition and dietetics workforce. *J Hum Nutr Diet.* 2010;23:244–253. doi:10.1111/j.1365-277X.2010.01069.x

58. World Health Organization. Violence Prevention Alliance. *The ecological framework.* 2019. https://www.who.int/violenceprevention/approach/ecology/en

2

NUTRITION EPIDEMIOLOGY PRINCIPLES

ERIN BOULDIN, KAREN GRIMMER, AND RONNY A. BELL

LEARNING OBJECTIVES

1. Understand the basics of epidemiology with reference to nutrition.
2. Identify different sources of research evidence.
3. Understand the limitations around each research evidence source.
4. Determine the research evidence required to make informed healthcare decisions.

INTRODUCTION

Epidemiology and Role in Public Health Nutrition

Health is a fundamental human right (www.who.int/healthsystems/topics/equity/en). Health is measured in a range of ways, and it is not just the absence of **disease**.

In this chapter, the term "disease" is used in epidemiological terms, as an umbrella term for a disease diagnosis, death, a poor health outcome (for instance, high body mass index [BMI] or low back pain), and problematic health event (like a car crash). The term **exposure** is used ubiquitously for any factor that may be associated with disease. There is an array of factors, but common ones include biological, familial/genetic, chemical, physical, occupational, psychosocial, socioeconomic, geographic, travel-related, educational, cultural, and nutrition.[1]

Public health is the "science and art of preventing disease, prolonging life and promoting human health through organized efforts and informed choices of society, organizations, public and private, communities and individuals."[2] An alternative definition of public health is provided by the Centers for Disease Control and Prevention (CDC) Foundation in the United States as "the science of protecting and improving the health of people and their communities. This work is achieved by promoting healthy lifestyles, researching disease and injury prevention, and detecting, preventing and responding to infectious diseases."[3] The traditional core disciplines of public health are biostatistics, epidemiology, health policy and management, social and behavioral sciences, and environmental health. However, public health is informed and carried out by a number of other disciplines, including health services, community health, behavioral health, health economics, mental health, sexual and reproductive health, gender issues in health, and occupational safety.[4] Information combined from these areas of practice underpins public health knowledge, priorities, and decisions.[5]

Epidemiology is the study of health in populations.[6,7] Epidemiology encompasses a set of methods by which population health (public health) and the threats to it are assessed and monitored.[6]

LET US CONSIDER PUBLIC HEALTH FIRST

The term "public" in "public health" is variably interpreted, depending on circumstances and the health challenges being dealt with.[2] "Public" reflects the group of interest, which can be a defined group of people faced with a particular threat to health, a whole town, one region in a country, a whole country, or many countries. "Health" takes into account physical, mental, and social well-being and thus is not merely the absence of disease or infirmity.[8] Modern public health practice requires multidisciplinary teams comprising epidemiologists, biostatisticians, medical assistants, public health nurses, midwives, medical microbiologists, economists, sociologists, geneticists, and data managers. Depending on the problem, additional support may be required from environmental health officers, public health inspectors, bioethicists, veterinarians, gender experts, and sexual and reproductive health specialists.[5]

Public health aims to improve populations' quality of life through surveillance of existing cases and health indicators and by promoting healthy environments and behaviors.[5] Examples of public health interests are ensuring healthy and sufficient drinking water, appropriate sanitation, vaccinations for childhood communicable diseases, appropriate nutrition, and prevention of transmissible diseases.

Ten essential services of public health were proposed in 1994 by the CDC Core Public Health Functions Steering Committee.[9] These services link to the four core functions of public health: assessment, policy development, quality assurance, and research:

Assessment:

1. Monitor health status to identify and solve community health problems.
2. Diagnose and investigate health problems and health hazards in the community.

Policy Development:

3. Inform, educate, and empower people about health issues.
4. Mobilize community partnerships and action to identify and solve health problems.
5. Develop policies and plans that support individual and community health efforts.

Assurance:

6. Enforce laws and regulations that protect health and ensure safety.
7. Link people to needed personal health services and assure the provision of healthcare when otherwise unavailable.
8. Assure a competent public and personal healthcare workforce.
9. Evaluate effectiveness, accessibility, and quality of personal and population-based health services.

Research:

10. Investigations for new insights and innovative solutions to health problems.

Public health and the essential component services listed previously are interlinked by equity principles and **social determinants of health (SDOH)**; see Figure 2.1. Equity is defined by the World Health Organization (WHO) "as the absence of avoidable or remediable differences among

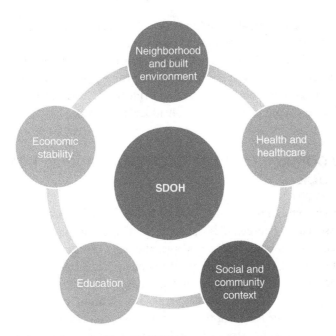

FIGURE 2.1 Social determinants of health (SDOH).

Source: From Office of Disease Prevention and Health Promotion. *Social Determinants of Health.* 2019. https://www
.healthypeople.gov/2020/topics-objectives/topic/social-determinants-of-health

groups of people, whether those groups are defined socially, economically, demographically, or geographically, and where there is opportunity for everyone to attain their full health potential regardless of demographic, social, economic or geographic strata."[10] Health inequities usually involve more than inequality with respect to health determinants; they also involve access to the resources needed to improve and maintain health or health outcomes. Whitehead, an early researcher in equity, noted that "the term 'inequity' has moral and ethical dimensions. This refers to differences which are unnecessary and avoidable, and also unfair and unjust."[11] The Cochrane Collaboration promotes the use of the PROGRESS Plus checklist for researchers to ensure that research questions and their underpinning methods are appropriately planned so that sampling and data collection identifies and addresses relevant issues of equity.[12,13] The PROGRESS Plus mnemonic describes categories of social differentiation as **P**lace of residence; **R**ace/ethnicity/culture/language; **O**ccupation; **G**ender/sex; **R**eligion; **E**ducation; **S**ocioeconomic status; and **S**ocial capital. **Plus** refers to (a) personal characteristics associated with discrimination (e.g., age, disability); (b) features of relationships (e.g., smoking parents, excluded from school); and (c) time-dependent relationships (e.g., leaving the hospital, respite care, other instances when a person may be temporarily at a disadvantage). SDOH relate to the health risks associated with places where "people live, learn, work, and play."[14] SDOH include people's neighborhood and built environment; economic stability; education; health and healthcare, and social and community contexts.[15]

Public health nutrition is a quickly growing area, but it is currently variably defined. The Giessen Declaration defined nutrition science as the study of food systems, foods and drinks and their nutrients and other constituents, and their interactions within and between all relevant biological, social, and environmental systems.[16] Lawrence and Worsley built on this definition and contend that public health nutrition is concerned with promoting and maintaining the nutritional health of populations and is a fundamental resource for the social, cultural, and economic well-being of local, national, and global communities.[17] On the other hand, The Nutrition Society in the United Kingdom "defines public health nutrition as the application of nutrition and physical activity to the promotion of good health, the primary prevention of diet-related illness of groups, communities, and populations (not individuals)."[18] This differentiates public health nutrition from clinical nutrition and medical nutritional practices.

LET US NOW CONSIDER EPIDEMIOLOGY AS A PUBLIC HEALTH BUILDING BLOCK

As noted earlier, epidemiology is a fundamental public health building block that estimates the strength of association between disease and its potential causes. The word "epidemiology" comes from Greek: *epi* = among, *demos* = people, and *logos* = study. Epidemiological research is often observational and, as such, may not deliberately intervene in people's environments to manipulate their circumstances. Epidemiological research may also include intervention research (trials/experiments), in which deliberate intervention into people's environments or behaviors is the core research component. Epidemiological research capitalizes on natural occurrences and the fact that humans make choices, or have different opportunities to encounter exposures, that might cause them to contract diseases or experience poor health outcomes. Epidemiological research is an appropriate way of studying population choices and behaviors or the impact of specific events (changes to country's laws or natural disasters), particularly when it is impractical or unethical to intervene in a population to produce disease. Thus, epidemiology is the research method of choice to examine situations in which diseases occur naturally in specific locations or might be the result of exposures such as occupational hazards, cigarette smoking, or poor diets.

Clinical epidemiology goes hand in hand with biostatistics because the underpinning tenet of epidemiology is the capacity to measure exposures and disease accurately, to understand their relationships, and to take account of potentially confounding and modifying factors.[7] Biostatistics, which applies statistical concepts to the field of human and population health, offers a set of tools to evaluate the quality of measures and to construct models that enable us to compare health outcomes across populations and exposures. This does not suggest that epidemiological inferences can be made by simply examining associations between measures in a dataset (data mining) and then proposing theories to explain what has been found. Any epidemiological investigation requires careful a priori hypothesis setting and considering the underlying rationale for the proposed exposures to be linked with disease outcomes. *A priori* (Latin for "from the former") means ideas that formed or conceived beforehand.[19] More about this is discussed later.

Common reasons to apply epidemiological principles include

- Understanding cause and effect (for instance, disease causality or whether disease occurs differently in different populations)
- Defining population characteristics that could inform future experimental research
- Understanding important subgroups or combinations of factors that impact health

Many epidemiologists argue that no one should attempt to conduct an intervention study (experiment/trial) without first exploring all that is known about the epidemiology of the condition and its determinants.[6,19,20] It is particularly important to ensure that good statistical principles are followed when an experiment is conducted, for instance, when establishing that there is no difference at baseline between trial arms. Unless epidemiological research has identified important confounders (important variables that might obscure the true relationship between an exposure and disease), testing for homogeneity at baseline may fail to identify the impact of important characteristics of subjects or the environment.

HISTORY OF EPIDEMIOLOGY

Epidemiology is generally considered to be a "'young" research area in that it has really only emerged in research importance in the Western literature in the past 50 or so years. Indeed, epidemiological methods, understandings, and mechanics have improved exponentially since the early 1980s as it has become easier to share knowledge nationally and internationally, surveillance mechanisms have become more accurate, understanding of the biology of disease has improved, and software and computing capacity has developed and refined. Such is the importance of the area that acquiring some understanding of epidemiological and biostatistical principles is considered essential to the curricula in health training programs, if not in undergraduate programs, then certainly in graduate and postgraduate programs.

However, epidemiological observations have been reported for centuries, and some of the most impactful findings about disease causality have occurred by keen observation, well before computers or even recognition of the germ theory of disease. Early epidemiological research could be termed "forensic epidemiology," as it was usually associated with determining causes of diseases which were posing serious and immediate threats to health. Observation and critical thinking are what epidemiology is all about, underpinned by careful a priori consideration of biological rationale and reasoned deductions on available evidence. One often-cited example of historical observational epidemiology is the story of the Broad Street well in Soho, London, and the cholera outbreak, involving an early epidemiologist and public health activist, Dr. John Snow, in 1854 (see Box 2.1). John Snow is credited with challenging the predominant "miasma theory" with detailed evidence of cause and effect regarding the spread of cholera via the water in the well. The miasma theory was widely proposed by learned people at the time, who believed that diseases were spread through "bad air," in which particles from decomposed matter become part of the air and cause the spread of disease.[21]

Another historical example of epidemiological enquiry is that of rickets (called the English disease), for which there are over 400 years of medical observations and theories. This disease largely affects babies and young children and is evidenced by retarded bone growth—particularly leg bones, spine, skull, and ribs—and abnormal postural development. Zhang et al. provide a comprehensive overview of the history of rickets diagnosis and epidemiology.[22] There were many proposed causes of rickets in the 1600s and 1700s, including evil spirits, the pressure of swaddling clothes, and miasma (again). Now, it is well understood that inadequate diet, particularly vitamin D, and exposure to sunlight are key causes of rickets. Zhang et al. warn of a resurgence of rickets because of modern day environmental and social factors such as poverty; inadequate (or restricted) diet on cultural or religious grounds, or because of nutrition beliefs; pollution; and child neglect.[22]

BIOSTATISTICAL PRINCIPLES IN EPIDEMIOLOGY

Epidemiological data are usually collected or interpreted in binary form (1 = disease is present; 0 = disease is absent; 1 = exposure is present; 0 = exposure is absent). Epidemiological theory suggests that any sample (or population) can be divided into four groups: those with or without

BOX 2.1

JOHN SNOW'S DISEASE OUTBREAK MAP OF CHOLERA DEATHS AROUND LOCAL WATER PUMPS

In 1854, a major cholera outbreak occurred in Soho in London, England. In the space of a week, 127 people died, diagnosed with cholera. By the next week, a further 500 people had died. John Snow, who was also credited with breaking down religious, medical, and ethical opposition by administering chloroform to Queen Victoria for the births of Prince Leopold and Princess Beatrice, was called in to try to identify the cause of the cholera outbreak. He mapped the geography of the neighborhood, watched what people did, and gathered verbal evidence from anyone who would talk to him about their daily activities and those of their neighbors. He was seeking something that would link these cholera deaths together (he was thinking as an epidemiologist). An issue that emerged again and again was the water pump on Broad Street. All but 10 of the cases lived close to the pump, and it was their main water source. Of the 10 cases that did not live close to the pump, eight also used the pump. Snow mapped out the cholera deaths on the streets surrounding the pump to validate his thinking. This mapping was perhaps one of the most important legacies he made to future epidemiologists, the production of data to underpin his observations. He proposed to the local council that there was something wrong with the water from the Broad Street pump (not found in any others nearby), and it was a reason for the cholera outbreak. Although there was resistance in the council to this finding, there was agreement to remove the pump handle, and the spread of cholera halted. Snow later pointed out that there was no real evidence that this action stopped the disease, as its incidence may have been declining. However, the end result was that the events of new cholera cases dramatically declined.

Source: Data from https://www1.udel.edu/johnmack/frec682/cholera/cholera2.html

disease and exposure. The common way of organizing epidemiological data in a population is by a 2 × 2 table, which includes two columns denoting disease presence (1) or absence (0) and two rows denoting exposure presence (1) or absence (0) (Exhibit 2.1).

EXHIBIT 2.1

COMMON EPIDEMIOLOGY DATA ORGANIZATION: THE 2 × 2 TABLE

	DISEASE	NO DISEASE	
Exposed	A	B	Exposed Total
Not Exposed	C	D	Not Exposed Total
	Disease Total	No Disease Total	

People in Cell A are classified as 1,1 (they have both disease and exposure of interest) and people in Cell D are classified as 0,0 (they have neither disease nor exposure of interest). The people in Cell B have the exposure of interest but not the disease (classified 0,1), and conversely, the people in Cell C have the disease of interest but not the exposure (classified 1,0). The coding 1, 0 is reflective of the way that early epidemiological measures were taken and recorded (Yes = 1 = people have the disease or exposure; No = 0 = people do not have the disease or exposure). So if we take the example of John Snow's cholera outbreak and drinking the water in the Broad Street well (Box 2.1), he may well have constructed a 2 × 2 table as follows: People in Cell A are classified 1,1 if they have a diagnosis of cholera and a history of drinking water from the Broad Street well; People in Cell D would be classified as 0,0 if they have neither a diagnosis of cholera nor a history of drinking water from the Broad Street well. The people in Cell B have the exposure of interest (they drank the Broad Street well water but do not have a cholera diagnosis; classified 0,1). Conversely, the people in Cell C have a cholera diagnosis but no history of drinking water from the Broad Street well (classified 1,0).

The 2 × 2 table is a helpful tool to evaluate whether the exposure is related to disease. Specifically, it enables the calculation of the strength of association between the disease columns and exposure rows, which is usually expressed as relative risk or risk ratio (RR).

- The RR is a ratio of two probabilities. The probability of a disease event occurring in the exposed group is $a/(a + b) = R1$, and similarly, the probability of a disease event occurring in the nonexposed group is $c/(c + d) = R2$. The risk of disease occurring in the exposed group (R1) is then compared to the risk of disease occurring in the unexposed group (R2). The ratio of these two probabilities (RR) R1/R2 is calculated as $[a/(a + b)]/[c/(c + d)]$.

- Although the RR is the preferable measure of the association between exposure and outcome because it is based on the probability of disease, it is not always possible to calculate directly, given the study design or analytical approach used. Therefore, epidemiologists may use an odds ratio (OR) to approximate the RR. The OR is the ratio of the odds of a disease event occurring in the exposed group, compared with the odds of a disease event occurring in the nonexposed group. The odds of a disease event are calculated as the number of disease events divided by the number of nondisease events (equivalent to the probability of a disease event divided by the probability of a nondisease event). Odds are often written as $P/(1 − P)$. The formula for OR is $(a × d)/(b × c)$.

RR and OR can take on any value from 0 to infinity. Because both measures represent a ratio, the value is 1.0 when the probability (or odds) of disease is exactly the same in the exposed and unexposed groups. The farther the value moves from 1, the more strongly the exposure is related to the disease. For example, an RR of 2.0 means that people who are exposed are twice as likely (or 100% more likely) to develop disease compared to people who are not exposed.

If we take a very simplistic nutrition example, a population study might be concerned with amounts of saturated fats in a population's diet and how this links to high blood pressure, because high blood pressure is the precursor for cardiovascular diseases (heart attack, stroke, etc.). These diseases are expensive to manage in the acute and secondary health sectors, and require costly ongoing care for individuals and society, particularly when they influence the individual's capacity to work or study. If blood pressure is lowered by conservative means (for instance, decreasing fat intake in the diet), events of heart attack and stroke may decline and costs to the individual, society, and health sectors will decrease.

Epidemiology and public health are intrinsically linked because epidemiology describes the health of populations. Public health interventions (such as promotion of particular food, or patterns of eating, or exercise interventions) are based on population-based evidence of cause and effect. For instance, epidemiological studies have shown repeatedly that people who have a high saturated fat intake have higher risks of high blood pressure than people who eat lower amounts of saturated fat. Considering the 2 × 2 table in Exhibit 2.1, Cell A would contain the people who have a high saturated fat intake and high blood pressure; Cell D would contain the people who have low saturated fat intake and normal blood pressure; Cell B would contain the people who have a high saturated fat intake but normal blood pressure; and Cell C would contain the people who have a low saturated fat intake but high blood pressure.

This example raises issues of measurement, which will be discussed later, concerning putting appropriate "cut points" in the data to define high and low and good and bad.

Confidence Intervals (CIs)

It is essential to estimate variability (precision) of the ORs and RRs in order to determine how strong the association actually is. Significance in biostatistics is identified when 95% CIs do not encompass 1 (1 means no association). To calculate the CI, the log odds ratio, $\log(OR) = \log(a^*d/b^*c)$, is used to calculate its standard error: $se(\log(OR)) = \sqrt{1/a + 1/b + 1/c + 1/d}$.

The CI is calculated as $\exp(\log(OR) \pm Z\alpha/2^*\sqrt{1/a + 1/b + 1/c + 1/d})$, where $Z\alpha/2$ is the critical value of the normal distribution at $\alpha/2$ (e.g., for a confidence level of 95%, α is 0.05 and the critical value is 1.96). The ease of calculating CIs around ORs and RRs has increased exponentially with the advent of increasingly sophisticated software in the past 30 years.

Confounding

Not taking account of confounding can lead to spurious and incorrect associations between exposure and disease. A confounder is usually associated with both the exposure and disease being studied, but it need not be a risk factor for the disease. The confounding variable can either inflate or deflate the true association, and it must be unequally distributed between subjects with and without disease/exposure.[7]

In experimental research, random selection of subjects from a known reference population and random allocation to study arms are undertaken largely to minimize the influence of potential confounders (i.e., theoretically, confounders have been distributed equally across study arms).[23] Thus, when testing for homogeneity at baseline, researchers are assuring themselves that before the intervention commences, there is no real difference between the cohorts allocated to intervention or control arms. The best way to identify confounders is to undertake epidemiological research, where the notion of confounding is embraced and tested.

Prior to conducting an epidemiological study, a causal pathway is generally designed, consisting of the exposure, the disease measure of choice, interim disease outcomes (which might provide alternative measures of disease), any antecedent factors that may have led to the exposure, and potential confounding variables (see Figure 2.2).[24] In the process of designing a causal pathway, epidemiologists can ensure that they have considered (as well as possible) the best way to test their hypothesis and the best measurements to take.

A number of statistical methods can be applied to control for potential confounding factors. Potential confounding factors should first be identified theoretically, either from findings of previous studies or because the factor may be considered as biologically plausible.[25] A simple way to determine whether a variable is a confounder is to determine whether there is a difference between the crude OR and the adjusted OR of 10% of greater. To do this, researchers compute the measure of association for the different levels of the confounder and then recombine the data, standardizing it by the denominator for each level of the confounder. If the difference between the crude and adjusted measures of association is 10% or more, then confounding is present. If it is less than 10%, then there was little, if any, confounding. This

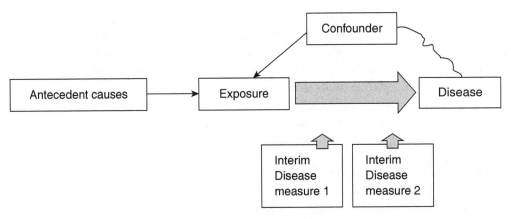

FIGURE 2.2 Causal pathway.

Source: Data from Kirkwood BR, Sterne JC. *Essential Medical Statistics.* 2nd ed. New York, NY: Blackwell Science; 2003. https://pdfs.semanticscholar.org/2de1/78e7e19a6641d48caa0ed935743ed07d409e.pdf

uses a data management approach called stratification. Software design has made testing for confounding very much simpler than it was 30+ years ago. Usually, potential confounders are first identified as being strongly associated with the exposure and with the disease (using OR calculated from 2 × 2 tables or from univariate logistic regression analyses). The potential confounder is then added to a multivariate model, which tests its influence on the association between exposure and disease. Given that the data are generally in binary form, multiple logistic regression models are used and a confounder is identified if it accounts for a significant amount of variance (adjustment) in the crude association. The potential confounder must be checked in a priori biological terms to ensure that it is not a proxy for either exposure or disease.[25] Significant associations are identified when 95% CI do not encompass 1. Another approach to identifying a confounder is to create a causal diagram, similar to the causal pathway outlined earlier. A causal diagram, namely a directed acyclic graph (DAG), seeks to identify all causal pathways between exposure and disease and also between potential confounders included in the diagram. Then, in order to identify which confounders should be included in a statistical model, one seeks to identify any paths from the exposure to the disease that do not emanate directly from the exposure itself.[26]

Effect Modification (Interaction)

Another benefit of examining potential confounders in subgroups of the data is that effect modification can be detected. This occurs when the effect of an exposure is different among different subgroups and may require different interventions. For instance, if women are suspected as having a different biological causal path for obesity and blood pressure than men, the association between obesity and blood pressure will be significantly different for women than for men.[7] This will be shown by stratification of the association between obesity and blood pressure (for women and for men) and testing the difference in ORs between the subgroups.

STUDY TYPES AND ORGANIZATION

Observational epidemiological studies may be **cross-sectional studies**, **cohort studies**, or case–control studies.

Cross-sectional studies are distinguished from other types of observational studies because they occur at a single point in time and therefore represent a cross-section of the respondent's life experience. Data for cross-sectional studies frequently come from surveys or surveillance systems, which collect information on a variety of health behaviors and health outcomes across members of a population. For example, one might be interested in knowing whether obesity is more common among children who live in households experiencing poverty than in households above the poverty threshold. In this case, a cross-sectional study could be conducted to compare the prevalence of childhood obesity in households below and above the poverty threshold, adjusting for potential confounding factors, using data from a state or national health surveillance system.

The advantages of cross-sectional studies include the fact that often data are already collected and available, often as part of routine public health practice, and therefore these types of studies are relatively inexpensive and quick to conduct. A primary disadvantage of cohort studies is that the temporal (time) sequence of an exposure–disease relationship is unclear. In other words, because we measure both exposure and outcome simultaneously, it can be difficult to determine which came first. This is the primary reason why cross-sectional studies generally are not sufficient for us to make causal inference about an exposure–disease relationship. Imagine, for example, that we are interested in understanding whether fish consumption influences the likelihood of being obese based on a person's BMI. We might survey people about their fish consumption and their height and weight, or perhaps even be able to use data from an existing health survey to make this comparison. Even if we observe that people with higher fish consumption tend to be classified as obese less often than people with lower fish consumption, it would be difficult to establish whether the fish consumption caused people to have a lower BMI or whether the person's BMI influenced the likelihood of eating fish. In some cases, it is possible to ask questions in such a way that we can be relatively confident that the exposure preceded the outcome. However, these approaches will always rely on a respondent's memory because we are asking about historical exposures, and therefore we may have misreporting in our data, which can result in misclassification and potentially bias. Other biases that can occur in cross-sectional studies include sampling and selection bias (in that people may self-nominate or investigators may seek out particular types of people to participate), information bias (in terms of attenuation of information that is provided, which participants might perceive to be less than acceptable), and recall bias.[27]

Cohort studies are those in which a group of people is recruited, typically at one place or time point, and are divided into an exposed subgroup and an unexposed subgroup. All members of the cohort must be free of the disease of interest at the start so that the incidence (development) of disease can be compared in the exposed and unexposed groups. A cohort may be prospective, in which the development of disease is followed in real time, or retrospective, in which records are used to determine past exposure levels and follow-up for disease incidence. A cohort is potentially likely to have been exposed to the same type of factors (environmental, nutritional, personal) and to have similar risks of exhibiting (or developing) a disease.[6]

There is no perfect way of undertaking epidemiological research or recruiting samples, probably because of the very nature of researching people! Fletcher et al. provide a list of advantages and disadvantages of cohort studies.[6]

Advantages include:

- It is the only way of establishing incidence directly.
- They follow the same logic as clinical questions (if a person is exposed, do they get the disease?).

- Exposure can be elicited without the bias that might occur if outcome was already known.
- Researchers can assess the relationship between exposure and many diseases.

Disadvantages include:

- They are inefficient. More subjects need to be enrolled than experience the event of interest; therefore, cohort studies are not useful for rare diseases.
- They are expensive because of resources necessary to study people over time.
- Results may not be available for some time.
- They can only assess the relationship between disease and exposure to relatively few factors.

A retrospective cohort study is a study in which disease is known and the exposure is hypothesized. People with the disease usually come to the attention of clinicians first, and when concerns are raised by astute clinicians that something is not right (i.e., the prevalence or presentation of the disease is unusual), epidemiologists track back in time to establish the exposure and to identify other cases with disease that may not have been identified or in which disease may not yet have occurred. There are many examples of retrospective cohort studies around the world, with a range of diseases and historical exposures, and varying periods of latency of disease presentation.

One area that has attracted worldwide interest is the Wittenoom study in Western Australia of the effect of blue asbestos on miners and their families living in Wittenoom during the period 1940–1970s. The first case of mesothelioma in a Wittenoom worker was diagnosed in 1960, despite fears for more than 10 years by respiratory physicians that the town's asbestos industry would spawn an epidemic of serious lung disease among its workers. By the time a report of the late mill worker's fatal cancer was published in the *Medical Journal of Australia* 2 years later, about 100 miners and millers at Wittenoom already had serious lung damage. In 1975, a retrospective cohort study was instigated to identify who among the workers at Wittenoom were most at risk of developing lung disease and the length of time between their first exposure to blue asbestos and when the disease was first detected. The researchers obtained access to workers' records and air quality data, and attempted to trace the 6,505 men employed at Wittenoom between 1943 and 1966. Armed with the names of workers (the Wittenoom cohort), the researchers then scoured electoral rolls, drivers' licenses, hospital records, and death certificates to find out what had happened to the men. Of the 6,200 workers whom the research team traced, 220 (3.5%) had pneumoconiosis, or serious lung damage, and 26 had mesothelioma. Sixty men had already died from respiratory cancer—nearly twice the mortality rate for all Western Australian males. The study reported a strong relationship between intensity of asbestos exposure and these diseases. There have been more than 50 papers published to date on the study, and another wave of research is now investigating women and children who lived in Wittenoom around this time.[28–30]

There are many biases inherent in retrospective cohort studies, mostly relating to sampling and measurement. If old records are accessed (as in the Wittenoom study), data integrity or completeness may be questionable. If data are missing, there may be no other source of information, particularly if "dead" cases are being counted (people who died prior to the study commencement, and who may have died of the disease of interest, but it may not have been diagnosed as such at the time).

Retrospective studies in nutrition are notoriously flawed by recall bias in self-reporting. Recall bias is

a systematic error that occurs when participants do not remember previous events or experiences accurately or omit details: the accuracy and volume of memories may be influenced by subsequent events and experiences. . . . Bias in recall can be greater when the study participant has poorer recall in general, and when [the time interval being asked about is longer]. Other issues that influence recall include age, education, socioeconomic status and how important the [disease] is to the patient. [Added to this], undesirable habits such as smoking or eating unhealthy foods tend to be underreported, and are therefore subject to recall bias. Pre-existing beliefs may also impact on recall of previous events.[31]

These studies hypothesize a (short-term) relationship between disease (poor outcome) and exposure such that they can both be measured within a short period of time (few hours or days); see Figure 2.3. An example of cause–effect hypotheses that might be appropriate for cross-sectional cohort study design is the relationship between eating different types of food at lunchtime (salads vs. baked dinner vs. rice vs. no lunch) on levels of energy 1 hour after lunch. This is a question that bothers many teachers and university professors when teaching postlunch classes to students who are in various states of sleepiness! One important reminder is that causality cannot be inferred from cross-sectional studies, so lecturers concerned that students are going to sleep in class after lunch cannot say that eating pasta (for instance) makes them sleepy.

Prospective cohort studies compile a cohort of subjects who are currently nondiseased and a mix of exposed and unexposed. Cohort members are then tracked for disease occurrence (incidence), as some are expected to make choices or assume different behaviors over time (exposures), which may contribute to disease occurrence (Figure 2.3).

Prospective (longitudinal) studies usually follow cohorts for years. They are expensive and challenging to conduct because the initial cohort needs to be tracked comprehensively to ensure minimal attrition and each member of the cohort needs to be reassessed regularly over time. If behaviors are being tracked, then the most accurate way of recording behaviors needs to be determined, and individuals in the cohort have to agree to ongoing data collection.

The Framingham Heart Study is an internationally known example of a prospective cohort study, examining cardiovascular disease occurrence in people living in Framingham, Massachusetts. The study began in 1948 with 5,209 adults, and is now on its third generation of participants.[32] Much of the now-common knowledge concerning heart disease (for instance, the

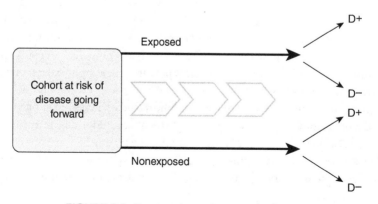

FIGURE 2.3 Prospective cohort study design.

impact of diet, exercise, aspirin) comes from this study. A number of cohort studies have resulted from this prospective study:

- The Original Cohort: The first cohort study began in 1948 with 5,209 participants ranging in age from 30 to 62. Participants were men and women with no history of stroke or heart attack.

- The Offspring Cohort: The next cohort study began in 1971. The 5,124 participants included children of the Original Cohort patients as well as the children's spouses.

- The Omni Cohort: This cohort study began in 1994 and focused on the growing diversity of the Framingham community. The 506 participants were recruited from different ethnic groups.

- The Third Generation Cohort: This cohort study started in 2002 with 4,095 of the children of the Offspring Cohort (many of whom were also grandchildren of the Original Cohort participants).

- The Omni Two Cohort: This cohort study started in 2003 with children of the Omni Cohort patients. There were 410 participants, making the Omni Two Cohort approximately 10% of the size of the Third Generation Cohort.[32]

There are a number of biases that can plague longitudinal studies, including loss to follow-up (subjects dropping out of the study), Hawthorne bias (behaviors change because of being observed), and measurement error (as in over- or underreporting).[33] If the cohort is recruited at the same point in time, then chronological bias is unlikely to play a role (when study participants are subject to different exposures or are at a different risk from participants who are recruited later).[31]

In *case–control studies*, cases are known (disease is already diagnosed) and control subjects are chosen from people who are similar but without the disease. A case–control study aims to select controls who represent the population that produced the cases (providing an estimate of the exposure rate in the population). Case–control studies are by nature retrospective because disease has already occurred in cases, and reasons for it are sought. Cases and controls are usually matched by factors that are considered to be potential confounders (e.g., age, gender, place of residence, socioeconomic factors). The feature that distinguishes case–control studies from cohort studies is that "cases have the outcome of interest at the time that information on risk factors is sought."[6] In other words, in a cohort study participants are sampled based on exposure and in a case–control study they are sampled based on outcome. Data collection integrity is essential in case–control studies so that researchers do not bias the way they elicit information. They must ensure that they ask each study participant the same questions in the same way so as not to influence their responses.

An example of a case–control study that significantly influenced hospital policy regarding education of mothers of newborn babies was the Tasmanian Sudden Infant Death study.[34] This was a population-based retrospective case–control study conducted between 1988 and 1991, during which time there were 62 sudden infant death syndrome (SIDS) cases. These cases were matched with babies of the same gender, date and place of birth, maternal age, and smoking status. Predictors of SIDS events were found to be sleeping prone, maternal smoking, a family history of asthma, and bedroom heating during last sleep. Protective factors were maternal age over 25 years and more than one child health clinic attendance. On the findings of this study, mothers of newborns were educated about placing their children on their sides or backs to sleep, no smoking, not heating the child's room, and using child health clinics as often as possible.[34]

Diagnostic accuracy is essential in case–control studies so that all cases included in the study are based on the same diagnostic criteria. Case–control studies may be biased by reporting biases or errors during data collection, and there may be differential reporting of exposure information between cases and controls, based on their disease status (recall bias). For example, in a case–control study of cancer, people with the disease may have thought more about their past diets and therefore report more accurately than people without disease, or they may have read about dietary components associated with developing cancer and therefore overreport their consumption of particular food items compared to people without disease. In either of these cases, recall bias would result, which could cause us to make the wrong conclusion about whether diet influences the risk of developing cancer. Other types of bias are also possible in case–control studies. Recording of exposure information may vary depending on the investigator's suspicion of disease status (interviewer/observer bias). Selection bias is inherent in case–control studies, in which it gives rise to noncomparability between cases and controls. Selection bias in case–control studies may occur when "cases (or controls) are included in (or excluded from) a study because of some characteristic they exhibit which is related to exposure to the risk factor under evaluation."[20] Therefore, selection bias may occur when those individuals selected as controls are unrepresentative of the population that produced the cases. Selection bias in case–control studies occurs when cases and controls are recruited from one site (hospital, school, workplace), as people in these sites may have different characteristics than the general population. If these characteristics are related to exposures under investigation, then estimates of exposure among controls may differ from the broader reference population.[20] Selection bias may be minimized by selecting controls from more than one source.[6]

Experimental studies, sometimes referred to as clinical trials, are considered the gold standard for epidemiologic inquiry. Unlike observational studies, experimental studies require the alteration by researchers of the natural history of study participants in order to test the effectiveness of an "exposure" or intervention on a disease outcome. These studies are generally not conducted without sufficient evidence from observational studies to justify such an approach.

Clinical trials, particularly drug trials, are conducted in phases designed primarily to assess safety, dosage, and efficacy/effectiveness. Information gathered in each phase is used to justify moving to the next phase. Phase 0 studies are exploratory in nature and are conducted in small groups of humans (approximately 10–20) to assess drug properties. Phase 1 studies are usually conducted with healthy volunteers (approximately 20–100) and focus on drug safety, metabolism, and excretion. Phase 2 studies gather preliminary data in a sample of approximately 100–300 participants on efficacy/effectiveness. When appropriate, these studies may include the use of an inert substance, or "placebo," to compare the impact on short-term outcomes. These studies also assess safety.

Phase 3 studies are generally the ones that are most popular in the media and are conducted across a variety of interventions. These studies primarily gather information from large study populations (300 or more) to assess safety and efficacy/effectiveness by studying different populations and levels of the intervention. The ideal scenario is for these studies to be conducted in such a manner that study participants are randomized into the intervention or placebo arms (or various levels of the intervention). It is also ideal for the study to be conducted, when feasible, for the study participants and researchers to not know which arm they are in, which is known as "double-blinded." For drug trials that show significant efficacy and are approved by the Food and Drug Administration (FDA), Phase 4 studies assess a drug's safety, efficacy, and optimal use after they have been released on the market for a period of time.

There are many advantages to experimental studies, including being the only true test of the efficacy of an intervention, the ability to control the exposure of the study participants to the intervention and adjust for confounding factors, and to simultaneously test for safety and dosage while assessing efficacy. Disadvantages of experimental studies include excessive time and costs, limited external validity and the potential that there will be loss to follow-up and minimal adherence to the protocol by study participants.

Experimental study designs can be used in nutrition research to assess the impacts of dietary patterns on chronic diseases (e.g., diabetes, cancer, cardiovascular disease) and chronic disease risk factors (e.g., glycemic control, blood pressure, blood cholesterol). Study participants can be randomized to follow a particular nutritional intervention versus their usual dietary intake. Adherence to the study protocol can be determined through self-reported dietary intake, nutritional biomarkers, and/or direct observation.[35,36]

Epidemiological Data

Data can be captured by a number of methods for epidemiological studies, and many studies use multiple forms of data capture. There is usually a lot of data required to ensure that important associations are identified and tested. Data can come from surveys (mailed, emailed, face to face, telephone), from registry data (for instance, chronic disease or registries, road accident records, hospital databases), and from objective measures captured face to face. Each method of data capture has its limitations, and before decisions are made to capture data in a particular manner, all possible methods should be considered. This may require systematic reviews of the literature to understand how others have captured similar data and to understand the degree of potential measurement error.[7,24]

Measures need to be valid to limit opportunities for misinterpretation of findings. They also need to be accurate, particularly because data are usually only collected once. When epidemiological data were captured in the early days of its history, there was little opportunity for error in disease—people were either dead (1) or alive (0) or they had cholera (1) or not (0), and they had a definitive exposure (they had drunk their water from the Broad Street well (1) or not (0)). These measures were valid and accurate and could reliably be made by another person.

However epidemiological measurements are not as simple now, and more thoughtful and sophisticated data capture and management may be required to ensure that people are correctly classified as diseased or exposed. For instance, take eating behaviors. If researchers are interested in testing the consumption of vegetables in relation to heart disease, subjects in a study might be asked about usual consumption (type of vegetable, portion, daily frequency; exposure) and heart disease status (defined from pathology tests; Yes = 1, No = 0). Vegetable consumption might then be collated into a type–portion–frequency index (a continuous variable). "Usual" consumption would need to be defined first, with a set time period (yesterday, on average in a week, etc.). The vegetable consumption index would range from 0 to the highest number (for people with high vegetable intake). This number would then need to be divided into binary form for analysis, particularly to be compared with heart disease outcomes (binary form; Yes = 1, No = 0). The usual way to divide continuous exposure data is to examine the distribution of the type–portion–frequency index, and divide it at the median value. The hypothesis under consideration would probably be that low vegetable intake is associated with heart disease (1); thus the risk level of vegetable intake would be the lower end of the index (coded 1). This means that the 2 × 2 table would be designed so that 1,1 identified people with low vegetable intake and heart disease, and 0,0 identified people with high vegetable intake and no heart disease. Other more fancy ways of identifying the appropriate cut point might be to apply an approach in which the exposure variable was divided into smaller portions (say tertiles, quartiles, and even quintiles) and the differential association between exposure categories and disease was tested using independent exposure categories in logistic regression models.[1,7] Thus, determining appropriate measures of dietary exposure can be complex, and much thought needs to go into data capture methods before the study gets off the ground.

Similar situations may arise with capture of disease data. All the elements of the disease may need to be considered, in terms of chronicity of symptoms, patterns of severity (frequency, intensity), and nature of symptoms. Take headache or low back pain, which can vary in presentation, frequency, and impact on the individual. An index of low back pain is often produced, and the same principles applied to determine low back pain occurrence that has high and low classifications. Often in situations such as this, the sample may be divided into three classifications: those with no low back pain (0) and two "diseased" groups (those with low index of low back pain and those with high index of low back pain). Three comparisons can then be made between diseased groups and potential risk factors (high index of low back pain compared with none; low index of low back pain compared with none; high index of low back pain compared with low index). This type of approach may identify different causal pathways and may identify dose–response relationships.

CONCLUSION

The constructs of epidemiology must be considered prior to designing any research, as these constructs underpin the methods inherent in all scientific endeavors. Epidemiological principles provide a framework for understanding and determining best measures and ways of applying them and for identifying cause and effect on causal pathways. Epidemiological principles underpin not only the conduct of good research but also its reporting and the implementation of research findings into real-world practices. The value of using a framework of epidemiology in public health nutrition is yet to be fully explored, as not only is good nutrition intrinsic to people's health but it also is integral to the way people operate within their cultures and languages, their social structures, their familial roles, and their family economics. The development of epidemiological principles has correlated with better quality research over the past 30 years, and it has produced better educated and more critical researchers, healthcare providers, and policy-makers.

KEY CONCEPTS

It is important for students, researchers, clinicians, and policy-makers to understand the components of causality and the epidemiology of nutrition when designing interventions. There are different types of research evidence and they provide different pieces of information. The causality of disease in specific circumstances should underpin understanding of effective interventions as well as outcome measures. It is important that end users understand the ways in which this evidence is produced and the limitations of each research evidence source.

CASE STUDY: 56-YEAR-OLD WHITE FEMALE PRESENTS WITH WORSENING OSTEOPENIA

Michelle is a 56-year-old White female. She is 5′6″ tall and weighs 120 pounds (BMI 19.4). She is postmenopausal and is not taking hormone-replacement therapy. She is very active; she runs approximately 50 miles a week and also does strength training exercises. She has a history of melanoma and so she tries to limit her direct exposure to sunlight. Despite her physical activity level, she has been diagnosed with osteopenia, which has gotten worse in recent years. Her doctor has advised her to spend more time outside and increase her consumption of vitamin D and calcium. She is reluctant to increase her sunlight exposure given her history of melanoma, and she does not like many foods that include vitamin D and calcium. She is also on a limited budget; so she has not been willing to purchase nutritional supplements.

Case Study Questions

1. What advice would you give Michelle to try to avoid her declining bone health?

2. What other concerns might Michelle consider in her overall health?

3. What type of study design might you use to answer the questions that Michelle might have to help make informed decisions about her health?

SUGGESTED LEARNING ACTIVITIES

1. Consider every public health nutrition issue with which you are faced, in terms of likely exposures (including antecedent causes) that may contribute to the disease (outcome), and the confounders that may be at play.

2. Consider how you would apply observation and clinical reasoning, which are essential skills for every epidemiologist, and nothing is too basic or simple to consider.

3. Consider how individual choice and health literacy influence exposures and disease outcomes.

4. Identify which exposures and confounders are mutable (can be changed) and which are not.

5. Do not seek to intervene to change nutritional outcomes until you have a clear understanding of cause and effect; there is no point in applying an intervention that may not be relevant to the cause–effect model.

6. Identify the strongest exposures for disease outcomes and focus interventions on them for optimum effect.

REFLECTION QUESTIONS

1. How might research be used to help address the impact of the SDOH and enhance equity in populations in various venues?

2. What challenges might be found in conducting nutritional epidemiological research in rural communities? In urban communities?

3. How might technology be used in epidemiological research to better enhance the potential to collect high-quality data?

CONTINUE YOUR LEARNING RESOURCES

Nutritional Epidemiology is a journal focused on nutrition research in disease prevention. https://www
.frontiersin.org/journals/nutrition/sections/nutritional-epidemiology

Take a look at the EPIC study on the WHO website. It is one of the largest prospective studies in which nutritional data have been collected from over 500,000 people in 10 European countries in which hundreds of studies have been published demonstrating an evidence basis for existing hypotheses for the development of nutrition recommendations to prevent disease. https://epic.iarc.fr/research/
activitiesbyresearchfields/nutritionalepidemiology.php

Review this article on the relationship between nutritional epidemiology and food policy along with those cited in the article. https://www.ncbi.nlm.nih.gov/pmc/articles/PMC4288279

GLOSSARY

Clinical epidemiology: A field of study that involves designing and managing clinical trials, maintaining disease registries, and conducting studies to evaluate the usefulness of diagnostic and screening tests in clinical practice.

Cohort studies: Studies in which a group of people is recruited, typically at one place, or time point, and is divided into an exposed subgroup and an unexposed subgroup. All members of the cohort must be free of the disease of interest at the start so that the incidence (development) of disease can be compared in the exposed and unexposed groups. A cohort may be prospective, in which the development of disease is followed in real time, or retrospective, in which records are used to determine past exposure levels and follow-up for disease incidence. A cohort is potentially likely to have been exposed to the same type of factors (environmental, nutritional, personal) and to have similar risks of exhibiting (or developing) a disease.

Cross-sectional studies: Distinguished from other types of observational studies because they occur at a single point in time and therefore represent a cross-section of the respondent's life experience. Data for cross-sectional studies frequently come from surveys or surveillance systems, which collect information on a variety of health behaviors and health outcomes across members of a population. For example, one might be interested in knowing whether obesity is more common among children who live in households experiencing poverty than in households above the poverty threshold. In this case, a cross-sectional study could be conducted to compare the prevalence of childhood obesity in households below and above the poverty threshold, adjusting for potential confounding factors, using data from a state or national health surveillance system.

Disease: The term "disease" is used, in epidemiological terms, as an umbrella term for a disease diagnosis, death, a poor health outcome (for instance, high BMI or low back pain), or problematic health event (like a car crash).

Epidemiology: The study of health in populations. Epidemiology encompasses a set of methods by which population health (public health) and the threats to it are assessed using biostatistics and monitored.

Exposure: The term "exposure" is used ubiquitously for any factor that may be associated with disease. There is an array of factors, but common ones include biological, familial, chemical, physical, occupational, psychosocial, socioeconomic, travel, educational, cultural, and nutrition.

Public health: The "science and art of preventing disease, prolonging life and promoting human health through organized efforts and informed choices of society, organizations, public and private, communities and individuals."[2]

Social determinants of health (SDOH): These relate to the health risks associated with places where "people live, learn, work, and play."[14] SDOH comprise people's neighborhoods and built environment, economic stability, education, health and healthcare, and social and community contexts.[15]

REFERENCES

1. Kelsey JL, Thompson WD, Evans AS. Methods in observational epidemiology. In: *Monographs in Epidemiology and Biostatistics.* Vol. 10. New York, NY: Oxford University Press; 1986.
2. Winslow CA. The untilled field of public health. *Mod Med.* 1920;2:183–191.

3. CDC Foundation. *What is public health?* https://www.cdcfoundation.org/what-public-health

4. Porta M. *A Dictionary of Epidemiology.* 6th ed. New York, NY: Oxford University Press; 2014.

5. Joint Task Group on Public Health Human Resources; Advisory Committee on Health Delivery & Human Resources; Advisory Committee on Population Health & Health Security. *Building the Public Health Workforce for the 21st Century.* Ottawa, Canada: Public Health Agency of Canada; 2005.

6. Fletcher RH, Fletcher SW, Wagner EH. *Clinical Epidemiology: The Essentials.* Baltimore, MA: Wilkins & Wilkins; 1988.

7. Rothman KJ. *Modern Epidemiology.* Boston, MA: Little, Brown & Co; 1986.

8. World Health Organization. *Public health surveillance.* https://www.who.int/topics/public_health_surveillance/en 2019

9. Centers for Disease Control and Prevention. *The public health system & the 10 essential public health services.* https://www.cdc.gov/publichealthgateway/publichealthservices/essentialhealthservices.html

10. World Health Organization. *Gender, Equity and Human Rights.* 2020. https://www.who.int/gender-equity-rights/understanding/equity-definition/en

11. Whitehead M. The concepts and principles of equity and health. *Health Promot Int.* 1991;6(3):217–228. doi:10.1093/heapro/6.3.217

12. Ueffing E, Tugwell P, Welch V, et al. *Equity Checklist for Systematic Review Authors.* Version 2012-10-02. http://equity.cochrane.org/sites/equity.cochrane.org/files/uploads/EquityChecklist2012.pdf

13. Oliver S, Kavanagh J, Caird J, et al. *Health Promotion, Inequalities and Young People's Health: A Systematic Review of Research.* London, UK: EPPI-Centre, Social Science Research Unit, Institute of Education, University of London; 2008. http://eppi.ioe.ac.uk

14. Office of Disease Prevention and Health Promotion. *Social Determinants of Health.* 2019. https://www.healthypeople.gov/2020/topics-objectives/topic/social-determinants-of-health

15. Commission on Social Determinants of Health. *Closing the Gap in a Generation: Health Equity Through Action on the Social Determinants of Health.* Geneva, Switzerland: World Health Organization; 2011. http://www.who.int/ social_determinants/en

16. Beauman C, Cnnon G, Elmadfa I, et al. The Giessen Declaration. *Public Health Nutr.* 2005;8(6A):783–786. doi:10.1079/phn2005768

17. Lawrence M, Worsley A. *Public Health Nutrition: From Principles to Practice.* Crow's Nest, Australia: Allen & Unwin; 2007:512.

18. Uauy R. Understanding public health nuttrition. *Lancet.* 2007;370(9584):309–310. doi:10.1016/S0140-6736(07)61145-3

19. Dictionary by Merriam-Webster. https://www.merriam-webster.com/dictionary

20. Hennekens CH, Buring JE. *Epidemiology in Medicine.* Philadelphia, PA: Lippincott Williams & Wilkins; 1987.

21. Ramsay MAE. John Snow, MD: anaesthetist to the Queen of England and pioneer epidemiologist. *Baylor Univ Med Cent Proc.* 2006;19(1):24–28. doi:10.1080/08998280.2006.11928120

22. Zhang M, Shen F, Petryk A, et al. "English disease": historical notes on rickets, the bone–lung link and child neglect issues. *Nutrients.* 2016;8(11):722. doi:10.3390/nu8110722

23. Sackett DL, Rosenberg WM, Gray JA, et al. Evidence-based medicine: what it is and what it isn't. *BMJ.* 1996;312:71–72. doi:10.1136/bmj.312.7023.71

24. Kirkwood BR, Sterne JC. *Essential Medical Statistics.* New York, NY: Blackwell Science; 2003.

25. Hill A. The environment and disease: association or causation?. *Proc R Soc Med.* 1965;58:295–300.

26. Greenland S, Pearl J, Robins JM. Causal diagrams for epidemiologic research. *Am J Epidemiol.* 1999;10(1):37–48. doi:10.1097/00001648-199901000-00008

27. Yu IT, Tse SL. Clinical Epidemiology Workshop 6—sources of bias in cross-sectional studies; summary on sources of bias for different study designs. *Hong Kong Med J.* 2012;18:226–227.

28. Armstrong BK, de Klerk NH, Musk A, Hobbs MH. Mortality in miners and millers of crocidolite in Western Australia. *Br J Ind Med.* 1988;45(1):5–13. doi:10.1136/oem.45.1.5

29. Berry G. Prediction of mesothelioma, lung cancer, and asbestosis in former Wittenoom asbestos workers. *Br J Ind Med.* 1991;48:793–780. doi:10.1136/oem.48.12.793

30. Reid A, de Klerk NH, Magnani C, et al. Mesothelioma risk after 40 years since first exposure to asbestos: a pooled analysis. *Thorax.* 2014;69:843–850. doi:10.1136/thoraxjnl-2013-204161

31. Catalogue of Bias Collaboration, Spencer EA, Brassey J, Mahtani K. Recall bias. In: *Catalogue of Bias.* 2017. https://www.catalogofbias.org/biases/recall-bias

32. Mahmood L, Vasan W. The Framingham Heart Study and the epidemiology of cardiovascular disease: a historical perspective. *Lancet.* 2013;383(9921):999–1008. doi:10.1016/S0140-6736(13)61752-3

33. Lissner L, Skoog I, Andersson K, et al. Participation bias in longitudinal studies: experience from the population study of women in Gothenburg, Sweden. *Scand J Prim Health Care.* 2003;21(4):242–247. doi:10.1080/02813430310003309-1693

34. Ponsonby AL, Dwyer T, Kasl SV, Cochrane JA. The Tasmanian SIDS Case-Control Study: univariable and multivariable risk factor analysis. *Paediatr Perinat Epidemiol.* 1995;9(3):256–272. doi:10.1111/j.1365-3016.1995.tb00141.x

35. Friedman LM, Furberg CD, DeMets D, Reboussin DM, Granger CB. *Fundamentals of Clinical Trials* (5th ed.). New York, NY: Springer International Publishing; 2015.

36. Willett W. *Nutritional Epidemiology* (3rd ed.). Oxford: Oxford University Press; 2012.

NUTRITION EPIDEMIOLOGY RESEARCH METHODS

ERIN BOULDIN, KAREN GRIMMER, JAMIE GRIFFIN, M. MARGARET BARTH, AND RONNY A. BELL

LEARNING OBJECTIVES

1. Understand the objective of **nutritional epidemiology** research.

2. Explain types of study designs that are used in nutritional epidemiological research.

3. Describe the usefulness and limitations of different epidemiological study designs for research in nutritional epidemiology.

4. Describe the strengths and limitations of different methods of measuring diet and identify when specific dietary methods may be most appropriate.

5. Explain the statistical methods commonly used in nutritional epidemiology to analyze diet–disease associations.

INTRODUCTION

Nutritional epidemiology is the study of how diet affects health and **disease** in human populations, and it is also referred to as the science of public health nutrition. The overarching goals of nutritional epidemiological research include investigation of the relationship between dietary and nutrition intake of a person and his or her health and/or disease risk; identification of groups of people at risk for developing disease as a result of their dietary and/or nutrition intake; and development and evaluation of interventions to improve or maintain healthful dietary patterns. This chapter provides an overview of research methods employed in nutritional epidemiology and applied in the field of public health nutrition. Methodologies included in the design, implementation, analysis, and interpretation of nutrition epidemiological studies to evaluate the relationship between nutritional status, diet, and disease are reviewed. **Nutrition assessment** tools commonly used in conducting nutrition assessments and in nutritional epidemiological research are described along with some of their strengths and limitations.

RESEARCH METHODS AND STUDY DESIGNS IN PUBLIC HEALTH NUTRITION

Current State of Play in Epidemiology

The science and study of **epidemiology** is continually evolving, with new areas of epidemiology emerging (such as genetics). The evolution of epidemiology is linked to the evolution of biostatistical principles and capacities as computing capacity grows and software programs are refined. Advances in epidemiology have largely occurred in conjunction with statistical software development. The Centers for Disease Control and Prevention (CDC) disease surveillance program, Epi Info, is one example; see Box 3.1.

Building the Case for Exposures Associated With Disease

Sir Austin Bradford Hill, a British statistician, proposed nine criteria to provide epidemiological evidence of a causal relationship between a presumed cause and an observed effect.[1] These criteria are immensely useful in thinking through what is known about proposed associations between **exposure** and disease so that data collection and analysis can test well-reasoned hypotheses. They are outlined in Box 3.2.

Considering these criteria, any budding epidemiologist would understand that preparation is essential. Before undertaking any inquiry, researchers (including clinicians and policy-makers) should be aware of the literature that has been previously published in the area (preferably by undertaking a literature review conducted systematically and thoroughly), summarize and reflect

---

BOX 3.1

EPI INFO: EPIDEMIOLOGICAL SOFTWARE FROM THE CDC

In 1985, the CDC produced the first version of this groundbreaking epidemiological software to chart disease outbreaks, designed specifically for clinicians, health scientists, and epidemiologists working at the coalface to identify **exposures** potentially associated with disease quickly and accurately. Epi Info originally used MS-DOS programming and was distributed on 5.25″ floppy discs. It would be fair to say that this program revolutionized epidemiological data collection and analysis and enabled epidemiologists to test cause–effect hypotheses more efficiently and accurately than ever before. Because it only took up a small amount of hard drive capacity and storage space, Epi Info ran easily on early computers and was ideal for field work. Epi Info supports epidemiological inquiry from data collection (questionnaire development, validation of data fields, data entry, and validation of entered data) through to basic epidemiological analysis. It also provides useful sample size calculators, and excellent tutorials in the use of each of its features, with worked examples. Epi Info was upgraded in 2001 to run on a Windows platform, and it is now in its seventh version. Moreover, Epi Info is free and regularly updated. Any budding epidemiologist would be advised to download a copy and use the excellent tutorials: https://www.cdc.gov/epiinfo/support/downloads.html.

CDC, Centers for Disease Control and Prevention.

Source: Data from Centers for Disease Control and Prevention. *The Epi Info™ Story.* 2019. https://www.cdc.gov/epiinfo/story.html

BOX 3.2

BRADFORD HILL'S CRITERIA FOR CAUSALITY

1. Known strength (or risk) of the causal association (What have others found about how large the relative risk or odds ratio is?)

2. Consistency (Has previous epidemiological research found the same relationship?)

3. Specificity (Is disease limited to specific types of people?)

4. Temporality (Does exposure clearly precede disease?)

5. Dose/response curve (Does more exposure result in more disease?)

6. Plausibility (Does it make sense biologically, clinically, and socially?)

7. Coherence (Is the knowledge from different sources pointing in one direction?)

8. Experimental evidence (Is it possible to intervene successfully in the cause to reduce the disease?)

9. Analogy with other circumstances (Are there other situations that could be used to explain the cause–effect hypothesis?)

Source: Data from Hill BA. The environment and disease: association or causation? *Proc R Soc Med.* 1965;58:295–300. doi:10.1177/003591576505800503

on what has already been reported, organize the potential causes into strengths of association to assess for potential size of effect, to determine whether all findings are similarly positive (or negative), and to consider whether there is a dose–response relationship (the more the exposure, the more the disease).

One trap for young epidemiologists is deciding on what data items to collect (core [essential] and nice to have [optional]). Core data items are those that you must have, or else the study will be pointless. Optional items are those that are nice to have but that you could do without if your funding is limited. It is wise to learn from what others have done (and reported in the literature) because it is easier to replicate and build on others' work than to potentially make the same mistakes that they made because you did not look for efficiencies.

Before undertaking any epidemiological inquiry, it is important to consider whether any "cause" (exposure) that you believe is strongly related to a disease (your hypothesis) can be altered by an intervention from an experiment. This type of reflection will assist with choosing appropriate study measures. More about this is discussed later; however, an example is provided in Box 3.3 to start you thinking.

Fields of Epidemiology

As outlined in the history of epidemiology (Chapter 2, Nutrition Epidemiology Principles), this science had its genesis in disease measurement, and identification of causes of disease, to enable targeted interventions that are likely to be effective. As techniques and methods advance, epidemiology has diversified into different fields. The science of methodology (design of research and disease outbreak investigations) is now widely recognized, and few health teams would not have a member with epidemiology skills.

BOX 3.3

DETERMINING APPROPRIATE STUDY MEASURES RELATED TO POTENTIAL CAUSALITY

After having conducted your literature review, you believe that you have evidence that older age could be a strong predictor for a particular health state (such as a chronic disease). Measuring age alone (by years of life) in your observational study will not give you the type of answer that you can do anything with. You cannot stop people getting older no matter how hard you try, and no funding body is going to support this type of inquiry if you have collected age in years as the only age marker.

First of all, you need to think about what "older age" means, and you should identify and measure features of "older age" that are amenable to change so that if your hypothesis is supported by your epidemiological inquiry, you will have the information you need for a subsequent intervention study.

Consider what "older age" means. Is there likely to be a linear function if you compare age and chronic disease state (the older a person is, the more diabetes he or she has)? Is there a threshold effect? For instance, do people entering their 60s have more likelihood of suffering this chronic disease than people aged in their 50s? Do people in their 70s have more likelihood of suffering this chronic disease than people aged in their 60s? Does something amazing happen when someone turns 60 or 70 to increase their susceptibility for disease? Or is change insidious, and each year of life incurs subtle changes that culminate at some point in disease detection?

For instance, as people age, their metabolism may change; so age-related physiological factors might be appropriate to measure (perhaps blood pressure, heart rate, oxygenation, or biomarkers through blood tests). Another approach is that for many people, their diet changes as they age, depending on a multitude of factors such as appetite, financial capacity to purchase healthy food, dental health, physical activity, living arrangements, and mental health. Thus study measures of these features may be useful, along with age, to ensure that you have captured as much relevant information about how aging is affecting the individual.

Forensic epidemiology is the enginehouse of investigations mounted by disease control units in government health departments. Forensic epidemiologists often need to act quickly once a disease outbreak is alerted and be responsive to ways of identifying potential causes. They need to understand the biological rationale underpinning the disease, the likely causes of this, and then capture accurate measures of potential causes as quickly as possible to identify the true cause and recommend a public health intervention to attenuate the disease outbreak. Forensic epidemiology truly is multidisciplinary, involving input from methodologists, statisticians, public health specialists, pathologists, biologists, community healthcare providers (particularly, general medical practitioners), water quality specialists, and often veterinarians (where animal–human transfer of organisms is suspected).

John Snow's cholera outbreak investigation is a good example of early forensic inquiry and subsequent (effective) public health intervention. In forensic epidemiology inquiries, the disease state is usually known before the cause is identified. The disease is usually identified when its prevalence is higher than expected (epidemic). John Snow was called in when cholera cases were at epidemic proportions in Soho in 1885. After his careful mapping of cases, consideration of local evidence, and testing his hypothesis that cholera was associated with drinking water from the Broad Street well, he provided evidence to the local council of the likelihood of the association between drinking the Broad Street well water and developing cholera. The local council acted by removing the pump handle (public health intervention), and the frequency of new cholera cases decreased (because of the intervention, because the outbreak was self-limiting, or because there were no more people available to get the disease).

A real-world example of forensic epidemiology occurred in South Australia in 1994–1995. This example changed the face of food production standards in Australia and also set legal precedents for redress from disease outbreaks. The health crisis (hemolytic uremic syndrome [HUS]) resulted in the death of one 4-year-old child and the hospitalization of 24 others with HUS. Most of these children required dialysis, and 22 years later, many have ongoing health issues. The cause of the child's death, as stated in the coroner's court, was the result of eating mettwurst from a local smallgoods producer (the company's name is replaced in this example as Smallgoods producer X) believed to contain *Escherichia coli* 0111. *E. coli* 0111 is a special gut bacterium that produces a potent toxin called Shiga-like toxin. It is a rod-shaped bacterium 2 μm long. It is commonly found in the intestines of livestock and so, potentially, can contaminate meat during the slaughter process. Human infection is caused usually by eating contaminated meat or dairy products that have not been adequately cooked or processed. Once in the intestines, the organism multiplies, producing a toxin and causing diarrhea. The toxin is also absorbed into the bloodstream and attacks the kidney and cells lining the small blood vessels, resulting in HUS. The chronology of the disease outbreak is summarized in Box 3.4.[2]

BOX 3.4

CHRONOLOGY OF SOUTH AUSTRALIAN HUS OUTBREAK, 1994–1995

December 31, 1994: The first case of HUS disease is hospitalized (normally two a year, no cause for any public health concern).

January 16, 1995: Second and third cases of HUS reported. Public officers become involved as this is now higher than normal prevalence. Public health officials believe an epidemic may be occurring, and intensive investigations begin. Extensive data started to be collected on each patient but not enough information can be gleaned from children to pinpoint a single common source of infection (water, food, other). The initial common ingredient appears to be fritz (a form of precooked meat sausage eaten cold).

January 17, 1995: Sought information from Australian Paediatric Surveillance Unit on numbers of HUS cases notified from around Australia. Answer: seven in the past 6 months. A fourth case is notified. Meeting held between public health officials, IMVS, Agricultural Department, and WCH. Water is eliminated as the possible source. Food is more likely the source. IMVS to letter-drop 700 surgeries alerting general practice doctors. Samples of HUS victims from homes taken. Questionnaire for interviewing victims drafted.

January 18, 1995: Health departments and communicable disease network notified nationally by this time. MI pathology laboratories informed and asked to send specimens to WCH for special testing. Minister informed. General medical practitioners informed. Fifth and sixth cases notified.

(continued)

BOX 3.4

CHRONOLOGY OF SOUTH AUSTRALIAN HUS OUTBREAK, 1994–1995 (*CONTINUED*)

January 19, 1995: Calls from general medical practitioners about possible cases. Laboratory confirmation that *E. coli* was responsible for HUS. Special testing facilities set up at IMVS for testing food samples. IMVS tests various meat samples including Smallgoods producer X garlic mettwurst. Fifth case (South Australian source) found in New South Wales. Seventh and eighth cases notified. Information suggesting some victims had consumed large quantities of fritz, burgers, mettwurst, and hot dogs.

January 20, 1995: All major hospitals asked to check whether other cases may be misdiagnosed and actually HUS. Press release issued warning of symptoms and warned source likely to be a meat product and said meat should be cooked properly. Asked general medical practitioners for prompt notification.

January 22, 1995: Fritz still most likely suspect. Still uncertain whether this is a coincidence or the actual source of contamination.

12.40 p.m. WCH suggests connection made by two families of eating same brand of mettwurst.

1.30 p.m. IMVS say blind testing showed Smallgoods producer X sample proved positive. Fritz samples prove negative.

1.35 p.m. Parents interviewed by public health officials again. Asked if Smallgoods producer X rang any bells. Asked where it had been bought so that it could be confirmed that was what was bought. Initial media coverage targeting processed meats. Another sample of Smallgoods producer X mettwurst was in the process of being tested and could confirm new lead the next day (Monday). (Test process takes 3 days.)

January 23, 1995: Brand names checked with histories of victims. IMVS confirms second sample of mettwurst has toxin late morning. Smallgoods producer X is notified of link with their product. Smallgoods producer X ceases production of all mettwurst. No further mettwurst has been manufactured. Media conference is called at 3.30 p.m. with acting minister Lucas in which Smallgoods producer X is named and particular batch of mettwurst specified. Smallgoods producer X inspection of premises indicates no product left and prohibition not required. Request for immediate recall of specified mettwurst. Smallgoods producer X officially indicates they are moving to remove the product from sale and agree to recall by means of phone and visits, as well as by advertisement in *The Advertiser* (the local Adelaide newspaper).

January 24, 1995: Local government notified of public health concerns and naming of Smallgoods producer X and specific mettwurst. Local government organizes official notices. At the same time, Smallgoods producer X contacts distribution outlets. Public health officials meet with Smallgoods producer X. Tenth case hospitalized.

January 25, 1995: Communicable diseases national network teleconference. Health Commission informs local government to ensure specified mettwurst is removed from local retail outlets. Samples taken of mettwurst from a variety of manufacturers for testing.

January 27, 1995: Inspection of Smallgoods producer X premises. Request for all information regarding meat sources, quality assurance procedures and production procedures, ingredients, etc. Smallgoods producer X refuses until legal advice was sought. Notification of similar epidemic in the United States originating from mettwurst/salami.

(continued)

BOX 3.4

CHRONOLOGY OF SOUTH AUSTRALIAN HUS OUTBREAK, 1994–1995 (*CONTINUED*)

January 30, 1995: Public health officials raise concerns that not all products removed from retail outlets. Follow-up letter sent to local councils advising them to ensure inspection of retail premises. Further inquiry made regarding Smallgoods producer X. Smallgoods producer X says still getting advice.

January 31, 1995: Smallgoods producer X asks for, and gets, meeting with Smallgoods producer X lawyers and public health officials. Agree to supply information only if request made in writing.

February 1, 1995: At 8.30 a.m., a 4-year-old child dies from HUS in WCH. Notification of 20th HUS case. All cases so far have been from ingestion of contaminated material prior to or on date of public announcement pinpointing Smallgoods producer X source. Press conferences by WCH and Minister for Health. Smallgoods producer X provides some of requested information. IMVS results of testing of sample of meat that was claimed by Smallgoods producer X to be used in contaminated batch of mettwurst proves positive for *E. coli* responsible for HUS epidemic.

February 2, 1995: Smallgoods producer X instigates recall of all mettwurst products.

HUS, hemolytic uremic syndrome; IMVS, Institute of Medical and Veterinary Science; MI, myocardial infarction; WCH, Women's and Children's Hospital.

Source: From Kriven S. *Media Release, Minister for Health.* Adelaide. South Australia. 1995. http://www.agrifood. info/review/1995/Kriven.html#Epidemic%20chronology%20of%20events

---

It took until 2017 for all legal challenges to be completed and for the ongoing health and social needs of the HUS survivors to be monitored and recompensed for projected lifetime health costs. Smallgoods producer X was bankrupted and went out of business within 12 months of the HUS outbreak.

Clinical epidemiology is the arm of epidemiology usually involved in designing and managing clinical trials, maintaining disease registries, and conducting studies to evaluate the usefulness of diagnostic and screening tests in clinical practice. Clinical epidemiologists will often be linked to a specific clinical unit in a hospital or health department, and may support clinicians and policy-makers in evidence-based clinical or policy decision-making. Their role is to maintain sampling processes (for instance, concealed allocation to treatment arms or random sampling), data integrity, and accuracy in clinical trials; ensure that the unit stays up to date with currently published research; and to be vigilant that biases do not creep into data collection, analysis, or reporting.

Disease registries are accumulative collections of secondary data from specific subgroups of people in the population for tracking prevalence, clinical care and outcomes of conditions, surgical or medical interventions, or disease. Most high- and middle-income countries have well-established disease registries for prevalent and potentially preventable chronic diseases (stroke, diabetes, coronary artery disease, asthma), and registries have been established for many cancers. Results of routine population screening (such as Pap smears) can be logged on registries to assist in surveillance of screening outcomes and population compliance.[3] Registries are useful for postmarketing surveillance of pharmaceuticals (tracking prescribing practices, adverse events).[4] The number and focus of registries are regularly changing. For instance, registries have been established for joint replacements (such as the American Joint Replacement Registry) and surgical procedures (for instance, New York State CABG Registry to track all cardiac bypass surgeries performed in the state of New York.[5,6]

Registries collate data on common conditions that may be amenable to wide-scale public health interventions (such as diabetes, stroke, heart disease), but they also can monitor rare conditions that are difficult to research because sampling is challenged by low prevalence (e.g., juvenile idiopathic arthritis [STRIVE trial, which is supported by a dedicated registry]).[7] Registers of patients with rare conditions improve capacity to efficiently contact them, which assists with research sampling, and efficient dissemination of new treatment information.

Clinical epidemiologists are well placed to manage data registries as they understand sampling and measurement issues, data quality, updating databases, and maintaining data integrity. High-quality data in disease registries is essential to ensure its believability; to maintain ongoing use by policy-makers, clinicians, and researchers; and to attract ongoing funding for its upkeep. Recruitment and data collection processes are critical to the success of a registry. To be credible, people listed on the registry need to reflect as complete a sample as possible of people with the problem, collated from all available data sources. Data can be obtained from multiple sources (e.g., hospital admission registers, health insurance data, pathology tests, communicable disease surveillance processes, clinician records), and data collection processes need to be routine. Disease-specific registers often have inclusion and exclusion criteria, which need to be strictly adhered to. Ensuring that registers capture consecutive, eligible people diagnosed with specific conditions or provide particular medical interventions is challenging, and requires vigilance. We discuss sampling in more detail in a later section of this chapter.

Finally, clinical epidemiologists work to evaluate whether and how tests should be implemented in clinical practice to identify disease. Virtually all tests have a chance of resulting in a false positive or false negative result. Both of these situations are potentially harmful; a false positive may lead to someone undergoing unnecessary procedures while a false negative would delay needed treatment. Therefore, epidemiological principles are employed to design studies that help us determine under what circumstances the outcome of a disease is improved by conducting a test. These studies are then used to develop recommendations like the age at which women should begin receiving mammograms or whether men who have a family history of prostate cancer should be screened for disease at a given time. The details of these studies and the measures used in them—including sensitivity, specificity, and positive and negative predictive values—are beyond the scope of this chapter, but are detailed elsewhere.[8]

Theoretical epidemiology is the third arm of epidemiology, which has largely been responsible for advancing skills and knowledge in research methods and improving rigor of evidence production and reporting. The focus of theoretical epidemiologists is on improving the quality of available research evidence, translating it into practice, and implementing appropriate evidence for individual patient's needs. Theoretical epidemiologists are often also involved in the conduct and reporting of secondary evidence research (systematic reviewing, conducting meta-analyses) and in designing, conducting, and writing clinical practice guidelines.

ROLE OF EPIDEMIOLOGY IN INFORMING EVIDENCE-BASED PROGRAMS

Nomenclature

There is ongoing debate in the world of theoretical epidemiologists regarding nomenclature. There are three general terms in current use.

1. *Evidence-based medicine (EBM):* The well-accepted definition of EBM is that it is "the conscientious, explicit, and judicious use of current best evidence in making decisions about the care of individual patients. The practice of evidence based medicine means integrating individual clinical expertise with the best available external clinical evidence from systematic research."[9] In the early days of the evidence-based practice (EBP) movement, the term EBM was used because doctors (and medicine) were the focus of evidence production. Nowadays, it is more common to use the term *evidence-based practice,* which recognizes the care provided by all types of healthcare providers.

2. *Evidence-informed practice* is a term that is being used more commonly than EBP to reflect the impact of four main issues on evidence production and implementation:

   - The lack of certainty in the findings of much research evidence[10]

   - The potential differences between clinicians in the way they interpret evidence and incorporate it into their clinical reasoning[11]

   - The potential for disconnect between the three traditional circles of EBP, particularly the lack of congruence between research and clinician input, compared with what patients actually understand and/or need[12]

   - The importance of considering context when interpreting evidence (what works in one place may not work equally well in another), an issue that is particularly important when developing evidence-informed policy[13-15]

3. *Practice-informed research* is of interest particularly to the more qualitative health fields (social work, speech and language pathology, nutrition), where there can be a problematic disconnect between available evidence, clinical practice, and patient need. It reflects the translation of evidence developed from groups of people, for application to one person, whose needs may not be reflected in the group from which the evidence was derived. The question commonly asked is: "To what extent is research influenced by practice?"[15] The basic foundation of practice research is building theory from practice and not only from academia. Practice-informed research should be a combination of research methodology, field research, and practical experience. "The challenge from practice to research is to support or provoke research to become more creative in understanding practice built on complexity, and to act flexibly instead of constructing a paradigm suitable for research."[16]

Practice-informed research is the (often unrecognized) approach used by clinical practice guideline developers to establish consensus practice or context points when there is inadequate, insufficient, poor quality, or simply no research evidence on which to base a recommendation.[17,18] It is of note in the debate about the value of evidence that these practice points are reflected on some hierarchies of evidence as the lowest ranking, termed "expert opinion." This recognizes the value of "practice-based" information to inform current recommendations. These practice points also flag areas in which research could be conducted in order to strengthen the research evidence base.

ASSESSING NUTRITION STATUS IN EPIDEMIOLOGICAL RESEARCH

Reasons to Assess Nutrition Status

Nutritional epidemiology studies how diet (what a person regularly eats and drinks) and nutrition (the overall macro- and micronutrient composition and makeup of the diet) impact a person. The goal of nutritional epidemiological research is to (a) investigate the relationship between dietary and nutrition intake of a person and his or her health and/or disease risk, (b) identify groups of people at risk for developing disease(s) due to their dietary and/or nutrition intake, and (c) develop and evaluate interventions to improve or maintain healthful dietary patterns.

Nutrition Assessment in Epidemiology Studies

Choosing the type of nutrition assessment to use depends on what the researcher is studying. Nutrition assessment tools are categorized based on whether they capture short-term intake or long-term intake and whether they are interviewer-administered or self-administered.

Short-term intake assessments provide a snapshot of a person's actual eating pattern and intake of certain food groups. This assessment type looks at a person's daily food consumption. Short-term intake assessments include food recalls and food records. Food recalls rely on a person's memory and therefore require a trained dietary interviewer to accurately collect food and beverage intake. Food recalls do not require a high literacy level. Food records rely on the person to record in real time all foods and beverages consumed over a 3- to 7-day period. Food records do not rely on memory. Food records do, however, require a higher literacy level. They are also subject to underreporting due to miscalculation of portion sizes as well as recall bias due to intentional "forgotten reporting" of some foods and beverages

Long-term intake assessments provide information on usual or average food consumption over time, providing information on average or habitual daily intake of a food or nutrient. The most commonly incorporated long-term intake assessment tool is the Food Frequency Questionnaire (FFQ).[19,20] FFQs are widely used in epidemiology studies to determine long-term diet versus short-term dietary intakes. FFQs estimate average nutrient intake. FFQs also help determine the frequency of consumption of certain foods and food intake behaviors.

Interviewer-administered (direct measure) nutrition assessments involve highly trained researchers or interviewers to administer 24-hour recalls and FFQs.[21] The advantage of this type of assessment is that it provides a more quantitative and objective measure of a person's intake. Multiday 24-hour food recalls ranging from 3 to 7 days can account for an individual's day-to-day diet variation. Interviewer-administered assessments reduce measurement errors by verifying portion sizes, food brand and type, combination foods, and additional sauces or condiments. They do not require the individual to have a higher literacy level. Disadvantages include the cost associated with training and employing interviewers and the requirement for coding reported food and drinks.[21]

Self-administered (indirect measure) assessments, also known as self-report, are completed by the person without assistance. Self-administered assessments include food records, automated self-administered 24-hour recall, and automated self-administered FFQ.[21] Advantages of this type of assessment are that it is easy and fast to administer, relatively inexpensive, and less burdensome on the respondent. Disadvantages include random and systematic errors, recall errors such as over- or underreporting, failure to identify daily variations in diet, inconsistencies in measuring portion sizes, intentional misreporting of some foods, inability of food composition databases to accurately calculate intake, and the need for higher literacy.[20,22,23]

Self-Report Data and Nutrition Assessment

Self-report data form the cornerstone of nutritional assessment in epidemiology studies. Self-report data are also associated with many challenges, as discussed previously.

How can we overcome these disadvantages? One current recommendation is for studies to use internal validation methods. For example, a study using an FFQ as the main instrument should also use another self-report reference instrument such as a 24-hour recall or multiple-day food record.[20]

Many self-report instruments are available for nutrition assessment. The National Cancer Institute Epidemiology and Genomics Research Program has compiled a list of evidence-based dietary assessment methods and dietary monitoring resources, which are available at epi.grants. cancer.gov/dietary-assessment/resources.html.[24]

Biological Markers (Biomarkers) and Nutrition Status

Over the past few decades, biomarkers have been incorporated into nutritional epidemiology studies as an objective measure of dietary intake or indicator of nutrition status. Several studies support that biomarkers provide a source validation and accurate assessment.[22,25] Biomarkers associated with dietary intake are compared to a person's reported intake to help validate studies using FFQ and food recalls.

Biomarkers most commonly used in nutrition research measure intakes of salt, protein, sucrose/fructose, potassium (measured through 24-hour urine samples), energy expenditure (measured through double labeled water), carotenoids (measured through resonance Raman spectroscopy), and fatty acid intake (measured through subcutaneous adipose tissue sample).[19,22,25-27] Advantages of biomarkers are that they are easily accessible using urine, feces, blood, and tissue samples. Disadvantages are that there may be other factors independent of a person's dietary intake that can affect a specific nutrient concentration in tissues of well-fed people.[22,25]

Table 3.1 summarizes the different dietary assessment methods[28-31]

BASING PRACTICE ON BEST AVAILABLE EVIDENCE (WHATEVER THAT IS)

Archie Cochrane is considered to be the father of EBM.[32] He promoted the notion of basing clinical decisions on methodologically sound research evidence rather than on opinion. He also proposed the importance of knowing what all primary studies in a particular clinical area have found first (a review) before undertaking another primary study in the area. He developed and promoted the use of systematic searching to ensure comprehensive collection of published papers to answer a particular question as well as the notion of bias. His work founded current systematic review methods and the current philosophy of EBM.[9] For many years, the randomized controlled trial (RCT; and systematic reviews of RCTs) was held to be the only reliable form of evidence. However, this has evolved as epidemiologists have realized that different research questions require different forms of evidence to best answer them, and the debate about what constitutes best evidence continues.

The term "evidence" means different things to different people. Sharing a common view of "evidence" is essential prior to conducting any research or implementing research findings. Guyatt et al. noted that any observation in nature comprises evidence, but it is the accuracy of inferences drawn about evidence that is the challenge for researchers and research implementers.[33]

The tension between prosaic evidence sources and evidence from beliefs is beautifully outlined in the exchange between Strephon and the Lord Chancellor in Act 1 of Gilbert and Sullivan's *Iolanthe*, where Strephon declares that Nature has given him all the evidence he needs to support his claims of affection for a young woman through "the bees — the breeze — the seas — the

TABLE 3.1 DIETARY ASSESSMENT METHODS IN EPIDEMIOLOGICAL STUDIES

ASSESSMENT TOOL	MEASURE (DIRECT/INDIRECT)	SHORT-TERM/ LONG-TERM INTAKE	PARTICIPANT LITERACY LEVEL	RELY ON MEMORY	GROUP SIZE	EXAMPLE
24-hr dietary recall	Direct	Short-term	Low	Yes	Small	
Dietary record	Indirect	Short-term	High	No	Small	
FFQ	Direct	Long-term	Low	Yes	Large	NHANES Food Frequency Questionnaire[28]
Self-administered 24-hr dietary recall	Indirect	Short-term	High	Yes	Small or large	USDA-AMPM[29] ASA24[30]
Self-administered FFQ	Indirect	Long-term	High	Yes	Small or large	NCI DHQ III[31]

ASA24, Automated Self-Administered 24-Hour; NCI DHQ, National Cancer Institute Diet History Questionnaire III; FFQ, Food Frequency Questionnaire; NHANES, National Health and Nutrition Examination Survey; USDA-AMPM, United States Department of Agriculture Automated Multiple-Pass Method.

BOX 3.5

EXCERPT FROM GILBERT AND SULLIVAN'S *IOLANTHE*

Lord Chancellor . . . my difficulty is that at present there's no evidence before the Court that chorused Nature has interested herself in the matter.

Strephon. No evidence! You have my word for it. I tell you that she bade me take my love.

Lord Chancellor. Ah! but, my good sir, you mustn't tell us what she told you — it's not evidence. Now an affidavit from a thunderstorm, or a few words on oath from a heavy shower, would meet with all the attention they deserve.

Strephon. And have you the heart to apply the prosaic rules of evidence to a case which bubbles over with poetical emotion?

Source: Excerpt from Sullivan A, Gilbert WS. *Iolanthe, Or, The Peer and the Peri: A New and Original Comic Opera in Two Acts.* New York, NY: J. M. Stoddart; 1882.

---

rooks — the brooks — the gales — the vales — the fountains and the mountains cry, 'You love this maiden — take her, we command you!'"[52] The Lord Chancellor is less than convinced however (see Box 3.5).

The Canadian Health Services Research Foundation proposed a definition of "evidence" that highlights its many elements:

> Evidence is information that comes closest to the facts of a matter. The form it takes depends on [the] context. The findings of high-quality, methodologically appropriate research are the most accurate evidence. Because research is often incomplete and sometimes contradictory or unavailable, other kinds of information are necessary supplements to or stand-ins for research. The evidence base for a decision is the multiple forms of evidence combined to balance rigour with expedience—while privileging the former over the latter.[34]

Determining the most believable form of evidence continues to challenge healthcare professionals. Evidence needs to relate to the individual patient, community, or healthcare system. The critical question about evidence is its believability and applicability to specific circumstances.

Sackett et al. proposed the now classic model of EBM (three intersecting circles of evidence as the most appropriate mechanism for arriving at EBP—combining evidence from research, evidence from patient perspectives and beliefs, and evidence from clinician experience); see Figure 3.1.[9]

Satterfield et al. expanded this model to propose the notion of uncertainty in transdisciplinary EBP, within a fourth circle of local context. The Satterfield model resonates with public health theory and practice because it also acknowledges the many sources of evidence for which there is little certainty (Figure 3.2).[10]

The Renaissance Movement

There is current questioning of the increasingly sophisticated EBP approach by the Renaissance Group.[35] This group includes people who have been leaders in the EBM world for many years. This group is expressing concerns about the utility of current high-quality evidence and the growing divide among evidence, clinical practice, and what patients want. (In fact, they indicate that

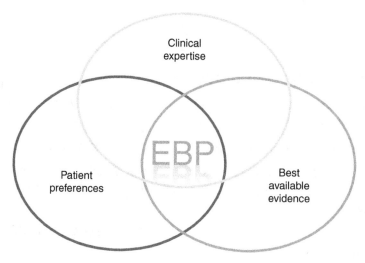

FIGURE 3.1 Classic EBP configuration.

EBP, evidence-based practice.

Source: From Sackett DL. Bias in analytic research. *J Chronic Dis.* 1979;32(1–2):51–63. doi:10.1016/0021-9681 (79)90012-2

research rigor is driving the separation between the research circle in the EBM model from the clinician and patient evidence circles.) This group argues that although EBM has benefited many and improved the quality of published research, it has had "some negative unintended consequences." The group's concerns include:

> The evidence based "quality mark" has been misappropriated by vested interests. The volume of evidence, especially clinical guidelines, has become unmanageable. Statistically significant benefits may be marginal in clinical practice. Inflexible rules and technology driven prompts may produce care that is management driven rather than patient centred. Evidence based guidelines often map poorly to complex multimorbidity.[35]

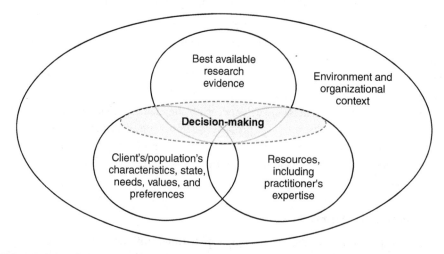

FIGURE 3.2 Satterfield model of decision-making and evidence uncertainty.

Source: From Satterfield JM, Spring B, Brownson RC, et al. Toward a transdisciplinary model of evidence-based practice. *Milbank Q.* 2009;87(2):368–390. doi:10.1111/j.1468-0009.2009.00561.x

This group argues for

a return to the movement's founding principles—to individualise evidence and share decisions through meaningful conversations in the context of a humanistic and professional clinician-patient relationship . . . . To deliver this agenda, evidence based medicine's many stakeholders—patients, clinicians, educators, producers and publishers of evidence, policy makers, research funders, and researchers from a range of academic disciplines—must work together.[35]

The importance of ensuring that public health nutrition targets areas of need in ways that will address this cannot be argued with. The proposals by the Renaissance Movement offer leadership in ensuring that all stakeholders in public health nutrition, and the epidemiological inquiries that underpin it, are engaged in determining what is important and how to address it.

Hierarchies of Evidence

A hierarchy of evidence helps end users to target evidence searches at the type of evidence that is most likely to provide a reliable answer for their question.[36]

There are two broad types of research:

- **Quantitative research** approaches a problem by generating measurements, using numeric data or data that can be transformed into numbers to which statistics can be applied and patterns uncovered. Quantitative data collection methods include direct measurement (objective), surveys, and systematic observations.[3] There are two types of quantitative study data (continuous/equal interval and categorical data). There is no one agreed hierarchy for qualitative or quantitative research.

- **Qualitative research** is exploratory research used to gain understanding of the way people feel and behave. It provides insights into a problem or helps to uncover trends in thought and opinions. Qualitative data collection methods vary using unstructured or semistructured techniques such as interviews, focus groups (group discussions), and participation/observations.[37] Qualitative data is derived from analysis of documents and is presented as words, phrases, themes, and exemplar quotations. There is no agreed hierarchy of evidence for qualitative or quantitative research.

Considering quantitative evidence, the historical EBM research largely dealt with intervention (treatment) studies because that is what doctors did (treat). The EBM theory proposed that RCTs provide the most believable evidence of effectiveness from primary studies. This hierarchy of evidence traditionally put the least biased evidence source at the top and the most biased source at the bottom. RCT designs are preferred because they attempt to minimize biases by randomizing selection of samples from reference populations and then randomizing and concealing allocation of subjects to study groups (see Figure 3.3). Systematic reviews and (if possible) meta-analyses of RCTs provide the most believable form of secondary evidence (evidence synthesis).

In the past few years, there has been an increasing recognition that different research questions and approaches require different hierarchies of evidence. For instance, an RCT might provide the best evidence for an intervention question, but it does not provide the best evidence for an epidemiological question. The Oxford Centre for Evidence-Based Medicine has been at the forefront of redesigning hierarchies of evidence. In 2009, this group proposed five different hierarchies of evidence relative to the research question: therapy/prevention, etiology/harm; prognosis; diagnosis; differential diagnosis, symptom prevalence; economic and decision analysis.

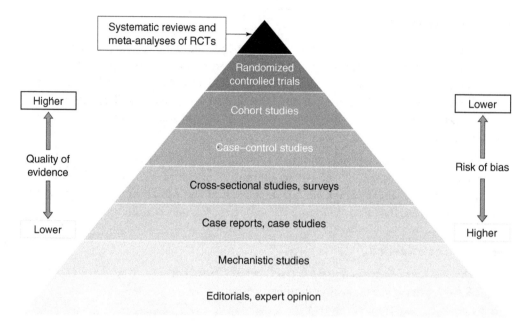

FIGURE 3.3 Traditional experimental hierarchy of evidence.

RCT, randomized controlled trial.

Source: From Yetley EA, MacFarlane AJ. Options for basing Dietary Reference Intakes (DRIs) on chronic disease endpoints: report from a joint US-/Canadian-sponsored working group. *Am J Clin Nutr.* 2017;105(1):249S–285S. doi:10.3945/ajcn.116.139097

Recently, the Oxford Centre for Evidence-Based Medicine revised its hierarchy of quantitative evidence, considering study designs relevant to clinician questions (www.cebm.net/wp-content/uploads/2014/06/CEBM-Levels-of-Evidence-2.1.pdf).

Nearly 25 years after this paper, the debate about best evidence in healthcare continues, and there remains little certainty about the best evidence upon which to make best healthcare decisions. In many ways, not much has changed since the 1999 *BMJ* Christmas spoof paper, in which Isaacs and Fitzgerald proposed seven alternative sources of evidence when none is available from research: "Eminence based medicine, Vehemence based medicine, Eloquence based medicine, Providence based medicine, Diffidence based medicine, Nervousness based medicine, Confidence based medicine".[38] This article appeared to resonate with many evidence skeptics, and in one of the several commentaries that subsequently appeared, an alternative evidence hierarchy was proposed that potentially reflects the ways that many healthcare decisions are made.

Class 0: Things I believe

Class 0a: Things I believe despite the available data

Class 1: Randomised controlled clinical trials that agree with what I believe

Class 2: Other prospectively collected data

Class 3: Expert opinion

Class 4: Randomised controlled clinical trials that don't agree with what I believe

Class 5: What you believe that I don't[39]

TABLE 3.2 COMMON QUALITATIVE RESEARCH DESIGNS

METHOD	FOCUS	SAMPLE SIZE	DATA COLLECTION
Ethnography	Context or culture	—	Observation and interviews
Narrative	Individual experience and sequence	1 to 2	Stories from individuals and documents
Phenomenological	People who have experienced a phenomenon	5 to 25	Interviews
Grounded theory	Develop a theory grounded in field data	20 to 60	Interviews, then open and axial coding
Case study	Organization, entity, individual, or event	—	Interviews, documents, reports, observations

Source: From Sauro J. *Qualitative Research*. 2015. https://measuringu.com/qual-methods

Qualitative research is used relatively infrequently, at the moment, in epidemiological research. Qualitative research methods have been described as five different types, each with a different purpose, and with different underpinning frameworks and methods (see Table 3.2).[40]

There is unresolved debate as to whether qualitative designs should be placed into a hierarchy of evidence because bias management is quite different for qualitative studies, compared with quantitative studies.[37] It is not within the remit of this chapter to enter into this debate, but for comparison with the quantitative hierarchies, we report a qualitative hierarchy proposed by Daly et al.; see Figure 3.4.[41]

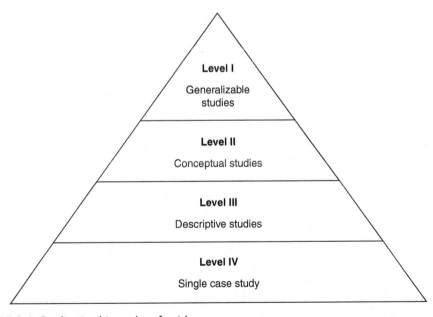

FIGURE 3.4 Qualitative hierarchy of evidence.

Source: From Daly J, Willis K, Small R, et al. A hierarchy of evidence for assessing qualitative health research. *J Clin Epidemiol*. 2007;60:43–49. doi:10.1016/j.jclinepi.2006.03.014

Mixed Methods Research

It is likely, with the increasing recognition by methodologists of the different information derived from qualitative and quantitative studies, that epidemiological research will include more mixed methods (or multimethods) research. This is where quantitative and qualitative studies are designed to understand different aspects of the research question, and the data is combined to comprehensively provide answers.[42] There are three ways that **mixed methods research** has been described.[31]

- *Explanatory sequential design*: An explanatory sequential design emphasizes quantitative analysis, which we follow with interviews or observation (qualitative measures) to help explain quantitative findings.[43]

- *Exploratory sequential design*: An exploratory sequential design starts with qualitative research and then uses insights gained to frame the design and analysis of the subsequent quantitative component. This approach is commonly used to develop questionnaire items and wording.[43]

- *Convergent parallel design*: Collect qualitative data and quantitative data simultaneously and independently, and then combine the results at the analysis phase. The analysis gives equal weighting to the different types of data collected in each study, and comparisons are made between the data findings to identify patterns, continuity, or contradictions.

Mixed methods is a research area that has much to offer future epidemiological research, and it has particular relevance to nutrition research, given the importance of understanding people's choices and the barriers to good nutrition.[44]

Quality Reporting and Checklists

As a result of advances in theoretical epidemiological principles, a number of international organizations have emerged, which are engaged in, and promote, such activities including Cochrane Collaboration (us.cochrane.org); Campbell Collaboration (campbellcollaboration.org); World Health Organization (WHO; www.who.int/publications/guidelines/en); and National Institute for Health and Care Excellence (NICE; www.nice.org.uk).

Advances in theoretical epidemiological methods have led to the production of resources such as checklists for researchers to ensure that biases are accounted for in the design and reporting of studies (EQUATOR Network [Enhancing the QUAlity and Transparency Of health Research]; www.equator-network.org). This repository includes regularly updated checklists for the conduct of different study designs (systematic reviews [PRISMA], experimental studies [CONSORT]; observational [epidemiological] studies [STROBE], study protocols [SPIRIT, PRISMA-P]; diagnostic/prognostic studies [STARD, TRIPOD]; case reports [CARE]; clinical practice guidelines [AGREE, RIGHT]; qualitative research [SRQR, COREQ]; quality improvement studies [SQUIRE] and economic evaluations [CHEERS]).

Critical appraisal of methods and reporting of studies is also recommended for end users (clinicians, policy-makers, funders). A range of critical appraisal tools has been developed to assist end users, including design-specific tools in the Critical Appraisal Skills Program (CASP), Physiotherapy Evidence Database (PEDro) designed for RCTs, and the McMaster University generic qualitative and quantitative tools.[45–47]

The purpose of author checklists is to improve the quality of research conduct and reporting and ensure that biases are managed as best as possible. The purpose of reader checklists is to use reading time wisely and to identify the best quality (least biased) evidence to translate into clinical practice. Sackett, one of the early leaders of the EBP movement, wrote a seminal paper in 1979 on biases that could impact on the quality of quantitative research. This work became the first draft of a catalog of biases "which may distort the design, execution, analysis and interpretation of research."[48] In this paper, Sackett cataloged 35 biases that arise in sampling and measurement, in the context of clinical trials, and listed 56 biases potentially affecting case–control and **cohort studies**. He proposed the continued development of an annotated catalog of bias as a priority for research, the challenge of which has been taken on by the Catalogue of Bias Collaboration at the Oxford Centre for Evidence Based Medicine (see www.cebm.net/wp-content/uploads/2014/06/CEBM-Levels-of-Evidence-2.1.pdf).[49] This group's website provides information on how to detect and attenuate the effect of biases, with the most commonly viewed biases to date being detection bias, ascertainment bias, attrition bias, confounding by indication, observer bias, recall bias, perception bias, selection bias, misclassification bias, and confounding.

CONCLUSION

Nutritional epidemiology has made a tremendous contribution to our understanding of the relationships between diet and disease. The future of nutritional epidemiology is bright, yet it has some challenges. However, with a comprehensive understanding of the discipline along with the strengths and limitations of nutrition assessment and research methodologies, key insights on diet and health outcomes can be obtained, resulting in improved dietary recommendations to reduce disease risk. Overall, nutritional epidemiology has made important contributions to the development of general dietary recommendations and guiding nutrition policy related to diet and health.

KEY CONCEPTS

- Nutritional epidemiology: the study of how diet affects health and disease.

- Nutritional status: process managed by the intake and utilization of nutrients in an individual. When bodily needs are met, it is referred to as normal nutritional status. If there is a lack or excess of nutrients or reduced utilization resulting in an imbalance, it is referred to as malnutrition.

- Nutrition assessment: the interpretation of subjective and objective data to assess nutritional status. Data collected include anthropometrics, biochemical, clinical observations, and dietary assessment results to determine the adequacy of nutrition intake in individuals and populations.

- Dietary guidelines: demonstration of healthy eating guidelines for promoting health and reducing disease.

- Quantitative research: method of collecting objective measurements and statistical analysis of data obtained through surveys and questionnaires used to quantify opinions, attitudes, and behaviors.

- Qualitative research: method of observation to collect non-numeric data. The three common types of qualitative research methods include observation, in-depth interviews, and focus groups used to gain understanding of opinions and trends.

- Mixed methods research: method for conducting research that integrates collecting and analyzing data from quantitative and qualitative research.

- Evidence-based practice: collecting, processing, and implementing research findings to improve clinical care. Information based on sound research and not on opinion.

CASE STUDY: ASSESSING POTENTIAL FACTORS OF INCREASING PREVALENCE OF ASTHMA IN CAMEROON THROUGH A VALIDATED FOOD FREQUENCY QUESTIONNAIRE

The Cameroon Ministry of Health is responsible for maintenance of all public health services in Cameroon. Respiratory health is a significant health concern among Cameroonian children (~6%), and the Ministry of Health has identified an increasing prevalence of asthma among children in both urban and rural areas over the past two decades. The ministry is interested in looking at respiratory health (asthma) and diet as a protective factor among children (6–7 years old). They have proposed initiating a prospective longitudinal cohort study of children (6–7 years old). You have been asked to consult on the development of an FFQ for assessing dietary intakes at baseline in the children. A validated FFQ does not currently exist in this country. Even though you may not agree with the selection of the FFQ as the dietary assessment tool, it is all that the Ministry of Health can afford at this time. Thus, you are tasked with the development of an FFQ for this country to assess dietary intakes and estimate energy and nutrient intakes of the children and design a study to validate it.

Case Study Questions

1. Conduct a brief review of the literature and discuss the following:

   a. FFQs as a successful dietary assessment instrument for examining the relationships between health and diet

   b. Appropriateness of an FFQ as the primary dietary assessment instrument in large, prospective studies

2. Develop a proposal for how you will develop the FFQ for this country and a study to validate it that includes the following:

   a. Design of the FFQ instrument

      i. Selection of the type of FFQ (see National Cancer Institute website for additional insights on FFQs: dietassessmentprimer.cancer.gov/profiles/questionnaire)

      ii. Consider any seasonal or regional differences in food availability and access in this country

      iii. Instrument that provides measures of the major antioxidant nutrients, zinc, vitamin D, and other nutrients to support respiratory health outcomes (reducing risk for infections, wheezing, asthma) in this age group

   b. Design of the study to validate the FFQ instrument

      i. Review the literature on study designs for validating FFQs (e.g., National Cancer Institute website : dietassessmentprimer.cancer.gov/profiles/questionnaire/validation.html)

    ii.   Compare and contrast FFQ validity studies based on objective biomarker recovery studies versus the second class of validity studies based on comparison of the FFQ results with other self-reported instruments such as the 24-hour recall

    iii.   Describe the study design that you propose along with the method of data analysis

  c.   Share your proposals

SUGGESTED LEARNING ACTIVITIES

1. **Dietary assessment research methodologies**: Satija et al. reported that

> [t]he exposure of interest in nutritional epidemiology is human diet, which is a complex system of interacting components that cumulatively affect health. Consequently, nutritional epidemiology constantly faces a unique set of challenges and continually develops specific methodologies to address these. Misunderstanding these issues can lead to the nonconstructive and sometimes naive criticisms we see today.50

Review the article (www.ncbi.nlm.nih.gov/pmc/articles/PMC4288279) and prepare the following: summarize three key points on how we can reliably measure dietary intakes in populations; outline the set of strengths and limitations unique to each method to make it appropriate for use in specific applications.

2. **Portion size estimation aids (PSEAs) for assessment of nutrient intake and dietary composition**: Schnefke et al. reported that

> [c]urrent dietary recall methods used in low-resource settings are prone to errors in portion size estimation. This study investigated the preference for, ease of use perceptions, and accuracy of visual variables in portion size estimation aids (PSEAs) for dietary recall in Malawi. Visual variables tested included food shapes compared with photos, number of portion size options, photo angle, and simultaneous compared with sequential portion size image presentation.51

Review the article (academic.oup.com/cdn/article/2/11/nzy045/5048991) and prepare the following: your response to the results of participant preference and ease of use perceptions across photos, photo angles, and simultaneous presentation of the PSEAs among the Malawi community members; which PSEAs provided a more accurate portrayal of the actual gram weight of the meal; and how you believe the use of PSEAs could be optimized to improve participant's experiences and enhance the accuracy of the dietary recall.

3. Complete a 24-hour recall, a diet record, an FFQ, and a fruit/vegetable screener found at:

  a.   Automated web-based 24-hour recall: https://deets.feedreader.com/asa24demo .westat.com (input at least two meals)

  b.   Diet record/diary: use format shown here: www.nhlbi.nih.gov/health/educational/ lose_wt/eat/diary.htm (input at least one large meal, noting ingredients in as much detail as possible [oils, condiments, etc.])

    c.   Food frequency questionnaire (the NCI Diet History Questionnaire III): https://epi.grants.cancer.gov/dhq3/ Then go to the DHQ III Web Demo https://www.dhq3.org/study/demo/ (complete in full)

    d.   F&V screener: riskfactor.cancer.gov/diet/screeners/fruitveg/allday.pdf (complete in full)

    4.   Review selected topics of interest in the Nutrition Evidence Library (www.nel.gov).

REFLECTION QUESTIONS

1.   Why is nutritional epidemiological research important in influencing life expectancy and disease prevalence?

2.   What are some of the primary strengths and weakness of the various types of dietary assessment instruments used in nutrition epidemiology research?

3.   What are some of the different types of studies that public health nutritionists use to study diet–disease relationships?

4.   Exploring the National Health and Nutrition Examination Survey (NHANES; at www.cdc.gov/nchs/nhanes/about_nhanes.htm), how does the primary research method differ from other large, population-based studies?

CONTINUE YOUR LEARNING RESOURCES

Nutritional Epidemiology. https://www.frontiersin.org/journals/nutrition/sections/nutritional-epidemiology

Illner AK, Freisling H, Boeing H, et al. Review and evaluation of innovative technologies for measuring diet in nutritional epidemiology. *Int J Epidemiol.* 2012;41(4):1187–1203. doi:10.1093/ije/dys105.

Thompson FE, Subar AF. Dietary assessment methodology. In: Coulston AM, Boushey CJ, Ferruzzi MG, Delahanty LM, eds. *Nutrition in the Prevention and Treatment of Disease.* 4th ed. St. Louis, MO: Elsevier; 2017:5–30.

Scagliusi FB, Polacow VO, Artioli GA, et al. Selective underreporting of energy intake in women: magnitude, determinants, and effect of training. *J Am Diet Assoc.* 2003;103(10):1306–1313. doi:10.1016/s0002-8223(03)01074-5.

Boeing H. Nutritional epidemiology: new perspectives for understanding the diet-disease relationship? *Eur J Clin Nutr.* 2013;67(5):424–429. doi:10.1038/ejcn.2013.47.

Willett W. *Nutritional Epidemiology.* 3rd ed. New York, NY: Oxford University Press; 2012.

Stote KS, Radecki SV, Moshfegh AJ, et al. The number of 24 h dietary recalls using the US Department of Agriculture's automated multiple-pass method required to estimate nutrient intake in overweight and obese adults. *Public Health Nutr.* 2011;14:1736–1742. doi:10.1017/S1368980011000358.

Diep CS, Hingle M, Chen TZ, et al. A validation study of the Automated Self-Administered 24-Hour Dietary Recall for Children (ASA24-Kids) among 9 to 11-year-old youth. *J Acad Nutr Diet.* 2015;115(10):1591–1598. doi:10.1016/j.jand.2015.02.021.

GLOSSARY

Clinical epidemiology: Designing and managing clinical trials, maintaining disease registries, and conducting studies to evaluate the usefulness of diagnostic and screening tests in clinical practice.

Cohort studies: Studies in which a group of people is recruited, typically at one place, or time point, and is divided into an exposed subgroup and an unexposed subgroup. All members of the cohort must be free of the disease of interest at the start so that the incidence (development) of disease can be compared in the exposed and unexposed groups. A cohort may be prospective, in which the development of disease is followed in real time, or retrospective, in which records are used to determine past exposure levels and follow-up for disease incidence. A cohort is potentially likely to have been exposed to the same type of factors (environmental, nutritional, personal) and to have similar risks of exhibiting (or developing) a disease.

Disease: The term "disease" is used, in epidemiological terms, as an umbrella term for a disease diagnosis, death, a poor health outcome (for instance, high body mass index or low back pain), and problematic health event (like a car crash).

Epidemiology: The study of health in populations. Epidemiology encompasses a set of methods by which population health (public health) and the threats to it are assessed using biostatistics and monitored.

Exposure: A term used ubiquitously for any factor that may be associated with disease. There is an array of factors, but common ones include biological, familial, chemical, physical, occupational, psychosocial, socioeconomic, travel, educational, cultural, and nutrition.

Forensic epidemiology: Forensic epidemiologists often need to act quickly once a disease outbreak is alerted and be responsive to ways of identifying potential causes. They need to understand the biological rationale underpinning the disease, the likely causes of this, and then capture accurate measures of potential causes as quickly as possible to identify the true cause, and recommend a public health intervention to attenuate the disease outbreak. Forensic epidemiology truly is multidisciplinary, involving input from methodologists, statisticians, public health specialists, pathologists, biologists, community healthcare providers (particularly, general medical practitioners), water quality specialists, and often veterinarians (where animal–human transfer of organisms is suspected).

Mixed methods research: Quantitative and qualitative studies are designed to understand different aspects of the research question, and the data are combined to comprehensively provide EBM.

Nutrition assessment: An evaluation of both subjective and objective data to provide an assessment of a population's nutritional status. Data collected can include dietary intake, biochemical results, anthropometric measures, and clinical observations related to nutrient deficiencies.

Nutrition epidemiology: The approach to studying the relationship between nutrition and disease in human populations. This approach has primarily focused on dietary intake and disease. However, it can involve the classic areas of nutrition assessment including dietary intake, biochemical, anthropometric, and clinical parameters. This has also been referred to as the science of public health nutrition.

Qualitative research: Exploratory research used to gain understanding of the way people feel and behave. It provides insights into a problem or helps to uncover trends in thought and opinions. Qualitative data collection methods vary using unstructured or semistructured techniques such as interviews, focus groups (group discussions), and participation/observations. Qualitative data are derived from analysis of documents and are presented as words, phrases, themes, and exemplar quotations.

Quantitative research: Studies a problem by generating measurements, using numeric data or data that can be transformed into numbers to which statistics can be applied and patterns uncovered. Quantitative data collection methods include direct measurement (objective), surveys, and systematic observations.. There are two types of quantitative study data (continuous/ equal interval and categorical data). There is no one agreed-upon hierarchy for qualitative or quantitative research.

Theoretical epidemiology: Largely responsible for advancing skills and knowledge in research methods and improving rigor of evidence production and reporting. The focus is on improving the quality of available research evidence, translating it into practice, and implementing appropriate evidence for individual patient's needs.

REFERENCES

1. Hill BA. The environment and disease: association or causation? *Proc R Soc Med.* 1965;58:295–300. doi:10.1177/003591576505800503
2. Kriven S. *Media Release, Minister for Health.* Adelaide. South Australia; 1995; http://www.agrifood.info/review/1995/Kriven.html#Epidemic%20chronology%20of%20events
3. National Guideline Clearinghouse | Guideline Synthesis: Screening for Cervical Cancer. https://elbiruniblogspotcom.blogspot.com/2012/01/national-guideline-clearinghouse_4960.html
4. McNeil, JJ; Piccenna, L; Ronaldson, K; et al. The value of patient-centered registries in Phase IV Drug Surveillance. *Pharm Med.* 2010;24(5):281–288. doi:10.1007/bf03256826
5. American Joint Replacement Registry. *Improving Orthopaedic Care Through Data.* 2016. ajrr.net.
6. Hannan EL, Racz MJ, Walford G, et al. Long-term outcomes of coronary-artery bypass grafting versus stent implantation. *N Engl J Med.* 2005;352(21):2174–2183. doi:10.1056/NEJMoa040316
7. Juvenile Idiopathic Arthritis (JIA) Registry (STRIVE). U.S. National Library of Medicine. 2008. https://clinicaltrials.gov/ct2/show/NCT00783510
8. Weiss NS. *Clinical Epidemiology: The Study of the Outcome of Illness.* 3rd ed. New York, NY: Oxford University Press; 2006.
9. Sackett DL. Bias in analytic research. *J Chronic Dis.* 1979;32(1–2):51-63. doi:10.1016/0021-9681(79).90012-2
10. Satterfield JM, Spring B, Brownson RC, et al. Toward a transdisciplinary model of evidence-based practice. *Milbank Q.* 2009;87(2):368–390. doi:10.1111/j.1468-0009.2009.00561.x
11. Seidel BM, Campbell S, Bell E. Evidence in clinical reasoning: a computational linguistics analysis of 789,712 medical case summaries 1983–2012. *BMC Med Inform Decis Mak.* 2015;15:19. doi:10.1186/s12911-015-0136-8
12. Elwyn G, Edwards A, Thompson R, eds. *Shared Decision Making in Health Care: Achieving Evidence Based Patient Choice.* 3rd ed. New York, NY: Oxford University Press; 2016.
13. Bowen S, Zwi AB. Pathways to "evidence-informed" policy and practice: a framework for action. *PLoS Med.* 2005;2(7):e166. doi:10.1371/journal.pmed.0020166
14. Rycroft-Malone J. Evidence-informed practice: from individual to context. *J Nurs Manag.* 2008;16:404–408. doi:10.1111/j.1365-2834.2008.00859.x
15. Shanahan JO, Liu X, Manak J, et al. Research-informed practice, practice-informed research: the integral role of undergraduate research in professional disciplines. *Counc Undergrad Res.* 2015;35(4):6–16.
16. Uggerhøj L. What is practice research in social work—definitions, barriers and possibilities. *Social Work Soc.* 2011;9(1):45–59. https://www.socwork.net/sws/article/view/6
17. Kredo T, Bernhardson S, Young T, et al. Guide to clinical practice guidelines: the current state of play. *Int J Qual Health Care.* 2016;28(1):122–128. doi:10.1093/intqhc/mzv115
18. Grimmer K, Dizon JM, Louw AQ, et al. South African Guidelines Excellence (SAGE): efficient, effective and unbiased clinical practice guideline teams. *S Afr Med J.* 2016;106(5):440–441. doi:10.7196/SAMJ.2016.v106i5.10770

19. Freedman L, Commins J, Moler J, et al. Pooled results from 5 validation studies on dietary self-report instruments using recovery biomarkers for energy and protein intake. *Am J Epidemiol.* 2014;180:172–188. doi:10.1093/aje/kwu116

20. Freedman L, Commins J, Willet W, et al. Evaluation of the 24-hour recall as a a reference instrument for calibrating other self-report instruments in nutritional cohort studies: evidence from the validation studies pooling project. *Am J Epidemiol.* 2017;186:73–82. doi:10.1093/aje/kwx039

21. Thompson F, Dixit-Joshi S, Potischman N, et al. Comparison of eninterviewer-administered and automated self-administered 24-hour dietary recalls in 3 diverse integrated health systems. *Am J Epidemiol.* 2015;181:970–978. doi:10.1093/aje/kwu467

22. Brennan L, Hu F. Metabolomics-based dietary biomarkers in nutritional epidemiology—current status and future opportunities. *Mol Nutr Food Res.* 2019;63:1701064. doi:10.1002/mnfr.201701064

23. Naska A, Lagiou A, Lagiou P. Dietary assessment methods in epidemiological research: current state of the art and future prospects. *F1000Research.* 2017;6:926. doi:10.12688.f1000research.10703

24. National Institute of Health, National Cancer Institute. *Dietary Assessment Research Resources.* 2018. https://epi.grants.cancer.gov/dietary-assessment/resources.html

25. Jenab M, Slimani N, Bictash M, et al. Biomarkers in nutritional epidemiology: applications, needs and new horizons. *Hum Genet.* 2009;125:507–525. doi:10.1007/s00439-009-0662-5

26. Bingham S. Biomarkers in nutritional epidemiology. *Public Health Nutr.* 2002;5:821–827. doi:10.1079/PHN2002368

27. Mayne S, Cartmel B, Scarmo S, et al. Noninvasive assessment of dermal carotenoids as a biomarker of fruit and vegetable intake. *Am J Clin Nutr.* 2010;92:794–800. doi:10.3945/ajcn.2010.29707

28. Centers for Disease Control and Prevention. *NHANES Food Frequency Questionnaire.* 2004. https://www.cdc.gov/nchs/data/nhanes/nhanes_03_04/tq_fpq_c.pdf

29. U.S. Department of Agriculture Agricultural Research Service. *USDA Automated Multiple-Pass Method.* 2016. https://www.ars.usda.gov/northeast-area/beltsville-md-bhnrc/beltsville-human-nutrition-research-center/food-surveys-research-group/docs/ampm-usda-automated-multiple-pass-method

30. National Institute of Health National Cancer Institute. *Automated Self-Administered 24-Hour (ASA24) Dietary Assessment Tool.* 2019. https://epi.grants.cancer.gov/asa24

31. National Institute of Health National Cancer Institute. *Diet History Questionnaire III (DHQ III).* 2019. https://epi.grants.cancer.gov/dhq3/index.html

32. Cochrane AL. *Effectiveness and Efficiency: Random Reflections on Health Services.* London, UK: Nuffield Provincial Hospitals Trust; 1973.

33. Guyatt GH, Haynes RB, Jaeschke RZ, et al. Users' guides to the medical literature: XXV. Evidence-based medicine: principles for applying the users' guides to patient care. Evidence-Based Medicine Working Group. *JAMA.* 2000;284(10):1290–1296. doi:10.1001/jama.284.10.1290

34. Canadian Health Services Research Foundation. *Annual Report 2005.* Ottawa, Canada: Canadian Health Services Research Foundation; 2005:9. https://www.cfhi-fcass.ca/Migrated/PDF/AnnualReports/2005_e.pdf

35. Greenhalgh T, Howick J, Maskrey N, Evidence Based Medicine Renaissance Group. Evidence-based medicine: a movement in crisis? *Br Med J.* 2014;348:g3725. doi:10.1136/bmj.g3725

36. Howick J, Chalmers I, Glasziou P, et al. *Explanation of the 2011 Oxford Centre for Evidence-Based Medicine (OCEBM) Levels of Evidence (Background Document).* Oxford Centre for Evidence-Based Medicine. 2016; https://www.cebm.net/index.aspx?o=5653

37. Patton MQ. *Qualitative Research & Evaluation Methods: Integrating Theory and Practice.* Thousand Oaks, CA: Sage Publications; 2014.

38. Isaacs D, Fitzgerald D. Seven alternatives to evidence based medicine. *Br Med J.* 1999;319:1618. doi:10.1136/bmj.319.7225.1618

39. Mariotto A. Alternatives to evidence based medicine. *Br Med J.* 2000;321:239. doi:10.1136/bmj.321.7255.239

40. Sauro J. *Qualitative Research.* 2015. https://measuringu.com/qual-methods.

41. Daly J, Willis K, Small R, et al. A hierarchy of evidence for assessing qualitative health research. *J Clin Epidemiol.* 2007;60:43–49. doi:10.1016/j.jclinepi.2006.03.014

42. Johnson RB, Onwuegbuzie AJ. Mixed methods research: a research paradigm whose time has come. *Educ Res.* 2004;33(7):14–26. doi:10.3102/0013189x033007014

43. Sauro J. *3 Ways to Combine Quantitative and Qualitative Research*. 2015. https://measuringu.com/mixing-methods

44. Ghiara V. Disambiguating the role of paradigms in mixed methods research. *J Mix Methods Res*. 2020;14(1):11–25. doi:10.1177/1558689818819928

45. de Morton NA. The PEDro scale is a valid measure of the methodological quality of clinical trials: a demographic study. *Aust J Physiother*. 2009;55:129–133. doi:10.1016/S0004-9514(09)70043-1

46. Law M, Stewart D, Pollock N, et al. *Critical Review Form–Quantitative Studies*. Hamilton, ON, Canada: McMaster University; 2007. https://www.unisa.edu.au/siteassets/episerver-6-files/global/health/sansom/documents/icahe/cats/mcmasters_quantitative-review.pdf

47. Letts L, Wilkins S, Law M, et al. *Critical Review Form—Qualitative Studies*. Hamilton, Ont. Canada: McMaster University; 2007. https://monash.rl.talis.com/items/766BE0A2-0957-B9B8-ACEC-8CDE5564E516.html

48. Sackett DL, Rosenberg WM, Gray JA, et al. Evidence based medicine: what it is and what it isn't. *Br Med J*. 1996;312:71–72. doi:10.1136/bmj.312.7023.71

49. Catalogue of Bias Collaboration, Spencer EA, Brassey J, Mahtani K. Recall bias. In: *Catalogue of Bias*. 2017. https://www.catalogofbias.org/biases/recall-bias

50. Satija A, Yu E, Willett WC, Hu FB. Understanding nutritional epidemiology and its role in policy. *Adv Nutr*. 2015;6(1):5–18. doi:10.3945/an.114.007492

51. Schnefke CH, Kantukule CT, Muth MK, et al. Nutritional epidemiology. *Curr Dev Nutr*. 2018;2(11):nzy045. doi:10.1093/cdn/nzy045

52. Sullivan A, Gilbert WS. *Iolanthe, Or, The Peer and the Peri: A New and Original Comic Opera in Two Acts*. New York, NY: J. M. Stoddart; 1882.

BEHAVIORAL ASPECTS OF PUBLIC HEALTH NUTRITION

KAREN CHAPMAN-NOVAKOFSKI AND KRISTEN N. DIFILIPPO

LEARNING OBJECTIVES

- Explain the role of behavior in public health nutrition using key constructs from eight behavior theories.
- Understand the role that **behavioral economics** plays in behavior change.
- Apply behavior theory to the development of public health nutrition interventions.

INTRODUCTION

Many forces work together to impact health outcomes for populations. As discussed in previous chapters, public health nutrition considers social determinants of health and biology. Social determinants of health is a topic area within Healthy People 2020 with the goal of establishing social and physical environments that support good health for everyone.[1] Social determinants of health include factors related to the individual, such as literacy, language, and culture, as well as factors about resources and access to resources (Figure 4.1). Resources might include safe housing, food markets, healthcare services, transportation, and technology. Access to these resources and the quality of the resources are very important. Health equity is a core theme when discussing the social determinants of health, especially when considering the structural or policy-level issues of health. A social gradient is evident where one's social position is linked to health, and one's social position is influenced by economic, social, and political factors.[2]

Another component determining health is human behavior. Many behaviors impact health and nutrition outcomes, and many interventions focus on changing these behaviors. Public health nutrition initiatives target numerous behaviors such as increasing fruits and vegetables, selecting whole grains and low-fat dairy, increasing activity, and decreasing saturated fat and sodium. On the surface, it may appear that education on what behaviors are beneficial would result in improved health; however, behavior change is a complex process. An individual may know exactly what behavior he or she needs to engage in, but still not be able to execute the change process. Behavior theories provide frameworks for understanding why and how people change, as well as what barriers prevent change. These theories are useful for identifying targets

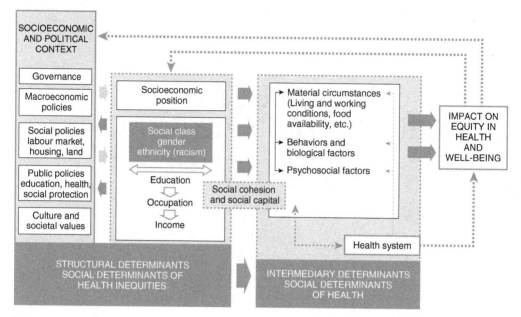

FIGURE 4.1 Framework for social determinants of change and health.

Source: From Solar O, Irwin A. A conceptual framework for action on the social determinants of health. *Social Determinants of Health Discussion Paper 2 (Policy and Practice)*. Geneva: World Health Organization; 2010.

of education in public health nutrition interventions as well as for understanding why a program may have failed to change behavior.

Theorizing how behavior changes requires understanding the numerous internal and external forces that contribute to human behavior. Personal characteristics such as genetics, preferences, and personality all play a role in the behaviors people engage in. However, these individual characteristics are not the only predictor of behavior. The environment also directly and indirectly influences behavior. Environment can be broken down into many levels, such as the home environment, the community, the social environment, and even policy and cultural factors. Different theories focus on these varying levels of influence. Understanding each level of influence and how these levels interact is critical to creating effective interventions.

LEVELS OF BEHAVIOR THEORY

Individual

Individual qualities impact behavior patterns. The biological and psychological traits exhibited by a person play a role in the behaviors one will engage in or avoid. Multiple theories examine individual factors as primary constructs of behavior change. For example, the **Health Belief Model** (HBM) centers around an *individual's perceptions* as primary predictors of behavior.[3,4] The **Theory of Planned Behavior** (TPB) also focuses on individual attitudes and perception of control as primary to predicting intention to change.[5] When using these constructs to predict behavior or target behavior change, the central focus is characteristics of the individual. External factors are also examined from the perspective of the influence on the individual. For example, in the HBM, **cues to action** may be external (information from media or healthcare providers) as well as internal (pain, symptoms). Socioeconomic status is considered as it impacts individual perceptions. In the TPB, subjective norm or perceived social pressures are also external factors that predict behavior change based on how the individual perceives them.

Social and Environmental

Behavior change can also be examined with social constructs as a primary focus. **Social Cognitive Theory** (SCT) examines the social forces that impact learning and behavior.[6,7] In this theory, individual behaviors and personal factors are shown as reciprocal with both each other and the social environment. Social determinants of health, while not a specific theory, play a role in determining health outcomes. These include the neighborhood and built environment, availability of healthcare, the community context, education, and economic stability (social determinants of health). While many theories focus on individual choices, the policy and cultural environment can have direct impacts on behavior and should be considered while targeting behavior change interventions.

Social-Ecological Models

Social-ecological models are useful tools for visualizing how the individual as well as the environmental context determines behavior outcomes. Brofenbrenner's ecological framework considers the interrelatedness of individual, community, and population characteristics to behavior.[8] Social-ecological models are characterized by levels of influence starting with individual factors and then expanding to family context, community, and the larger cultural and political environment. For each level added, the models consider that all lower levels are impacted. For example, the community impacts both the family and the individual.

Many models have been created based on the target behavior being studied. One example is shown in the 2015–2020 Dietary Guidelines for Americans.[9] Social-ecological models always position the individual at the center, with expanding layers of influence. In this example, social and cultural norms and values are shown as the outermost layer of influence impacting sectors, settings, and individuals. Social-ecological models are used to identify potential targets of interventions, especially when considering complex problems. Using the Food and Physical Activity Decisions Social-Ecological Model (health.gov/dietaryguidelines/2015/guidelines/chapter-3/social-ecological-model/#figure-3-1-a-social-ecological-model-for-food-and-physical-activ), an intervention targeting child eating patterns might focus on home, childcare, or school settings, or the policies impacting those settings. In the latter case, the purpose of changing policy would be to change the environment and as a result to change food-related behaviors of a population of individuals.

BEHAVIOR THEORIES AND APPLICATIONS

Behavioral theories can help us understand the reasons *why* an intervention or program works or not. Knowing why a program is successful or not can help to develop better, more tailored programs. However, it is sometimes not practical to measure all possible influencers of a particular behavior change. In addition, audiences change, and what has been influential with one group may not be true for another. Time, effort, and financial considerations are important in program development and evaluation. Nevertheless, having a theoretical framework for program development and evaluation provides some structure and insight into a program's outcome. There are many behavioral theories and models. This chapter focuses on four: the HBM, the SCT, the **Social-Ecological Model** (SEM), and the **Diffusion of Innovation**.

Health Belief Model

The HBM is a health behavior change model developed by Irwin M. Rosenstock for studying and promoting the uptake of health services. The model was further developed by Becker and colleagues in the 1970s.[3,4,10] The basic components of the HBM include **perceived susceptibility**, **perceived severity**, **perceived benefits**, and **perceived barriers**. The first two consider an individual's perceptions regarding a health outcome. The latter two focus on perceptions regarding health behaviors. Cues to action are factors within the HBM that can cause a person to change. These may be internal or external. Internal cues to action include noticing symptoms of a disease or condition. People may be motivated to change their physical activity habits if they realize they are having difficulty climbing the stairs or playing with their child. External cues to action are environmental, such as receiving a reminder card to schedule a checkup or a text reminder to log more steps. **Self-efficacy** has been added to the original model, and it is the **belief** that one can accomplish change (Table 4.1).

An example of the HBM in action is reflected in this scenario:

Lucy's mother has osteoporosis and so did her grandmother. Lucy fears she is also *susceptible* to this condition. Her grandmother had terrible pain and several fractures that compromised her quality of life. Her mother doesn't mention pain, but has become shorter with some curvature of the spine. As a result, she doesn't like the way some of her clothes fit any longer. Lucy's *perceived severity* of osteoporosis ranges from annoyance to quite severe. Lucy feels that improving her diet and physical activity habits would be a clear *benefit* in reducing her risk of osteoporosis. She *perceives the barriers* to changing diet and physical activity habits to be mostly related to time for planning meals more carefully and managing more minutes per day being active. Lucy's mother falls from a stepladder while reaching a top closet shelf. This *cue to action* motivates Lucy to make changes.

TABLE 4.1 HEALTH BELIEF MODEL: A BEHAVIOR CHANGE MODEL FOR STUDYING ACCEPTANCE AND APPLICATION OF HEALTH SERVICES

	AN INDIVIDUAL'S EVALUATION OF:	EXAMPLE QUESTIONS
Perceived susceptibility	The risk of getting the condition	How likely do you think you are to develop this health issue?
Perceived severity	The seriousness of the condition and its potential consequences for them as individuals; consequences may be health related or social	How serious are the consequences for you if you develop this condition?
Perceived benefits	Positive consequences of adopting a behavior related to the health condition	How powerful are the potential positive consequences of adopting this behavior?
Perceived barriers	Difficulties in adopting a behavior related to the health condition	How powerful are the potential difficulties related to adopting this behavior?
Cues to action	The impact of the stimulus to accept the recommended action	How powerful is the stimulus related to adopting this behavior?
Self-efficacy	The person's confidence on ability to successfully perform the behavior	How powerful is their confidence to successfully adopt this behavior?

In a study of 232 Chinese adults with hypertension, the HBM was used to predict medication adherence. A questionnaire reflecting the HBM factors in relation to antihypertension medication use was administered as well as a section related to self-efficacy for taking medication as prescribed. Results indicated that those with higher levels of perceived susceptibility, cues to action, and self-efficacy and a lower level of perceived barriers were significantly associated with better adherence to their antihypertensive medication prescription. The authors suggested that focusing counseling on these four factors could improve medication adherence in Chinese patients.[11]

Studies have shown that some factors are stronger than others in a given targeted behavior, depending on the behavior itself, the target audience, and context. In a cross-sectional study of college students ($n = 476$), the perceived benefits of eating a healthful diet and engaging in physical activity were the strongest predictors within the HBM for body mass index.[12] In a study of 170 women in Appalachia, perceived barriers predicted frequency of mammography, but other HBM variables did not fit well in the statistical models.[13]

Although the HBM is fairly easy to understand and apply, it does not necessarily take into account habits, attitudes, or emotions such as fear or denial. However, expansion of the HBM can include threat, action, and outcomes assessment, as well as antecedents such as demographics and health history, social influences, emotional responses, and intentions.[14] At times, the HBM has been "expanded" to include factors from other theories, such as stage of readiness and knowledge.[15] The HBM can be used with programs promoting decreasing disease risk, but does not adapt easily to nondisease-related nutrition behaviors, such as general healthy nutrition and MyPlate adoption or school nutrition programs.

Social Cognitive Theory

The SCT was developed in the 1960s by Bandura, and it was referred to at that time as the Social Learning Theory.[6,7] The SCT has four concepts: **competencies** and **skills**; **expectancies** and beliefs; **evaluative standards**; and personal goals. Competencies involve both declarative and procedural knowledge. **Declarative knowledge** is facts, such as knowing which foods are high in sodium. **Procedural knowledge** is knowing how to do something, such as knowing how to eat during the day to keep sodium levels below 2,300 mg. Being able to act upon both declarative and procedural knowledge reflects a person's skill. Expectancies and beliefs frame what people think will happen if a situation occurs, such as a health issue. For instance, some people may believe that if they are diagnosed with cancer, they will die. Others may believe managing cancer will be a struggle, but do not believe death would be imminent.

Evaluative standards are one's own moral or social standards that may change with different situations or challenges. For instance, a person may feel that a plant-based diet is the "best" choice, but do not feel badly if they do not eat that pattern every day. Reflection on one's own behavior and evaluating this behavior leads to **self-regulation** and goal attainment. Personal goals help to establish behavioral priorities and contribute to self-regulation. In a systematic review of online dietary interventions, the most often used behavior change techniques were goal setting and self-monitoring, which have also been reported for face-to-face interventions focused on diet and physical activity.[16,17]

A key component in SCT is **observational learning** and modeling, recognizing that we can learn and adapt by modeling the behavior of others. Thus, skill can be developed through declarative and procedural knowledge, as well as by observational learning. For instance, reading a recipe can supply both declarative (ingredients) and procedural knowledge (recipe directions), but watching a cooking demonstration can enhance that skill (observational learning). Figure 4.2

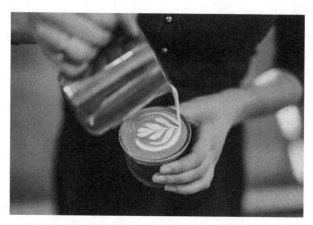

FIGURE 4.2 Demonstration of making latte art as an example of observational learning.
Source: Photo by Tyler Nix on Unsplash.

shows someone making latte art. A video showing latte art would be more informative, but the observational component of a skill is evident. Self-efficacy is embedded within these concepts. Both observational learning and practice can add to skill development and enhance one's self-efficacy. Factors that can affect observational learning include both the status of the model and how similar the model is to the learner. The model should have some status to influence the learner, but not so much that he or she cannot identify with the model. For instance, watching a chef demonstrate a recipe might intrigue or challenge the learner, but it may also provide little reinforcement to the learner that he or she can create the dish. However, having a nutrition educator demonstrate the recipe can provide both status and comparability.

The SCT includes a process called **reciprocal determinism**. This process recognizes that personal, behavioral, and environmental factors are intertwined and influence each other in a dynamic manner. For example, a person whose brother was killed in an alcohol-related accident (personal factor) may choose not to drink at a social event (behavioral factor). If the event includes nonalcoholic beverages, the environmental factors would support this behavior. However, if the event did not serve nonalcoholic beverages, and the person requests nonalcoholic beverages for the next year, the individual would be influencing the environment. The behavior of not drinking alcohol at a social event may influence others' attitudes or behaviors. Thus, the personal, behavioral, and environmental factors influence one another in a reciprocal manner.

Although the SCT is flexible and broad, this may be a limitation as well as an advantage. The fluidity of the interactions may make it difficult to use effectively in a focused program. Although the SCT is often cited as the framework for nutrition and physical activity interventions, and many are successful, most do not directly test the effects of SCT aspects on the behavioral outcome in a statistically meaningful way. For instance, a program to improve vegetable intake may be effective when measured by postprogram intake minus preprogram intake as compared to a control group; but the program leaders may not have reported whether measures of self-efficacy or goal setting statistically affected vegetable intake. This type of analysis is important but requires higher level statistics.

Theory of Planned Behavior

The Theory of Reasoned Action (TRA) provided the framework for the TPB.[5,18] Both focus on the intention to perform a behavior and the various factors that might influence one's intention. The intention to complete a behavior is purported to be highly correlated with the actual behavior. Three basic mediators of intention within this theory are attitudes, subjective norms (those people who influence a person), and perceived behavioral control (whether behaviors can be under one's own control).

Attitudes are favorable or unfavorable judgments about a given behavior and may be further divided into cognitive or evaluative factors and affective factors. Examples of cognitive or evaluative factors within attitudes are "eating fruit would be good/bad" or "eating fruit would be healthy/unhealthy." An example of the affective factors within attitudes is "if I ate fruit, I would feel good/bad."

Subjective norms relate to whether most people who are important to you approve or disapprove the behavior or are supportive or not of the behavior. These may be different people in different situations. For instance, for a young adult, the subjective norms would include friends, coworkers, and perhaps supervisors or teachers for behaviors related to how they dress, whereas for behaviors related to what they eat, supervisors and teachers might not be important. Subjective norms include normative beliefs about what friends or influential people may think, as well as a motivation to comply with what those people may think.

Perceived behavioral control relates to the beliefs that one can control external factors as well as the person's perceived power. Perceived power has been thought of as self-efficacy, or the belief that one can achieve the behavior. An example of control beliefs is "I (always . . . never) have access to vegetables I like to eat." An example of perceived power is "I (am extremely certain . . . extremely uncertain that I) can eat two servings of vegetables each day."

The TPB assumes a causal chain of factors leading to the intention to perform the behavior and then to the behavior itself. The TPB works best with concrete, singular behaviors that are under a person's volitional control. For instance, drinking milk is a behavior that is concrete, singular, and under volitional control; whereas eating a healthy meal is ambiguous without specific criteria, could include multiple behaviors (drinking milk, eating vegetables, choosing lower fat foods), and would also be under volitional control.

Within a systematic review and meta-analysis of 42 journal articles, the TPB variable with the strongest association with intention to consume certain food choices was attitudes.[19] However, the influence of TPB factors on intentions varied with whether the food choices were health promoting or health compromising and whether the individuals were younger or older.

When using the TPB to direct a program or intervention, formative work to determine which factors are most related to the behavioral intention is needed since these influential factors may change with each audience and each behavior. Figure 4.3 illustrates the results of a study to evaluate whether gender or ethnicity changed the influence of TPB factors related to fruit and vegetable intake according to the 5-A-Day promotion. The data supported the concept that neither gender nor ethnicity influenced the TPB factors, and so future programs would not need to consider these demographics specifically.[20]

Stages of Change

The Stages of Change (SOC) or Transtheoretical Model includes personal categorizations of where a person might be in the behavior change process (Table 4.2), as well as Processes of Change, Context of Change, and Markers of Change. Identifying where a person might be in the behavior change process provides clues as to what activities or programs would be helpful in moving the person toward behavior maintenance.[21] In the precontemplation stage, raising awareness of the need for behavior change is appropriate. In the contemplation stage, assisting

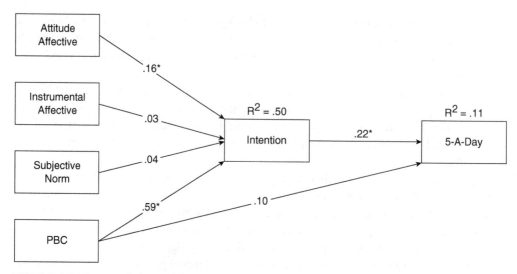

FIGURE 4.3 Theory of Planned Behavior structural coefficients for the combined sample.
PBC, perceived behavioral control.

Note: *p < .05; R^2 = variance explained.

Source: From Blanchard CM, Fisher J, Sparling PB, et al. Understanding adherence to 5 servings of fruits and vegetables per day: a theory of planned behavior perspective. J Nutr Educ Behav. 2009;41(1):3–10. doi:10.1016/j.jneb.2007.12.006

with the decision-making process and discussing the advantages and disadvantages of making a change can help move to the preparation stage at which the person takes some small step or action. Providing options for taking this small step might facilitate action completion. In the action stage, acknowledgment and support for a person's efforts are important, as they are also in the maintenance stage. Behavior change is not always linear, and people may move back and forth or relapse.

TABLE 4.2 STAGES OF CHANGE CATEGORIES

	DEFINITION, STATE IN WHICH. . .	EXAMPLE QUESTION
Precontemplation	Little or no consideration of change	Do you know you should or how often do you use a separate cutting board for meats and for vegetables? Didn't know/Never do this
Contemplation	Some thought has been given to the change	Have heard of that/Don't really do this
Preparation	Some task has been completed or some behavior related to the goal behavior change has occurred	Knew that/Bought another board
Action	A behavior plan is implemented to achieve the behavior goal	Knew that/Began using two boards
Maintenance	The behavior has been sustained for a given amount of time	Yes, knew/Always do this

An example of SOC is as follows:

Brenna is planning to start a running club for the Health Education Department at her university. She discusses the program with a group of her friends and finds that they have very different responses to her goal. John quickly tells her that he doesn't understand why anyone would want to run anywhere (precontemplation). James explains that he has often thought about running, but has no idea how to get started (contemplation). Hilary says she used to run in high school, but has not run in a long time. She asks how to sign up for the program and orders new running shorts and downloads a running app (formerly action/maintenance, currently preparation). Rita explains that she just started running. Although it is hard to stay motivated, she has consistently been running 2 to 3 days a week for the last month (action). Brenna, who has been running consistently for years (maintenance), realizes she would need to use a different strategy to motivate each of her friends.

The Processes of Change include both cognitive and behavioral aspects. Cognitive Processes of Change include activities that increase awareness either with facts or with emotional arousal. Marketing strategies often use these tactics. For example, in marketing a new phone, companies may provide information about the phone, but also show situations that are fun and inviting, hoping that the potential buyer will associate fun with the phone and then buy the phone. Behavioral Processes of Change include using substitutions for a behavior and rewarding oneself for a small behavior change step. For instance, if the overall goal is weight loss, substituting thin-crust pizza for thick-crust pizza and then rewarding oneself with a movie would be substitution and self-reward Behavioral Processes of Change.

The Context of Change reflects the need to consider a more holistic approach to changing behavior. People's life situation, beliefs and attitudes, and interpersonal relationships can all influence whether a behavior change occurs and if it will be sustained. Personal characteristics might also be important to consider as well as the larger social and cultural context.

Using the SOC Model can be helpful in tailoring a program or initiative toward a particularly predominant stage. Many public health messages target the precontemplation stage by increasing awareness of a health issue and prioritizing the behavior. However, when used in a class or program, some in the audience will not be at the stage the program is targeting and could be left out. The SOC Model is also useful for one-on-one counseling.

Health Action Process Approach

The **Health Action Process Approach** is a framework that distinguishes between motivation factors that influence the intention to change a behavior and postintentional volition factors that influence the actual behavior change.[22] Motivation factors that can result in an intention to change include perceived risk, perceived task self-efficacy, and positive outcome expectancies. Postintentional volition factors include planning, action control, social support, and perceived task maintenance self-efficacy. Planning includes the where, what, and how of an action or behavior, whereas action control includes self-regulation and awareness of internal standards or goals. The approach also includes staging of the individual in that he or she is either in the preintention stage, the intention stage, or the action stage.[23]

One program designed to address all three stages of the Health Action Process Approach to improve health outcomes for those with type 2 diabetes reported the approach to be useful in predicting outcomes, but the program was not successful in changing those outcomes. The researchers noted that the intensity or duration of the program may need to be increased. A limitation was having individuals at three stages and the program for all three stages may not match the program and the individuals appropriately.[24]

Social-Ecological Model

The HBM primarily focuses on the individual. The SCT includes the individual as well as the influence of other people and environmental factors. The SEM has a broader view of behavior change.[25] Whereas the SEM includes the individual, it also reflects interpersonal factors; institutional, organizational, or community influences; and policy and systems approaches to behavior change. The individual is focused on to change an individual's behavior through attitudes, knowledge, and skills. Interpersonally focused programs may also target those educators who in turn attempt to modify the individual's behavior. Interpersonal factors may also include programs focusing on peers or the family. Modifying the workplace cafeteria offerings, the facilities offered for breastfeeding mothers, and development of home-delivered meal services are all examples of a focus on the institution, organization, or community. Modifying the school snack policies, the taxes on sugar-sweetened beverages, and laws requiring measuring students' body mass indices with reports to parents are examples of policy or systems change.

A cross-sectional study of women examined whether women engaged in self-directed learning to understand menopause.[26] Because this issue is complex, the SEM was used to interpret findings. Figure 4.4 illustrates how the SEM can be used to better examine complex issues. For instance, at the intrapersonal level, embarrassment or reliance on healthcare providers was identified. At the interpersonal level, mothers and friends were helpful in finding information about menopause. At the institutional level, healthcare providers were not helpful in supporting women. At the community level, frustration at hormonal therapy being an "answer" to menopause and common references to hot flash jokes were issues with a broader landscape. Although women had the least to say about issues within the policy level, some identified the need for additional research funding and including menopause information in health education. The study concluded that these results highlighted the need for the normalization of menopause within our culture and identified issues throughout the SEM that might be addressed to achieve this goal.

Policy, Systems, and Environmental Change

A model related to the SEM is the **Policy, Systems, and Environmental (PSE) Change Approach**. As in the SEM, policy changes include those at the organization, institution, or community level as well as national legislation policy. Systems change supports policy change. Systems change refers to a change in rules or procedures. Environmental change may encompass physical, social, and economic environments. For example, within a school district, changing the rules about having recess before or after lunch may support a policy change in both school meals and physical activity. Adding more lunchroom space and additional physical activity equipment would represent an environmental change. The overall goal is a healthier diet and appropriate physical activity for students.

Most communities or programs adopting a PSE approach focus primarily on the policy and environmental aspects. Unfortunately, the PSE terms are not rigorously defined, so there may be overlap among policy, environment, and systems. In addition, many PSE approaches have not documented the impact on the individual's behavior or health. Nevertheless, many federal agencies and nonprofit organizations believe that focusing more broadly on population health is an important public health strategy.

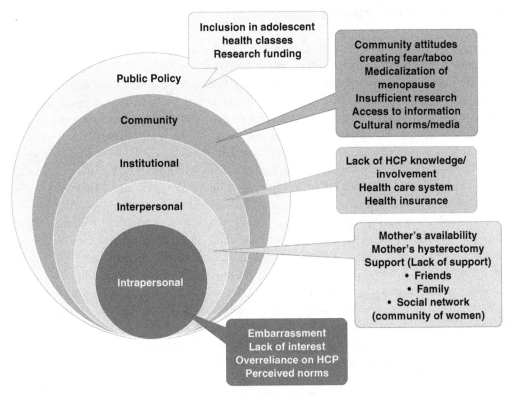

FIGURE 4.4 The socio-ecological factors influencing the SDL actions of women. This figure illustrates the levels of environmental determinants of behavior that influenced women's ability to be self-directed in their search for information about menopause.

HCP, healthcare personnel; SDL, self-directed learning.

Source: From Cooper J. Examining factors that influence a woman's search for information about menopause using the socio-ecological model of health promotion. *Maturitas.* 2018;16:73–78.

Diffusion of Innovation Theory

The Diffusion of Innovation Theory (DIT) provides a perspective on *which* new ideas are adopted by people, *who* primarily adopts these new ideas, and *how*.[27] As the public evaluates innovations, ideas, or even behaviors, they should seem new, easy, and compatible with the person's beliefs or lifestyles in order to be adopted. They should be able to be tried on a limited basis and have observable results. The theory posits that there are five categories of people in regard to adopting a new idea: innovators, early adopters, early majority adopters, late majority adopters, and laggards. People can be influenced by their peers, important others, and marketing.

The DIT can be applied to both food producers and food consumers, and they may influence each other. For instance, developing and marketing organic food products must first be adopted by food producers before consumers can buy and consume them. If food producers see this as new, fitting within their product development plan with some ease, and having a tangible result in sales, then innovators and early adopters may be followed by additional companies. Consumer innovators may be the first to purchase, wanting something new that fits with their beliefs. Social pressure may promote the sales to early and late adopters. This growth in sales may increase the number of organic products on the market as well as the number of companies producing organically labeled food.

BEHAVIORAL ECONOMICS

Behavioral economics is a term that reflects reasons that a person might buy something. Behavioral economics often focuses on environmental issues. In the case of food purchases, availability and cost are key components. In terms of availability, interventions might provide salad bars at schools, farmer's markets in neighborhoods, or remove sugar-sweetened beverages from school vending machines. In terms of cost, interventions might offer coupons for healthier foods, points within an insurance plan, or a tax on alcohol or sugar-sweetened beverages.

In the area of increasing healthier food intake, strategies that appear most promising are using incentives paired with healthy options; changing the default option to the healthier choice (choice architecture or nudges); and decreasing energy-dense food intake. An example of using incentives paired with healthy food options is the Double Up Food Bucks Program (DUFB), which provides a dollar-for-dollar match of Supplemental Nutrition Assistance Program (SNAP) dollars in about 24 states (www.doubleupfoodbucks.org/national-network). In Utah farmers' markets, DUFB participants increased their fruit and vegetable intake significantly with this program.[28] In a supermarket setting in Michigan, DUFB participants increased their vegetable expenditures, but the authors believed the impact was not persistent and not as large as other incentive programs.[29]

Choice architecture has also been described as nudges or environmental changes that modify behavioral choice by nudging the individual in the desired direction. For instance, vegetables and fruits are placed in a cafeteria serving line or the default meal option includes fruit instead of chips and fat-free milk instead of sugar-sweetened beverage. However, studies have not consistently shown the effectiveness of these techniques, and more research is needed to determine which nudges produce the desired effects and in what settings.[30] Strategies to decrease energy-dense food intake include smaller portions of the energy-dense food or replacement of the energy-dense food with a lower energy food.

In the area of increasing physical activity, strategies that include decreasing sedentary time by altering the physical environment or social environment through peer support might be effective. Signage to suggest taking the stairs instead of the elevator or wearable devices to alert individuals that it is time to move rather than sit are both examples of strategies to decrease sedentary behavior. Both online and in-person peer support of increased activity have been effective.

Within a community or organization, framing may prove useful. For example, the label on a food may influence choice as in regular, large, supersize, or value size. Labels or indicators of healthfulness (green, yellow, red) might also influence choice. Posting of caloric information within vending machines and on restaurant menus is another behavioral economic strategy.

When using behavioral economics in counseling, behavioral contracts or pledges are sometimes employed. This strategy has been used with smoking, alcohol use, food intake, and physical activity. Incentives can provide feedback to reinforce the desired behavior.

ISSUES IN BEHAVIORAL THEORY APPLICATIONS AND TESTING IN RURAL, URBAN, AND GLOBAL COMMUNITIES

Applying behavior theories in diverse settings requires additional considerations for the theories to be used effectively and for the programs or interventions to be effective. Knowing your audience is important in program planning or behavior theory selection, but this can be complex. For instance, although most of the United States can be considered **rural**, most U.S. citizens live in **urban** settings. Indeed, "rural" and "urban" are terms that have different definitions, depending on the reason for using these terms. For instance, counties may be defined as urban or rural, or areas/territories of land. Counties may have both urban and rural areas, whereas territories cross counties. County, state, and national policy-makers may look at all of these statistics. Metro–nonmetropolitan (**metro**) is a term that also may be used to evaluate economic and environmental trends. Metro areas have 50,000 or more people and may include adjacent counties if 25% or more of the workforce commutes to the metro county. Land use, economics, and administrative units might differ depending on whether a county or area is isolated, or connected to a metro area. In any case, areas with fewer than 2,500 people are generally considered rural and **nonmetro**.[31]

Behavior theory application may be different for rural versus urban areas, especially if the behavior theory includes environmental aspects. For instance, access to food, food security, access to healthcare, Internet access, physical activity opportunities and influencers, and health beliefs may differ. However, rural differences in using health technology, as well as the availability and accessibility of Internet infrastructure, appear to be modified by educational and economic differences between rural and urban groups.[32]

Access to food and **food deserts** have been studied in both rural and urban settings. Food deserts also have many definitions. The term may relate to how many stores, how many employees in stores, how far away stores are from home or work, the economics of the area, or the quality of food available.[33] Transportation differs in rural versus urban markets, and may also present challenges to food access. People may travel farther to find better quality food, obtain lower prices, or use federal food assistance benefits. Indeed, people may not shop at the stores closest to their home for a variety of reasons.

Access to healthcare in rural areas continues to be a primary issue,[34] often because of fewer providers in rural areas. However, those in rural areas are more likely to engage in risky health behaviors, be uninsured, have chronic conditions, and be less likely to receive screening and diagnostic tests. While telemedicine may reduce the burden of fewer providers, challenges include bringing technology to rural areas, technology acceptance by rural residents, and insurance/Medicare reimbursement for such services.

In addition, the people and their beliefs may differ between rural and urban settings. For the rural individual, good health has been defined as being able to work, have social relationships, and remain independent. Rural residents may see death as natural whereas urban residents resist the idea of death.[35] These types of beliefs can have a profound impact on willingness to change health-related behaviors. Rural and urban issues are discussed more thoroughly in Chapter 6, Cultural Aspects of Public Health Nutrition, and Chapter 7, Promoting Nutritional Health, Healthy Food Systems, and Well-Being of the Community.

These concepts are more pronounced when working in global communities (discussed more thoroughly in Chapter 9, Urban Health and Urbanization: Acting on Social Determinants in Urban Settings). Culture impacts people's perceptions, outcome expectations, beliefs, and behavior. When culture is ignored, the public health initiative will not be effective. Getting to know a multicultural or global audience takes time, an openness to others, and careful attention to the dynamics of diversity. Knowing yourself and your own potential biases is also important. Being blind to differences among people is not being culturally competent. Understanding, embracing, and modifying programs and policies to suit different cultures reflect the cultural competency concepts (discussed more thoroughly in Chapter 5, Public Health and Food Policy: Role in Public Health Nutrition).

Attention to differences in people and place is inherent in certain behavior theories. **Social Marketing Theory** includes **Exchange Theory**, whereby consumers or audiences must perceive benefit from participating; **audience segmentation**, in which similarities are identified; the **marketing mix** of price, product, place, and promotion; **customer orientation**; and monitoring of process and results.[36] An example of Social Marketing Theory can be found within the Centers for Disease Control and Prevention's project VERB! It's what you do![37] For audience segmentation, planners focused on four racial or ethnic groups (American Indian and Native Alaskan, African American, Hispanic, Asian American) within the 9- to 13-year age range, with additional targets on tweens who did not engage in much physical activity. Planners spent a year branding the campaign for the marketing mix and developed tangible goods to enhance the perceived benefit. For the customers in this age range, being social, fun, and cool was part of the customer orientation. Monitoring of the processes and results culminated in over 30 published articles.[38]

All of these considerations create a challenge for the practitioner or researcher when adapting programs or interventions from one type of community to another. **Formative research** represents the time and effort taken to really know your target audience and their environmental, personal, or behavioral perspectives. This might be the time to pilot-test a program or gather information about the needs or beliefs of your community. Generalizations gathered from the literature can help mold the program, but spending time with the community is necessary for a well-developed project. Issues in program planning are discussed more thoroughly in Chapter 11, Community Assessments in Public Health Nutrition.

CONCLUSION

The complex process of behavior change involves numerous internal and external factors. These include the characteristics of the individual as well as the environments, systems, and policy influencing that individual. Understanding the process of behavior change is crucial for public health nutrition professionals who are working to influence nutrition behaviors. The theories discussed in this chapter provide frameworks for describing human behavior. Each theory provides a different approach for understanding and modifying behavior. The theory that is best for a project depends on the factors that are influencing the behavior that needs to be changed.

Behavior theories are useful for program design and evaluation in public health nutrition. During program design, theories provide context for identifying strategies to influence behavior change. In evaluating programs, theories provide structure for explaining some of the complex reasons projects experience success or failure. The proper use of behavior theories by public health nutrition professionals provides a valuable structure for addressing the complexity of nutrition behavior change.

KEY CONCEPTS

1. Behavior change is complex in terms of factors influencing behavior change both internally and externally and in terms of the process of behavior change.

2. Understanding these factors is important so that programs can provide a robust approach to influencing behavior.

3. Beyond the individual, systems, policy, and the environment may need to change to support individual behavior change.

CASE STUDY 1: IMPROVING CLIENT CARE PLANS AND STAFF MORALE AT A COMMUNITY HEALTH CENTER

Staff at a community health center have noticed that many of their clients say that they do not have the time or money to improve their family's meals. At a staff meeting of the physicians, nurses, pharmacist, social worker, and nutritionist, they admit that they are bored and frustrated with making suggestions that are quickly rejected by the client. Many end up handing the client a sheet of money-saving tips and noting in the care plan that this was the action step.

Both for the morale of the staff and health of the clients, an administrator sets a 3-month challenge: form a work group of at least three staff, brainstorm a project, and try it for 3 months. The work group with the most positive reflection on the project from their own perspective as well as the clients' perspective will receive recognition at the center, free parking for 3 months, and a pass to the local gym or pool for the summer.

Case Study Questions

1. Describe a social marketing campaign that a work group might develop.
2. Describe a program based on the SCT that a work group might develop.
3. This case study can be visually described by the SEM. Draw a figure to represent the case scenario.

CASE STUDY 2: DEVELOPING HEALTH AND WELLNESS PROGRAMS FOR A STUDENT HEALTH ORGANIZATION

The student health organization works on campus to promote a healthy environment, guide policy on student health priorities, deliver health and wellness activities and events, and offer health and wellness programs to student groups. The organization includes both undergraduates and graduate students, primarily from kinesiology, nutrition, community and public health, and healthcare management.

With diverse backgrounds and interests, it has been a challenge to narrow their focus for program planning for the next academic year. Some were most concerned with overweight and obesity issues and others with excessive alcohol intake. Sexual health was a priority, and bullying continued to be a problem. After much discussion, the group decided a common element among all of these topics was stress. They decided to plan the year's activities and programs around managing stress. Knowing that programs are most effective if framed within a theory, they decided to use parts of the HBM in their programming.

Case Study Questions

1. The first semester will be focused on raising awareness of the impact that stress can have. The committee wants to target perceived severity of stress and perceived susceptibility of stress. Although posters and flyers could be used, they want to be more engaged with the students. In a small group or individually, brainstorm ideas that engage the students and convey the message.
2. The second semester will be focused on management, especially the perceived benefits of managing stress and the perceived barriers to managing stress. What skills could be taught in a short workshop to address these two topics?

3. Someone in the group feels that flyers and posters could be effective cues to action. Create a flyer or poster that could be an effective cue to action for managing stress.

SUGGESTED LEARNING ACTIVITIES

Case: Mark and Gloria are both premed students in biology who have enrolled in a study abroad class during the summer. They will be working and learning in the public clinics in the city of Gaborone in Botswana. Because English is spoken, they feel comfortable about being able to communicate on some level with the staff and patients. However, they do not feel they know much about the health beliefs or practices of those they are going to be serving.

Complete the following:

1. Gloria feels that as long as they remember basic first aid and follow the lead of the healthcare providers that they will be fine. She also thinks they might be able to teach the staff and patients from her recent experience in a U.S. well-baby clinic. As a group, discuss the implications of Gloria's beliefs.

2. Mark is enthusiastic as well, and he wants to develop a physical activity program that the elders at the clinic could participate in to help flexibility, joint pain, and stiffness. He has worked in an assisted care facility part-time, and got to know the physical therapist quite well. As a group, discuss the advantages and disadvantages of Mark's plan.

REFLECTION QUESTIONS

1. Do you think you are susceptible to a chronic disease? Do you think your grandparents are susceptible? How do social determinants of health influence this perceived health susceptibility and health outcome?

2. A person can influence the environment, and the environment can influence a person's behavior. Can you describe a situation in which both of these scenarios are true?

3. Self-efficacy can be important to behavior change. For instance, if you do not believe you can make a change, you are unlikely to be successful. Describe a time when you or someone you know improved their self-efficacy. Could this be replicated in a program?

4. Being aware of a health risk is necessary before behavior to decrease that risk can occur. Describe the stages of change in terms of first becoming aware and then following through the stages. Which stages might be most difficult to move through?

5. Certain people adopt behaviors more readily, according to the DIT. Reflect on someone you know who has this personality. Did they influence you to adopt the behavior? Why or why not?

CONTINUE YOUR LEARNING RESOURCES

Contento I. *Nutrition Education: Linking Research, Theory, and Practice.* 3rd ed. Burlington, MA: Jones and Bartlett; 2016.

Coreil J, ed. *Social and Behavioral Foundations in Public Health.* Thousand Oaks, CA: Sage; 2009.

DiClemente RJ, Crosby RA, Kegler MC. *Emerging Theories in Health Promotion and Practice Research.* 2nd ed. San Francisco, CA: Jossey-Bass; 2009.

DiClemente RJ, Salazar L, Crosby RA. *Health Behavior Theory for Public Health.* Burlington, MA: Jones and Bartlett; 2013.

U.S. Department of Health and Human Services, National Institutes of Health, National Cancer Institute. *Theory at a Glance: A Guide for Health Promotion.* 2005. https://cancercontrol.cancer.gov/brp/research/theories_project/theory.pdf.

GLOSSARY

Audience segmentation: Dividing people into subgroups based on similar characteristics, such as gender, age, or how often they use a product or service.

Behavioral economics: The study of why people buy products, especially related to cost and availability.

Belief: What a person thinks will happen as a result of a behavior; how a person feels the world works.

Competencies: Behavioral capabilities (skills) or cognitive capabilities (knowledge).

Cues to action: Internal or external factors that cause a person to change behavior or want to change behavior.

Customer orientation: Actions taken to align the product or service with what the target audience perceives their wants or needs to be.

Declarative knowledge: Facts or information stored in memory.

Diffusion of Innovation: A theory that tries to explain how and why new ideas, use of new products or services, or changes in behavior spread.

Evaluative standards: Internal or external benchmarks against which behavior or outcomes are compared.

Exchange Theory: How a person weighs the "pros" and "cons" or risks and rewards of a behavior.

Expectancies: What a person thinks will occur as a result of a specific behavior.

Food deserts: An area where it is difficult to buy food, sometimes related to buying high-quality food, sometimes to distance, and sometimes to cost.

Formative research: Information gathered to design an intervention or program that includes the needs and characteristics of the targeted population.

Health Action Process Approach: Framework of factors that relate to developing an intention to change and those factors influencing intention to develop into action.

Health Belief Model: A framework used to predict or modify health-related behavior focused on perceived barriers and benefits to change; perceived susceptibility for and severity of the condition; and cues to action and self-efficacy toward changing behavior.

Marketing mix: Factors that may promote a product or service, specifically product, price, promotion, and place.

Metro: Generally refers to an urban area.

Nonmetro: Generally refers to a rural or nonurban area.

Observational learning: Learning by watching others perform a behavior or skill.

Perceived barriers: What someone thinks the "cons" of changing a behavior may be.

Perceived benefits: What someone thinks the "pros" of changing a behavior may be.

Perceived severity: What someone thinks the potential impact a condition may have on himself or herself.

Perceived susceptibility: How likely someone believes they may develop a condition.

Policy, Systems, and Environmental (PSE) Change Approach: An ongoing, long-term plan to change behaviors by addressing factors external to the individual.

Procedural knowledge: Understanding how to do something.

Reciprocal determinism: A key tenant of the Social Cognitive Theory in which personal factors, the environment, and personal behavior are influenced by and can influence each other.

Rural: Generally sparsely populated areas but can also include isolation from larger population areas.

Self-efficacy: The belief that one can achieve a set goal or behavior change.

Self-regulation: Internal reflection on behavior that influences future behavior.

Skills: Capacity to perform certain functions.

Social Cognitive Theory: A theory used to predict behavior or model interventions that will change behavior that includes reciprocal determinism concepts, observational learning, self-efficacy, and self-regulation.

Social-Ecological Model: A framework used to develop programs or interventions that include a focus on the individual, intrapersonal behavior, organizational and community factors, and policy.

Social Marketing Theory: Mass communication or advertising theory used to promote a product, service, or behavior.

Theory of Planned Behavior: A theory that posits that subjective norms, attitudes, and behavioral control explain the variance in intention to perform a behavior, which in turn is associated with performing that behavior.

Urban: Area of dense population.

REFERENCES

1. Office of Disease Prevention and Health Promotion. *Healthy People 2020: Social Determinants of Health.* https://www.healthypeople.gov/2020/topics-objectives/topic/social-determinants-of-health
2. Lucyk K, McLaren L. Taking stock of the social determinants of health: a scoping review. *PLoS One.* 2017;12(5):e0177306. doi:10.1371/journal.pone.0177306
3. Rosenstock IM. Historical origins of the Health Belief Model. *Health Educ Monogr.* 1974;2(4):328–335. doi:10.1177/109019817400200403
4. Rosenstock IM. The Health Belief Model and preventive health behavior. *Health Educ Monogr.* 1974;2(4):354–386. doi:10.1177/109019817400200405
5. Ajzen I. From intentions to actions: a theory of planned behavior. In: Kuhl J, Beckmann J, eds. *Action Control: From Cognition to Behavior.* Berlin, Heidelberg: Springer-Verlag; 1985.
6. Bandura A. *Social Learning Theory.* Englewood Cliffs, NJ: Prentice-Hall; 1977.
7. Bandura A. Social cognitive theory of self-regulation. *Organ Behav Hum Decis Processes.* 1991;50:248–287. doi:10.1016/0749-5978(91)90022-L
8. Brofenbrenner U. Ecological models of human development. In: Postlethwaite TN, Husen T, eds. *International Encyclopedia of Education.* Vol. 3. 2nd ed. Oxford: Elsevier; 1994.
9. U.S. Department of Health and Human Services and U.S. Department of Agriculture. *2015–2020 Dietary Guidelines for Americans.* 8th ed. Washington, DC: U.S. Department of Health and Human Services and U.S. Department of Agriculture; 2015. https://health.gov/dietaryguidelines/2015/guidelines
10. Becker MH, ed. The health belief model and personal health behavior. *Health Educ Monogr.* 1974;2:324-473. doi:10.1177/109019817400200407

11. Yue Z, Li C, Weilin Q, Bin W. Application of the Health Belief Model to improve understanding of antihypertensive medication adherence among Chinese patients. *Patient Educ Couns.* 2015;98:669–673. doi:10.1016/j.pec.2015.02.007

12. McArthur LH, Riggs A, Uribe F, Spaulding TJ. Health Belief Model offers opportunities for designing weight management interventions for college students. *J Nutr Educ Behav.* 2018;50(5):485–493. doi:10.1016/j.jneb.2017.09.010

13. VanDyke SD, Shell MD. Health beliefs and breast cancer screening in rural Appalachia: an evaluation of the Health Belief Model. *J Rural Health.* 2017;33(4):350–360. doi:10.1111/jrh.12204

14. Burns AC. The Expanded Health Belief Model as a basis for enlightened preventive health care practice and research. *J Health Care Mark.* 1992;12(3):32–45.

15. Sohler NL, Jerant A, Franks P. Socio-psychological factors in the Expanded Health Belief Model and subsequent colorectal cancer screening. *Patient Educ Couns.* 2015;98(7):901–907. doi:10.1016/j.pec.2015.03.023

16. Young C, Campolonghi S, Ponsonby S, et al. Supporting engagement, adherence, and behavior change in online dietary interventions. *J Nutr Educ Behav.* 2019;51:719–739. doi:10.1016/j.jneb.2019.03.006

17. Greaves CJ, Sheppard KE, Abraham C, et al. Systematic review of reviews of intervention components associated with increased effectiveness in dietary and physical activity interventions. *BMC Public Health.* 2011;11:119. doi:10.1186/1471-2458-11-119

18. Fishbein M, Ajzen I. Attitudes toward objects as predictors of single and multiple behavioral criteria. *Psychol Rev.* 1974;81:59–74. doi:10.1037/h0035872

19. McDermott MS, Oliver M, Svenson A, et al. The theory of planned behavior and discrete food choices: a systematic review and meta-analysis. *Int J Behav Nutr Phys Act.* 2015;12:162. doi:10.11/86/s12966-015-0324-z

20. Blanchard CM, Fisher J, Sparling PB, et al. Understanding adherence to 5 servings of fruits and vegetables per day: a theory of planned behavior perspective. *J Nutr Educ Behav.* 2009;41(1):3–10. doi:10.1016/j.jneb.2007.12.006

21. Prochaska JO, DiClemente CC. Stages and processes of self-change of smoking: toward an integrative model of change. *J Consult Clin Psychol.* 1983;51(3):390–395. doi:10.1037/0022-006X.51.3.390

22. Schwarzer R. Modeling health behavior change: how to predict and modify the adoption and maintenance of health behaviors. *Appl Psychol.* 2008;57:1–29. doi:10.1111/j.1464-0597.2007.00325.x

23. Schwarzer R, Lippke S, Luszczynska A. Mechanisms of health behavior change in persons with chronic illness or disability: the Health Action Process Approach (HAPA). *Rehabil Psychol.* 2011;56(3):161–170. doi:10.1037/a0024509

24. MacPhail M, Mullan B, Sharpe L, et al. Using the health action process approach to predict and improve health outcomes in individuals with type 2 diabetes mellitus. *Diabetes Metab Syndr Obes.* 2014;7:469–479. doi:10.2147/DMSO.S68428

25. Sallis JF, Owen N, Fisher EB. Ecological models of health behavior. In: Glanz K, Rimer B, Viswanath K, eds. *Health Behavior and Health Education: Theory, Research, and Practice.* 4th ed. San Francisco, CA: Jossey-Bass, 2008:464–485.

26. Cooper J. Examining factors that influence a woman's search for information about menopause using the socio-ecological model of health promotion. *Maturitas.* 2018;16:73–78. doi:10.1016/j.maturitas.2018.07.013

27. Rogers E. *Diffusion of Innovations.* 5th ed. New York, NY: Simon and Schuster; 2003.

28. Durward CM, Savoie-Roskos M, Atoloye A, et al. Double Up Food Bucks participation is associated with increased fruit and vegetable consumption and food security among low-income adults. *J Nutr Educ Behav.* 2018;51(3):342–347. doi:10.1016/j.jneb.2018.08.011

29. Steele-Adjognon M, Weatherspoon D. Double Up Food Bucks program effects on SNAP recipients' fruit and vegetable purchases. *BMC Public Health.* 2017;17:946. doi:10.1186/s12889-017-4942-z

30. Szaszi B, Palinkas A, Palfi B, et al. A systematic scoping review of the choice architecture movement: toward understanding when and why nudges work. *J Behav Decis Making.* 2018;31:355–366. doi:10.1002/bdm.2035

31. Economic Research Service. *Rural Economy Populations, Rural Classifications.* https://www.ers.usda.gov/topics/rural-economy-population/rural-classifications/what-is-rural. Updated October 23, 2019.

32. Haggstrom DA, Lee JL, Dickinson SL, et al. Rural and urban differences in the adoption of the new health information and medical technologies. *J Rural Health*. 2019;35:144–154. doi:10.1111/jrh.12358

33. Walker RE, Keane CR, Burke JG. Disparities and access to healthy food in the United States: a review of food deserts literature. *Health Place*. 2010;16:876–884. doi:10.1016/j.healthplace.2010.04.013

34. Bolin JN, Bellamy GR, Ferdinand AO, et al. Rural Healthy People 2020: new decade, same challenges. *J Rural Health*. 2015;31:326–333. doi:10.1111/jrh.12116

35. Gessert C, Waring S, Bailey-Davis L, et al. Rural definition of health: a systematic literature review. *BMC Public Health*. 2015;15:378. doi:10.1186/s12889-015-1658-9

36. Grier S, Bryant CA. Social marketing in public health. *Annu Rev Public Health*. 2005;26:319–339. doi:10.1146/annurev.publhealth.26.021304.144610

37. Wong F, Huhman M, Heitzler C, et al. VERB—a social marketing campaign to increase physical activity among youth. *Prev Chronic Dis*. 2004;1(3):A10.

38. Huhman M, Kelly RP, Edgar T. Social marketing as a framework for youth physical activity initiatives: 1 10-year retrospective of the legacy of CDC's VERB campaign. *Curr Obes Rep*. 2017;6:101–107. doi:10.1007/s13679-017-0252-0

PUBLIC HEALTH AND FOOD POLICY: ROLE IN PUBLIC HEALTH NUTRITION

LINDSEY HAYNES-MASLOW AND STEPHANIE BELL JILCOTT PITTS

LEARNING OBJECTIVES

1. Examine U.S. and global public health nutrition and agriculture policy.

2. Describe the purpose and functions of the major federal food and nutrition assistance programs.

3. Understand the policy development process in the United States.

4. Explain how public health nutrition policy can influence the community and consumer food environments.

5. Describe the links among the food environment, **food security**, and **health disparities**.

INTRODUCTION

Prior to delving into the complex nature of U.S. food policy and the intersection with U.S. public health policy, it is critical to review the basic principles of government in the United States, which many of us may have last discussed in a high school course. As you might recall, in the United States, we are a constitutional representative democracy that functions with a federalism form of governing. We have three levels of government, including the federal, state, and local levels. Each level of government is provided authority and guidance by the U.S. constitution. At both the federal and state levels, there are three coequal branches of government: legislative (elected congressional representatives); executive (elected president/governor and agencies/appointed agency heads); and judicial (the appointed and elected judges). The branches are expected to provide a system of checks and balances over each other. The majority of public health authority, as delegated by the 10th amendment to the U.S. constitution, lies at the state level. However, federalism promotes a sharing of power between the federal and state levels, and thus, much of the regulatory action and funding at the state level is directed by the federal government. At the end of the day, most public health activities, including nutrition services, are delivered at the local county/parish level, with funding support from both the federal and state levels. In the following sections, we further describe the federal departments and agencies involved in the U.S. food system, along with a summary of the major federal food and nutrition programs.

FEDERAL DEPARTMENTS AND AGENCIES INVOLVED IN U.S. AGRICULTURE AND PUBLIC HEALTH POLICY

The federal government is organized into departments, independent establishments, and commissions and corporations. Federal departments can consist of federal agencies.[1] The U.S. agricultural system involves more than 10 federal departments and organizations. Because food touches many areas of the government, different aspects of the food system are overseen by different agencies. A brief overview of the federal agencies and organizations that include food provisions is listed in the following:

1. U.S. Department of Agriculture (USDA)[2]
   - The USDA is the main federal agency overseeing U.S. food and agricultural policy. It consists of 29 agencies and numerous departments and programs that oversee marketability, sustainability, quality, and safety of agricultural commodities. The organizational structure of the department includes several agencies that offer a variety of programs, many of which are provided as a service to agricultural industries. The USDA is explained in detail later in this chapter.

2. U.S. Department of Health and Human Services[3]
   - The Food and Drug Administration (FDA)[4] is the primary regulatory agency impacting the food industry with regard to food safety, food adulteration, and food labeling or misbranding. It protects consumers against impure, unsafe, and fraudulently labeled products. The FDA is also responsible for the safety of drugs, medical devices, biologicals, animal feed and drugs, cosmetics, and radiation emitting devices.
   - The National Institutes of Health (NIH)[5] is composed of several highly specialized research and education based bodies, termed institutes and centers.
   - The Centers for Disease Control and Prevention (CDC)[6] leads federal efforts to gather data on foodborne illnesses, investigate foodborne illnesses and outbreaks, and monitor the effectiveness of prevention and control efforts in reducing foodborne illnesses. The CDC also plays a key role in building state and local health department epidemiology, laboratory, and environmental health capacity to support foodborne disease surveillance and outbreak response.

3. U.S. Environmental Protection Agency (EPA)[7]
   - The EPA is housed under the Department of the Interior. It is primarily involved with protecting human health and safeguarding the natural environment. The EPA is responsible for regulating the use of pesticides in food. The EPA, in cooperation with the states, carefully regulates pesticides to ensure that their use does not compromise food safety.

4. U.S. Department of Homeland Security[8]
   - The Department of Homeland Security works to ensure that our country is able to respond quickly and effectively to an attack on the food supply, major disease outbreak, or other disasters affecting the national food infrastructure.

5. U.S. Department of Commerce (DOC)[9]
   - The primary role of the DOC is to regulate industrial commerce and to prevent illegal stock market profiteering practices. The DOC agencies that most impact the food industry (directly or indirectly) include the National Institute of Standards and Technology (NIST),[10] which works cooperatively with federal agencies and

departments (e.g., FDA, USDA) in regulating standards, weights, and measures as they pertain to food products; and the National Oceanic and Atmospheric Administration (NOAA), which is primarily involved in conservation and management of marine and coastal resources.

6. U.S. Department of Justice (DOJ)[11]

   ▣ The federal court system is involved in the prosecution of food manufacturers and/or individuals suspected of violating food safety regulations.

   ▣ Under the DOJ, the Bureau of Alcohol, Tobacco, Firearms and Explosives (ATF)[12] is responsible for regulating the manufacture and sale of alcoholic beverages. The ATF National Laboratory Center tests new food products. Additionally, they determine whether any products currently sold in the market pose a health risk to consumers.

7. Federal Trade Commission (FTC)

   ▣ The FTC,[13] while technically not a federal department, enforces a variety of laws that protect consumers from unfair, deceptive, or fraudulent practices. The agency's food-related activities primarily involve preventing misleading advertising on food and dietary supplement packages.

8. U.S. Department of Labor (DOL)

   ▣ The DOL[14] is responsible for overseeing labor-related regulations. Additionally, food processing and handling facilities are covered by regulations regarding worker safety administered by the Occupational Safety and Health Administration (OSHA).[15] OSHA's mission is to ensure the safety and health of America's workers by setting and enforcing standards; providing training, outreach, and education; establishing partnerships; and encouraging continual improvement in workplace safety and health.

9. U.S. Department of Defense (DOD)

   ▣ The DOD[16] has a variety of functions and activities that impact the food industry. DOD works cooperatively with the FDA with regard to emergency food supplies and conducts research activities on military food rations. The U.S. Army Veterinary Corps[17] audits, inspects, and approves food and water supplies and manufacturing facilities for military bases and military personnel.

10. Department of the Treasury

   ▣ The Department of the Treasury[18] operates the U.S. Customs Service, which works with other federal agencies to ensure that importing or exporting foods is done in accordance with U.S. laws and regulations. For imported foods, the U.S. Customs Service regulations require that the country of origin be identified.

11. Department of Transportation (DOT)

   ▣ The DOT[19] regulates food products being shipped across state lines. As needed, in the event of a natural or intentional food contamination, the DOT works with the FDA and other agencies in food recalls, seizures, and tracebacks to where the food originated.

Major Federal Food and Nutrition Programs

The U.S. Department of Agriculture Food and Nutrition Service (USDA-FNS) has a goal to end hunger and obesity through the administration of a variety of federal nutrition assistance programs.[20] The USDA-FNS mission is to "increase food security and reduce hunger by providing children and low-income people access to food, a healthful diet and nutrition education in a way that supports American agriculture and inspires public confidence."[20] In what follows, we provide a brief description of each program administered by the USDA-FNS. More information about the programs is available on the National Conference of State Legislatures website.[21]

The **Supplemental Nutrition Assistance Program (SNAP**, formerly the Food Stamp Program) is administered by the USDA-FNS, and provides funding through the use of electronic benefit transfer cards to supplement low-income recipients' ability to purchase foods. The benefit amount varies by household size, income, and expenses. To be eligible, families must meet income requirements and have liquid assets less than $2,250 or less than $3,500 if elderly.

The National School Lunch Program (NSLP) provides federal assistance, in the form of cash and commodities, to schools that provide lunch to students. The National School Breakfast Program (SBP) provides federal cash assistance for schools that provide breakfast to students. Students are eligible to receive free school breakfasts and lunch if their family income is below 130% of federal poverty guidelines, or if they receive Temporary Assistance for Needy Families (TANF) or SNAP benefits or services, or if they are migrants, runaways, homeless, or are in foster care. Children are eligible to receive reduced-price school breakfasts and lunch if the household income is between 130% and 185% of federal poverty guidelines. Schools with 40% or more students eligible for free meals may serve free meals to all students at the school.

The **Special Supplemental Nutrition Program for Women, Infants, and Children (WIC)** provides supplemental, nutrient-rich foods; nutrition education and counseling; and breastfeeding promotion and support to low-income women, infants, and children. WIC benefits can be used to purchase from a list of nutrient-rich foods. Individuals are eligible if they are pregnant, postpartum, or breastfeeding women, infants, and children up to age 5 with household income at or below 185% of the federal poverty level (FPL).

The WIC Farmers' Market Nutrition Program (FMNP) provides grants to participating states to offer vouchers to WIC participants that may be used in farmers' markets and other approved venues to purchase fresh produce. All WIC participants are eligible to participate.

The Child and Adult Care Food Program (CACFP) provides cash subsidies to participating childcare centers, family day-care homes, after-school programs, and nonresidential adult-care centers for the meals and snacks they serve. In childcare centers and nonresidential adult-care settings, per-meal/snack subsidy payments are the same as those for school meals. In childcare centers, eligibility for free and reduced-price meals and snacks is the same as for school meals programs. *Elderly or chronically disabled persons* attending participating nonresidential adult-care centers are eligible for free or reduced meals based on income guidelines that are the same as for school meals programs.

The Summer Food Service Program (SFSP) provides federal cash assistance and some commodity foods to local public and private nonprofit institutions that run summer youth programs, camps, or other recreation sites that serve low-income children during summer break or lengthy school-year breaks. Individuals are eligible if they are 18 years old or younger and live in a low-income area where at least 50% of the children are in households below 185% of federal poverty guidelines or who are enrolled in a program in which 50% of the children are from families with incomes below 185% of federal poverty guidelines.

The Senior Farmers' Market Nutrition Program (SFMNP) provides grants to participating states to offer vouchers to low-income seniors for use at farmers' markets and other approved venues to purchase fresh produce. Individual eligibility is determined by states but all participants must be at least 60 years old, with a household income less than 185% of the FPL.

The Fresh Fruit and Vegetable Program provides grants to schools to purchase fresh fruit and vegetable snacks to be provided during the school day. The program operates in select schools nationwide, with priority to schools with a high proportion of children who are eligible for free and reduced-price meals.

The Special Milk Program provides public or nonprofit schools or childcare institutions that do not participate in other federal meal programs with a per half pint reimbursement for part of the cost of milk served to children. Any child at a participating school or childcare institution can participate.

The Emergency Food Assistance Program (TEFAP) provides cash supports, food commodities, and distribution costs to emergency feeding organizations such as food banks and soup kitchens. States establish income standards for individual eligibility.

The Commodity Supplemental Food Program (CSFP) provides monthly food packages to low-income elderly persons over the age of 60 years who have access to a local CSFP project and have a household income below 130% of the FPL.

Food Distribution Program on Indian Reservations (FDPIR) provides a food package of USDA commodities to low-income households on Indian reservations and to Native American families residing in Oklahoma or in designated areas near Oklahoma. In addition to geographic eligibility requirements, FDPIR has income requirements similar but not identical to those for SNAP. A household cannot participate in both SNAP and FDPIR.

The Older Americans Act (OAA) Nutrition Programs are not included. These programs are part of the Administration on Aging within the Administration for Community Living, and provide funding for nutrition services for older people throughout the country. The OAA Nutrition Programs include the Congregate Nutrition Program and the Home-Delivered Nutrition Program. The goals of these programs center around making community-based nutrition services available to older, at-risk adults.[22]

POLICY DEVELOPMENT AND PROCESS ACROSS GOVERNMENTAL LEVELS

The **farm bill** is known as the primary agricultural and food law run by the federal government. This comprehensive **bill** is passed every 5 years by the U.S. **Congress**. This is referred to as the "reauthorization process" and deals with both agriculture and nutrition. The farm bill is overseen by the USDA. Every 5 years, when the farm bill is reauthorized, Congress proposes, debates, and votes on the farm bill in hopes that it will be signed into law by the president. The last farm bill, the Agricultural Act of 2014, was signed into law on February 7, 2014 and expired on September 30, 2018.[23]

Topics in the farm bill include nutrition and food assistance programs, farm crop prices and income supports, agricultural conservation, farm credit, trade, research, rural development, bioenergy, and foreign food aid. However, because it is reauthorized every 5 years, the farm bill provides an opportunity for policy-makers to adjust, remove, and address specific agricultural and food issues. Because the farm bill covers so many topics (from nutrition to farming to conservation), in recent years, more parties have become involved in the debate, including national farm groups, commodity associations, state organizations, nutrition and public health officials, and advocacy groups representing conservation, recreation, rural development, faith-based interests, local food systems, and certified organic production.[23]

The farm bill was first passed in 1933 as part of President Franklin Delano Roosevelt's New Deal legislation. It was created in response to the economic downturn that arose from the Great Depression and environmental crises caused by the Dust Bowl, in which drought and unsustainable farming practices led to soil turning to dust. Its goals were to (a) keep food prices fair for farmers and consumers, (b) create an adequate food supply so that Americans would not go hungry, and (c) protect and sustain the country's natural resources.[23]

Since then, farm bills traditionally have focused on farm commodity crop program support for primarily corn, soybeans, wheat, cotton, rice, dairy, and sugar. These support programs, often in the form of subsidies, evolved through the 1960s, when President Lyndon B. Johnson's Great Society reforms drew attention to food assistance programs such as the SNAP, formerly known as food stamps. The 1973 farm bill was the first "omnibus" farm bill; it included not only farm supports but also food stamp reauthorization to provide nutrition assistance for needy individuals. Subsequent farm bills expanded in scope, adding titles for formerly stand-alone laws such as trade, credit, and crop insurance. New conservation laws were added in the 1985 Farm Bill, organic agriculture in the 1990 Farm Bill, research programs in the 1996 Farm Bill, bioenergy in the 2002 Farm Bill, and horticulture and local food systems in the 2008 Farm Bill.[24]

The farm bill is an extremely large and complex piece of legislation. It is divided into various sections called "titles."[23] The 2014 Farm Bill had 12 titles. A brief summary of what each title includes, according to the National Sustainable Agriculture Coalition, is listed in the following:

- **Title 1: Commodities.** This title covers price and income supports for the farmers who raise "commodity crops," which are widely grown and traded crops in the United States and abroad. They include crops like corn, soybeans, wheat, and rice as well as dairy and sugar.

- **Title 2: Conservation.** This title covers programs that help farmers implement resource conservation efforts on their land as well as land retirement programs, and easement programs that protect agricultural land. The title also helps institutions and community organizations provide farmers with conservation technical assistance.

- **Title 3: Trade.** This title covers trade, including food exports to other countries and international food aid programs.

- **Title 4: Nutrition.** This title covers nutrition and food assistance programs to help low-income Americans purchase food for their families and educate them about healthy eating. These programs include SNAP (formerly known as "food stamps"), SNAP-Education, SNAP-Outreach, the Expanded Food and Nutrition Education Program (EFNEP), and the Food Insecurity Nutrition Incentive (FINI) Program.

- **Title 5: Credit.** This title covers federal loan programs for farmers to help them get access to loans and financial tools they need to purchase land and equipment and continue their farming operations.

- **Title 6: Rural Development.** This title covers help to boost economic growth in rural communities through rural business and community development (including farm businesses), housing, and infrastructure improvement.

- **Title 7: Research, Extension, and Related Matters.** This title supports agriculture and food research, education, and extension programs. This title helps train and educate the next generation of farmers.

- **Title 8: Forestry.** This title supports conservation efforts in forest-specific settings. It also provides incentives and programs that help farmers and rural communities protect forest resources.

- **Title 9: Energy.** This title includes programs that encourage farmers to grow and process crops for biofuel. It also helps farmers with installing renewable energy systems on their land and supports research related to energy.

- **Title 10: Specialty Crops & Horticulture.** In the farm bill, the term "specialty crops" refers to fruits, vegetables, nuts, and nursery crops (such as flowers, trees, and plants). This title supports farmers' market and local food programs, as well as funding for research and infrastructure specific to those specialty crops. Last, it includes funding for organic research and organic certification programs.

- **Title 11: Crop Insurance.** This title provides payments in the form of "premium subsidies" to farmers as well as payments in the form of "subsidies" to crop insurance companies who sell federal crop insurance to farmers. It also gives the USDA's Risk Management Agency the authority to research, develop, and change insurance policies.

- **Title 12: Miscellaneous.** This title includes many topics, including outreach programs for beginning, socially disadvantaged, and veteran farmers and ranchers; agricultural labor safety and workforce development; and livestock health.

How the Farm Bill Becomes a Law

How does the farm bill become law? The first step is to reauthorize the farm bill. This happens approximately every 5 years. It begins with farm bill hearings, also known as "listening sessions" where members of Congress take input from the public, industry, and advocates about what they want to see in a new bill. These hearings take place in Washington, DC, and in cities across the country. Hearings can take up to several months.

After the hearings, the **House of Representatives** (House) and Senate Agriculture Committees each write ca draft of their own farm bill and debate, amend, and change it (this process is referred to as "marking up"). These House and Senate agricultural committees can write farm bills that look very different. Once each agricultural committee is ready for the House or **Senate** to vote on their bill, it will go up for a full "floor vote." That means the entire House or Senate members debate the bill, make amendments, and vote on it.[23]

After both the full House and Senate have passed their version of the farm bill—which can take months and may require the farm bill being sent back to the agricultural committee for more work—the two separate House and Senate farm bills go to a smaller group of senators and House members called a "conference committee." In the conference committee, these members will work to combine the two separate House and Senate farm bills into one farm bill. This process often requires a great deal of compromise between the House and Senate conference committee members.[23]

Once the conference committee agrees on a single farm bill, it goes back to the House and Senate floors for a vote. Once the House and Senate vote to approve the farm bill, they send it to the president. The president can sign it into law or can veto it (and send it back to Congress to make additional changes).[23] Figure 5.1 details the process by which a bill becomes law.

Farm Bill Spending by Major Programs

Another component of passing the farm bill has to do with funding (also known as "appropriations"). The cost of the farm bill has grown over time, though relative proportions across the major program groups have shifted. Since the 1990s, conservation program spending has steadily risen

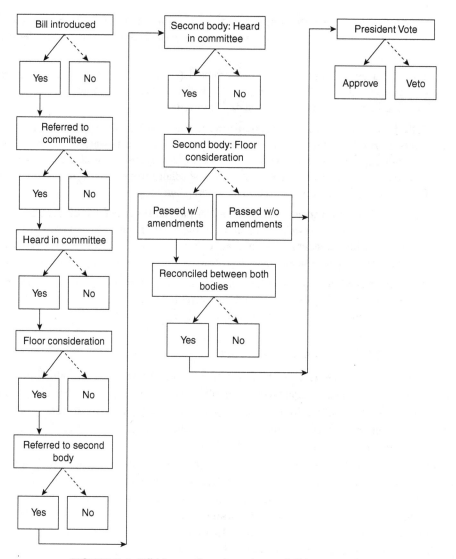

FIGURE 5.1 Bill history flowchart: how a bill becomes law.

as conservation programs have expanded. Farm commodity program spending has both risen and fallen in response to market prices. Crop insurance program costs have increased steadily to cover more commodity crops and they have become a primary strategy for risk management. Nutrition assistance programs in the farm bill rose sharply after the economic recession in 2009, in which President Obama approved stimulus funding to increase aid to families suffering in the economic downturn. However, funding for nutrition assistance programs has slightly declined since the economy has improved.[24]

Currently, nearly 80% of the farm bill's funding goes to nutrition programs. Crop insurance programs are approximately 9%. Conservation and commodity crop programs are approximately 5% to 6% of the farm bill funding, and all other programs account for approximately 1% of the farm bill's budget.

The 5-year reauthorization of the farm bill was signed by President Trump on December 20, 2018. The $867 billion reauthorization will help support county economies and provide critical investments to rural and underserved communities. The farm bill conference agreement protects the SNAP (formerly known as food stamps) by maintaining existing eligibility and work requirements for SNAP recipients. It contains reforms that encourage approaches to job training and other employment-related activities proven effective by the SNAP Employment and Training (SNAP E&T) pilot programs. The farm bill conference agreement would establish a new National Accuracy Clearinghouse to prevent individuals from simultaneously receiving SNAP benefits in multiple states. Finally, it would eliminate an awards program that gave states up to $48 million a year in federal funding for high performances related to program access and payment accuracy. The projected savings from these changes will be reinvested into food banks and other nutrition assistance programs.

THE CHILD NUTRITION ACT

One other major piece of federal legislation that impacts nutrition among children is the Child Nutrition Act. It includes funding for programs that serve food to preschool, school-based, and out-of-school settings. The most prominent programs under the Child Nutrition Act are the NSLP, SBP, and WIC.[25] In the following, we provide a brief overview of these programs:

- ▨ NSLP[26]: NSLP was started in 1946 in response to military needs stemming from World War II, when the U.S. government found that 40% of young adults who were not qualified for service were malnourished. Schools participating in NSLP make decisions about how to design meals and set prices. Schools receive cash subsidies and commodity foods from the USDA. The USDA dictates operational rules and implementation process. To help provide food to low-income children, schools participating in the NSLP are required to offer free meals to children from families with incomes less than 130% of the FPL and reduced-price meals to children less than 185% FPL.

- ▨ SBP: First piloted in 1966[27] and later passed into law in 1975, the SBP provides cash assistance to schools and childcare institutions operating nonprofit breakfast programs. Like the NSLP, schools receive cash subsidies and commodity foods from the USDA to operate the program. To help provide food to low-income children, children can be determined to be "categorically eligible"[28] to receive free meals if they participate in SNAP, are enrolled in Head Start program, and live in households with families with incomes less than 130% of the FPL.

- ▨ WIC: Established in 1974,[29] the WIC provides federal funding to states for supplemental foods, healthcare referrals, and nutrition education for low-income pregnant, breastfeeding, and non-breastfeeding postpartum women, and to infants and children up to age 5 who are found to be at nutritional risk.

Like the farm bill, the Child Nutrition Act is reauthorized every 5 years. Each time it is reauthorized, it is given a new name. In 2010, the Child Nutrition Act was called the "Healthy Hunger-Free Kids Act." The Child Nutrition Act was supposed to be reauthorized by Congress in 2015, but the House and Senate failed to agree on a final bill. Therefore, this act has been operating in the interim under 2010 rules.

U.S. AGRICULTURAL TRADE

With the election of President Donald J. Trump in 2016, one core tenet of his presidential campaign was to promote American goods and products, including food. To accomplish this, in 2018 the White House administration imposed tariffs on multiple other country's goods being imported into the United States. Generally, tariffs are a tax or fee collected by a government on imported goods from another country.[30] While tariffs can raise revenue for a country (i.e., tariffs can encourage consumers to buy domestic products), they also have the potential to harm domestic business if other countries also decide to impose tariffs. In the spring of 2018, after a round of tariffs imposed on other countries, such as China and Canada, these countries also imposed their own tariffs on U.S. goods, including agricultural products such as soybeans, dairy, pork, beef, and many fruits, vegetables, and nuts. It is important to understand that promoting domestic products through tariffs has both advantages and disadvantages.

GLOBAL HEALTH AND AGRICULTURAL ORGANIZATIONS

In addition to other countries' agricultural government agencies or programs, there are global health organizations that work to promote access to food for low-income and vulnerable populations. The most prominent include the World Health Organization (WHO), World Food Programme (WFP), United Nations Children's Fund (UNICEF), and Food and Agriculture Organization (FAO) of the United Nations. These organizations work across various countries. In the following, a brief explanation of each is listed:

1. World Health Organization: WHO was established after World War II in 1948.[31] Currently WHO works across six regions and more than 150 countries. Their mission is to achieve better health for all individuals. One of their main issue areas is nutrition.[32] The organization focuses on malnutrition and food insecurity, breastfeeding child nutrition, solving the obesity epidemic, dietary recommendations, the role that micronutrients play in health, and the impact nutrition has on infectious and chronic disease.

2. World Food Programme: The WFP was created in 1961 in response to President Dwight Eisenhower's request to create an experimental food aid program through the United Nations system.[33] The WFP focuses on emergency food assistance, relief and rehabilitations, development aid, and special operations. A majority of their work is done in countries that are malnourished. They work with approximately 80 countries assisting 80 million individuals each year.[34]

3. UNICEF: Created in 1964, the UNICEF works to promote children and adolescents' health, defend their rights, and help them with upward mobility in society.[35] The UNICEF works in 190 countries with multiple programs, one of them focused on nutrition. The UNICEF focuses on breastfeeding, solving micronutrient deficiencies, using nutrition to assist with chronic disease, addressing emergency food assistance situations, improving child and maternal nutrition, and preventing overweight and obesity.[36]

4. FAO of the United Nations: The FAO was started in 1945. The FAO is an agency within the United Nations that works to address international hunger and food insecurity. The organization works in over 130 countries to ensure that all individuals have access to high-quality food.[37]

UNDERSTANDING THE ROLE OF PUBLIC HEALTH POLICY IN INFLUENCING THE FOOD ENVIRONMENT

In the United States, it often costs more to eat healthy foods than to eat unhealthy foods,[38,39] and neighborhood residents who have lower socioeconomic status often have less access to healthy foods.[40] A variety of public health policies can influence the availability of healthy and less healthy foods and beverages in communities. For the purposes of this chapter, we compartmentalize the food environment into the *community* and *consumer* food environments.[41] The *community food environment* includes the types of food venues in a community, and is usually measured using distance to or density of "healthy" (supermarkets and farmers' markets) versus "unhealthy" (fast food and convenience stores) food venues.[42] The *consumer food environment* includes the foods and beverages available, the price of available foods and beverages, and the quality of products available in food venues, and is measured using food observation/audit tools, such as the Nutrition Environment Measures Survey in Stores (NEMS-S),[43] Farmers' Market Audit Tool,[44] and the Bridging the Gap Food Store Observation Form.[45]

PUBLIC HEALTH NUTRITION POLICY AND THE COMMUNITY FOOD ENVIRONMENT

The community and consumer food environments are influenced by public health policy in that policy can influence what is available in each setting. Two policy options for increasing availability of healthy foods and beverages in the community food environment include encouraging grocery stores to locate into communities that lack access to healthy food, and restricting the number of fast-food or drive-through restaurants that can be located in communities through the use of zoning laws.

Encouraging Grocery Stores to Locate Into Communities That Lack Access to Healthy Food

The Healthy Food Financing Initiative (HFFI) is a federal policy initiative that was modeled after the 2004 Pennsylvania Fresh Food Financing Initiative.[46] The HFFI is a $400 million initiative to entice food retailers (e.g., supermarkets) into food deserts to promote greater availability, purchase, and consumption of healthy foods in U.S. food deserts.[46] The goal was to eliminate urban and rural food deserts within 7 years.[46] There have been evaluation studies of some of these initiatives, demonstrating that neighborhood residents' perceptions of availability of healthy foods in their neighborhoods may improve,[47] but diet does not necessarily improve as a result of residents shopping in the new supermarkets.[47–50]

Restricting the Number of Fast-Food or Drive-Through Restaurants That Can Be Located in Communities Through the Use of Zoning Laws

Another example of the way that policy can influence the community food environment includes zoning to limit fast-food restaurants in a community. Zoning laws are defined as those that determine "what can and cannot be built on parcels of land" within communities' districts.[51] Zoning laws have two main purposes in regulating "what" can be built: (a) the height and design of a building and (b) the use of the building (i.e., what activities are permissible).[52] Zoning laws to limit the presence of fast-food restaurants in their community fall under one of two themes: banning and restricting. Under the first theme, local governments can ban fast-food restaurants entirely; ban certain types of fast-food restaurants, such as chain or franchise restaurants (also known as a "formula" restaurant); or ban restaurants from locating in certain areas, such as neighborhoods or historic districts. Under the second theme, local governments can restrict fast-food restaurants based on the number of fast-food restaurants in a certain area (also known as quota); restrict the number of fast-food restaurants per unit space (also known as density); or restrict fast-food restaurants from locating near places with specific uses, such as schools, parks, or hospitals.[52] While zoning restrictions for fast-food and formula restaurants have occurred in several municipalities, the "Fast Food Ban" in Southern Los Angeles, California, is the first that was presented as a health measure and for a large municipality.[53] It was a zoning regulation that restricted opening or expanding a "stand-alone fast-food restaurant" in Baldwin Hills, Leimert Park, and portions of South Los Angeles and Southeast Los Angeles.[54]

Governments can use scientific studies, epidemiological reports, and public health data to support the argument that zoning laws are needed to protect and promote the public's health and safety.[55] However, although there is much data to support that obesity is *correlated* with fast-food consumption, fast-food restaurant density, and proximity to neighborhoods and schools, there is limited data to support a *causal* link between obesity and fast-food restaurants.[56]

PUBLIC HEALTH NUTRITION POLICY AND THE CONSUMER FOOD ENVIRONMENT

There are several examples of ways that policy influences the consumer food environment, including changes to federal food assistance programs, such as the WIC and SNAP, taxes on unhealthy foods and beverages, and menu labeling in restaurants.

WIC Food Package Policy Changes

The 2009 WIC food package policy included revisions to the food package to bring it more into alignment with the Dietary Guidelines for Americans, and also included minimum stocking requirements for stores that accepted WIC benefits.[54] The 2009 food package policy change resulted in healthier items within stores that accepted WIC benefits,[57-59] better prices,[60,61] and improved dietary behaviors among WIC participants.[62,63]

SNAP Retailer Rule

Another federal policy that may lead to an improved consumer food environment is the new SNAP retailer rule, which includes a requirement for all food retail stores that accept SNAP benefits to include minimum depth of stock for healthier foods. The policy is closed for public comments related to the definition of "variety" and small food retailers may face many barriers to meeting the minimum stocking requirements.[64,65]

Taxes and Tariffs on Unhealthy Foods and Beverages

Sugar-sweetened beverage taxes can influence the price and availability of sugary beverages, ultimately decreasing consumption.[66,67] A 2014 tax on sugar-sweetened beverages in Mexico was associated with a 9.7% reduction in consumption of these products in 2015, with steeper declines in lower income households.[66,67] Additional taxes have been enacted in several U.S. municipalities; however, there are limited evaluation studies on changes in consumption as a result of these taxes.[68] At an international level, trade policy can influence the pricing and availability of various types of foods: For example the Pacific Islands, which experience high levels of obesity, have imposed tariffs on sugary beverages and other obesity-promoting foods and beverages, ultimately making them less available.[69]

Menu Labeling in Restaurants

Required by the Affordable Care Act, menu labeling in restaurants is another way in which policy can influence the consumer food environment. Restaurants with more than 20 stores under the same name must post calories on menu boards. One 2014 review article found that menu labeling with calories alone did not have the intended effect of decreasing calories selected or consumed.[70] Adding interpretive nutrition information on menus could help consumers in the selection and consumption of fewer calories, and females (versus males) tended to use the information to select and consume fewer calories.[70]

Policy Change and the School Food Environment

While not directly related to the community or consumer food environments, school food policies have a critical impact on the foods and beverages served in U.S. public schools. The 2010 Healthy Hunger Free Kids Act tightened nutrition standards in schools, requiring schools to serve more fruits, vegetables, and whole grains, and less sugar, salt, and fat.[71] These standards also redefine portion sizes and apply calorie counts (by grade level) designed to maintain a healthy weight, and schools are provided an additional 6 cents per lunch for meeting these updated standards.[71] In general, policies to improve the school food environment have resulted in healthier dietary behaviors among students and, in some cases, improvements in students' weight status.[72-74]

Food Environments, Food Security, Health Disparities, and Other Food Policy Drivers

Healthy food environments can be compartmentalized into healthy community and healthy consumer food environments. A healthy community food environment includes being closer to food outlets that offer several healthier foods and beverages, such as supermarkets and farmers' markets, and a less healthy food environment is defined by living or working closer in proximity to food outlets with fewer healthy options, including fast food and convenience stores. The Retail Food Environment Index (RFEI)[75] and modified RFEI (mRFEI; CDC) take density of both healthier food outlets and unhealthy food outlets into consideration in one index. The RFEI is calculated as the ratio of fast-food retailers and convenience stores to grocery stores and supermarkets. In a cross-sectional analysis, the RFEI in California was associated with diabetes and obesity, such that individuals living in a less healthy environment had a higher likelihood of having diabetes and obesity.[75] There are several cross-sectional studies demonstrating that healthier elements of the food environment (e.g., supermarkets, farmers' markets) are associated with lower body mass index (BMI) and more fruit and vegetable consumption.[76-78] A healthy consumer food environment includes stocking healthier foods at an affordable price, and marketing such foods in appealing ways for consumers.[79,80] As mentioned previously, changes in the consumer food environment in response to the revised WIC food package policy have resulted in improved dietary behaviors among WIC participants.[62,63]

Poor Food Environments and Health Disparities

A poor food environment can be conceptualized as a food swamp or food desert. *Food swamps* can be classified in several ways. Cooksey-Stowers et al.[81] used three measures to quantify food swamps: (a) RFEI; (b) Expanded RFEI, which included fast food, convenience stores, and supercenters in the numerator and supermarkets/grocery stores, farmers' markets, and specialty food stores in the denominator; and (c) fast food and convenience stores in the numerator and supermarkets/grocery stores, farmers' markets, specialty food stores, and supercenters in the denominator. All three food swamp measures were positively associated with county-level obesity rates, controlling for food deserts, fitness/recreation centers, natural amenities, low-fat milk price to soda price ratio, county size in square miles, and sociodemographic indicators.[81] *Food deserts* are areas with limited access to affordable and nutritious food.[82,83] Although the original 2010 report indicated that distance to healthy food retail venues, such as supermarkets, was critical, the report has since been updated,[84] illustrating the importance of individual-level factors, such as transportation and cost of healthier foods, in determining food purchase and consumption.

Associations Among Food Deserts, Food Swamps, RFEI and mRFEI and Food Insecurity, and an Unhealthy Diet

Zenk et al. used a longitudinal design to examine whether the proximity of food outlets, by type, was associated with BMI changes between 2009 and 2014 among 1.7 million veterans in 382 metropolitan areas, finding no evidence that either absolute or relative geographic accessibility of supermarkets, fast-food restaurants, or mass merchandisers was associated with changes in an individual's BMI over time.[85] Cooksey-Stowers et al.[81] found that all three measures of food swamps were associated with county-level obesity rates. In a longitudinal study, Lamb et al. found that BMI changes among women were not associated with changes in access to fast-food restaurants.[86] In a California-based study, participants lost 1 pound for each standard-deviation improvement in their food environment.[87]

Efforts to Improve the Community Food Environment

Efforts to improve elements of the community food environment include establishing farmers' markets in underserved areas,[88] building new supermarkets in underserved areas,[47,48,50] and zoning to restrict fast-food restaurants,[53] all with limited effectiveness. A recent study of food shopping behaviors indicates that individuals with very low food security are more likely to shop at convenience/corner stores compared to those with greater food security.[89] Findings such as these indicate that access to healthy and unhealthy foods is not the only factor that influences consumers' purchasing and dietary choices.

Efforts to Improve the Consumer Food Environment

Efforts to improve the consumer food environment include healthy corner stores,[79,90,91] point-of-purchase labels in supermarkets to denote healthier foods,[92] and cost offset community supported agriculture (CSA) programs.[93] More evaluation studies are needed to determine the effectiveness of such efforts.

There are several "little p policies," such as the Baby Friendly Hospital Initiative to support breastfeeding[94] and Partnerships for Healthier American Healthy Hospital Initiative,[95,96] which improve the food environment in worksite and other community settings. Jacobson et al. offer policy strategies to reduce diet-related disease in the United States: (a) tax sugary beverages, (b) reduce sodium levels in processed foods, (c) require effective front-of-package nutrition labels, (d) eliminate marketing of unhealthy food to children, (e) increase subsidies to low-income people for the purchase of healthy foods, (f) improve restaurant meals, and (g) mount campaigns to promote healthier diets.[67] It is noteworthy that all of these suggestions are consumer-level or supply-level, versus community-level.

Most of what we have discussed is related to U.S. food security and food environment. Internationally, efforts are underway to improve the food environment in low- and middle-income countries. A review of various interventions to improve food security and the household environment includes agricultural interventions (e.g., home gardening, animal husbandry), air quality interventions (e.g., improved cook stoves), water quality interventions (e.g., water filters), and nutritional interventions (e.g., nutrition education).[97]

Health Policy Advocacy and Infrastructure in Rural, Urban, and Global Communities

The role of funding and partnerships in advocacy success is invaluable: For example, states receiving funding from the CDC's Nutrition, Physical Activity, and Obesity program enacted more obesity-related state legislation than states without funding and those with high partnership involvement implemented more local policies compared to states with low partnership involvement.[98] Holding retreats to reach consensus on the most critical policy advocacy efforts to focus efforts is one way to ensure that funding is used efficiently and that partnerships are maximized to achieve common goals.[99] The Healthy Food Environment Policy Index (Food-EPI) is one tool to assess the extent of implementation of recommended food environment policies by national governments compared to international best practice.[100] The utility of the Food-EPI is the potential to increase accountability to implement widely recommended food environment policies and reduce the burden of diet-related diseases.[100]

INFLUENCING FOOD SYSTEMS AT THE COMMUNITY LEVEL

Community Food Assessments

Community food assessments can be used to inform healthy food policies in local communities. For example, examining zoning ordinances in a local municipality may reveal inequities in opportunities to establish healthier food venues such as farmers' markets.[101,102] If such inequities are revealed, community nutrition practitioners and advocates can lobby for more equitable zoning ordinances.

Food Policy Councils

Food policy councils are often coalitions of food system stakeholders interested in advocating and developing improvements in the food system.[103] In a survey of food policy councils, a majority reported participating in the policy process through problem identification (95%) and education (78%), though few mentioned evaluating their policy work.[104]

CONCLUSION

In this chapter, we described the federal agencies responsible for food and nutrition policy in the United States, including the USDA, the FDA, and the Department of Health and Human Services. Actions of these agencies influence food and nutrition policy in the United States. We also provided an overview of various food and nutrition-related programs to assist families in need, including the SNAP and the WIC. We described the policy process as it relates to the farm bill and Child Nutrition Act, which both influence many of these agencies and programs. In addition, global agencies such as WHO, WFP, UNICEF, and the FAO of the United Nations work to promote access to food for low-income and vulnerable populations.

Later in this chapter, we provided an overview of how the food environment is defined and measured at the community and consumer levels. We also described how policies at the federal, state, and local levels can influence the food environment, as well as individual-level nutrition- and obesity-related outcomes. Such policies can range from changes to the WIC food package and changes to the National Lunch Program, as well as "Fast Food Bans" and sugar-sweetened beverage taxes. We concluded the chapter with metrics related to assessing policies that affect food and nutrition-related policies globally.

As you can see, individual-level food consumption is influenced by a complex dynamic of global, federal, state, and local policies, which influence what is available in our food environment for consumption.

KEY CONCEPTS

1. There are several food-policy-related organizations in the United States and globally.

2. The nutrition policy development process in the United States is built upon the U.S. farm bill and the Child Nutrition Act.

3. Public health nutrition policy can influence the community and consumer food environments in several ways.

4. There are associations among various aspects of the food environment, food security, and health disparities.

CASE STUDY 1: PUBLIC HEALTH NUTRITION EDUCATOR: INCREASING THE NUMBER OF LOCAL FARMERS' MARKETS

You are a public health nutrition educator in a local health department who wants to increase the number of districts in the municipality that have zoning ordinances that allow farmers' markets.

Case Study Questions

1. Where would you find out how districts are currently zoned?

2. Describe a strategy for engaging the planning department to work together to change the zoning ordinance to allow more farmers' markets.

CASE STUDY 2: NONPROFIT THINK TANK: EDUCATING FEDERAL POLICY-MAKERS ABOUT LOCAL FRUIT AND VEGETABLE PRODUCTION

You are working in Washington, DC, for a nonprofit think tank, interested in educating federal policy makers about the positive health and economic benefits of local fruit and vegetable production and consumption.

Case Study Questions

1. What types of information would you put on a 1-page policy brief about the topic?

2. How would you go about disseminating the policy brief?

SUGGESTED LEARNING ACTIVITIES

Learning activity #1:
Write a 1-page letter to your legislator about a food-related policy issue.

Learning activity #2:
Create an infographic about a food-related policy issue. Please see this example: www
.ucsusa.org/food-agriculture/expand-healthy-food-access/infographic-lessons-lunchroom#
.W3BUqi2ZO1I.

Learning activity #3:
Start following a food policy Twitter handle.

Learning activity #4:
Pick a food-related policy issue and write a 1-page brief that you could share with a hypothetical
political stakeholder. Address the following questions: (a) What is the current status of the issue?
(b) What are you asking for? (c) Why are you asking for it? (d) Why should they care? and (e)
What is the result if they end up choosing the option?

Learning activity #5:
Policy playing field exercise: Congress has been holding hearings to address concerns that current SNAP policies may be contributing to the growing obesity rates among low-income SNAP
participants. The House Committee on Agriculture has asked you to analyze whether the SNAP
program should be amended to prohibit the use of SNAP benefits to purchase unhealthy food
products (such as sugar-sweetened beverages, chips, cookies, and other junk foods). As part of
your policy analysis, please:

- Describe the pros and cons of the proposed policy.
- List which stakeholders will support it and which will oppose it. What arguments will
  they use to defend their position?
- Prepare a stakeholder analysis to identify the likely positions of (a) low-income advocates (such as anti-hunger groups), (b) public health officials, and (c) the food industry. If you are unable to identify the public positions of the different interest groups
  for each of these policies, present what you think the interest group's position will be
  (given their positions on other similar proposals).

Learning activity #6:
Conduct a NEMS-S food store audit in three local supermarkets and Nutrition Environment
Measures Survey for Corner Stores (NEMS-CS) in three local convenience or corner stores (www
.med.upenn.edu/nems/measures.shtml). Describe the methods you use to select the stores and
describe your results.

Learning activity #7:
Map out all the food stores, farmers' markets, and restaurants in your county on Google maps.
Describe any spatial patterns you see in the geographic distribution of these venues. Would you
advocate for any changes? If so, what types of changes would you suggest?

REFLECTION QUESTIONS

1. Each time the farm bill is updated, there are many national conversations and contro-
    versies regarding funding decisions for various aspects of the farm bill. Based on what

you read for this chapter, what would you say are some of the key debates? Based on where you would like to practice nutrition in the future, on which side of the debate do you think the majority of individuals you work with would align? Please describe some reasons for your answer.

2. Which federal programs described in the chapter do you think best address food insecurity? Please describe reasons for your response. Are there ways these programs could be improved to help families even more who are struggling to provide food for themselves and their children?

3. There are several elements of the food environment that influence food and beverage consumption at an individual level. Please describe how you personally are influenced by your food environment at the community or organizational level, and describe a policy you think could be enacted in order to address the food environment to make it more conducive to healthier eating in your community or organization.

CONTINUE YOUR LEARNING RESOURCES

Read about the 5-year reauthorization of the farm bill, signed by President Trump on December 20, 2018: https://www.naco.org/blog/president-signs-five-year-farm-bill-reauthorization-containing-several-key-wins-counties

Read the Food Research & Action Center (FRAC) report of the final farm bill: https://frac.org/wp-content/uploads/2018-farm-bill-conference-report-analysis.pdf

Read about the development of the RFEI: https://escholarship.org/content/qt9zc7p54b/qt9zc7p54b.pdf

GLOSSARY

Bill: "The primary form of legislative measure used to propose law."[105] The proposed measure is discussed and voted on by a government or legislative body.

Congress: "The United States Congress is made up of the Senate and the House of Representatives, which is a body of elected officials who represent individual districts in their home states."[106]

Farm bill: The primary agricultural and food law run by the federal government. This comprehensive bill is passed every 5 years by the U.S. Congress. Topics in the farm bill include nutrition and food assistance programs, farm crop prices and income supports, agricultural conservation, farm credit, trade, research, rural development, bioenergy, and foreign food aid.[24]

Food security: The USDA defines four categories of food security:[107]

- "High food security: no reported indications of food-access problems or limitations.

- Marginal food security: one or two reported indications—typically of anxiety over food sufficiency or shortage of food in the house. Little or no indication of changes in diets or food intake.

- Low food security: reports of reduced quality, variety, or desirability of diet. Little or no indication of reduced food intake.

- Very low food security: Reports of multiple indications of disrupted eating patterns and reduced food intake."

Health disparities: "Preventable differences in the burden of disease, injury, violence, or opportunities to achieve optimal health that are experienced by socially disadvantaged populations."[108]

House of Representatives: Referred to as the "lower house," the House of Representative members vote on and pass laws; the number of House members is determined by state population, and a representative's term is 2 years.[105]

Special Supplemental Nutrition Program for Women, Infants, and Children (WIC): "The Special Supplemental Nutrition Program for Women, Infants, and Children (WIC) provides Federal grants to States for supplemental foods, healthcare referrals, and nutrition education for low-income pregnant, breastfeeding, and non-breastfeeding postpartum women, and to infants and children up to age five who are found to be at nutritional risk."[29]

Supplemental Nutrition Assistance Program (SNAP): "SNAP offers nutrition assistance to millions of eligible, low-income individuals and families and provides economic benefits to communities. SNAP is the largest program in the domestic hunger safety net. The Food and Nutrition Service works with State agencies, nutrition educators, and neighborhood and faith-based organizations to ensure that those eligible for nutrition assistance can make informed decisions about applying for the program and can access benefits. FNS also works with State partners and the retail community to improve program administration and ensure program integrity."[109]

U.S. Senate: "The upper house of the United States Congress." Each state elects two senators, who serve a term of 6 years.[106]

REFERENCES

1. Schmidt RH, Archer DL, Olexa MT. *Federal Regulation of the Food Industry—Part 2: Federal Regulatory Agencies*. 2018. http://edis.ifas.ufl.edu/fs121
2. *U.S. Department of Agriculture. About the U.S. Department of Agriculture*. 2018. https://www.usda.gov/our-agency/about-usda
3. *U.S. Department of Health and Human Services. About HHS*. 2018. https://www.hhs.gov/about/index.html
4. *Food and Drug Administration. About FDA*. 2018. https://www.fda.gov/AboutFDA/default.htm
5. *National Institutes of Health. What We Do*. 2018. https://www.nih.gov/about-nih/what-we-do
6. *Centers for Disease Control and Prevention. CDC Organization*. 2018. https://www.cdc.gov/about/organization/cio.htm?CDC_AA_refVal=https%3A%2F%2Fwww.cdc.gov%2Fabout%2Forganization%2Findex.html
7. *Environmental Protection Agency. About EPA*. 2018. https://www.epa.gov/aboutepa
8. *Homeland Security Presidential Directive / HSPD-9*. 2004. https://fas.org/irp/offdocs/nspd/hspd-9.html
9. Department of Commerce. 2018. https://www.commerce.gov
10. National Institute of Standards and Technology. 2018. https://www.nist.gov
11. *Department of Justice. About Department of Justice*. 2018. https://www.justice.gov/about
12. Bureau of Alcohol, Tobacco, Firearms and Explosives. 2018. https://www.atf.gov/alcohol-tobacco
13. Federal Trade Commission. *What We Do*. 2018. https://www.ftc.gov/about-ftc/what-we-do
14. U.S. Department of Labor. *About Us*. 2018. https://www.dol.gov/general/aboutdol
15. *Occupational Safety and Health Administration. About OSHA*. 2018. https://www.osha.gov/about.html
16. Grasso VB. *Department of Defense Food Procurement: Background and Status*. Washington, DC: Congressional Research Service; 2013. Report No.: RS22190.
17. U.S. Army Medical Department: Veterinary Corps. 2018.
18. *U.S. Treasury. Role of the Treasury*. 2018. https://home.treasury.gov/about/general-information/role-of-the-treasury
19. U.S. Department of Transportation. *About Us*. 2018. https://www.transportation.gov/mission/about-us
20. U.S. Department of Agriculture Food and Nutrition Service. *FNS Nutrition Programs*. https://www.fns.usda.gov/programs

21. National Conference of State Legislatures. *Chart of Federal Nutrition Programs*. http://www.ncsl.org/research/human-services/federal-nutrition-programs-chart.aspx. Published March 15, 2018

22. Administration for Community Living. *Older Americans Act Nutrition Programs*. https://acl.gov/sites/default/files/news%202017-03/OAA-Nutrition_Programs_Fact_Sheet.pdf. Published 2016

23. *National Sustainable Agriculture Coalition. What is the Farm Bill?* 2018. http://sustainableagriculture.net/our-work/campaigns/fbcampaign/what-is-the-farm-bill

24. Johnson R, Monke J. *What Is the Farm Bill?* Washington, DC: Congressional Research Service; 2018. Report No.: 7-5700.

25. USDA Food and Nutrition Service. Child Nutrition Act of 1966. https://www.fns.usda.gov/child-nutrition-act-1966

26. *U.S. Department of Agriculture Food and Nutrion Service. National School Lunch Program.* 2018. https://www.fns.usda.gov/nslp/national-school-lunch-program-nslp

27. *U.S. Department of Agriculture Food and Nutrion Service. National School Breakfast Program.* 2018. https://www.fns.usda.gov/sbp/program-history

28. *U.S. Department of Agriculture. School Breakfast Program Fact Sheet.* https://www.fns.usda.gov/sbp/fact-sheet. Updated March 31, 2019.

29. USDA Food and Nutrition Service. The Special Supplemental Nutrition Program for Women, Infants, and Children (WIC Program). https://www.fns.usda.gov/wic

30. *International Trade Theory and Policy: Import Tariffs.* 2008. http://internationalecon.com/Trade/Tch10/T10-1.php

31. *World Health Organization. About WHO.* 2018. http://www.who.int/about/who-we-are/en

32. World Health Organization. *Nutrition Topics.* 2018. http://www.who.int/nutrition/topics/en

33. World Food Programme. *History.* 2018. http://www1.wfp.org/history

34. World Food Programme. *Overview.* 2018. http://www1.wfp.org/overview

35. UNICEF. *What We Do.* 2018. https://www.unicef.org/what-we-do

36. UNICEF. *Nutrition.* 2018. https://www.unicef.org/nutrition

37. Food and Agricultural Organization of the United Nations. *About FAO.* 2018. http://www.fao.org/about/en

38. Monsivais P, Drewnowski A. The rising cost of low-energy-density foods. *J Am Diet Assoc.* 2007;107(12):2071–2076. doi:10.1016/j.jada.2007.09.009

39. Drewnowski A, Moudon AV, Jiao J, et al. Food environment and socioeconomic status influence obesity rates in Seattle and in Paris. *Int J Obes.* 2014;38(2):306–314. doi:10.1038/ijo.2013.97

40. Larson NI, Story MT, Nelson MC. Neighborhood environments: disparities in access to healthy foods in the US. *Am J Prev Med.* 2009;36(1):74–84.e10. doi:10.1016/j.amepre.2008.09.025

41. Glanz K, Sallis JF, Saelens BE, Frank LD. Healthy nutrition environments: concepts and measures. *Am J Health Promot.* 2005;19(5):330–333. doi:10.4278/0890-1171-19.5.330

42. Sharkey JR. Measuring potential access to food stores and food-service places in rural areas in the US. *Am J Prev Med.* 2009;36(4):S151–S155. doi:10.1016/j.amepre.2009.01.004

43. Glanz K, Sallis JF, Saelens BE, Frank LD. Nutrition environment measures survey in stores (NEMS-S): development and evaluation. *Am J Prev Med.* 2007;32(4):282–289. doi:10.1016/j.amepre.2006.12.019

44. Byker Shanks C, Jilcott Pitts S, Gustafson A. Development and validation of a farmers' market audit tool in rural and urban communities. *Health Promot Pract.* 2015;16(6):859–866. doi:10.1177/1524839915597899

45. Rimkus L, Powell LM, Zenk SN, et al. Development and reliability testing of a food store observation form. *J Nutr Educ Behav.* 2013;45(6):540–548. doi:10.1016/j.jneb.2013.02.005

46. Holzman DC. White House proposes healthy food financing initiative. *Environ Health Perspect.* 2010;118(4):A156. doi:10.1289/ehp.118-a156

47. Dubowitz T, Ghosh-Dastidar M, Cohen DA, et al. Diet and perceptions change with supermarket introduction in a food desert, but not because of supermarket use. *Health Aff (Millwood).* 2015;34(11):1858–1868. doi:10.1377/hlthaff.2015.0667

48. Elbel B, Mijanovich T, Kiszko K, et al. The introduction of a supermarket via tax-credits in a low-income area: the influence on purchasing and consumption. *Am J Health Promot.* 2017;31(1):59–66. doi:10.4278/ajhp.150217-QUAN-733

49. Elbel B, Moran A, Dixon LB, et al. Assessment of a government-subsidized supermarket in a high-need area on household food availability and children's dietary intakes. *Public Health Nutr.* 2015;18(15):2881–2890. doi:10.1017/S1368980015000282

50. Pitts SBJ, Wu Q, McGuirt JT, et al. Impact on dietary choices after discount supermarket opens in low-income community. *J Nutr Educ Behav.* 2018;50(7):729–735. doi:10.1016/j.jneb.2018.03.002

51. Feldstein LM. *General Plans and Zoning: A Toolkit for Building Healthy, Vibrant Communities.* Sacramento, CA: California Department of Health Care Services; 2007.

52. Mair JS, Pierce MW, Teret SP. *The Use of Zoning to Restrict Fast Food Outlets: A Potential Strategy to Combat Obesity.* Washington, DC: Johns Hopkins and Georgetown Universities; 2005. http://www.jhsph.edu/center-for-law-and-the-publics-health/research/Z

53. Sturm R, Hattori A. Diet and obesity in Los Angeles County 2007–2012: is there a measurable effect of the 2008 "fast-food ban"? *Soc Sci Med.* 2015;133:205–211. doi:10.1016/j.socscimed.2015.03.004

54. Institute of Medicine. *WIC Food Packages: Time for a Change.* Washington, DC: National Academies Press; 2006.

55. Ashe M, Jernigan D, Kline R, Galaz R. Land use planning and the control of alcohol, tobacco, firearms, and fast food restaurants. *Am J Public Health.* 2003;93(9):1404–1408. doi:10.2105/AJPH.93.9.1404

56. Lydon CA, Rohmeier KD, Sophia CY, et al. How far do you have to go to get a cheeseburger around here? The realities of an environmental design approach to curbing the consumption of fast-food. *Behav Soc Issues.* 2011;20:6–23. doi:10.5210/bsi.v20i0.3637

57. Zenk SN, Odoms-Young A, Powell LM, et al. Fruit and vegetable availability and selection: federal food package revisions, 2009. *Am J Prev Med.* 2012;43(4):423–428. doi:10.1016/j.amepre.2012.06.017

58. Andreyeva T, Luedicke J, Middleton AE, et al. Positive influence of the revised Special Supplemental Nutrition Program for Women, Infants, and Children food packages on access to healthy foods. *J Acad Nutr Diet.* 2012;112(6):850–858. doi:10.1016/j.jand.2012.02.019

59. Andreyeva T, Luedicke J, Middleton AE, et al. *Changes in Access to Healthy Foods after Implementation of the WIC Food Package Revisions.* New Haven, CT: Rudd Center for Food Policy and Obesity, Yale University; 2011.

60. Zenk SN, Powell LM, Odoms-Young AM, et al. Impact of the revised Special Supplemental Nutrition Program for Women, Infants, and Children (WIC) food package policy on fruit and vegetable prices. *J Acad Nutr Diet.* 2014;114(2):288–296. doi:10.1016/j.jand.2013.08.003

61. Lu W, McKyer ELJ, Dowdy D, et al. Evaluating the influence of the Revised Special Supplemental Nutrition Program for Women, Infants, and Children (WIC) food allocation package on healthy food availability, accessibility, and affordability in Texas. *J Acad Nutr Diet.* 2016;116(2):292–301. doi:10.1016/j.jand.2015.10.021

62. Kong A, Odoms-Young AM, Schiffer LA, et al. The 18-month impact of special supplemental nutrition program for women, infants, and children food package revisions on diets of recipient families. *Am J Prev Med.* 2014;46(6):543–551. doi:10.1016/j.amepre.2014.01.021

63. Schultz DJ, Shanks CB, Houghtaling B. The impact of the 2009 special supplemental nutrition program for women, infants, and children food package revisions on participants: a systematic review. *J Acad Nutr Diet.* 2015;115(11):1832–1846. doi:10.1016/j.jand.2015.06.381

64. Haynes-Maslow L, Andress L, Pitts SJ, et al. Arguments used in public comments to support or oppose the US Department of Agriculture's Minimum Stocking Requirements: a content analysis. *J Acad Nutr Diet.* 2018;118:1664–1672. doi:10.1016/j.jand.2017.12.005

65. Ross A, Krishnan N, Ruggiero C, et al. A mixed methods assessment of the barriers and readiness for meeting the SNAP depth of stock requirements in Baltimore's small food stores. *Ecol Food Nutr.* 2018;57(2):94–108. doi:10.1080/03670244.2017.1416362

66. Colchero MA, Rivera-Dommarco J, Popkin BM, Ng SW. In Mexico, evidence of sustained consumer response two years after implementing a sugar-sweetened beverage tax. *Health Aff.* 2017;36(3):564–571. doi:10.1377/hlthaff.2016.1231

67. Jacobson MF, Krieger J, Brownell KD. Potential policy approaches to address diet-related diseases. *JAMA.* 2018;320:341. doi:10.1001/jama.2018.7434

68. Backholer K, Blake M, Vandevijvere S. Sugar-sweetened beverage taxation: an update on the year that was 2017. *Public Health Nutr.* 2017;20(18):3219–3224. doi:10.1017/S1368980017003329

69. Snowdon W, Thow AM. Trade policy and obesity prevention: challenges and innovation in the Pacific Islands. *Obes Rev.* 2013;14:150–158. doi:10.1111/obr.12090

70. Sinclair SE, Cooper M, Mansfield ED. The influence of menu labeling on calories selected or consumed: a systematic review and meta-analysis. *J Acad Nutr Diet.* 2014;114(9):1375–1388.e15. doi:10.1016/j.jand.2014.05.014

71. Welker E, Lott M, Story M. The school food environment and obesity prevention: progress over the last decade. *Curr Obes Rep.* 2016;5(2):145–155. doi:10.1007/s13679-016-0204-0

72. Alaimo K, Oleksyk SC, Drzal NB, et al. Effects of changes in lunch-time competitive foods, nutrition practices, and nutrition policies on low-income middle-school children's diets. *Child Obes.* 2013;9(6):509–523. doi:10.1089/chi.2013.0052

73. Terry-McElrath YM, O'Malley PM, Johnston LD. Potential impact of national school nutritional environment policies: cross-sectional associations with US secondary student overweight/obesity, 2008-2012. *JAMA Pediatr.* 2015;169(1):78–85. doi:10.1001/jamapediatrics.2014.2048

74. Micha R, Karageorgou D, Bakogianni I, et al. Effectiveness of school food environment policies on children's dietary behaviors: a systematic review and meta-analysis. *PloS One.* 2018;13(3):e0194555. doi:10.1371/journal.pone.0194555

75. Babey SH, Diamant AL, Hastert TA, Harvey S. *Designed for Disease: The Link Between Local Food Environments and Obesity and Diabetes.* Los Angeles, CA: UCLA Center for Health Policy Research; 2008.

76. Jilcott Pitts SB, Wu Q, McGuirt JT, et al. Associations between access to farmers' markets and supermarkets, shopping patterns, fruit and vegetable consumption and health indicators among women of reproductive age in eastern North Carolina, U.S.A. *Public Health Nutr.* 2013;16(11):1944–1952. doi:10.1017/S1368980013001389

77. Jilcott SB, Keyserling T, Crawford T, et al. Examining associations among obesity and per capita farmers' markets, grocery stores/supermarkets, and supercenters in US counties. *J Am Diet Assoc.* 2011;111(4):567–572. doi:10.1016/j.jada.2011.01.010

78. Laska MN, Hearst MO, Forsyth A, et al. Neighbourhood food environments: are they associated with adolescent dietary intake, food purchases and weight status? *Public Health Nutr.* 2010;13(11):1757–1763. doi:10.1017/S1368980010001564

79. Laska MN, Pelletier J. *Minimum Stocking Levels and Marketing Strategies of Healthful Foods for Small Retail Food Stores.* Durham, NC: Healthy Eating Research; 2016.

80. Karpyn A, DeWeese RS, Pelletier JE, et al. Examining the feasibility of healthy minimum stocking standards for small food stores. *J Acad Nutr Diet.* 2018;118:1655–1663. doi:10.1016/j.jand.2017.12.006

81. Cooksey-Stowers K, Schwartz MB, Brownell KD. Food swamps predict obesity rates better than food deserts in the United States. *Int J Environ Res Public Health.* 2017;14(11):1366. doi:10.3390/ijerph14111366

82. Walker RE, Keane CR, Burke JG. Disparities and access to healthy food in the United States: a review of food deserts literature. *Health Place.* 2010;16(5):876–884. doi:10.1016/j.healthplace.2010.04.013

83. Ver Ploeg M. *Access to Affordable and Nutritious Food: Measuring and Understanding Food Deserts and Their Consequences: Report to Congress.* Collingdale, PA: Diane Publishing; 2010.

84. Ver Ploeg M, Dutko P, Breneman V. Measuring food access and food deserts for policy purposes. *Appl Econ Perspect Policy.* 2014;37(2):205–225. doi:10.1093/aepp/ppu035

85. Zenk SN, Tarlov E, Wing C, et al. Geographic accessibility of food outlets not associated with body mass index change among veterans, 2009-14. *Health Aff.* 2017;36(8):1433–1442. doi:10.1377/hlthaff.2017.0122

86. Lamb KE, Thornton LE, Olstad DL, et al. Associations between major chain fast-food outlet availability and change in body mass index: a longitudinal observational study of women from Victoria, Australia. *BMJ Open.* 2017;7(10):e016594. doi:10.1136/bmjopen-2017-016594

87. Laraia BA, Downing JM, Zhang YT, et al. Food environment and weight change: does residential mobility matter? The Diabetes Study of Northern California (DISTANCE). *Am J Epidemiol.* 2017;185(9):743–750. doi:10.1093/aje/kww167

88. Evans AE, Jennings R, Smiley AW, et al. Introduction of farm stands in low-income communities increases fruit and vegetable among community residents. *Health Place.* 2012;18(5):1137–1143. doi:10.1016/j.healthplace.2012.04.007

89. Ma X, Liese AD, Hibbert J, et al. The association between food security and store-specific and overall food shopping behaviors. *J Acad Nutr Diet.* 2017;117(12):1931–1940. doi:10.1016/j.jand.2017.02.007

90. Gittelsohn J, Laska MN, Karpyn A, et al. Lessons learned from small store programs to increase healthy food access. *Am J Health Behav.* 2014;38(2):307–315. doi:10.5993/AJHB.38.2.16

91. Jilcott Pitts SB, Wu Q, Truesdale KP, et al. Baseline assessment of a healthy corner store initiative: associations between food store environments, shopping patterns, customer purchases, and dietary intake in Eastern North Carolina. *Int J Environ Res Public Health.* 2017;14(10):1189. doi:10.3390/ijerph14101189

92. Katz DL, Njike VY, Rhee LQ, et al. Performance characteristics of NuVal and the Overall Nutritional Quality Index (ONQI). *Am J Clin Nutr*. 2010;91(4):1102S–1108S. doi:10.3945/ajcn.2010.28450E

93. Seguin RA, Morgan EH, Hanson KL, et al. Farm Fresh Foods for Healthy Kids (F3HK): an innovative community supported agriculture intervention to prevent childhood obesity in low-income families and strengthen local agricultural economies. *BMC Public Health*. 2017;17(1):306. doi:10.1186/s12889-017-4202-2

94. Philipp BL, Merewood A, Miller LW, et al. Baby-friendly hospital initiative improves breastfeeding initiation rates in a US hospital setting. *Pediatrics*. 2001;108(3):677–681. doi:10.1542/peds.108.3.677

95. Jilcott Pitts S, Graham J, Mojica A, et al. Implementing healthier foodservice guidelines in hospital and federal worksite cafeterias: barriers, facilitators and keys to success. *J Hum Nutr Diet*. 2016;29(6):677–686. doi:10.1111/jhn.12380

96. Partnership for a Healthier America [Internet]. 2018. Retrieved from https://www.ahealthieramerica.org

97. Gaihre S, Kyle J, Semple S, et al. Type and extent of trans-disciplinary co-operation to improve food security, health and household environment in low and middle income countries: systematic review. *BMC Public Health*. 2016;16(1):1093. doi:10.1186/s12889-016-3731-4

98. Hersey J, Lynch C, Williams-Piehota P, et al. The association between funding for statewide programs and enactment of obesity legislation. *J Nutr Educ Behav*. 2010;42(1):51–56. doi:10.1016/j.jneb.2009.05.005

99. Holton-Hodson R, Brousseau R. Strengthening a state's health advocacy infrastructure. *Health Aff*. 2006;25(3):856–859. doi:10.1377/hlthaff.25.3.856

100. Vandevijvere S, Mackay S, Swinburn B. Measuring and stimulating progress on implementing widely recommended food environment policies: the New Zealand case study. *Health Res Policy Syst*. 2018;16(1):3. doi:10.1186/s12961-018-0278-0

101. Pitts SBJ, Acheson MLM, Ward RK, et al. Disparities in healthy food zoning, farmers' market availability, and fruit and vegetable consumption among North Carolina residents. *Arch Public Health*. 2015;73(1):1. doi:10.1186/s13690-015-0085-9

102. Mayo ML, Pitts SB, Chriqui JF. Associations between county and municipality zoning ordinances and access to fruit and vegetable outlets in rural North Carolina, 2012. *Prev Chronic Dis*. 2013;10:E203. doi:10.5888/pcd10.130196

103. Schiff R. The role of food policy councils in developing sustainable food systems. *J Hunger Environ Nutr*. 2008;3(2–3):206–228. doi:10.1080/19320240802244017

104. Scherb A, Palmer A, Frattaroli S, Pollack K. Exploring food system policy: a survey of food policy councils in the United States. *J Agric Food Syst Community Dev*. 2016;2(4):3–14. doi:10.5304/jafscd.2012.024.007

105. Legislative Glossary. 2020. https://www.congress.gov/help/legislative-glossary

106. Vocabulary.com Dictionary. 2020. https://www.vocabulary.com/dictionary/House%20of%20Representatives

107. *U.S. Department of Agriculture Economic Research Service. Definitions of Food Security*. 2018. https://www.ers.usda.gov/topics/food-nutrition-assistance/food-security-in-the-us/definitions-of-food-security.aspx

108. Centers for Disease Control and Prevention. *Community Health and Program Services (CHAPS): Health Disparities Among Racial/Ethnic Populations*. Atlanta: U.S. Department of Health and Human Services; 2008.

109. Supplemental Nutrition Assistance Program (SNAP). 2018. https://www.fns.usda.gov/snap/supplemental-nutrition-assistance-program-snap

II

CULTURAL ASPECTS OF PUBLIC HEALTH NUTRITION

FOOD AND CULTURE IMPORTANCE IN PUBLIC HEALTH NUTRITION

CAROL ANNE HARTWICK-PFLAUM, JOHN COVENEY, DAVID N. COX, AND CLAUDE FISCHLER

LEARNING OBJECTIVES

1. Discuss the ways in which culture manifests as different **foodways**.

2. Describe some of the major differences in food cultures and the associated public health issues.

3. Describe ways of achieving public health nutrition goals and being respectful to cultural differences.

INTRODUCTION

Culture is now recognized to be a foundational imperative for food choice and food identity. The endurance of culture is embedded in the everyday experiences of individuals, groups, and societies. It is visible in habits, choices, morals, and codes of practice that unite people. Although cultures may have very similar roots, they can often differ significantly in material expression. The sociologist Pierre Bourdieu is famous for noting that class structures—working class, middle class, and so on—are actually cultural structures, with each class having its own means of expressing habits. Bourdieu's book *Distinctions: A Social Critique of the Judgement of Taste* describes the ways in which class is an expression of culture. For food habits, culture plays a significant role in food and dietary choices. Sometimes these roles are only visible when one culture is compared with another, revealing stark differences and contrasts. These distinctions are often overlooked when public health nutrition programs are planned, developed, and executed. Furthermore, the appreciation of cultural distinctions requires knowledge and skills that are often missing from the capacities with public health nutrition teams. More recently, talent from social sciences and anthropology has been incorporated into the development of public health nutrition programs to capture the role played by culture and social class. Multidisciplinary approaches addressing problems of diet-related diseases are now believed to have the best chances of meeting aims and objectives. Unfortunately, however, the need to acknowledge cultural distinctions is overlooked and programs developed in one jurisdiction are often imported into another without recognition of cultural difference. Part of this chapter describes the ways in which culture played an important role in the success of a public health nutrition program, which was developed in one culture and was introduced into another without recognition of cultural differences. The lessons learned are also discussed.

Cultural Vignette*

*We met as planned at Lunel station. I thought the train would be late and would upset our plans to shop at **Les Halles** in Lunel central. But no, it arrived right on time. Louis was standing at the platform, looking for my familiar face. It was good to see him there. We greeted each other in the familiar southern France manner and headed over to his car. As we climbed in, we offered each other the usual salutations: "how well are you going" and "how is life right now." For Louis, this is always a tricky question. He is an architect, and his life is influenced by his work, which comes in peaks and troughs. So his response is often unexpected, when he tells you how good (plentiful) or not good (bleak) is his workload.*

Sunday morning in Lunel central is wonderful. Always very crowded, with the pavement cafes full of folk sunning themselves in the morning sunshine. But being crowded brings its own problems, especially with parking and finding somewhere to put the car. Louis's familiarity with Lunel meant that he fell back on experience, which gave him the chance to find something others would not have noticed. Lunel is probably typical of small to medium towns in southern France. A main square with lots of cafes, shops, official buildings taking up most of the space.

Out of the car and into the food hall. Bags in hand. First stop, the poissonnerie (fish stall) for ingredients of an entrée we would be eating at lunch. Oyster, prawns, periwinkles. I watch Louis's trained eye move slowly over the offerings. I saw his nose twitch as he sniffed the air that told him how long the shellfish had been out of water. His eyes moved on to an adjacent stall selling much the same products, and to my untrained eye, what looked to be very similar degrees of freshness. But Louis obviously saw differently. A look of satisfaction told me he was more satisfied with offerings over here. Similar experience at the fruit and vegetable stalls. He seems to know what is available and where. He also seems to know what is in season and thus what is to be bought and thus cooked. At an earlier visit, I expressed an interest in cardoons, which I had never eaten. Louis told me this was the cardoon season and toured the local fruit and vegetable shops arriving eventually at one with reliable supply, which then comprised the central dish that evening. I offered to buy the cheese. What would be reliable and suitable for our meal which we would cook and eat together later? The aged Cantal would be good and some soft goat cheese. That will do just fine. Back to the car with bags heaving. Homeward bound.

What was obvious here was the sense of experience, trust in decisions, and engagement directly with the food that we were buying. Louis seemed to bring all his senses to the experience of deciding what to eat and choosing the best ingredients. Because most of the food came unprocessed even unwrapped, there were not signatures or signposts on labels that could be used to guide choice or purchase. What mattered here was the direct engagement with the food and bringing to that the years of observation, experience, and with this a confidence in food purchasing. But not only in the buying of food because in the kitchen later the same levels of experience and know-how were also on show.

The dominance of the central fridges, cold cabinets, and the racks and shelves of packaged food products—and a strange yet familiar odour—was the hallmark of the shopping experience with Katy. We agreed to meet at the entrance to a large shopping mall and go off to the supermarket together. Katy was fitting our meeting into her busy architect practice schedule and was shopping for a family of four, including two children under 10 years old, and one of them—the 4-year-old—in tow. Katy made it clear that food shopping was not her favourite activity, especially with an accompanying child. So there was a need to be efficient and well organized. But, hey, no cutting corners and going

---

* This vignette was first published in Coveney J, Booth S, eds. *Critical Dietetics and Critical Nutrition Studies.* New York, NY: Springer Publishing Company; 2019 and is reproduced here with permission.

for the quick and dirties because like most parents and food providers, Katy wanted to ensure that family meals were healthy and tasty. After cruising through the fruit and vegetable section, near the entrance, like almost all supermarkets, we find ourselves at the fridges. Katy finds that the shelves with her usual brands of yoghurt and cheese are empty. So she is in the process of finding others. Her eyes scanning the alternative offerings Katy finds herself choosing between one product over another. The labels of each are replete with information about contents and provenance. But the most import-ant decision maker is the Health Star Rating[†] that occupies almost a third of the front of pack. No need to dwell on the decision for too long because the one with 4 stars is a clear winner over the oth-ers, 3 star and 3.5 star, respectively. Katy finds herself applying this logic, based on science, to almost all her food purchasing decisions. That is to say, she relies on a scientific appraisal of the food, relayed through the **Health Star Rating system,** *to inform her about the quality of the food she is purchasing. "Quality" here meaning nutritional contents.*

We are out of the supermarket in super quick time, and back to her car where we load up the boot with our bought items.

So, we have descriptions here of two shopping expeditions separated by geographical distance, culture, and language. But the main separation is between an appraisal of food quality relying on experience, familiarity, and know-how. Or rather, different types of experience, familiarity, and know-how. For Louis, his repository of knowledge about food, accumulated over years of shoul-dering the family responsibility for food provisioning, is employed to seek out and choose what he understood to be quality. His knowingness of and familiarity with the offerings at Les Halles allowed him to be in command of his food purchases. For Katy, there is another kind of knowingness; one informed by nutritional science, and ipso facto, requiring deciphering to make it intelligible for the majority of shoppers. Katy needed to have the nutrition facts and figures concentrated into one visual representation: the Health Star Rating system. But there is another difference between the two shopping experiences. Louis's culture, that of the French food culture, will have supplied him with the products of centuries of savoir and connaissance: know-how and know-what. The Cantal cheese, the goat cheese, and many of the other purchases come from a long historical line of food production and food manufacturing. Granted some of these may have been modernized and industrialized. But even so one can see elements of an unchanging process; like the chestnut leaves that are wrapping the goat cheese, a practice that harks back to the time when these cheeses were wrapped and stored over winter months. That is to say, Louis lives in a deep food culture. Deep in terms of its history and its tradition.

Coming from a **"soft" food culture,** *Katy relies on very different senses and sensibilities. With no roots to anchor her food practices into history and tradition, Katy uses modern methods of knowl-edge—based on scientific, more modern rationalities—to inform her decision-making processes. In this way, she is reliant less on her own innate experiences and expertise, and more on the scientific knowledge embedded in and displayed by the Health Star Rating system. She is by this fact, a more passive shopper.*

CONTEXT OF CULTURE

Although Louis and Katy are attached to similar cultural roots, the preceding example demon-strates that they derive from different cultures and one of the most noticeable features of a culture is its ability to define and protect its food culture.

[†] For a full description of Health Star Ratings in Australia and New Zealand, see: http://healthstarrating.gov.au/internet/healthstarrating/publishing.nsf/Content/About-health-stars

CULTURE AND FOODWAYS

To notice that different cultures eat different foods is to observe the ways in which human populations have sought different sources of food as their culture. It becomes obvious that what some
cultures regard as food, other cultures see as nonfood. We call this kind of division "food classification." Helman[1] has usefully described this and other classifications:

- Food versus nonfood
- Sacred versus profane foods
- Food as medicine and medicine as food
- **Social foods** (which designate various social status and occupation groupings)

Food Versus Nonfood

The observation by some that different cultures eat different foods suggests that there is some
functionality in the decision to eat this and not that. For example, some cultures eat the meat from
dog, and many others do not. The reason for not eating dog is, it is often suggested, because in
non–dog-eating cultures dogs play a useful role in protection, hunting, and even companionship
and, as such, are not valued for their meat. However, this "functionalist" argument only goes so
far, and falls apart when cultures that value live dogs, or indeed other animals, also see them as
food. For example, camels are valued in northern Saharan Africa for the transport and other functions they serve. And camel meat is available for purchase in all marketplaces where the camel is
a transport animal. Quite why some foods are nonfoods is still a cultural mystery.

Sacred Versus Profane Foods

The term "profane" here is used to indicate it is outside the edible considerations for some religious communities. For example, pork is forbidden (taboo or harem) in Islamic and Jewish cultures. Some Hindu cultures eschew cow meat. Others, Jains, forbid consumption of all flesh and
other animal products, such as dairy foods. Some cultures follow a rule of fasting during certain
periods, for example, Ramadan in the Islamic culture and Easter in Greek Orthodox. In a study
of different faith-based foodways, we noticed that the admission or prohibition of various foods
by particular religious groups is a way of creating "in" and "out" communities. That is to say, food
choice was a marker of belonging and community.[2]

TRADITIONAL AND THERAPEUTIC USES OF FOODS IN RURAL, URBAN, AND GLOBAL COMMUNITIES

Food as Medicine and Medicine as Food

The relationship between food and medicine is one that is evident in most if not all human cultures. In Western culture, for example, early writings by the Greeks and Romans indicate that
food was medicine and medicine was food. Treating various maladies required attention to diet
and dietetics ("diete"—the daily regime). This was never so apparent as in the theory of humors,
which dominated Western medicine until relatively recently. The system was based on a belief
that the body relied on four fluids, or humors, that circulated throughout the system. The fluids
had independent properties, but they also had a relationship with each other, so careful balance
of the humors was required. The humoral fluids were blood, yellow bile (or choler), black bile,

and phlegm. Each of these was credited with having different and distinctive effects on the body, making it more or less vulnerable to various sicknesses. So having too much of one humor could create a susceptibility to particular diseases.

Many cultures still adhere to the humoral version (or similar) of the creation of health and sickness. For example, in a study of Vietnamese women who were breastfeeding,[51] we noticed that mothers obeyed rules concerning foods considered to be "heating" (but not temperature-wise) and foods thought to be "cooling" (again, not temperature-wise). The food characteristics of heating and cooling were considered to help or hinder the quality of breast milk. Similar observations have been made in other cultures.

Social Foods (Which Designate Various Social Status and Occupation Groupings)

As Mary Douglas and Mike Nicod found out in a foundational research project,[3] food and meals follow a particular "language" and format within particular social groups. Formal meals, for example, have a sequence that is common and recognized with different courses following one after another. It is also possible to see different subgroups within social classes. For example, in one research project on "food in the family setting,"[4] we noticed that parents in more socially advantaged groups used the language of nutritional sciences (vitamins, minerals, calories) when describing some of the concerns they harbored about fussy eating habits in children. On the other hand, in parents in less advantaged groups, we noticed that the vocabulary was more about children being "fit," "active," and "robust" in relation to food choice. These examples demonstrate that working with communities in which there are different cultural and social groupings, a one-size-fits-all approach is likely to be inappropriate and even disrespectful. Public health nutrition programs need to be tailored with their respective cultural groups. The next section describes how this is best achieved.

Development of Culturally Appropriate Programs and Interventions in Diverse Communities

The development of programs in one culture and transferring to another culture is a frequent finding in the area of public health nutrition and health promotion. Indeed, the robustness of a methodology or an analytical framework has often been measured by the ability to transfer to another setting, often in a different culture. However, several works have highlighted methodological issues to consider when conducting research cross-culturally. For example, Triandis and Brislin[5] outline some of the issues that often limit cross-cultural research.

First, similar concepts may have different meanings across cultures. For example, Fischler and Masson[6] demonstrate that the notion of "eating well" may have a nutritional meaning in some cultures compared to a social meaning in others. On this point, Sekaran[7] believes that ensuring functional equivalence is a major methodological goal, arguing that it requires ensuring that the behavior in question developed in different cultures in response to similar problems is shared by the different social or cultural groups.

In our research, we have explored the triggers for specific behaviors in each culture under examination, and therefore we not only studied behaviors such as eating or learning about food; rather, we observed these habits within their cultural contexts in order to understand the issues they respond to. For example, in research on a program called **EPODE (Ensemble, Prevenons l'Obesite Des Enfants)** and its genesis in France, we explored its transference to Australia, where it was called **OPAL (Obesity Prevention and Lifestyle)**. We found that, although both EPODE and OPAL were created in response to a believed obesity epidemic in each jurisdiction, the French program holds a primary focus on the preservation of cultural and traditional habits, while the Australian program sought to disrupt current eating habits by replacing so-called nonhealthy with healthier food choices.

Second, Sekaran raises the issue of language and translation. She claims that vocabulary, idiomatic, grammatical, and experiential equivalences should be verified in instrument development.[7] Triandis and Brislin state that the translation of research tools or data leaves room for discrepancies due to the subjective interpretation of meanings or differences in the range of vocabulary from one language to another. The French language, for example, has a much richer vocabulary and different expressions around food and eating than English does. Whereas English speakers say, "I'm full" when they would like to stop eating, the French say, "Je n'ai plus faim" (*I am not hungry anymore*). In the research reported on EPODE and OPAL, we met this challenge through the primary researcher's proficiency in both languages. Interviews were conducted directly in French and English, and French transcripts were translated by the researcher who conserved French expressions in parentheses when it was felt that the meanings of respondent discourses were compromised.

Third, failure to combine research methods and approaches to analyses to cross-check findings also makes cross-cultural research a challenge. In light of the challenges that cross-cultural research holds, extra precautions should be taken to verify the validity of the cross-cultural data collected[5] and to base data analyses on multivariate techniques.[7] Exploring the same phenomenon through different means allows for this. In the EPODE and OPAL programs, although our research focused primarily on the interviews conducted with selected participants, the researcher conducted situational observations and dedicated several months to exploring and experiencing herself the EPODE and OPAL programs within their respective cultural contexts.

Fourth, the issue of timing of data collection is essential to cross-cultural research.[7] In order to ensure response equivalence, the research should be conducted at equivalent times for each group.[7] We could broaden this point to consider the environments within which obesity prevention initiatives are implemented. When transferring obesity prevention methodologies cross-culturally, it is important to consider the relevance of the messages for the specific time and place in the host context.

Finally, Leung and Bond[8] raise the important point that the samples should be representative of the population and comparable. Of course, when conducting cross-cultural research, ensuring comparability is not easy and special precautions should be taken. What follows is an examination of the EPODE and OPAL programs in depth to illustrate the points made earlier.

Global Childhood Obesity Prevention

Nutrition and health programs for the prevention of childhood obesity have been developed in abundance in the past 10 to 20 years, and some global strategies have been explored. Borys and colleagues claim that "universal community interventions are the most effective in terms of obesity prevention on the condition that a methodological framework is used."[9] Following the World Health Organization (WHO) Ottawa Charter for health promotion published in 1986, there has been a change in emphasis from individual behavior focus to public policy, communities, environments, and health services.[10] This chapter reports on research conducted in two different jurisdictions, France and Australia, and compares and contrasts methodologies, outcomes, and consequences.

Evidence shows that obesity prevention and treatment are more effective in childhood than on adults.[11-15] The most important prevention strategy is believed to be a public health model that focuses on school children and individuals at a young age.[16,17]

Childhood obesity is a serious global problem. In 2004, according to the International Obesity Task Force (IOTF; now known as World Obesity Clinical Care) criteria, it was estimated that ~10% of children worldwide aged 5 to 17 years were overweight.[18] Nutrition and health programs for the prevention of childhood obesity have been developed in the past 10 to 20 years and some global strategies have been explored. Some prevention models include programs that have been developed in one country and transferred and implemented in others, such as **L.E.A.D.** (for Locate the evidence, Evaluate the evidence, Assemble the evidence, and inform Decisions) and ANGELO (Analysis Grid for Elements Linked to Obesity), EPODE models.[19-22] The conditions for the successful cultural transfer of these programs are currently unknown.

Community-Based Childhood Obesity Prevention

Reviews have examined the determinants of healthy lifestyles and support models that address childhood obesity prevention from a community perspective.[23,24] Holistic approaches to childhood obesity prevention consider the collective characteristics of a society and its norms that influence individual behavior.[25] Kumanyika et al. claims that "education alone is not sufficient to change weight-related behaviours. Environmental and societal intervention are also required to promote and support behaviour change."[26]

Davison and Birch[27] argue the usefulness of the **Ecological Systems Theory** (EST) to incorporate all factors involved in the development of childhood overweight and obesity. Such a community-focused model should include "children's dietary and activity patterns, parenting practices that shape children's dietary and activity practices, the environment in which parenting takes place" and "child characteristics, such as gender and age, that influence parenting practices and moderate the impact of risk factors on the development of overweight."[27] They suggest that this comprehensive model would facilitate the development of effective obesity prevention strategies within communities.

Swinburn and colleagues divide the community food environment into three categories in an attempt to understand and dissect the obesogenic environment: physical (what is available), economic, political (what the costs are), and sociocultural (what the rules, attitudes, and beliefs are).[17] Ecological models for health promotion show that education-based interventions associated with social support and environmental changes minimize the barriers to healthy food and lifestyle habits have a higher potential for change.[21,28-30]

Community-based childhood obesity prevention models using environmental and nutrition interventions, for example, are designed to "alter food environment determinants of excessive weight gain in children within an interdependent population in a society before obesity arises."[31] These programs function as the composition of community, political, physical, and economic, food environment interventions and appear effective over a period of 2 months to 3 years in generating significant community food behavior change that contributes to the reduction in the prevalence of childhood obesity.[31] Swinburn and colleagues claim that although more evidence is needed for environmental approaches to obesity prevention, the strength in the approach lies in its ability to easily reach large numbers of people through even modest environmental impacts.[17]

In France, community-based obesity prevention interventions are prevalent, and the country is characterized by the overarching presence of the national educational campaign on nutrition and health (known as PNNS). The French EPODE program, which was informed by the PNNS, has been franchised and exported into several communities globally, including to Australia.

In Australia, community-based obesity prevention programs have been developed in different states. One of the best known examples is the Eat Well Be Active communities, which have a goal of contributing to the healthy weight of children and young people in two communities in South Australia.[32] The program used a community development and community capacity building approach to place the intervention community at the center of the program's implementation.[33] It adopted the **Social-Ecological Model**, highlighting the interrelationships between individuals and their environment and the importance of influencing both to stimulate sustainable change.[34]

To summarize so far, childhood is regarded to be the most effective part of the life course with which to engage for the prevention of obesity, and a number of childhood-focused programs exist. The most effective program models appear to be community-based, and many examples of community-based models exist and there has been adoption of programs from one cultural milieu to another.

CONCLUSION

This chapter provides examples of the ways in which culture operates to influence food choice and eating habits. It provides a number of examples that compare and contrast food cultures demonstrating that even within the same cultural roots, food habits can be very difference. Last, the chapter describes the importance of careful adaptation of public health programs so as to appreciate cultural differences.

KEY CONCEPTS

1. Culture as a marker of differences and distinctions
2. Foodways as examples of the ways in which different food habits are expressed
3. Cross-cultural approaches as forms of inquiry that privilege socio/cultural differences

CASE STUDY: COMPARING THE EPODE PROGRAM IN FRANCE AND THE OPAL PROGRAM IN AUSTRALIA

There is contention about the extent to which programs developed in one jurisdiction can be transported and transplanted in another and remain effective. An example is the EPODE program developed in France and franchised internationally and, specifically for the research reported here, in Australia. As such, we wanted to identify the conditions for cultural transfer of the EPODE program to OPAL, its Australian equivalent. Our objectives were therefore to:

1. Examine the methods, practices, and principles of EPODE and OPAL programs.
2. Compare and contrast how the programs were deployed on the ground.
3. Identify the considerations important for cross-cultural transfers in public health.

Findings

EPODE

EPODE methodology

The EPODE methodology is based on four main pillars:

1. A strong political will, thanks to the involvement of political representatives

2. A coordinated organization and approach based on social marketing methods

3. A multilevel, multistakeholder approach, involving public and private partners

4. Sound scientific background, evaluation, and dissemination of the program[9]

These pillars are used to inform the execution of EPODE and give it sustainability and conformity.

One of the defining characteristics of the EPODE methodology in France is its focus on food and eating as sensory and social experiences. Children are taught to experience foods using the five senses and to share all food experiences as a group. Activities around taste, flavor, and texture are the program's most important components, along with hands-on workshops around the country's culinary traditions. EPODE coordinators are in charge of developing activities for children around the EPODE social marketing themes decided upon by the national coordination.

Importantly the EPODE program exists within the French cultural context of what is known as the so-called French Food Model, here taken to mean the structured food and eating events that take place throughout the day. We recognized that EPODE reinforces the education already provided in the school, family, and the community. These environments have been shown to stimulate children's curiosity and an appreciation for the pleasure, which can be associated to food and which is vital to the French culture and tradition.[35] This early childhood discovery and appreciation for food continues throughout adulthood and is believed to be the precursor to general preferences among the French for natural, quality foods and social eating experiences.[36]

We noted very uniform recounts of habits based on rules and structure, the importance of tradition, pleasure, taste, food quality, and conviviality. French respondents explained clearly that organized meals were the standard eating practice and were essential to family relationships, well-being, and daily life in general—whether at school, at home, or in community contexts in general. Even though the French often take for granted the specificity of their own cultural practices in comparison with other cultures, respondents described them very easily and with great detail, demonstrating that the structures are well defined and widely respected and were noticeable within our population group.

The themes identified by our analysis are consistent with research conducted by the Research Centre for the Study and Observation of Life Conditions in France[37] and other research which has studied and defined the French Food Model and which has provided information on the population's compliance with it.[6,37–42] Participants explained their habits easily, highlighting the structures in place for reinforcement and control: public policy in schools, media, industry, healthcare, and so on.

As part of the work that has defined the French Food Model, Mathé and colleagues at the Centre for Research and Observation of Consumption (CREDOC), France, conducted nationwide research to identify the current norms of the French around food. The findings concluded that the model is a very structured one, controlled and maintained by family, schools, and public policy (government regulation of advertising, school canteens, etc.).[37] EPODE is a good example of how schools and public policy contribute to the maintenance of the model that is introduced first within families.

Perceived EPODE Outcomes

Parents, school staff, and EPODE coordinators were asked to discuss the outcomes of the program for their family, school, and community. Most parents and teachers describe EPODE by its actions (presentations, fruit tasting, etc.) rather than as a broader community program. Thus, when they were asked to discuss their perception of the program's impact, they primarily spoke about the impact of these activities rather than of the program as a whole. School staff members were able to offer most information about EPODE's impact as they are closely involved in the implementation of the program and are more aware about it than the parents. Only EPODE coordinators spoke about the impact of EPODE on the community in general.

Parents and school staff generally praised the EPODE program for its contribution to children's food education. The program was most often referred to as a complement to the education offered at school and within the home. As one respondent noted,

> By doing [the EPODE program] in a group, they [children] saw the others and their reactions, and so it was a little more coherent with what we said at home. Because they don't really have the desire to listen to what the parents say. . . . So I think that it reinforced the things that were said at the house. It reinforced what was done. Especially for my daughter. She heard the messages and she manages to put them into action. (Françoise, nurse, mother of two)

Teachers and teacher assistants also perceive EPODE to impact children's taste preferences and food choices. A respondent said:

> Well, when we started the fruit tasting, we had the impression that it was more of a constraint. We obliged [the children] and they had to taste and it wasn't always a positive experience. Now it's true that they beg us for them. They're happy when it's the fruit period! [. . .] I think that it has had a very positive effect on the families. . . . The program has had a positive impact on their health as well because I assume that, if they ask for fruits at school, that they must ask at home too. (Olivia, teacher)

A teacher assistant explains her perception of EPODE and the impact on children's habits at the canteen:

> Well, I think that it is super good, it's super! Yes, I have seen that the children eat more fruit since this activity started. For example, the watermelon, before they didn't know what it was but now, well, when there is some at the canteen they jump all over it! (Anne-Sophie, teacher assistant)

At another school, teachers spoke about EPODE's impact on children's preference for fruit:

> I find that we, in terms of the children, we can see an evolution among the children in their responses. When there aren't any fruits – when we're not in the EPODE period of fruits, they're like 'wooow, there aren't any fruits?'. They ask for them back. (Danielle, school director)

Interviewee responses also reveal that school staff noticed the impact of EPODE on families and parents' efforts to send children with healthy after-school snacks and picnics. A teacher assistant illustrates this finding:

We especially see their picnics when we go on outings. When we go out we see what they bring and yesterday we had a picnic.... And there were some children who had little carrot sticks or cherry tomatoes and others had cucumber sticks. We really see an evolution concerning the picnics. The parents make a real effort. (Clémence, teacher assistant, canteen and classroom)

A teacher expressed the same opinion:

It's true that, in comparison with other schools that I have known that didn't work with EPODE, we do see that the parents and the children are much more careful about the quality of the snacks. You wouldn't see children coming with a packet of cookies, with chips or other ... here Coca and Orangina, etc. are forbidden in any case. (Marc, teacher)

Participant responses show that the EPODE program has made an impact on school's food and physical activity policies. Several teachers mentioned school policies around food, implemented with the help of EPODE:

We forbid the cans. We encourage them as much as possible to drink water or, when we have breakfast, when we have a snack here we ask them to bring fresh products ... a fresh orange juice or, at least, without adding sugar. (Marc, teacher)

A school director explained the impact that the EPODE program has had on school food policies:

Before there was a snack in the morning and now there's no snack before 16h30. At 16h30, on the other hand, they can have the snack that they want. There are no restrictions, aside from candies that are forbidden and the sweet drinks. Only water is authorized. (Danielle, school director)

A teacher from the same school explained that the program has changed the school culture: "I would say that the values of EPODE have really penetrated into the school culture. It works well." (Danielle, school director)

In summary, participants in France were able to talk positively about the effects of EPODE on children's eating preferences and attitudes to eating in a more structured way and preferring high-quality snacks. EPODE also allowed for the introduction into schools of policies that limited the availability of what were perceived to be unhealthy food products, such as soft drink and energy-dense nutrient poor snacks.

OPAL

OPAL in Australia

Methodology

The EPODE European Network (now called the EPODE International Network) allowed and supported the development of the program in other contexts provided that it be adapted and supported locally. In Australia, the federal government announced the National Partnership Agreement on Preventive Health in 2008. The program "aims to address the rising prevalence of lifestyle related chronic disease by laying the foundations for healthy behaviors in the daily lives of Australians through settings such as communities, early childhood education and care environments, schools and workplaces, supported by national social marketing campaigns."[43] It was under this scheme that the OPAL program was partially funded by the federal government starting in 2009. Furthermore, South Australian state and South Australian local governments partnered to fully fund the program and support its operations on all levels, avoiding the sourcing of any private funds (in contrast to the EPODE methodology). The EPODE international coordination team was contracted to provide support in the adaptation and implementation of the OPAL program over the next 4 years.

The South Australian Health Department placed a priority on developing the OPAL program in 2009, emphasizing that it would target "all levels of the environment and community including micro, meso and macro systems."[30,44,45]

However, while the EPODE methodologies were adapted in South Australia, differences between the Australian and French versions of EPODE were acknowledged.[45] These differences were, first, that the OPAL program was different from EPODE in that it was implemented on a much wider scale, with 20 South Australian councils having commenced the program (including nearly one quarter of the population). Each community had 5 years and the equivalent of $1 million invested to positively influence the social norms around physical activity and healthy eating.[45] The political commitment to OPAL, according to Jones and Williams, was also shown through the intervention period being set to 5 years and not 3 as per the usual policy cycle.

Second, the social marketing approach of OPAL made the program unique in comparison with other community-based programs in Australia. It uses a thematic approach, meaning that a central coordination unit decides and develops communication for all OPAL communities around simple key messages (e.g., "Think feet first"). Jones and Williams[45] state that the themes are developed upon the most relevant available evidence, although there remain challenges around sourcing adequate evidence for specific intervention activities and applying the evidence to local settings, each with their own specific priorities and issues.

Third, as promoted by WHO, this program targets childhood obesity not only by improving knowledge and skills but also by reducing the effects of environmental contributions to the issue.[47] According to Jones and Williams, OPAL differentiates itself through its seven strategy areas, which use these two ways among others. The following are the seven strategy areas. Importantly, unlike the prescribed EPODE methodology, there is no mention of partnerships including public and private parties:

1. Coordination and partnerships—to increase connectedness between programs and organizations in order to improve access and efficiency

2. Social marketing—to use social marketing strategies to positively change social norms

3. Policy, planning, and legislation—to positively influence relevant policy, planning, and legislation

4. Infrastructure and environment—to develop and maintain supportive environments

5. Targeted community programs and services—to support and develop targeted programs

6. Taskforce development—to increase the skills and knowledge of those working in OPAL communities

7. Research and evaluation—to contribute to the knowledge base and the effectiveness of community-based obesity prevention programs[45]

Finally, OPAL distinguishes itself from EPODE through its firm commitment to forming a solid evidence base and evaluation program. This commitment arguably responds to gaps in the literature around community-based obesity prevention program evaluation.[46] Indeed, Daniel and McDermott raise the question of how France's EPODE functioned to produce positive outcomes on childhood obesity.[48] When considering the international dissemination of the program, these authors express their concerns about the Fleurbaix–Laventie study that preceded the development of the EPODE methodology.[48] Similarly, Swinburn et al. highlight the need for more significant priority to be placed on appropriate designs and rigorous evaluations for obesity prevention programs.[49] It has been claimed that OPAL's evaluation program is designed to take into account these concerns through the implementation of a quasi-experimental research design with group matched data. It uses mixed methods (both quantitative and qualitative) and includes process, impact, and outcome measures.[45]

OBSERVED OPAL OUTCOMES

Evaluation data shows that, after 4 years in action, the OPAL program has developed and sustained effective community engagement around the program themes and messages. OPAL has been present in all departments of South Australian local government and major community organizations in order to change the mind-sets of the influencers and impact their commitment to driving sustainable changes in the community. Community stakeholders are well aware of the program's aim and are very invested in contributing. Evaluation data suggests that this is where the real impact of OPAL lies.

An OPAL coordinator expressed her perception of OPAL's impact on these structural relationships and the necessary foundations for sustainable change:

> I think we've done some really good things and hopefully they'll last, but it's only the surface. I mean I feel like we've just scratched the surface. We've got really good networks in schools; we have relationships with people that are really on solid foundations, so there is nothing that we couldn't set out to do now that we couldn't achieve because the foundations that have been created are really rock solid. (Denise, OPAL Coordinator)

Denise discussed an activity of OPAL that illustrates the usefulness of these local partnerships:

> If I choose [the most successful] project it would have to be Plant Your Own Fresh Snack and that's because we've been able to develop a relationship with Housing SA, and of course Housing SA house the most disadvantaged group. (Denise)

Denise goes on to say:

> I mean Plant Your Own Fresh Snack has really been successful because – and it's not about the fruit and the vegetables and the garden box and the seedlings, it's actually about the mentor and it's also about the extended circle of influence around that tenant. So there's the mentor, there's OPAL, there's Housing SA, there's Skills for All regional development, Into Work, AC Care, Lifeline. All of these people sort of come in and out of their lives and suddenly they're being stimulated to do other things and it's human connection. (Denise)

Furthermore, the OPAL program has successfully influenced school and community environments in order to promote healthier habits. OPAL coordinators mentioned environmental changes made within the community thanks to the OPAL program:

> Well obviously there's a lot of water fountains have been installed so community will be able to use them. Assistance with playgrounds and that obviously children and parents use them. Outdoor gym equipment, that's utilised by the public as well. Free city bike hire which OPAL supported with the City of Mt Gambier and tourists and locals use the bikes. Bike lanes have been put in place so it's a lot safer for people to ride bikes on the road. (Jenny, OPAL coordinator)

Evaluation data gives very weak evidence to suggest, however, that the OPAL program had serious, lasting impacts on children's weight or health status. Evaluation data does suggest that a great deal of families were made aware of the OPAL messages and that they were encouraged to make changes in their lives in order to follow the advice: "I do know a little bit about [OPAL]. I think it's awesome. I've seen the signs, like the electronic signs and a few things like that" (Nancy, mother of three).

Most parents also said that their children speak to them about OPAL activities:

There was a breakfast the other morning, pop, peel and pour [. . .]. And something was on at the council too and I know we've also had something at work, some little brochures that have come through – water is nature's soft drink, something like that. (Melinda, dental nurse, mother of two)

Rachel, like other parents, said that her child recites OPAL's social marketing messages: "Yeah every morning my youngest will be just like 'peel, pour, pop'. Yeah it's on the fridge" (Rachel, mother of two).

Another parent explained that the OPAL increased her family's awareness around nutrition:

Yeah they do the pyramids at home all the time. Every single OPAL thing that they've brought home is on our fridge or on a wall somewhere. . . . Yeah, a massive impact for the kids to actually notice different things in the pyramid of 'okay, this is good but this is better.' (Linda, mother of four)

An OPAL coordinator supported this finding:

If you look at the individual factors around knowledge, motivation skills, attitudes, then we've definitely impacted on those. We've seen changes again through our surveys, our telephone based surveys, where parents are describing changes in behaviour and changes in knowledge and understanding so we know there have been those changes. (Michael)

Some parents, like John, explained that OPAL's impact on families is limited due to the difficulties of relying on children to pass messages on to families and parents:

Our kids see us eat and they follow us. I don't know how successful it would be for kids in reception year one to learn about it at school and then go home and try and influence the family diet because the parents. . . . (John, father of four)

Some respondents explained that OPAL's impact on families is limited due to low socioeconomic status:

I think there's a genuine desire to think about their health and wellbeing and their changes. It's certainly driven by socio-economic circumstances. The more means you have, the more likely you are to be in a much healthier lifestyle. The less means you have, the less likely you are to be living a healthy lifestyle. (Glenn, OPAL coordinator)

Although OPAL also makes efforts to influence school environments and provide educational activities to children and school staff, the lack of control over the school environment and children's habits has limited OPAL's ability to challenge fundamental issues such as policy and informing parents and children about health. OPAL can improve infrastructures to encourage physical activity; it can provide school gardens and healthy fruits and vegetables to children although it cannot influence the rules (or lack thereof) that govern children's school mealtimes, frequency, or the composition of their lunch boxes. School directors also mentioned that it was difficult to ensure behavior change due to differences in socioeconomic status and restrictions to food:

It is, it's hard, and a lot of our parents are very low socio-economic and often the dearer food is the healthy food so they opt for the cheaper stuff, but if we can keep just giving them ideas at school it helps I think. (Caroline, school director)

Given that the OPAL program centered its efforts primarily on the community stakeholder relationships, which are at the foundation of sustainable community changes, the impact of the program on schools was less evident for children, parents, and school staff. Some school directors showed a willingness to commit to improving the school environment in terms of children's food and lifestyle habits, although there were serious limits of OPAL's impact on school environments as Australian governments and the Department of Education have practically no control over children's food habits during their time at school. An OPAL coordinator specifically suggested that OPAL help lobby for governments to provide children with lunch meals daily and a pleasant dining experience:

It would be great to have the policies change within all schools so that children sit down and have a lunch all together and it's provided by the school and it's only healthy options, that parents don't actually provide the food, it's all incorporated into school fees and that there's no junk available. (Jenny, OPAL coordinator)

Similarly, another OPAL coordinator suggested the same:

I would do those big picture policy changes in the education department and so, yeah, I'd extend school hours for children so that it suits a working mother but also if lunches are provided, you know, that's a huge shift I think. (Melissa, OPAL coordinator)

Finally, we acknowledge that the OPAL brand is known by general community members, although its impact on their habits is not clear today. The data allowed us to understand that OPAL's greatest actions lie in its cross-governmental approach of creating relationships and encouraging community capacity building through bringing together different community actors around the same cause. These efforts contribute to the building of a foundation within which sustainable actions will be grounded and, later, sustainable behavior changes can be stimulated on individual and family levels.

Consequences of Differences Observed Between EPODE and OPAL

Our findings demonstrated that EPODE and OPAL programs differed in terms of aims and objectives, the implementation of the four pillars of the EPODE methodology, and also in terms of their outcomes for families, communities, and schools.

Generally speaking, our findings provide evidence to suggest that the EPODE program is characterized by it being complementary to the education provided in the home, reinforcing the French Food Model. The OPAL program, on the other hand, seems to be characterized by its widespread social marketing community presence and its focus on the factors that have been identified to specifically contribute to obesity in Australia: namely, nutrition and physical activity.

In summary, France's EPODE was a program that was designed to reinforce key messages based on existing principles founded in culture and tradition. The principles promoted by the program are widely communicated and known by the French population—adults and children—through the National Nutrition and Health Program and others. EPODE in France therefore acts as a support in promoting the same messages that are first promoted within the home and second through the widespread government program. The PNNS provides guidelines and nutritional recommendations adapted to the culture where the EPODE program offers hands-on experiences for children to live them and find a link with what they observe and learn at home. The EPODE program, therefore, uses a food appreciation approach to equip children, through fun activities, with the practical experiences they need to learn and develop healthier preferences (e.g., cooking, gardening, experimenting with taste).

Australia's OPAL plays a different role in preventing childhood obesity. The key findings highlighted earlier show that the OPAL program has implemented the four pillars of the EPODE methodology although, given the contextual differences around food and lifestyle habits, the program looks very different and promotes different messages. In contrast to the EPODE program, the OPAL program promotes habits outside current Australian behavioral norms. France's EPODE, on the other hand, reinforces messages already communicated by family tradition and a general public health campaign. Our observations showed that OPAL has the role of creating new dynamics within the community, building capacity among local actors, facilitating the organization of communication campaigns, and adapting all interventions to local needs.

We want to argue that our research suggests that there are cultural and contextual differences between France and Australia, and that these become the conditions for the successful transfer of the EPODE methodology. We would also suggest that in transferring ideas from one culture to another, full attention must be paid to context and content. Even something as common as health and illness has a cultural context, and assumptions and generalities cannot be made without careful evaluation of the cultural differences.[50]

Case Study Questions

1. What are the features of the most effective public health nutrition programs addressing childhood obesity?

2. What are the most appropriate and effective ways of bringing experience gained in one culture into a different cultural environment?

3. What steps need to be taken to ensure fidelity of a program developed in one jurisdiction and applied to another of a different culture?

SUGGESTED LEARNING ACTIVITIES

1. Go to this website and follow the links to the story about "cow sharing" as a means of accessing raw (unpasteurized) milk: https://www.faganfamilyfarm.com/what-is-a-dairy-herd-share-program.

    The story raised a number of issues concerning food cultures (visible as "belief systems") within an Australian community: one that supports access to raw milk and the other that regulates raw milk for public health reasons. Make a list of the "for" and "against" statement: "People should be able to have access to raw milk for their own and their family's consumption."

2. Go to this website from EPODE: epodeinternationalnetwork.com/events.

    Click on the video that looks at the views of a variety of individuals on public–private partnerships (PPPs) to tackle nutrition-related problems. Divide the responses into for PPPs and against PPPs. Sum up the main arguments of each. Discuss these summary responses in light of the following statement: "Public–private partnerships, where resources from the private sector are used by the public sectors for public good, are the best solution to current nutrition-related problems."

REFLECTION QUESTIONS

1. What are the most effective ways of understanding cultural differences and consequent influences on food choice?

2. When transferring a program developed in one culture into another culture, what are the best ways of ensuring respect for the host and the home culture?

3. Why would qualitative research approaches be more appropriate methods for understanding culture than surveys and questionnaire-based research?

CONTINUE YOUR LEARNING RESOURCES

For a number of resources on food and culture, follow this link to a website on food and culture: https://www.faganfamilyfarm.com/what-is-a-dairy-herd-share-program.

This website contains a number of current and future projects relevant to food and culture: https://www.foodculturehealth.com.

For more information about OPAL (Australia), go to this website: https://www.sahealth.sa.gov.au/wps/wcm/connect/public+content/sa+health+internet/healthy+living/healthy+communities/local+community/opal/opal.

GLOSSARY

Ecological systems theory: Can be defined as a framework in which community psychologists examine individuals' relationships within communities and also the wider society.

EPODE (Ensemble, Prevenons l'Obesite Des Enfants): An obesity prevention program developed in France, now franchised into many jurisdictions.

Foodways: The visible habits and patterns that confer particular food attributes to groups of people.

Health Star Rating systems: Health Star Rating systems are common in many jurisdictions. In Australia and New Zealand, Health Star Ratings provide a front-of-pack label that summarizes the nutritional quality of the food; see healthstarrating.gov.au/internet/healthstarrating/publishing.nsf/Content/About-health-stars.

L.E.A.D.: Is defined as Locate the evidence, Evaluate the evidence, Assemble the evidence, and inform Decisions. A model for the prevention of childhood obesity.

Les Halles: Indoor food hall, where individual stalls and counters sell a variety of food and produce, which is common throughout France.

OPAL (Obesity Prevention and Lifestyle): An obesity prevention program introduced into South Australia, based on the French EPODE model.

Social-Ecological Model (SEM): The SEM is a theory-based framework for understanding the multifaceted and interactive effects of personal and environmental factors that determine behaviors and for identifying behavioral and organizational leverage points and intermediaries for health promotion within organizations. There are five nested, hierarchical levels of the SEM: individual, interpersonal, community, organizational, and policy/enabling environment.

Social foods: How some foods convey social status or lack thereof.

Soft food culture: Describes the ways in which some cultures have strong and traditional roots that endure despite waves of social change (hard food cultures). On the other hand, soft food cultures—not having strong roots or traditions—are more easily changed through trends and fashion.

REFERENCES

1. Helman C. *Culture, Health and Illness*. London: Butterworths; 1990.
2. Neth J, Henderson J, Coveney J, et al. Consumer faith: a qualitative exploration of religion and trust in food. *Food, Cul Soc*. 2013;16(3):421–436. doi:10.2752/175174413x13673466711840
3. Douglas M, Nicod M. Taking the biscuit: the structure of British meals. *New Soc*. 1974;30:744–747.
4. Coveney J. A qualitative study of socio-economic differences in parental lay knowledge of food and health: implications for public health nutrition. *Public Health Nutr*. 2005;8(3):290–297. doi:10.1079/phn2004682
5. Triandis H, Brislin R. Cross-cultural psychology. *Am Psychol*. 1984;39(9):11.
6. Fischler C, Masson E. *Français, Européens et Américains face à l'alimentation*. Paris: Odile Jacob; 2008.
7. Sekaran U. Methodological and theoretical issues and advancements in cross-cultural research. *J Int Bus Stud*. 1983;14(2):13.
8. Leung K, Bond MH. On the empirical identification of dimensions for cross-cultural comparisons. *J Cross Cult Psychol*. 1989;20(2):133-151.
9. Borys J, Le Bodo Y, De Henauw S, et al. *Preventing Childhood Obesity: EPODE European Network Recommendations*. Cachan, France: Lavoisier; 2011.
10. Hancock T. The evolution, impact and significance of the healthy cities/healthy communities movement. *J Public Health Policy*. 1993;14(1):5–18.
11. Berenson GS. Health consequences of obesity. *Pediatr Blood Cancer*. 2012;58(1):117–121. doi:10.1002/pbc.23373
12. Dehghan M, Akhtar-Danesh N, Merchant AT. Childhood obesity, prevalence and prevention. *Nutr J*. 2005;4(1):24. doi:10.1186/1475-2891-4-24
13. Downey AM, Frank GC, Webber LS, et al. Implementation of "Heart Smart:" a cardiovascular school health promotion program. *J Sch Health*. 1987;57(3):7. doi:10.1111/j.1746-1561.1987.tb05378.x
14. Glenny A-M, O'Meara S, Melville A, et al. The treatment and prevention of obesity: a systematic review of the litterature. *Int J Obes*. 1997;21:23. doi:10.1038/sj.ijo.0800495
15. Hayman LL, Williams CL, Daniels SR, et al. Cardiovascular health promotion in the schools: a statement for health and education professionals and child health advocates from the committee on Atherosclerosis, Hypertension, and Obesity in Youth (AHOY) of the council on cardiovascular disease in the young, American Heart Association. *Circulation*. 2004;110(15):2266–2275. doi:10.1161/01.cir.0000141117.85384.64
16. Ells LJ, Campbell K, Lidstone J, et al. Prevention of childhood obesity. *Best Pract Res Clin Endocrinol Metab*. 2005;19(3):14. doi:10.1016/j.beem.2005.04.008
17. Swinburn B, Egger G. Preventive strategies against weight gain and obesity. *Obes Rev*. 2002;3:289–301. doi:10.1046/j.1467-789x.2002.00082.x
18. World Obesity Federation. *Childhood Obesity*. World Obesity; 2015. Retrieved from https://www.worldobesity.org/about/about-obesity/prevalence-of-obesity
19. Simons-Morton B, Greene WH, Gottlieb NH. *Introduction to Health Education and Health Promotion*. 2nd ed. Long Grove, IL: Waveland Press; 1995:510.
20. Kumanyika S, Parker L, Leslie J. *Bridging the Evidence Gap in Obesity Prevention: A Framework to Inform Decision Making*. Washington, DC: National Academies Press; 2010.
21. Swinburn B, Egger G, Raza F. Dissecting obesogenic environments: the development and application of a framework for identifying and prioritizing environmental interventions for obesity. *Prev Med*. 1999;29:563–570. doi:10.1006/pmed.1999.0585
22. World Health Organization. *Interventions on Diet and Physical Activity: What Works*. Geneva, Switzerland: World Health Organization; 2009.
23. Kumanyika SK, Gary TL, Lancaster KJ, et al. Achieving healthy weight in African-American communities: research perspectives and priorities. *Obes Res*. 2005;13(12):2037–2047. doi:10.1038/oby.2005.251
24. Raine KD. Determinants of healthy eating in Canada: an overview and synthesis. *Can J Public Health*. 2005;96(suppl 3):S8–S15. doi:10.1007/BF03405195
25. Rose N, Miller P. Political power beyond the state: problematics of government. *Br J Sociol*. 1992;43(2):33.
26. Kumanyika S, Jeffery R, Morabia A, et al. Obesity prevention: the case for action. *Int J Obes*. 2002;26:425–436. doi:10.1038/sj.ijo.0801938

27. Davison KK, Birch LL. Childhood overweight: a contextual model and recommendations for future research. *Obes Rev.* 2001;2(3):13. doi:10.1046/j.1467-789x.2001.00036.x

28. Booth SL, Sallis JF, Ritenbaugh C, et al. Environmental and societal factors affect food choice and physical activity: rationale, influences, and leverage points. *Nutr Rev.* 2001;59(3):S21–S39. doi:10.1111/j.1753-4887.2001.tb06983.x

29. Simon C, Wagner A, Platat C, et al. ICAPS: a multilevel program to improve physical activity in adolescents. *Diabetes Metab.* 2006;32:41–49. doi:10.1016/s1262-3636(07)70245-8

30. Egger G, Swinburn B. An "ecological" approach to the obesity pandemic. *Br Med J.* 1997;315:477–483. doi:10.1136/bmj.315.7106.477

31. Mayer K. Childhood obesity prevention: focusing on the community food environment. *Fam Community Health.* 2009;32(3):14. doi:10.1097/FCH.0b013e3181ab3c2e

32. Wilson A. Community-based obesity prevention initiatives in aboriginal communities: the experience of the eat well be active community programs in South Australia. *Health.* 2012;04(12):1500–1508.

33. Pettman T, McAllister M, Verity F, et al. *Eat Well Be Active Community Programs Final Report.* Adelaide, Australia: Department of Health; 2010:248.

34. Backett-Milburn K, Wills W, Roberts M-L, Lawton J. Food and family practices: teenagers, eating and domestic life in differing socio-economic circumstances. *Child Geogr.* 2010;8(3):303–314. doi:10.1080/14733285.2010.494882

35. Czernichow S, Martin A. *Nutrition et Restauration Scolaire, de la Maternelle au Lycée: Etat des Lieux.* Paris, France: Agence Française de Sécurité Sanitaire des Aliments; 2000.

36. Tessier S, Chauliac M, Descamps Latscha B. Éducation nutritionnelle à l'école: évaluation d'une méthode pédagogique «La Main à la Pâte». *Santé Publique.* 2010(2):229–238. doi:10.3917/spub.102.0229

37. Mathé T, Tavoularis G, Pilorin T. *La Gastronomie s'Inscrit dans la Continuité du Modèle Alimentaire Fançais.* Paris, France: Centre de Recherche pour l'Étude et l'Observation des Conditions de Vie; 2009.

38. Drewnowski A, Henderson SA, Shore A, et al. Diet quality and dietary diversity in France: implications for the French Paradox. *J Am Diet Assoc.* 1996;96(7):663–669. doi:10.1016/s0002-8223(96)00185-x

39. Dupuy M, Godeau E, Vignes C, Ahluwalia N. Socio-demographic and lifestyle factors associated with overweight in a representative sample of 11-15 year olds in France: results from the WHO-Collaborative Health Behaviour in School-aged Children (HBSC) cross-sectional study. *BMC Public Health.* 2011;11:442. doi:10.1186/1471-2458-11-442

40. Escalon H, Bossard C, Beck F. *Baromètre Santé Nutrition 2008.* Saint-Denis, France: Institut National de Prévention et d'Education pour la Santé; 2009.

41. Rozin P, Kabnick K, Pete E, et al. The ecology of eating: smaller portion sizes explain the French Paradox. *Psychol Sci.* 2003;14(5):5. doi:10.1111/1467-9280.02452

42. Tavoularis G, Mathé T. Le modèle alimentaire français contribue à limiter le risque d'obésite. *Consomm Modes Vie.* 2010;232:4.

43. Council of Australian Government. *National Partnership Agreement on Preventive Health.* Adelaide, South Australia: Australian Department of Health; 2013.

44. Economos CD, Irish-Hauser S. Community interventions: a brief overview and their application to the obesity epidemic. *J Law Med Ethics.* 2007;35:131–137. doi:10.1111/j.1748-720x.2007.00117.x

45. Jones M, Williams M. OPAL. *Public Health Bull.* 2010;7(3):15–19.

46. Healey BJ, Zimmerman RS. *The New World of Health Promotion: New Programme Development, Implementation and Evaluation.* Sudbury, MA: Jones and Bartlett; 2010.

47. World Health Organization. *Obesity: Preventing and Managing the Global Epidemic.* Geneva, Switzerland: World Health Organization; 2000.

48. Daniel M, McDermott R. Obesity prevention in France: yes, but how and why? *Public Health Nutr.* 2009;12(8):2.

49. Swinburn B, Bell C, King L, et al. Obesity prevention programs demand high-quality evaluations. *Aust N Z J Public Health.* 2007;31(4):305–307. doi:10.1111/j.1753-6405.2007.00075.x

50. Guillemin I, Marrel A, Arnould B, et al. How French subjects describe well-being from food and eating habits? Development, item reduction and scoring definition of the Well-Being related to Food Questionnaire (Well-BFQ©). *Appetite.* 2016;96:333–346. doi:10.1016/j.appet.2015.09.021

51. Reynolds B, Hitchcock N, Coveney J. A longitudinal study of Vietnamese children born in Australia: Infant feeding, growth in infancy and after five years. *Nutrition Research.* 1989;8:593.

PROMOTING NUTRITIONAL HEALTH, HEALTHY FOOD SYSTEMS, AND WELL-BEING OF THE COMMUNITY

ADAM HEGE, ALISHA FARRIS, AMY DAILEY, AND MARIA JULIAN

LEARNING OBJECTIVES

1. Describe the key concepts involved with nutritional health at a local level.
2. Understand the processes involved with developing a community food system.
3. Explain the barriers, disparities, and inequities commonly found in local communities.
4. Evaluate a community food system for inequities and future opportunities.
5. Apply a systems framework to promoting nutritional health and community wellness.

INTRODUCTION

Food and the manners by which it is produced and distributed across a community have profound implications for the livability and quality of life offered. In addition, health outcomes and economic viability are subsequently long-term outcomes of the food system that is created and maintained in a community. There is no doubt that community leaders and public health practitioners face a daunting task in seeking to meet the immediate needs of their citizens, while also having a forward vision for meeting future challenges. In this chapter, we seek to describe some of the key issues that are involved with food and nutritional health at the community level. Along the way, topics such as food security, food justice, community development, and systems thinking are detailed.

CONNECTION TO NATIONAL INITIATIVES (NATIONAL TO LOCAL)

Effectively promoting health at the community level requires an alignment of public health initiatives at all levels—national, state, and local. As discussed in previous chapters, national health initiatives are selected based on continuous nutrition monitoring and surveillance, and government organizations and health professionals should align their policies and programs to address those initiatives.

While the government bears a large responsibility for the public health promotion of national initiatives, local government, nongovernmental, and nonprofit organizations are vital for implementation at the community level. Effective and organized community efforts to promote health and healthy food systems and ensure the well-being of a community must involve all sectors of the community, including providers of healthcare services, local businesses, community organizations, the media, and the general public.

Federal Nutrition Programs Advance National Health Initiatives

As discussed previously, federal programs such as the U.S. Department of Agriculture (USDA) Food and Nutrition Service's Supplemental Nutrition Assistance Program (SNAP) and the Special Supplemental Nutrition Program for Women, Infants, and Children (WIC) help make healthy foods more accessible to limited-resource individuals and families.[1] While these programs are important in all areas of the United States, rural areas have higher rates of participation due to increased poverty levels.[2]

Connecting limited-resource individuals to national nutrition assistance programs that can alleviate hunger and influence diet and physical activity is impactful for promoting national health initiatives. This is an important and good first step in ensuring healthy communities. In addition to SNAP and WIC, nutrition programs available for rural children and older adults, which can be utilized by the public health practitioner, include the following.

Children:

- School Breakfast Program: www.fns.usda.gov/sbp/school-breakfast-program
- National School Lunch Program: www.fns.usda.gov/nslp
- Special Milk Program: www.fns.usda.gov/smp/special-milk-program
- Child and Adult Care Food Program: Afterschool Program: www.fns.usda.gov/cacfp/child-and-adult-care-food-program
- Summer Food Service Program: www.fns.usda.gov/sfsp/summer-food-service-program

Older adults:

- Nutrition Services: https://www.nutrition.gov/topics/food-assistance-programs/nutrition-programs-seniors
- Meals on Wheels: www.mealsonwheelsamerica.org
- Child and Adult Care Food Program: www.fns.usda.gov/cacfp/child-and-adult-care-food-program
- Senior's Farmers' Market Nutrition Program: www.fns.usda.gov/sfmnp/senior-farmers-market-nutrition-program

These programs are discussed in more detail in further chapters. However, it is important to discover where they exist and are offered in the local community so that information on accessing them can be disseminated.

Connecting National Initiatives to the Community

National health initiatives provide public health practitioners and community leaders with a road map for current and prevalent health issues in the United States. Public health practitioners are responsible for being aware of current national health initiatives and finding creative opportunities to implement initiatives on a community level. Most activities that public health practitioners engage in to influence behavior change include communication, education, and/or policy, systems, and environment strategies.[3]

Communicating National Initiatives at the Local Level

Health communication includes verbal and written strategies to influence and empower individuals, populations, and communities to make healthier choices. Public health practitioners can communicate national initiatives on a community level by tailoring national communication messages to their respective populations. For example, many health professionals utilize the *Core Nutrition Messages* developed by the USDA, Food and Nutrition Service, to communicate the key recommendations of the Dietary Guidelines for Americans to limited-resource audiences.[4] The *Core Nutrition Messages* are evidence-based messages, developed through extensive focus group discussions and survey research, and were developed and designed to resonate with limited-resource mothers and children. Some examples centered around child feeding include "Enjoy each other while enjoying family meals" and "Let them learn by serving themselves."

These types of national resources assist local community agencies in delivering consistent communication across the nation to a specific audience. Health professionals can choose which messages would resonate most with their respective populations and utilize the messages through verbal and written communication channels such as social media campaigns, billboards, newspaper articles and newsletters, television broadcasts, radio commercials, public service announcements, handouts, videos, digital and/or social media tools, health fairs, nutrition programs, and other media outlets.

When utilizing, adapting, or developing effective health communication strategies, several things should be considered by the public health practitioner:

- Are the messages evidence-based and appropriate to use in this community?
- What are the available and most effective channels of communication to reach the intended audience in this community?
- What cultural considerations, health literacy capacity, and social norms of the intended audience in this community should be considered?
- Does this communication strategy align with the goals and objectives of my employment organization?

Last, using multiple communication and media strategies will ensure a broader reach to your intended community audience. Consider how your organization might focus efforts to communicate only one or two messages across a broad range of channels.

Education of National Initiatives at the Local Level

Providing educational programming is one strategy for promoting health in a community. Public health practitioners should align the focus of educational programs and outreach with national health initiatives. Health education programs are tailored for their intended audience and can incorporate health communication messages through classes, seminars, webinars, workshops, and online modules.

Public health practitioners can conduct research to create evidence-based programs tailored for their intended audience, or they can utilize programs that are readily available, target national health initiatives, and can be tailored to an intended community audience. The SNAP-Ed program and Expanded Food and Nutrition Education Program (EFNEP) are federally funded programs that develop and provide evidence-based health education programming and evaluation.[5] These programs often provide access to programming through various channels. One such channel is the SNAP-Ed Strategies & Interventions Toolkit: An Obesity Prevention Toolkit for States, which was developed by USDA's Food and Nutrition Service, The Association of SNAP Nutrition Education Administrators (ASNNA), and the National Collaborative on Childhood Obesity Research (NCCOR), a partnership between the Centers for Disease Control and Prevention, the National Institutes of Health, the Robert Wood Johnson Foundation, and the USDA.[6] This online resource has many health intervention educational programs, all focused on national health initiatives such as healthy eating, overweight/obesity, and physical activity. For example, if your intended audience is children and your health initiative is childhood obesity, using the site you can locate the Coordinated Approach to Child Health (CATCH) program, an evidence-based program developed by the University of Texas School of Public Health, designed to prevent childhood obesity in school-age children.[7]

Other examples of national level resources that can be utilized to educate individuals at the community level include MyPlate, food labeling educational resources (USDA), and other educational tools from Team Nutrition (USDA), an educational resource library created by the USDA.[8-10] For example, MyPlate, the educational and visual representation of the Dietary Guidelines for Americans, can be used in a variety of settings from educating children in schools or adults in health education courses on eating well-balanced and appropriately portioned meals. These same institutions can make use of the food labeling guides and resources to teach individuals about reading food labels for dietary information, nutrition knowledge, and increasing self-efficacy when shopping for foods at the grocery store. Public health practitioners may also partner with other community organizations and businesses to provide or refer patients to cooking classes, meal programs, and other nutrition-related services and education. As with all educational resources, information should always be tailored to the intended community audience. For example, including culturally appropriate foods as part of MyPlate and food labeling demonstrations would be important to consider.

Policy, Systems, and Environmental (PSE) Changes at the Local Level That Support National Initiatives

For communication and educational strategies to be successful, policies, systems, and environments must also support and encourage healthy behaviors. PSE change strategies are designed to promote healthy behaviors by making healthy choices readily available and easily accessible in the community. Tackling the national health initiatives locally will require community-based efforts to increase the availability of healthy foods in local supermarkets, farmers' markets, corner and convenience stores, changes in national agricultural policy to encourage the availability of locally nutritious foods at reasonable costs, and regulation of food industry advertising to promote ethical marketing standards. Efforts to motivate individuals to be more active must be combined with strategies that create physical and social environments more conducive to physical activity. Some examples of community-based activities that would promote health through PSE changes and advance national initiatives locally include:

- Healthy vending. Establishing healthy food options in vending machines in public places (toolkit available from the Seattle and King County Public Health Department: www.kingcounty.gov/depts/health/nutrition/~/media/depts/health/nutrition/documents/healthy-vending-toolkit.ashx).

- Farmers' markets. Increase access to fresh and local produce while boosting the income of local farmers (toolkit available from the University of Minnesota Extension: extension.umn.edu/local-foods/power-produce-pop-club).

- Healthy retail. Partnering with local businesses to promote healthy food items or advocating for a state or regional tax on unhealthy food items (toolkit available from the Centers for Disease Control and Prevention: www.cdc.gov/nccdphp/dnpao/state-local-programs/pdf/Healthier-Food-Retail-guide-full.pdf).

- Green space. Increasing the number of parks, greenways, and trails in the community and/or making them more accessible (toolkit available from the Centers for Disease Control and Prevention: www.cdc.gov/healthyplaces/healthtopics/parks_trails_workbook.htm).

- School nutrition. Strengthening school wellness polices or working in schools to promote healthy food items (toolkits available from the USDA: www.fns.usda.gov/get-involved/toolkits).

- Farm-to-cafeteria initiatives. Working with local farmers to sell fresh produce directly to schools or worksites (toolkit available from the USDA: https://www.fns.usda.gov/cfs/farm-school-resources-1).

- Food environment. Increasing the availability of fresh, healthy foods in schools, restaurants, and other places where food is purchased (toolkit available from ChangeLab Solutions: www.changelabsolutions.org/publications/healthy-menus).

- Community-supported agriculture. Establishing or promoting partnerships between farmers and consumers to purchase weekly produce (toolkit available from the University of Connecticut Extension: www.ctfarmrisk.uconn.edu/documents/CSA-Guide.pdf).

- Creating social marketing campaigns to influence awareness and behavior change (toolkit available from the Community Tool Box, University of Kansas: www.ctfarmrisk.uconn.edu/documents/CSA-Guide.pdf).

Examples of PSE Change Interventions

- In North Carolina, the North Carolina Division of Public Health and Extension at North Carolina State University implements PSE changes through the Faithful Families Eating Smart and Moving More program. The program includes direct education curriculum on healthy eating and physical activity, training of community leaders, and environmental and policy changes chosen by the faith community such as healthy meeting policies and encouraging physical activity (Faithful Families Eating Smart and Moving More, faithfulfamilies.com).

- Healthy Kindergarten Initiative from The Food Trust is a direct education and PSE change intervention that integrates food choices with access. Families are connected to local, healthy foods through mobile farm markets or low-cost, community-supported agriculture; children are exposed to locally grown, healthy snacks at school; parents are involved through workshops or newsletters; and nutrition and physical activity education is integrated into the curriculum (*The kindergarten initiative: A healthy start to a healthy life*, thefoodtrust.org/uploads/media_items/the-kindergarten-initiative.original.pdf).

■ Blue Zones Project in rural Minnesota is a community-wide health initiative that implements PSE changes to increase healthy choices. Activities include the promotion of healthy foods at restaurants and schools, implementation of worksite health clinics, policies on tobacco use in public places, and increased walking/biking trails (*Blue Zones Project: Albert Lea, MN*, 2016, albertlea.bluezonesproject.com).

PSE strategies can have the greatest impact on the promotion of a healthy community because they target multiple levels of behavior influence. However, public health practitioners should be prepared to rely on other sectors of the community for successful planning and implementation, be considerate of the time required to implement changes, and develop a comprehensive plan to evaluate the effectiveness and impact of PSE changes on their communities.

Important Considerations

Public health practitioners cannot tackle every national health initiative. Understanding local needs, community resources, culture/social norms, and local values will assist in determining which health initiatives are a priority. The following can assist in deciding where to focus your communication, education, and PSE strategies.

Explore the local root causes of healthy or unhealthy behaviors. Consider the social determinants of health (e.g., socioeconomic status, housing, transportation)[11] that lead to reaching a person's full health capacity. Determine if there are strategies that could be implemented to effect change at the root level.

■ **Assess local needs and resources**. Consider what is feasible and which organizations could help implement changes for the greatest needs.

■ **Include the intended audience if at all possible**. Efforts to ensure that everyone has input in strategies that promote health can impact program effectiveness and increase community empowerment.

■ **Work together**. Consider and listen to what community members and stakeholders think are important issues. Collaborating with the community increases the ability of any program to effect change.

PROMOTION OF NUTRITIONAL HEALTH, FOOD SYSTEMS, AND COMMUNITY WELL-BEING THROUGH ADVOCACY AND COMMUNITY FOOD SECURITY ACROSS LIFE STAGES

Food Systems

Every food we consume has a complex history behind it. Before a food reaches our plate, it leaves its farmland or waterway origin and passes through the hands of producers, processors, transporters, storage operators, retailers, consumers, and handlers of waste. The term **food system** refers to all aspects of producing, buying, selling, eating, and disposing of food.[12] This includes production, processing and aggregation, distribution, marketing, consumption, and food waste recovery. A *local food system* encompasses a network of all of these components but is specific to a place. It can encompass a county, region, or an entire state. Every food system is based on the relationships among the people and resources involved at each point in the process.

A strong local food system can spur positive economic development and build community wealth.[13] It can protect water and soil quality and preserve agricultural land and waterways. By sustaining the viability of farm and fishery operations, a local food system can enhance the quality of life for both food producers and consumers.

The food system is extremely complex. Producers, consumers, processors, distributors, and retailers interact with people working in virtually every sector that exists in a community, from education to social services. As our food supply chains have become more globalized, the food system has become even more complex. Consumers now have more choices and greater access to food. Globalization of the food system has also created new opportunities and challenges for farmers, manufacturers, distributors, and policy-makers.[14]

Systems Thinking: The Natural World and Its Impact on Food

Improving a food system requires systems thinking, which is the ability to understand the way different things influence each other in a system. When we change one part of a food system— such as introducing pesticides to reduce the spread of insect-borne diseases—this change is likely to impact the other parts of the system. While use of pesticides can prevent disease and increase profits for farmers, it has led to problems such as pesticide resistance and harmful effects on humans and wildlife.[15,16] It is important to recognize the complex relationships that exist in any food system in order to avoid causing negative externalities to our health and the environment. The food system can also impact widespread issues such as chronic illness, infectious disease, social inequality, climate change, and environmental degradation.

The Growing Role of Food Systems

Nationwide, more aspects of a community are now focusing on the food system. Businesses, non-profits, universities, healthcare professionals, and policy-makers are recognizing the dynamic relationships that exist in the local food system among food access, health, income, economic development, and geography. Nontraditional partners—such as city planners and health insurance companies—are teaming up with traditional food stakeholders to impact the food system in new ways. Both private and public agencies are supporting the development of local food systems because of the positive economic and public health outcomes that can be achieved by building the infrastructure of a local food system. Consumers are also looking for a closer connection to their food producers. As a result, many local food systems have increased access to sustainable, organic farming.

Built Environment

A community's **built environment**—or human-made surroundings—has a strong effect on what and how people eat.[17] The type and location of food stores in a community, for example, are often associated with the diets of residents and their health.[18] People who live in areas with limited access, often referred to as "food deserts" or "food swamps," to healthy food tend to have poorer diets and suffer more from obesity and diabetes.[19,20] Food deserts generally refer to communities or neighborhoods where there is limited availability or access to healthy foods, whereas food swamps are where there is an abundance of fast, highly processed, and unhealthy food options available.[21]

Disparities in Food Access

Many differences in access to or availability of food, or **health disparities**, persist today. Healthy People 2020 defines a *health disparity* as "a particular type of health difference that is closely linked with social, economic, and/or environmental disadvantage."[22] Health disparities "adversely affect groups of people who have systematically experienced greater obstacles to health based on their racial or ethnic group; religion; socioeconomic status; gender; age; mental health; cognitive, sensory, or physical disability; sexual orientation or gender identity; geographic location; or other characteristics historically linked to discrimination or exclusion."[22] Many public health practitioners now advocate for the use of the term health inequities, which applies a justice and equity component to the very definition, rather than just highlighting differences. **Health equity** is the principle of pursuing elimination of health disparities because they are unjust. The term draws specific attention to the underlying social conditions that lead to higher health risks and poorer health outcomes for populations that are economically, socially, or environmentally disadvantaged.[23]

Disparities in access to healthy foods have affected low-income communities in both urban and rural areas.[24] Low-income and underserved communities often have fewer supermarkets and less access to stores that sell high-quality fruits and vegetables.[25] Rural communities often have a higher number of convenience stores, where healthy foods are less available than in larger, retail food markets.[26] African American and Hispanic neighborhoods are also more likely to be located in "food deserts," where fresh fruits, vegetables, and other healthful foods are not easily accessible.[25] This can often lead to higher prices, less variety, and lower quality of healthy foods for many neighborhoods.

Measuring health disparities by social stratification can be challenging. Factors such as education levels and household income are often used as indicators of social class, but they do not tell the whole story. In the United States, geographic areas, such as census tracts, zip codes, and counties, are often used to illustrate disparities by social strata. This kind of data can also help one visualize community-level food justice issues in ways that examining individual-level disparities does not. The map provided in Figure 7.1 visually displays food access disparities in the United States by county, representing the number of people in a county living more than 1 mile from a supermarket or large grocery store in an urban area or more than 10 miles in a rural area. Notice that this measure of food insecurity takes into account both the rural and urban contexts. In urban areas, there may be small corner stores within walking distance, but these stores do not usually carry much high-quality fresh produce. In rural areas, finding transportation to the nearest grocery store can be impossible.

Community leaders and public health practitioners are increasingly working to strengthen the local food system and combat food insecurity. One such strategy, the Healthy Corner Store Initiative, brings high-quality fruits, vegetables, and healthful foods into corner stores in lower income communities. Transportation improvements can also make it easier for low-income families, aging adults, and individuals with mobility challenges to access more sources of affordable, healthy food.[27]

Community Food Security

Social, economic, and/or environmental disadvantage is often linked to material disadvantages, particularly as it relates to food access. For example, families may not have enough material resources in the form of money to buy enough nutritious food for the entire family, or families may live in isolated areas without good grocery stores or transportation to those stores.

Easy access to fresh and affordable food is critical to positive health outcomes. **Food security** is defined by the United Nations Committee on World Food Security as the condition in which all people, at all times, have physical, social, and economic access to sufficient, safe, and nutritious food that meets their dietary needs and food preferences for an active and healthy life.

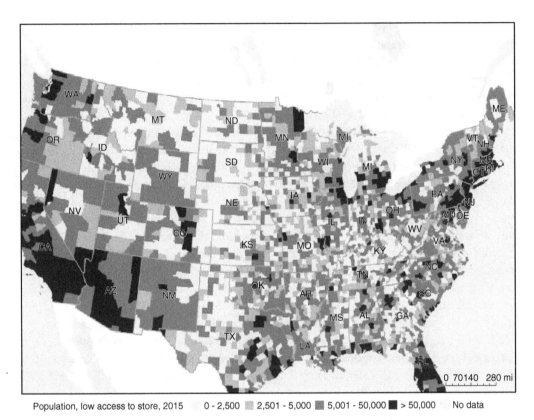

Population, low access to store, 2015   ☐ 0 - 2,500 ▨ 2,501 - 5,000 ▦ 5,001 - 50,000 ■ > 50,000   No data

FIGURE 7.1 Food access disparities in the United States by county.
Source: From U.S. Department of Agriculture, Economic Research Service. *Food Environment Atlas.* https://www.ers.
usda.gov/data-products/food-environment-atlas

The concept of food security began with the global food crisis of the mid-1970s, and the term has broadened over time to encompass more than combating hunger. Food security, as well as the role of nutrition within it, has been recognized as a major global concern since the mid-1990s.[28] The complex challenge of food security persists in many countries worldwide, including the United States. In 2016, an estimated one in eight Americans were food-insecure.[29] *Food insecurity* exists when people do not have adequate physical, social, or economic access to food. Food insecurity is a major social determinant of health.[30,31] Many American households have experienced chronic hunger and poverty for generations. Food insecurity has been associated with poor behavioral, emotional, and academic health outcomes for children.[32]

With over a billion people in the world living on less than $1.25 per day, malnourishment remains a significant global problem. This is not just a problem for low-income countries. In the United States, over 15 million households are considered food-insecure and the number of census tracts considered low-income and low-access has increased in the past decade.[29] Many households that do not qualify for government food assistance, because they make just above federal income requirements for SNAP, for example, or perhaps are undocumented individuals, are unable to meet the food needs of their families.

In the United States, food insecurity is not only unequally distributed by geographic areas but is also unequally distributed by race/ethnicity and nativity. A 2017 study of over 32,000 people, using many waves of the National Health and Nutrition Examination Survey, showed that after taking into account socioeconomic status, the significant food security divide between Whites and African Americans and Mexican Americans continues to be perpetuated.[33] This pattern held true for immigrants and U.S.-born individuals. This racial/ethnic inequity in food security is likely also related to geographic distributions of grocery stores. Racial/ethnic residential segregation remains highly prevalent in the United States, and this segregation is also associated with the limited access to grocery stores, as shown earlier.

Food insecurity is closely associated with disparities in health outcomes and other social justice issues. Food insecurity exacerbates susceptibility to diseases, mitigates the ability to fight diseases, and then contributes to the cycle of poverty by making it difficult for sick individuals to attend school and work. Food insecurity significantly contributes to infectious diseases, chronic conditions, and mental health issues. Access to cheap, highly caloric food, or food swamps, is a well-known contributor to the global obesity epidemic and related chronic conditions, such as diabetes, and is common in low-resource communities. Obesity and diabetes are both conditions that are strongly correlated with social gradients, with people of lower socioeconomic status at much higher risk. Individuals, particularly children, experiencing food insecurity and malnourishment can have difficulty in fighting off infectious and/or parasitic diseases. Harsh medications, such as complex antibiotic or antiretroviral regimens, can be difficult for malnourished bodies to tolerate, which then can lead to further susceptibility to other infectious diseases and can lead to problems with drug resistance. Mental health outcomes are also associated with food insecurity. A 2017 study showed that food insecurity was associated with poorer mental health outcomes across all global regions, even after taking into account other socioeconomic factors.[34]

The Future of Food Security

Many factors will continue to impact food security, such as the growing global population, rising food prices, and changing climate. By 2050, the demand for food is expected to be 60% greater than it is today.[35] Achieving food security and improved nutrition is one of the Sustainable Development Goals that the United Nations has set for the year 2030.

Access to affordable and healthy food should be included in the development of community health improvements. In addition to public health practitioners, food policy councils, local government officials, food retailers, and city planners are among the many stakeholders who can help ensure access to affordable and healthy food.

Food Sovereignty

As the food system becomes more complex and global food prices increase, the global movement for food sovereignty has challenged corporate food regimes and called for more equitable rights and participation in the food system.[36] **Food sovereignty** is the right for all people to choose healthy and culturally appropriate food that is produced through ecologically sound and sustainable methods. Food sovereignty focuses on the needs of those who produce, distribute, and consume food, rather than the demands of markets and corporations. The international peasant coalition, La Vía Campesina, introduced the concept of food sovereignty at the World Food Summit in 1996 to address ongoing global struggles over the control of food, land, water, and food producers. This movement calls for reviving small-scale farming as a public resource for food security and nutrition, while doing away with the monopoly of power from transnational corporations. The movement also calls for the democratization of community and regional food systems.[37]

The seven pillars of food sovereignty include the following:[38]

- Focuses on food for people: People have the right to food that is healthy and culturally appropriate. Food is not simply another commodity to be traded or speculated on for profit.

- Values food producers: Food sovereignty asserts the right of food producers to live and work in dignity, including women, who are the majority of food producers worldwide.

- Localizes food systems: Food must be seen primarily as sustenance for the community and only secondarily as something to be traded.

- Puts control locally: Food sovereignty places control over territory, land, grazing, water, seeds, and livestock and fish populations under local communities instead of outside corporate interests.

- Builds knowledge and skills: Food sovereignty approaches support the development of agricultural knowledge that is already being used, supplemented with new skills and appropriate technologies, rather than introducing costly new technology that can contribute to land loss for small farmers.

- Works with nature: Food sovereignty requires production and distribution systems that protect natural resources and reduce greenhouse gas emissions.

While the concepts of food security and food sovereignty both address global hunger and environmental degradation, food sovereignty is rooted in broad class and race struggles. It calls for respecting the rights of farmers and indigenous communities to make their own decisions around their food system. Food movements such as food security, food justice, and food sovereignty serve a critical role in applying social pressure for system change.

FOOD AND SOCIAL JUSTICE

Social justice generally refers to the fair and equal treatment of people. **Food justice** refers to food-related social justice matters and has been defined as "the struggle against racism, exploitation, and oppression taking place within the food system that addresses inequality's root causes both within and beyond the food chain."[39] These systemic matters have consequences at all levels of the **Social-Ecological Model (SEM)**, including individual, interpersonal, institutional, community, and societal levels resulting in significant health disparities or health inequities.

Many systems factors at local, state, national, and global levels contribute to the food justice issues that communities face. At the local level, even communities that have large agriculture economic sectors can suffer from lack of adequate access to healthy food. Growers can often get paid better prices to sell their products to large retailers or to higher end markets in wealthy urban areas, resulting in fresh food that is grown in localities, but exported elsewhere. Furthermore, state and national food policies can drive local growing patterns, prices, and access.

OPTIMIZING AVAILABLE RESOURCES: COMMUNITY ENGAGEMENT AND RESOURCE OPTIMIZATION

Critical to a socially just and effective community food system that reduces the risks for food insecurity and poor nutritional health opportunities are the elements of community engagement and community development. **Community engagement** refers to the *process* and actions of involving community members in decision-making that impacts the day-to-day quality of life offered in the community; furthermore, community engagement has consistently been shown to be a very effective strategy for engaging with and empowering vulnerable populations and reducing health inequities.[40-42] Often linked with community engagement as the goal outcome is an improved community development. **Community development** builds upon the engagement process and is focused on an improvement in *outcomes*, such as the physical environment, cultural norms, social and political actions, and enhanced educational and economic opportunities, to name a few.[43,44] The combination of the two can have sustainable positive outcomes. In the following section, we provide insight to the process, detail opportunities and challenges that can arise, and provide examples, as evidenced in the academic literature and the field of public health nutrition practice.

Community Engagement and Community Development in Public Health Nutrition Practice

As a practitioner in the field of public health nutrition, prior to embarking on a community engagement process for improved community nutrition, it is vital to understand the context (culture, demographics, etc.) and history of the community as this will assist in identifying key stakeholders to inform the decision-making process. **Stakeholders** are described as "any individual or group living within the community or likely to be affected by decisions or actions."[45] Whether it be a rural or urban community, key stakeholders involved in the food system includes an assortment of actors including agricultural workers/farmers, local government, nonprofit agencies and businesses, citizens, and most importantly from a public health perspective, those often overlooked and most vulnerable. With this understanding, many scholars advocate for a "bottom-up" approach in which citizens and farmers are given an increasingly larger voice in local food system decision-making—as opposed to the traditional top-down approach in which local leaders make all of the key decisions.[46] Nonetheless, engaging a wide array of stakeholders is imperative to the process.

Next, an important factor to consider with the goal of community development is the approach that is taken; as public health practitioners, we desire to build a sense of trust with our constituents and to come together over a common set of goals. We want to work with people, not on people! In doing so, over the past several decades, scholars from a variety of professional disciplines have shown that Asset-Based Community Development (ABCD) is a sound strategy for all contexts.[47] An ABCD approach focuses on what a community already has that can be capitalized upon, its assets, rather than the traditional needs-based approach, which first looks for what a community needs.[48,49] For example, what is often found in communities is that numerous individuals and groups are working to address food and nutrition issues (e.g., community gardens, food pantries), but they are doing so without the knowledge of each other's efforts. Our job as public health practitioners is frequently to bring all of those groups together and to help community members to work together in a more strategic manner—to work smarter, not harder. However, what so often occurs is that we center our attention on the limitations that our communities have with statements like, "If only we had more money or funding" or "What we need is...." Strategies grounded in the ABCD approach, or worldview, allow us to overcome these types of statements and to celebrate accomplishments and build upon successes.

Community-Based Coalitions and Faith-Based Initiatives

One of the great opportunities afforded through community engagement is the forming of coalitions. **Coalitions** are "groups of individuals and/or organizations with a common interest who agree to work together toward a common goal."[50] In effect, coalitions are "action oriented," "analyzing the issue," "identifying and implementing solutions," and "creating social change"—with the understanding that the best results occur when working collectively rather than individually.[51] When it comes to coalitions, there are three primary types: **grassroots**, professional, and community.[51,52] Grassroots coalitions are those organized by community members and advocates, professional coalitions are formed by professional associations (e.g., American Medical Association, American Nutrition Association, American Public Health Association), and community coalitions tend to blend the grassroots and professional stakeholders. For the most part, coalitions focused on nutrition at the local level are grassroots and community in spirit.

In keeping up with news and current events from around the world and in our communities, we all are familiar with grassroots initiatives rooted in coalitions. Grassroots movements are those that are organized by ordinary citizens to raise awareness about a cause(s) and to seek change. For example, on a national scale, here in the United States in recent years, we have seen the Tea Party and the Occupy Wall Street movements have success in building momentum for their respective causes. On a more local level, we witness communities everyday striving to improve food access and to improve nutritional health—all grounded in a grassroots mentality. Grassroots movements help to build excitement, and if done in a positive manner, can create a sense of community and lead to sustained change.

For local communities, one of the groups heavily involved in starting initiatives aimed at food justice and addressing food security and access needs are faith-based organizations. **Faith-based initiatives**, often underutilized and garnering little attention, are movements in which religious institutions such as churches or nonprofit agencies, either formally or informally, spearhead efforts and generally partner with public health agencies and the medical sector or an institution of higher education for community development and improved health.[53,54] These efforts can range from activities in policy and advocacy to health education to health promotion programming. With faith being a focal point of the culture and spirituality being a driving force in their communities, faith-based health promotion efforts have had a great deal of success in both rural and minority populations.[55–58]

When such efforts as grassroots and faith-based initiatives are coupled with professionals, such as health educators, registered dietitians, and other clinical and community health professionals, community coalitions are formed and the reach and ability to improve lives are increased exponentially. In Boone, North Carolina, where the Appalachian State University is located and where three of the authors of this chapter live and work, the Hunger and Health Coalition began in much this way over 35 years ago and continues to positively impact the northwestern region of the state each and every day. Exhibit 7.1 provides a brief history and a description of services and programs that are offered. Not only does a coalition such as the Health and Hunger Coalition provide much-needed services and programs but it also helps to connect residents to volunteer opportunities and partner with Appalachian State to engage in service learning and internships for students. This helps to build a sense of community pride, cohesion, and a commitment to service that every community needs in order to function effectively.

Community coalitions can also further elucidate strategies to highlight local agricultural efforts that can help to alleviate food security challenges. In Watauga County, North Carolina, some of the other initiatives that have sprung out of these and other efforts include F.A.R.M. Café; Watauga County Farmers' Market; Blue Ridge Women in Agriculture; and the High Country Food Hub. F.A.R.M. (which stands for Feed All Regardless of Means) Café is a local nonprofit agency centered on providing daily meals using local food sources; above all, it helps to build a sense of community, and visitors are always impressed by the hospitality and diversity that is found. As a result, F.A.R.M. Café was featured in *Our State Magazine* (www.ourstate.com/

EXHIBIT 7.1

THE HISTORY AND COMMUNITY IMPACT OF THE HUNGER AND HEALTH COALITION OF BOONE, NORTH CAROLINA

	Hunger and Health Coalition 141 Health Center Drive, Suite C, Boone, NC 28607 https://www.hungerandhealthcoalition.com
History	Began in January of 1982 in a closet at Boone United Methodist Church.
	Moved to a new and bigger location in 1989; at the same time, began to offer a free health clinic staffed by physicians from the local health department.
	In 1995, staff recognized that community members facing food security challenges often had to decide between food and prescription medications. As a result, a free pharmacy program was instituted.
	Now has grown to become a county-owned facility, providing both food and medical assistance to vulnerable populations in the area.
Services and programs/impact	Food Pantry (nearly 800,000 lbs of food to those in need in 2019)
	Fresh Produce Market (over 2,000 households received fresh food in 2019)
	Free Pharmacy (14,387 prescriptions at a value of $2,969,000 in 2019)
	Food Recovery Kitchen (families can receive a sandwich/soup combination or to-go meal for each member of the family)
	Helping Hands Wood Lot (brought firewood to 279 households in 2019)
	Backpack program (7,800 meals distributed in 2019)
	Simple Gesture (47,750 lbs of food donated to pantry in 2019)
	Snacks for Scholars/Healthy Start (1,768 snack bags given out in 2019)
	Sharing Tree (holiday gifts and meals to over 160 families and seniors in 2019)

Source: Data from Hunger and Health Coalition. https://www.hungerandhealthcoalition.com

at-boones-f-a-r-m-cafe-all-are-fed) as well as UNC TV (myhome.unctv.org/farm-cafe). Farmers' markets are found in many communities and are great ways for getting citizens connected to the local agriculture sources and to provide a way for farmers to serve the community and make a little money along the way. In recent years, farmers' markets, like the one found in Watauga County (www.wataugacountyfarmersmarket.org), have begun to accept SNAP and Electronic Benefits Transfer (EBT) benefits and have further worked to assist WIC and Senior Nutrition efforts. Blue Ridge Women in Agriculture (www.brwia.org) is a collaborative group of women farmers dedicated to improving the local food system to address health equity and hunger. In addition, the organization has a focus on educating consumers about farming and cooking practices to allow individuals to be more self-sufficient in their food practices. Last, in conjunction with the Watauga County Cooperative Extension offices, Blue Ridge Women in Agriculture has helped to create a local food hub, the High Country Food Hub (foodhub.brwia.org), for people to order food from local farms for pickup and to create a system in which farmers can further have their agriculture distributed at local food banks. In the end, these types of efforts help to bring people together, particularly when it comes to further advocacy efforts aimed at funding and policy causes.

Advocacy Efforts: Informed by Community Engagement and Supported by Coalitions

The process of community engagement and development along with the development of coalitions assists in moving advocacy efforts forward. **Advocacy** at the community level consists of "actions" intended to influence public policy for a particular cause, or to strengthen capacity and mobilize resources, or to decrease barriers to health.[59,60] Most public health advocacy strategies have been best informed by having a variety of perspectives involved and more voices to be heard—as the saying goes, "there is power in numbers." In a recent systematic review, the importance of understanding and engaging in the public policy process at all levels was deemed essential for the future of public health nutrition.[61] Needs for advocacy include (but are not limited to) more sustainable food production and practices aimed at protection of the environment;[62] structural and systems changes frequently leading to food insecurity and poverty;[63] unjust labor practices often used in agricultural production;[64] and adequate funding and capacity of public health systems.[65]

SYSTEMS THINKING FOR EFFECTIVE PUBLIC HEALTH NUTRITION AT THE COMMUNITY LEVEL

Many of us drive around in the latest and trendiest automobiles; all right, maybe some of us are just happy to have a car, any car, to get us around town and to travel to our intended destination. How many times, however, do we really stop to think about how complex an automobile is and how many intricate pieces are fit together to allow us to be able to get around so quickly? Or how about the organization that we work in, in which all of the staff members are completing their respective roles to allow the agency to perform? Or yet another example, what about all of the anatomy and physiology that allows us as human beings to perform daily activities? These three examples all have one thing in common: each is a system and when functioning at its highest ability, the system can be described as a "well-oiled machine."

Well, the same can be said of public health and the focus on public health nutrition. For a community to have optimal health and well-being, it is imperative that all of the pieces function as a system. In recent years, while borrowing from numerous other professional disciplines, public health has advocated for and adopted a systems thinking model in the pursuit of improved population health.[66–69] **Systems thinking** helps us to think about how the system is functioning collectively, rather than each individual or agency independently; with this there are new and innovative research strategies being utilized that are also leading to new forms of practice. This type of thinking and approach forces us to work in a collaborative and interdisciplinary way and to get out of our professional silos. In the following section, we delve into how this "thinking in systems" can help us to strengthen the field of public health nutrition. We also provide examples from the field and opportunities for how practitioners can make the most of this approach.

Systems Thinking for Public Health Nutrition

For the past several decades, the field of public health along with health promotion interventions has been informed by an ecological, or more precisely a social-ecological, perspective to address community health challenges, including nutrition and obesity.[70–72] This approach recognizes that health is influenced at multiple levels, driven by the combination of individual characteristics and social forces, often out of the control of the individual. Public health practitioners and researchers have had successes along the way, but what has often lacked is the integration of multiple levels into interventions. For example, nutrition education and cooking courses have been conducted with the best intentions, without foreseeing that when the participants have completed the course, they are going right back out into the environment that was present before—a food environment or social conditions that might not support an improved dietary intake. On the other hand, policies such as requiring restaurants to provide the caloric intake have been instituted, without providing supporting education to assist individuals in changing their nutritional habits. The point is that the system has not been integrative in nature.[73]

When we begin to think about the food system in this more integrative way, we recognize that it is a complex makeup of both natural and human-made systems, which can include such aspects as weather/climate, biology, transportation, the economy, and healthcare resources available.[74] There is no single cause for the system "breaking down," but it is more of the feedback loops that occur through all of the pieces at work. In addition, it makes us recognize that the "blaming the victim" mentality often found around food and other health issues, whether it be hunger and/or obesity, is lacking and uninformed. A systems approach in our thinking allows us to address and confront these preconceived, and often unconscious, biases that we as humans have toward the challenges that so many people face. Most important, systems thinking helps us to strengthen our public health and nutrition education efforts (see Box 7.1).

Maximizing Nutrition Education Through the Public Health, Interprofessional and Interdisciplinary Team

As public health practitioners focused on improving nutritional health, we have two main foci: making sure people have access to enough food (food security/hunger) *and* empowering people to use food and nutrition to maintain and improve their health. Up to this point, we have focused (for good reason) mainly on the former. However, it is also critically important to use an interprofessional and interdisciplinary approach to target nutrition education.

To maximize nutrition education for children in a community, many sectors of the community should be involved. Teachers, parents, and school administrators can invest in local community gardens, while school nutritionists can additionally provide education and learning opportunities for growing and eating healthy foods. The children (and parents) who attend those schools can be seen at the local health department or local pediatrics office and receive nutrition education from child health professionals. Grocery stores and farmers' markets can ensure availability of healthy options and offer incentives to purchase healthy food items, while community health educators can supply education and resources for shopping and preparing healthy meals at home. Restaurant owners can add healthy food choices to their menu items, and academic professionals can evaluate such activities to determine impact and effectiveness. All sectors working together will undoubtedly have a much larger impact on nudging toward healthy behaviors than just one sector working alone.

Marketing Programs in Communities: The Role of Communication and Health Literacy

One of the great challenges in public health is getting people to participate, and retaining them, in events and programs targeting improved health. There is not a much worse feeling than planning and developing an intervention—and then few, or none, are interested or actually able to participate. Therefore, it is critical to spend the proper time and attention toward how the program or intervention will be marketed and communicated to the public.

BOX 7.1

EXAMPLE FROM THE FIELD: FORMING THE ACFPC

The story of the *ACFPC* (www.adamsfoodpolicy.org) in Adams County, Pennsylvania, began in 2007 in a basement of an old school, where a community initiative, called Support Circles (see www.supportcircles .org/circles-model) met weekly to inspire and equip families and communities to end poverty. Low wage earners seeking to escape poverty, referred to as Support Circles Leaders, met to assess financial, emotional, and social resources; explore systemic barriers to escaping poverty; and connect with community allies who offered support through networking, listening, and guidance. As months went by, Support Circles Leaders made progress with new jobs and new living arrangements and some experienced new obstacles and setbacks. Cara, a single mom with two kids, was making fast progress—from a waitress making $10 an hour to a bank teller, making $16 an hour. One evening she said, "I am proud that I no longer receive SNAP benefits, but all we now eat is cereal." At over $15 an hour, Cara lost all SNAP benefits and would not break even again until she earned $20 an hour. Cara's experiences highlight a significant gap in self-sufficiency when benefits decrease with increased, but inadequate, wages. Watch this video that explains Cara's situation: https://www.adamsfoodpolicy.org/why-food-policy.

When all other expenses are fixed (e.g., housing, childcare, transportation), food is considered a flexible expense. As Cara, and other Support Circles Leaders, started to share their stories around town, people began to listen. Community-based food access initiatives started to independently take shape, including food recovery programs, famers' markets that accept SNAP benefits, community-supported agriculture, and community gardens. Connecting people at the head of these initiatives with major players in the food system became a new goal. The formal establishment of the ACFPC in 2008 brought together social service agencies, higher education, institutions, farmers, businesses, local government, and community members with a vision that all residents of Adams County, Pennsylvania, will have access to a safe, nutritious, affordable, and adequate food supply within a sustainable system that promotes the local economy. Focusing on a common community agenda has facilitated independent organizational shifts toward mutually reinforcing goals, influenced local policy changes, and promoted program development, particularly with respect to access to local fruits and vegetables for low-income families.

While each member organization independently prioritizes healthy food access within their own institutions, working toward the common community goal, the ACFPC also initiates collaborative programs. For example, since 2011, the ACFPC has administered *Healthy Options*, a food voucher program, which now serves 120 families and 60 seniors. Participants receive monthly vouchers to use at local farmers' markets and locally owned grocery stores. Many of the participants have now become Community Leaders, and have assumed administrative and social networking roles with the program. Results from a community-based participatory research and evaluation analysis showed that, in addition to increased access to healthy food, participation in the program also offers opportunities for social interaction and cross-cultural exchange. Healthy Options, largely funded by local donations, also supports local growers and the local economy, helping to realize the ACFPC vision of having a sustainable local food system.

ACFPC, Adams County Food Policy Council; SNAP, Supplemental Nutrition Assistance Program.

Source: From Dailey AB, Hess A, Horton C, et al. Healthy options: a community-based program to address food insecurity. *J Prev Interv Community.* 2015;43(2):83–94. doi:10.1080/10852352.2015.973248

The most widely utilized communication strategy in public health is diffusion of innovations. The Diffusion of Innovation Theory generally postulates that social change, or in this case involvement with a program, happens when communication occurs through a set of steps, including knowledge, persuasion, decision, implementation, and confirmation.[75] Additionally, this perspective recognizes that people fall into five categories in terms of how quickly they adopt an innovation or program: innovator, early adopter, early majority, late majority, and laggard.[76] With this thinking and framework, we as public health practitioners can formulate how best to reach our audiences, based on context and the populations targeted.

Connected to our ability to communicate and market community-level interventions and programs, two other important concepts to embed in our strategies include **health literacy** and **cultural competency**. Health literacy focuses on the general population's ability to access, comprehend, and utilize health information or services.[77] We have numerous citizens across our country with very low health literacy levels, and it is now a foundational principle for Healthy People 2030.[78] Cultural competency refers to one's ability to respect and value cultural differences and to one who strives to work effectively to address disparities that exist largely because of cultural differences—developing culturally competent public health professionals is vital to the pursuit of health equity.[79]

Collaborative Grantsmanship in Public Health Nutrition

It is widely recognized that most public health programming and interventions require adequate funding. Therefore, most public health professionals will be involved in developing grant proposals to obtain funding for their work—in fact, many employees are paid out of these grants. As such, to be competitive in funding pursuits, it is vital for public health nutritionists to use systems thinking and to seek out partnerships and collaborations for grant opportunities. When grant proposals are developed with multiple perspectives and expertise involved, much stronger proposals are submitted—and much better work is performed as a result. Fortunately, some funders have begun to support initiatives that prioritize systems change addressing health equity and food sovereignty from multiple perspectives of diverse stakeholders. For example, the W.K. Kellogg Foundation funded a 9-year Food and Fitness initiative focused on systems changes to address childhood obesity and health inequities. Two of the key takeaways from this process include recognizing the importance of deep engagement with people who bring diverse perspectives and lived experience and that sustainable systems change focused on equity requires community leadership and ownership.[80] As a result, many agencies that provide grant funding are now requiring that interdisciplinary collaborations are involved and that systems change is valued for improved health.

CONCLUSION

As discussed in this chapter, "it takes a village" to provide accessible and adequate nutrition to a community. Health equity and social justice are guiding principles of public health, and therefore, most of our public health nutrition efforts at the community level are centered on food justice and reducing food insecurity. To do so, it is paramount that we be the leaders in shaping food systems that allow this to occur. This includes engaging in the community, identifying key stakeholders, developing and maintaining partnerships, and using systems thinking to drive our work. Along the way, practitioners must practice cultural competency and continually develop and refine their communication skill sets. Thankfully, there are numerous models from the national level all the way down to the local level that can help to inform or improve our work. It is up to students, practitioners, and all of those involved in work at the community level to work side by side with members of the community and to never stop learning from each other—after all, community nutrition and health is a process that never stops!

KEY CONCEPTS

1. Public health, including nutrition, seeks to address root causes of poor health, social inequities, and health disparities at multiple levels.

2. Nutrition and food systems at the local community level are vastly influenced and affected by global and national level policies, programs, and events.

3. Food security and nutritional health should be at the forefront of overall community development initiatives.

4. It is vital that public health nutrition practitioners engage in the community and lead advocacy efforts aimed at PSE change.

5. The work of nutritional health at the local level is complex and requires a systematic, multidisciplinary, and evidence-based approach.

CASE STUDY: COMMUNITY FORUMS AND WORKING GROUPS: THE COMMUNITY ENGAGEMENT PROJECT OF MCDOWELL COUNTY, NORTH CAROLINA

The Community Engagement Project of McDowell County, North Carolina, is a public health intervention that holds frequent forums to hear directly from residents in order to better understand assets, needs, and challenges of the community with a focus on health equity. The program began in 2016 in West Marion, one of the rural towns in McDowell county, and it has now expanded as a joint project between the McDowell Health Coalition and McDowell Technical Community College to the rest of the county.

Over 70% of McDowell county is designated as rural Appalachia with high rates of poverty. In West Marion, where the project began, median household incomes are well below the county and national levels, with higher income disparities for African Americans and Latinos–Hispanics. Most residents have generational ties to the community.

Goals of the initial forum included:

- Engage an expert facilitator with skills and knowledge related to rural people and places.
- Create a local planning team to plan the forums and encourage the community to attend.
- Launch the first forum to identify priority issues and develop a vision for the future.

Goals of future forums and sustainability included:

- Host one-on-one outreach meetings between formal and informal leaders in the community.
- Invite resource partners to speak at the forum to share information and answer questions related to the community's issue areas.

- Create issue-based work groups, with goals, activities, and deadlines for future work.
- Support emerging leaders with coaching and training opportunities.
- Identify and hire a local coordinator to support the long-term sustainability of the forums.
- Apply for a grant to support local projects and activities.

Through the forums in West Marion, five target issues emerged. These issues led to the creation of working groups to address each issue in the community. The issues addressed a community garden, transportation, housing, childcare, and reviving the community. Each working group was tasked to create goals, activities, and timelines for improving their issue. Two of the working group successes are included in the following.

Working Group: Community Garden

An issue identified in the forum was a lack of access to fresh produce in the West Marion community. This group secured a grant from Resourceful Communities to support the formation of the garden. Community members brokered the land share, boy scouts built, and the city of Marion paid for the garden information board. In addition, a walking challenge was created to encourage people to get out and be active. Many surrounding churches joined in the challenge as a means to walk and share in fellowship. Youth in the area help maintain the garden and sell the produce at the local farmers' market. The extension has begun providing canning classes along with the garden.

Working Group: Transportation

In the West Marion community, residents lack transportation to the grocery store, medical appointments, government agencies, and much more. The working group secured a grant from the Kate B. Reynolds Charitable Trust to fund transportation for anyone in need in the West Marion community, specifically. In addition, the working group collected signatures to support a countywide transportation system.

Case Study Questions

1. Why do you think a community forum is a good or not good choice for the West Marion community?

2. Limited access to supermarkets, supercenters, grocery stores, or other sources of healthy and affordable food may impede the ability of some Americans to achieve a healthy diet. The Food Access Research Atlas (FARA) is a web-based mapping tool that allows users to investigate access to food stores at the census-tract level.[29] Go to FARA (www.ers.usda.gov/data-products/food-access-research-atlas) and find the McDowell County census tract. Compare food access to the rest of the state. Are there pockets in the state where people have more access to food stores than other areas? Hypothesize about what factors influence any observed disparity.

3. What national or local programs do you think are in place in McDowell County that assist in promoting health and wellness? Are there any barriers in McDowell County to accessing these programs?

4. What other sectors of the food system could be involved in the McDowell County Community Engagement Project to strengthen the community impact on promoting health, healthy food systems, and the well-being of the community? How would you expand or complement this project?

5. What strategies were used for policy, systems, and/or environmental changes in McDowell County?

SUGGESTED LEARNING ACTIVITIES

Activity #1: The Food Access Research Atlas (FARA)—The Use of Mapping to Understand Food Accessibility

"Limited access to supermarkets, supercenters, grocery stores, or other sources of healthy and affordable food may impede the ability of some Americans to achieve a healthy diet. The Food Access Research Atlas (FARA) is a Web-based mapping tool that allows users to investigate access to food stores at the census-tract level."[29] Go to FARA (www.ers.usda.gov/data-products/food-access-research-atlas) and find your census tract. Compare food access in your area of residence to the rest of the state. Are there pockets in the state where people have more access to food stores than other areas? Hypothesize about what factors influence any observed disparity.

Activity #2: Community Windshield Tour

A wonderful way to learn more about your community and to begin to understand root causes of nutritional and public health needs is to get out and either drive or walk through different neighborhoods within your town or community. The visual perspective gained through this experience can be powerful and give insight into the way of life for diverse populations found across the community. For this activity, go with a friend or a group of friends to take notes related to the physical and social conditions found in the neighborhoods that you visit. This could include (but is not limited to) grocery stores, gas stations, public transportation, restaurant selections, housing, churches/faith-based institutions, schools, and the people you see and the activities they are engaged in. Seek to visit these locations at different times of the day and different days of the week. In addition, seek to spend some time at one or more of these locations while taking notes (restaurant, grocery store, or another public place) and in areas that have contrasting socioeconomic statuses and economic opportunity. From this experience, compile a list of key attributes of each neighborhood. What was similar? What was different? What were some of the factors involved in the differences? How would these differences contribute to health disparities in relation to nutritional health?

REFLECTION QUESTIONS

1. What does an integrated food system look like at the community level?

2. In what ways do health disparities and food insecurity impact each other?

3. You are tasked with addressing nutritional needs in your community. Please describe how you would incorporate elements of food sovereignty, cultural competency, social justice, and systems thinking into your approach. What are the challenges and opportunities?

CONTINUE YOUR LEARNING RESOURCES

Food and Nutrition. U.S. Department of Agriculture. https://www.usda.gov/https://www.usda.gov/topics/food-and-nutrition.

Growing Food Connections. http://growingfoodconnections.org/about/community-food-systems-planning

Local Food Systems. U.S. Department of Agriculture. https://www.nal.usda.gov/afsic/local-food-systems

Journal of Agriculture, Food Systems, and Community Development. https://www.foodsystemsjournal.org/index.php/fsj

New Entry Sustainable Farming Project. https://nesfp.org/about

Food Security. U.S. Department of Agriculture. https://www.usda.gov/topics/food-and-nutrition/food-security

Feeding America. https://hungerandhealth.feedingamerica.org/understand-food-insecurity

Community Tool Box. https://ctb.ku.edu/en

Prevention Institute, Developing Effective Coalitions. https://www.preventioninstitute.org/publications/developing-effective-coalitions-an-eight-step-guide

Learning for Sustainability. http://learningforsustainability.net

U.S. Food Sovereignty Alliance. http://usfoodsovereigntyalliance.org/what-is-food-sovereignty

American Public Health Association. https://www.apha.org

The Nutrition Society, Public Health Nutrition. https://www.nutritionsociety.org/publications/public-health-nutrition

County Health Rankings. http://www.countyhealthrankings.org

Robert Wood Johnson Foundation. https://www.rwjf.org

The Community Guide to Preventive Services. https://www.thecommunityguide.org/topic/nutrition

Sustaining Community: Families, Communities, The Environment. https://sustainingcommunity.wordpress.com/2018/05/14/effective-engagement

NC State Extension (Local Food). https://localfood.ces.ncsu.edu/local-food-justice

GLOSSARY

Advocacy: Advocacy at the community level consists of "actions" intended to influence public policy for a particular cause, or to strengthen capacity and mobilize resources, or to decrease barriers to health.[59,60]

Built environment: A community's built environment—or human-made surroundings—has a strong effect on what and how people eat.[17] The type and location of food stores in a community, for example, are often associated with the diets of residents and their health.[18]

Coalition: Coalitions are "groups of individuals and/or organizations with a common interest who agree to work together toward a common goal."[50] In effect, coalitions are "action oriented," "analyzing the issue," "identifying and implementing solutions," and "creating social change"—with the understanding that the best results occur when working collectively rather than individually.[51]

Community development: Community development builds upon the engagement process and is focused on an improvement in outcomes, such as the physical environment, cultural norms, social and political actions, and enhanced educational and economic opportunities, to name a few.[43,44] This idea is often linked to that of community engagement.

Community engagement: Community engagement refers to the process and actions of involving community members in decision-making that impacts the day-to-day quality of life offered in the community; furthermore, community engagement has consistently been shown to be a very effective strategy for engaging with and empowering vulnerable populations and reducing health inequities.[40–42] This idea is often linked to that of community development.

Cultural competency: Cultural competency refers to one's ability to respect and value cultural differences and to one who strives to work effectively to address disparities that exist largely because of cultural differences—developing culturally competent public health professionals is vital to the pursuit of health equity.[79]

Faith-based initiative: Faith-based initiatives, often underutilized and garnering little attention, are movements in which religious institutions such as churches or nonprofit agencies, either formally or informally, spearhead efforts and generally partner with public health agencies and the medical sector or an institution of higher education for community development and improved health.[53,54] These efforts can range from activities in policy and advocacy to health education to health promotion programming. With faith being a focal point of the culture and spirituality being a driving force in their communities, faith-based health promotion efforts have had a great deal of success in both rural and minority populations.[55–58]

Food justice: Food justice refers to food-related social justice matters and has been defined as "the struggle against racism, exploitation, and oppression taking place within the food system that addresses inequality's root causes both within and beyond the food chain."[39,81]

Food security: The condition in which all people, at all times, have physical, social, and economic access to sufficient, safe, and nutritious food that meets their dietary needs and food preferences for an active and healthy life.

Food sovereignty: Food sovereignty is the right for all people to choose healthy and culturally appropriate food that is produced through ecologically sound and sustainable methods. Food sovereignty focuses on the needs of those who produce, distribute, and consume food, rather than the demands of markets and corporations.

Food system: The term food system refers to all aspects of producing, buying, selling, eating, and disposing of food. This includes production, processing and aggregation, distribution, marketing, consumption, and food waste recovery.

Grassroots: Grassroots movements are organized by ordinary citizens to raise awareness about a cause(s) and to seek change. For example, on a national scale, in the United States in recent years, we have seen the Tea Party and the Occupy Wall Street movements have success in building momentum for their respective causes. On a more local level, we witness communities everyday striving to improve food access and to improve nutritional health—all grounded in a grassroots mentality. Grassroots movements help to build excitement, and if done in a positive manner, can create a sense of community and lead to sustained change.

Health disparities: Healthy People 2020 defines a health disparity as "a particular type of health difference that is closely linked with social, economic, and/or environmental disadvantage. Health disparities "adversely affect groups of people who have systematically experienced greater obstacles to health based on their racial or ethnic group; religion; socioeconomic status; gender; age; mental health; cognitive, sensory, or physical disability; sexual orientation or gender identity; geographic location; or other characteristics historically linked to discrimination or exclusion."[22]

Health equity: Health equity is the principle of pursuing elimination of health disparities because they are unjust. The term draws specific attention to the underlying social conditions that lead to higher health risks and poorer health outcomes for populations that are economically, socially, or environmentally disadvantaged.[23]

Health literacy: Health literacy focuses on the general population's ability to access, comprehend, and utilize health information or services.[77] We have numerous citizens across our country with very low health literacy levels, and it is now a foundational principle for Healthy People 2030.[78]

Social-Ecological Model (SEM): The SEM is a theory-based framework for understanding the multifaceted and interactive effects of personal and environmental factors that determine behaviors and for identifying behavioral and organizational leverage points and intermediaries for health promotion within organizations. There are five nested, hierarchical levels of the SEM: individual, interpersonal, community, organizational, and policy/enabling environment.

Social justice: Social justice generally refers to the fair and equal treatment of people.

Stakeholders: Stakeholders are described as "any individual or group living within the community or likely to be affected by decisions or actions."[45] Whether it be a rural or urban community, key stakeholders involved in the food system include an assortment of actors including agricultural workers/farmers, local government, nonprofit agencies and businesses, citizens, and most importantly from a public health perspective, those often overlooked and/or most vulnerable.

Systems thinking: Systems thinking helps us to think about how the system is functioning collectively, rather than each individual or agency independently; with this, there are new and innovative research strategies being utilized that are also leading to new forms of practice. This type of thinking and approach forces us to work in a collaborative and interdisciplinary way and to get out of our professional silos.

REFERENCES

1. U.S. Department of Agriculture. *Programs and Services.* 2018. https://www.fns.usda.gov/programs-and-services
2. Mabli J. *SNAP Participation, Food Security, and Geographic Access to Food.* Washington, DC: Mathematica Policy Research; 2014.
3. Meit, M. *Final Report: Exploring Strategies to Improve Health and Equity in Rural Communities.* Bethesda, MD; Walsh Center for Rural Health Analysis; 2018. http://www.norc.org/PDFs/Walsh%20Center/Final%20Reports/Rural%20Assets%20Final%20Report%20Feb%2018.pdf
4. U.S. Department of Agriculture. *Core Nutrition Messages.* 2018. https://www.fns.usda.gov/core-nutrition/core-nutrition-messages
5. U.S. Department of Agriculture. *Supplemental Nutrition Assistance Program Education (SNAP-Ed).* 2018. https://www.fns.usda.gov/snap/supplemental-nutrition-assistance-program-education-snap-ed
6. U.S. Department of Agriculture. *SNAP-Ed Strategies and Interventions: An Obesity Prevention Toolkit for States.* 2016. https://snaped.fns.usda.gov/library/materials/snap-ed-strategies-interventions-obesity-prevention-toolkit-states
7. Hoelscher D, Springer A, Menendez T, et al. (2011). From NIH to Texas schools: policy impact of the Coordinated Approach to Child Health (CATCH) Program in Texas. *J Phys Act Health.* 2011;8(suppl 1):S5–S7. doi:10.1123/jpah.8.s1.s5
8. U.S. Department of Agriculture. *ChooseMyPlate.* 2018. https://www.choosemyplate.gov
9. U.S. Department of Agriculture. *Food Labeling.* https://www.nal.usda.gov/fnic/food-labeling
10. U.S. Department of Agriculture. *Team Nutrition.* https://www.fns.usda.gov/tn/team-nutrition
11. Centers for Disease Control and Prevention. *Social determinants of health: know what affects health.* https://www.cdc.gov/socialdeterminants/index.htm
12. Oxford Martin Programme on the Future of Food. *What is the food system?* https://www.futureoffood.ox.ac.uk/what-food-system

13. Shuman M. *The Local Economy Solution: How Innovative, Self-financing "Pollinator" Enterprises Can Grow Jobs and Prosperity.* White River, VT: Chelsea Green Publishing; 2015.

14. Hueston W, McLeod A. *Overview of the global food system: changes over time/space and lessons for future food afety. In: Institute of Medicine, ed. Improving Food Safety Through a One Health Approach: Workshop Summar.* Washington, DC: National Academies Press; 2012.

15. Bosch RVD. Public health advantages of biological insect controls. *Environ Health Perspect.* 1976;14:161–163. doi:10.1289/ehp.7614161

16. Devine G, Furlong, M. Insecticide use: contexts and ecological consequences. *Agric Hum Values.* 2007;24:281–306. doi:10.1007/s10460-007-9067-z

17. Prevention Institute. *Strategies for Enhancing the Built Environment to Support Healthy Eating and Active Living.* 2008. https://www.preventioninstitute.org/publications/strategies-for-enhancing-the-built-environment-to-support-healthy-eating-and-active-living

18. Glanz K, Sallis J, Saelens B, Franks L. Healthy nutrition environments: concepts and measures. *Am J Health Promot.* 2005;19(5):330–333. doi:10.4278/0890-1171-19.5.330

19. Babey S, Diamant A, Hastert T, Harvey S. *Designed for Disease: The Link Between Local Food Environments and Obesity and Diabetes.* Los Angeles, CA: UCLA Center for Health Policy Research; 2008.

20. Moore L, Roux AD, Nettleton J, Jacobs D. Associations of the local food environment with diet quality—a comparison of assessments based on surveys and geographic information systems. *Am J Epidemiol.* 2008;167(8):917–924. doi:10.1093/aje/kwm394

21. Cooksey-Stowers K. Schwartz MB, Brownell KD. Food swamps predict obesity rates better than food deserts in the United States. *Int J Environ Res Public Health.* 2017;14(11):1366. doi:10.3390/ijerph14111366

22. Office of Disease Prevention and Health Promotion. *Disparities.* https://www.healthypeople.gov/2020/about/foundation-health-measures/disparities.

23. Braveman P. What are health disparities and health equity? We need to be clear. *Public Health Rep.* 2014;129(1 suppl 2):5–8. doi:10.1177/00333549141291S203

24. U.S. Department of Agriculture Economic Research Service. *Ag and Food Statistics: Charting the Essentials/Food Security and Nutrition Assistance;* 2013. https://www.ers.usda.gov/data-products/ag-and-food-statistics-charting-the-essentials/

25. Hilmers A, Hilmers D, Dave J. Neighborhood disparities in access to healthy foods and their effects on environmental justice. *Am J Public Health.* 2012;102(9):1644–1654. doi:10.2105/AJPH.2012.300865

26. Morland K, Wing S, Roux AD, Poole C. Neighborhood characteristics associated with the location of food stores and food service places. *Am J Prev Med.* 2002;22(1):23–29. doi:10.1016/S0749-3797(01)00403-2

27. Vallianatos M, Shaffer A, Gottlieb R. *Transportation and Food: The Importance of Access.* Los Angeles, CA: Center for Food and Justice, Urban and Environmental Policy Institute; 2002.

28. Food and Agriculture Organization. *Rome Declaration on World Food Security and World Food Summit Plan of Action.* Rome: World Food Summit; 1996.

29. Coleman-Jensen A, Rabbitt A, Gregory A, Singh A. *Household Food Security in the United States in 2016.* Washington, DC: U.S. Department of Agriculture, Economic Research Service; 2017.

30. U.S. Department of Agriculture Economic Research Service. *Definitions of food security.* https://www.ers.usda.gov/topics/food-nutrition-assistance/food-security-in-the-us/definitions-of-food-security.aspx. Updated September 4, 2019.

31. International Food Policy Research Institute. *Food security.* https://www.ifpri.org/topic/food-security

32. Shankar P, Chung R, Frank D. Association of food insecurity with children's behavioral, emotional, and academic outcomes: a systematic review. *J Dev Behav Pediatr.* 2017;38(2):135–150. doi:10.1097/DBP.0000000000000383

33. Myers A, Painter M. Food insecurity in the United States of America: an examination of race/ethnicity and nativity. *Food Secur.* 2017;9(6):1419–1432. doi:10.1007/s12571-017-0733-8

34. Jones A. Food insecurity and mental health status: a global analysis of 149 countries. *Am J Prev Med.* 2017;53(2):264–273. doi:10.1016/j.amepre.2017.04.008

35. Food and Agriculture Organization. *Global Agriculture Towards 2050.* Rome: High Level Expert Forum: How to Feed the World in 2050; 2009.

36. Clendenning J, Dressler W, Richards C. Food justice or food sovereignty? Understanding the rise of urban food movements in the USA. *Agric Hum Values.* 2016;33:165–177. doi:10.1007/s10460-015-9625-8

37. McMichael P, Porter C. Going public with notes on cousins, food sovereignty, and food dignity. *J Agric Food Syst Community Dev.* 2018;8(suppl 1):207–212. doi:10.5304/jafscd.2018.08A.015

38. Food Secure Canada. *What Is Food Sovereignty.* 2018. https://foodsecurecanada.org/who-we-are/what-food-sovereignty

39. Glennie C, Alkon A. Food justice: cultivating the field. *Environ Res Lett.* 2018;13(7):073003. doi:10.1088/1748-9326/aac4b2

40. Cyril S, Smith B, Possami-Inesedy A, Renzaho A. Exploring the role of community engagement in improving the health of disadvantaged populations: a systematic review. *Glob Health Action.* 2015;8(1):29842. doi:10.3402/gha.v8.29842

41. O'Mara-Eves A, Brunton G, McDaid G, et al. Community engagement to reduce inequalities in health: a systematic review, meta-analysis and economic analysis. *Public Health Res.* 2013;1(4):1–526. doi:10.3310/phr01040

42. Swainston K, Summerbell C. *The Effectiveness of Community Engagement Approaches and Methods for Health Promotion Interventions.* 2008.

43. Phillips R, Pittman R. *An Introduction to Community Development.* 2nd ed. New York, NY: Routledge; 2014.

44. Phillips R, Wharton C. *Growing Livelihoods: Local Food Systems and Community Development.* New York, NY: Routledge; 2015.

45. Alexander M. Local communities and stakeholders. In: Alexander M. *Management Planning for Nature Conservation.* Dordrecht, The Netherlands: Springer; 2013.

46. Nelson C, Stroink M. Accessibility and viability: a complex adaptive systems approach to a wicked problem for the local food movement. *J Agric Food Syst Community Dev.* 2014;4(4):191–206. doi:10.5304/jafscd.2014.044.016

47. Mathie A, Cunningham G. From clients to citizens: asset-based community development as a strategy for community-driven development. *Dev Pract.* 2003;13(5):474–486. doi:10.1080/0961452032000125857

48. Ellis G, Walton S. Building partnerships between local health departments and communities: case studies in capacity building and cultural humility. In: Minkler M, ed. *Community Organizing and Community Building for Health and Welfare.* New Brunswick, NJ: Rutgers University Press; 2012.

49. Haines A. Asset-based community development. In: Phillips R, Pittman R, eds. *An Introduction to Community Development.* New York, NY: Routledge; 2014.

50. Doyle E, Ward S, Oomen-Early J. *The Process of Community Health Education and Promotion.* Long Grove, IL: Waveland Press; 2009.

51. Butterfoss F, Kegler M. A coalition model for community action. In: Minkler M, ed. *Community Organizing and Community Building for Health and Welfare.* New Brunswick, NJ: Rutgers University Press; 2012.

52. Feigherty E, Rogers T. *Building and maintaining effective coalitions.* Palo Alto, CA: Health Promotion Resource Center, Stanford Center for Research in Disease Prevention; 1990.

53. Levin J. Faith-based initiatives in health promotion: history, challenges, and current partnerships. *Am J Health Promot.* 2014;28(3):139–141. doi:10.4278/ajhp.130403-CIT-149

54. Levin J. Partnerships between the faith-based and medical sectors: implications for preventive medicine and public health. *Prev Med Rep.* 2016;4:344–350. doi:10.1016/j.pmedr.2016.07.009

55. Campbell M, Hudson M, Resnicow K, et al. Church-based health promotion interventions: evidence and lessons learned. *Annu Rev Public Health.* 2007;28:213–234. doi:10.1146/annurev.publhealth.28.021406.144016

56. Wilcox S, Laken M, Parrott A, et al. The faith, activity, and nutrition (FAN) program: design of a participatory research intervention to increase physical activity and improve dietary habits in African American churches. *Contemp Clin Trials.* 2010;31(4):323–335. doi:10.1016/j.cct.2010.03.011

57. Yanek L, Becker D, Moy T, et al. Project Joy: faith based cardiovascular health promotion for African American women. *Public Health Rep.* 2001;116:68–81. doi:10.1093/phr/116.S1.68

58. Yeary K. Rural church-based health promotion. In: Warren J, Smalley K, eds. *Rural Public Health: Best Practices and Preventive Models.* New York, NY: Springer Publishing Company; 2014.

59. Cohen B, Marshall S. Does public health advocacy seek to redress health inequities? A scoping review. *Health Soc Care Community.* 2017;25(2):309–328. doi:10.1111/hsc.12320

60. Loue S. Community health advocacy. *J Epidemiol Community Health*. 2006;60(6):458–463. doi:10.1136/jech.2004.023044

61. Cullerton K, Donnet T, Lee A, Gallegos D. Using political science to progress public health nutrition: a systematic review. *Public Health Nutr*. 2016;19(11):2070–2078. doi:10.1017/S1368980015002712

62. Freedman D, Bess K. Food systems change and the environment: local and global connections. *Am J Community Psychol*. 2011;47:397–409. doi:10.1007/s10464-010-9392-z

63. Allen P. Realizing justice in local food systems. *Cambridge J Reg Econ Soc*. 2010;3:295–308. doi:10.1093/cjres/rsq015

64. Neff R, Merrigan K, Wallinga D. A food systems approach to healthy food and agriculture policy. *Health Aff*. 2015;34(11):1908–1915. doi:10.1377/hlthaff.2015.0926

65. Bradley E, Canavan M, Rogan E, et al. Variation in health outcomes: the role of spending on social services, public health, and health care, 2000-09. *Health Aff*. 2016;35(5):760–768. doi:10.1377/hlthaff.2015.0814

66. Carey G, Malbon E, Carey N, et al. Systems science and systems thinking for public health: a systematic review of the field. *BMJ Open*. 2015;5:e009002. doi:10.1136/bmjopen-2015-009002

67. Leischow S, Best A, Trochim W, et al. Systems thinking to improve the public's health. *Am J Prev Med*. 2008;35(2):S196–S203. doi:10.1016/j.amepre.2008.05.014

68. Swanson R, Cattaneo A, Bradley E, et al. Rethinking health systems strengthening: key systems thinking tools and strategies for transformational change. *Health Policy Plan*. 2012;27(suppl 4):iv54–iv61. doi:10.1093/heapol/czs090

69. Wave TV, Scutchfield F, Honore P. Recent advances in public health systems research in the United States. *Annu Rev Public Health*. 2010;31:283–295. doi:10.1146/annurev.publhealth.012809.103550

70. Golden S, Earp J. Social ecological approaches to individuals and their contexts: twenty years of health education and behavior health promotion interventions. *Health Educ Behav*. 2012;39(3):364–372. doi:10.1177/1090198111418634

71. McLeroy K, Bibeau D, Steckler A, Glanz K. An ecological perspective on health promotion programs. *Health Educ Q*. 1988;15(4):351–377. doi:10.1177/109019818801500401

72. Stokols D. Translating social ecological theory into guidelines for community health promotion. *Am J Health Promot*. 1996;10(4):282–298. doi:10.4278/0890-1171-10.4.282

73. Hanlon P, Carlisle S, Hannah M, et al. A perspective on the future public health: an integrative and ecological framework. *Perspect Public Health*. 2012;132(6):313–319. doi:10.1177/1757913912440781

74. Lee B, Bartsch S, Mui Y, et al. A systems approach to obesity. *Nutr Rev*. 2016;75(S1):94–106. doi:10.1093/nutrit/nuw049

75. Haider M, Kreps G. Forty years of diffusion of innovations: utility and value in public health. *J Health Commun*. 2004;9:3–11. doi:10.1080/10810730490271430

76. Crosby R, DiClemente R, Salazar L. Diffusion of innovations theory. In: DiClemente R, Salazar L, Crosby R, eds. *Health Behavior Theory for Public Health: Principles, Foundations, and Applications*. Burlington, MA: Jones & Bartlett; 2013:211–230.

77. Batterham R, Hawkins M, Collins P, et al. Health literacy: applying current concepts to improve health services and reduce health inequalities. *Public Health*. 2016;132:3–12. doi:10.1016/j.puhe.2016.01.001

78. Office of Disease Prevention and Health Promotion. *Healthy People 2030 Framework*. Healthy People 2030; 2018. https://www.healthypeople.gov/2020/About-Healthy-People/Development-Healthy-People-2030/Framework

79. Cushman L, Delva M, Franks C, et al. Cultural competency training for public health students: integrating self, social, and global awareness into a master of public health curriculum. *Am J Public Health*. 2015;105(suppl 1):S132–S140. doi:10.2105/AJPH.2014.302506

80. Zurcher K, Doctor L, Imig G. Food & fitness: lessons learned for funders. *Health Promot Pract*. 2018;19(supp 1):9S–14S. doi:10.1177/1524839918783974

81. Hislop R. Reaping Equity Across the USA: FJ Organizations Observed at the National Scale. International Agricultural Development Graduate Group, University of California Davis; 2014.

8

RURAL HEALTH: IMPORTANCE OF INTERPROFESSIONAL APPROACH

KYLE L. THOMPSON, MELISSA GUTSCHALL, AND DOMINIQUE M. ROSE

LEARNING OBJECTIVES

1. Describe three standard definitions of the term **rural** and select the most appropriate definition for specific applications.

2. Compare and contrast similarities and differences regarding the rural environment versus the urban environment, including strengths and challenges of the rural environment.

3. Define healthcare access, quality, and equity as these issues impact rural residents, and be able to categorize common barriers to healthcare, including nutrition care, for rural residents.

4. Identify common nutrition-impacted health conditions associated with rural settings, including chronic diseases, substance abuse, and food security and associated outcomes.

5. List characteristics of healthcare professionals who choose to practice in rural settings and describe several common issues that rural public health nutrition practitioners (PHN practitioners) may face.

6. Describe basic skills of cultural competence and develop a plan for applying those skills in public health nutrition practice.

7. Describe the four components of the Rural Health Nutrition Practice Model (RHNPM) and categorize selected characteristics of a given rural population within the RHNPM.

8. Use the RHNPM to describe an interprofessional framework for rural public health nutrition practice.

9. Develop a plan for acquiring the necessary knowledge and skills to practice public health nutrition in a chosen rural setting.

INTRODUCTION

Much attention is currently focused on policy, strategies, interventions, funding sources, and methods for delivering effective public health nutrition interventions to **rural populations** in the United States.[1] Persons residing in rural areas often face challenges in accessing healthcare and safe, adequate food supplies.[2] Sociocultural factors including culturally based health beliefs and behaviors may impact rates of chronic disease, which are generally higher in rural than urban settings.[3] While urban populations, too, are affected by unique sociocultural and socioeconomic influences, **rurality** itself may exacerbate difficulties in accessing appropriate health and nutrition resources. This chapter examines the theory and practice of public health nutrition in rural health settings.

Throughout this chapter, it is of crucial importance for the reader to understand that when referring to "rural," there are no uniform characteristics of populations that live in rural parts of the country, and there is no monolithic "rural population." The challenges facing "coastal rural" are different from "mountain rural" or "frontier rural." In general, some issues are similar, for example, access to healthcare, food, and resources, but other issues, particularly cultural, are different. Thus, each rural population group is unique in its cultural distinctives and its nutrition needs.

WHAT IS "RURAL"?

What does it mean for a person, population, or facility in the United States to be *rural*? Is *rural* a subjective concept, existing in the mind of each individual as a particular mix of farms, fields, ranches, wilderness, mountains, forests, and wide open spaces?[4] Can *rural* be described by numbers? Is *rurality* dependent on the remoteness of the setting or on population density? And, if population numbers are the distinguishing characteristic of rurality, exactly what is the cutoff point that differentiates rural from urban settings? The fact that a number of different methods have been proposed for defining rurality indicates that *rural* is a complex concept, with many different aspects of the environmental and sociocultural setting influencing the categorization of a particular geographic area.

Rural settings can range from remote villages in Alaska accessible only by plane to ranches in Wyoming located hours by car from the nearest hospital, to mountainous regions of southern Appalachia where some residents still live in isolated **hollers**, to southern coastal areas, which have experienced catastrophic economic shifts resulting in high rates of poverty and poor access to healthcare, and to New England farms located in close proximity to major population centers. A majority of counties in the United States have both rural *and* urban areas. The rural environment in the United States is highly diverse, dynamic, and constantly changing.[5] Similarly, the people who live and work in rural areas are diverse, with an extensive range of differences in socioeconomic status, education levels, ability to access healthcare, and food and nutrition practices.[5]

Thus, there is no one definition of the term *rural*. Many definitions have been created over the years.[6] Specific definitions become important, however, when seeking funding for rural health programming such as public health nutrition programs.[6] The U.S. Department of Agriculture (USDA) Rural Information Center (RIC) continues to reference a seminal report, published by the U.S. General Accounting Office (GAO) in 1993, in providing three major federal definitions of the term *rural* that are commonly used in public health settings.[7] It is important to remember that the federal government considers *rural* to be defined by exclusion; that is, the boundaries or characteristics of urban areas are defined and described, and whatever is not *urban* is considered *rural*. The three primary federal definitions originate in the **U.S. Census Bureau (USCB)**, the Office of Management and Budget (OMB), and the U.S. Department of Agriculture Economic Research Service (USDA ERS):

1. *The USCB urban–rural classification:*

    The USCB does not utilize city or county boundaries when defining urban and rural areas, but rather delineates census tracts according to their concentrations of residents.[8] Thus, the USCB characterization of *rural* is primarily geographic, based on density of population and land use. The USCB recognizes two types of urban areas:

a. **Urbanized areas (UAs)** of 50,000 or more people

b. **Urban clusters (UCs)** of at least 2,500 but less than 50,000 people[9]

All persons, homes, and territory not located within a UA or a UC are considered rural.[8] As a result of the 2010 census, the USCB found that about 21% of the population, or 59.5 million people, and 95% of the land area of the United States is considered *rural*.[9] The USCB definition classifies a great deal of suburban area as *rural*, and thus may tend to *overestimate* the number of rural residents.[9]

2. *OMB delineation of metropolitan and nonmetropolitan statistical areas:*

In 1950, the Bureau of the Budget, which later became the OMB, established the concept of "standard metropolitan areas."[10] This designation has since been expanded and refined to include **core-based statistical areas** comprising *metropolitan* and **nonmetropolitan** counties, using county boundaries to provide a *metro* or *nonmetro* designation for each U.S. county.[10]

Metropolitan counties are usually divided into two types:

a. Metro counties are central counties containing a core, densely populated urban area with at least 50,000 inhabitants.

b. Counties designated as *metro* may also include those that are adjacent to a core urban county, and demonstrate a high degree of linkage with the core area as assessed by commuting patterns.[10]

Nonmetropolitan counties are subdivided into two types:

a. **Micropolitan** counties are those containing a core urban area with at least 10,000 but no more than 50,000 inhabitants, plus adjoining surrounding counties with a high degree of linkage with the core area as assessed by commuting patterns.

b. All remaining counties, which are often labeled **non-core rural counties** because they do not meet the core requirements for either a metropolitan or a micropolitan designation, are considered nonmetropolitan.[10]

Note that the OMB definitions of metro and nonmetro areas are not designed to specify whether a particular county is urban or rural. Rather, the only purpose for the OMB designations is to provide a consistent set of descriptions to be used to collect, analyze, and disseminate federal statistics for designated geographic areas.[10] The OMB definitions reflect a socioeconomic, labor-market perspective on rurality, and offer the ability to utilize accessible county data for a variety of indicators. Most rural researchers consider the nonmetropolitan designation to be more consistent with a rural classification since the designation of a town of 10,000 residents as a "core urban area" may be confusing. When using the OMB delineations, it is important to remember that because rurality is a continuum, and because a majority of U.S. counties contain both urban and rural areas, highly rural areas can be classified as "metro."[4] Thus, the OMB metro–nonmetro designations may tend to *underestimate* the numbers of rural residents and rural areas. For example, the Grand Canyon, arguably a remote area of the United States, is found in a metro county.

TABLE 8.1 RURAL–URBAN CONTINUUM CODES

CODE	DESCRIPTION
METRO COUNTIES	
1	Counties in metro areas of 1 million population or more
2	Counties in metro areas of 250,000 to 1 million population
3	Counties in metro areas of fewer than 250,000 population
NONMETRO COUNTIES	
4	Urban population of 20,000 or more, adjacent to a metro area
5	Urban population of 20,000 or more, not adjacent to a metro area
6	Urban population of 2,500 to 19,999, adjacent to a metro area
7	Urban population of 2,500 to 19,999, not adjacent to a metro area
8	Completely rural or less than 2,500 population, adjacent to a metro area
9	Completely rural or less than 2,500 population, not adjacent to a metro area

Source: From U.S. Department of Agriculture Economic Research Service. Rural-Urban Continuum Codes. 2013. https://www.ers.usda.gov/data-products/rural-urban-continuum-codes/documentation

3. *USDA definition of rural:*

The USDA, while officially utilizing no one definition of *rural*, recognizes both the USCB and the OMB definitions, noting that each definition is useful in specific contexts.[11] In order to enhance the utility of the OMB metro–nonmetro designations, the USDA ERS has developed two additional county-level classification systems utilizing OMB metro–nonmetro designation data. First, **Rural–Urban Continuum Codes (RUCCs)** have been prepared on the county level (Table 8.1).[11] The codes subdivide the OMB *metro* and *nonmetro* designations into three metro and six nonmetro categories, for a total of nine categories. The designations take into consideration the population numbers in metro counties. For nonmetro counties, the degree of urbanization and whether adjoining to metro counties are considered. The RUCCs allow researchers, government agencies, health professionals, and other interested parties to more specifically identify population groups of interest, and in the case of rural researchers, to better identify trends occurring in rural areas.[11] The second county-level classification system, Urban Influence Codes (UICs), offers 10 categories, two for metropolitan counties and eight for nonmetro counties. While similar to RUCCs, UICs offer greater distinctions among rural counties, and consider adjacency to both metropolitan counties and nonmetropolitan counties with a large town.[92]

At the census tract level, the **Federal Office of Rural Health Policy (FORHP)** has collaborated with the USDA ERS to develop **Rural–Urban Commuting Area (RUCA) Codes**.[9] RUCAs assign each census tract a code ranging from 1 to 10, based on standard USCB rural–urban census tract definitions plus commuting pattern data. RUCAs from 4 to 10 are considered "rural." The use of RUCA codes allows for the identification of rural areas (RUCAs 4–10) *within* metropolitan counties (RUCCs 1–3). Because most U.S. counties contain both urban and rural areas, the RUCA designation allows for a more nuanced assessment of the rurality of a given location. In the United States, there are 132 very large census tracts in which the RUCA codes are inconsistent, given low population density and long drives to access services; these areas have been designated "rural" even though their official RUCA code is 2 or 3.[9] RUCAs help to improve the accuracy of urban–rural classifications provided by the USCB, which tends to overestimate the rural population, and the OMB, which tends to underestimate the rural population.[9] A potential disadvantage of RUCA codes is that they are based on census tracts, which may change over time, while county boundaries in general remain fixed.

Rural Definitions and the PHN Practitioner

When choosing a definition of *rural* to use for research, securing funds for nutrition programs, or policy development, the PHN practitioner should consider the overarching purpose of the particular project. For example, a project designed to analyze the advance of suburbs into farmlands might be best served by using the USCB definition, because it is based on land use and distinguishes highly urbanized areas from nonurbanized locations. Similarly, the OMB definition is often used in applications examining socioeconomic factors and influences, because it reflects regional employment patterns based on the identification of economic centers of activity. If a researcher is interested in examining the commuting practices of nurses who work in rural critical access hospitals, the RUCAs may provide the most useful foundation for acquiring necessary data for analysis. Funding entities often mandate the particular rural definition to be used for specific grant applications; thus, the PHN practitioner should always confirm the correct definition to be used with the funding agency when seeking third-party resources.

Finally, the PHN practitioner should always keep in mind that there is no one clear definition of the word *rural*. Rural–urban classifications are not a clear dichotomy; rather, there is a rural–urban continuum.[11] A majority of Americans live in areas that comprise some mixture of urban and rural components.[11] Factors such as population, age, impairments, mean income, and access to healthcare resources may not be reflected in standard definitions and may require the identification of other data sources in order to acquire desired information.[12] The PHN practitioner should strive to avoid generalizations and should seek specific information on the location, demographics, social influences, cultural practices, and unique challenges of the rural population being served. By carefully studying the geography, **culture**, and resources of a given rural setting, including the area's federal rural/urban designations, PHN practitioners can most effectively intervene to improve the nutritional status of populations.

SIMILARITIES AND DIFFERENCES REGARDING THE RURAL VERSUS THE URBAN HEALTH ENVIRONMENT

Persons with a rudimentary understanding of rural America may come away from discussions of rural health and economic disparities with the thought, "Why don't rural people just move to places where greater opportunity is available?" A deeper investigation of rural issues reveals that in the broader context, strong and healthy rural regions are vital to the entire nation's well-being and security. All persons who value a ready food supply, adequate energy resources, and a viable national defense, among other benefits, should be concerned about the well-being of rural America. Indeed, rural and urban areas are highly interdependent, and the best interests of both are intertwined.

Rural America has many strengths and assets that can be leveraged to address challenges.[13] **Community assets** in rural areas encompass the collective strengths of rural individuals, organizations, and communities.[13] A first step toward identifying rural community assets may be listing those factors that make rural areas attractive places to live: friendly people, strong community ties, and an ethic of volunteerism and altruism among residents, among many others.[13,14] Rural communities may display a sense of interconnectedness that is evidenced in strong **social networks**. Observers of rural communities often note behaviors such as neighborliness and willingness to assist each other and the community in difficult circumstances.[14] Traits that are commonly valued in rural settings include independence, self-sufficiency, persistence, and **resilience** in the face of difficulties.[13] Rural residents often claim strong ties to the land based on family/community history; this sense of home and family can be motivating when the well-being and survival of that home is at stake, and creative thinking and a willingness to do things differently are needed. Interactions among rural residents and local organizations, such as schools and faith-based organizations, can result in strong networks for economic growth, community improvements, and individual support.[13,15] Rural community assets may also include natural resources, agricultural operations, manufacturing facilities, financial institutions, healthcare facilities such as hospitals and nursing homes, and other entities that provide opportunities for local and regional growth.[13] The development of effective models for enhancing the sustainability of community assets, which are not always under community control, is key to optimizing rural strengths.[13]

Public health nutrition professionals who work in rural areas will do well to begin with an assessment of **community strengths** and assets before assessing the barriers to implementing an intervention (even though the barriers may be daunting). The results of a strengths and assets assessment may reveal surprising possibilities and avenues for moving forward with positive change. Figure 8.1 provides a model for assessing rural strengths and assets.

Rural Environments Compared With Urban Environments

In recent years, the balance between rural and urban well-being in the United States has shifted toward metropolitan areas. Trends over the past three decades have indicated that by a variety of measures, rural U.S. populations' well-being has decreased while urban populations' well-being has increased.[16,17] Worsening statistics in regard to population decline, economic well-being, teen pregnancies, chronic disease rates, and poverty, among others, have been noted in rural America.[16] Another journalist described the phenomenon of younger residents leaving rural areas to migrate to urban locations as "the graying of rural America."[18] In some areas of the United States, rural population losses have been significant and have contributed to an increase in the average age of rural residents. Between July 2015 and July 2016, nonmetro counties as a whole showed an overall population loss of about 21,000 residents for the first time since data has been accumulated, although a number of nonmetro counties had been experiencing modest population losses for some time.[19] It should be noted that population loss figures are for the general nonmetro population; there is much variation among rural areas, and some have gained population within the described time frame. Wage and salary losses caused by shifts in economic centers over the past three decades have resulted in decreased economic opportunities for many rural dwellers.[18,20] In general, it appears that over the past several decades, many rural environments in the United States have become less viable places to build careers and lives.[20]

The challenges faced in accessing healthcare by persons who work and live in rural America may differ in kind, if not in severity, from difficulties encountered in urban settings. Both urban and rural low-income populations experience health disparities resulting in reduced life

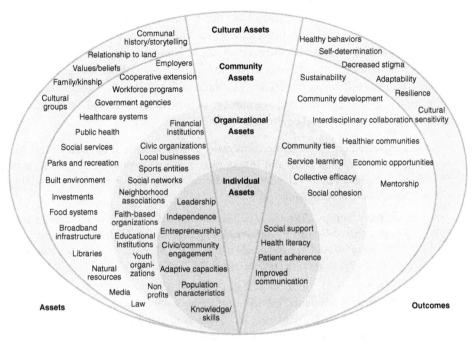

FIGURE 8.1 Rural assets map.

Source: From the Walsh Center for Rural Health Analysis, Meit M. *Final Report: Exploring Strategies to Improve Health and Equity in Rural Communities.* Bethesda, MD: Walsh Center for Rural Health Analysis; 2018. http://www.norc.org/PDFs/Walsh%20Center/Final%20Reports/Rural%20Assets%20Final%20 Report%20Feb%2018.pdf

expectancy and poor health outcomes. Data indicate that a greater number of healthcare providers and resources are available in urban areas.[21] Thus, accessibility issues for the urban poor tend to center on lack of financial resources and transportation to obtain care rather than geographic remoteness of care providers.[21] The urban poor may also live in closer geographic proximity to hospital EDs, where the federal Emergency Medical Treatment and Labor Act (EMTALA) requires that all persons must be provided with medical screening examinations and treatment for emergency conditions, including labor and delivery of babies, regardless of the ability to pay.[22]

Rural residents seeking healthcare face obstacles endemic to current reality in much of rural America: limited economic and educational opportunities, a dearth of infrastructure and dedicated resources based on lack of recognition by government entities, and, in many cases, geographic isolation.[2] The sheer distance that must be traveled to access facilities such as EDs, hospitals, clinics, and **full-service grocery stores** can become a daunting barrier to obtaining care and maintaining health. Rural environments often result in situations in which many rural Americans, especially low-income persons, face substantial health disparities, including nutrition disparities.[2,23–27]

Barriers to Healthcare Access and Equity That Impact Rural Residents

Both urban and rural health settings present challenges for the PHN practitioner. However, the distinctive elements of rural environments tend to present a unique set of difficulties for rural residents in regard to issues of access, quality, and equity. Lack of economic opportunities in rural areas can exacerbate access issues, as rural residents may not have employer-provided basic health insurance or insurance coverage for ancillary services such as dental or mental health treatments. Healthcare options available to rural residents may not be equivalent in quality to services provided in a more urban area. For a number of key indicators, data indicate worse outcomes for rural communities than urban communities.[23] The National Rural Health Association and other investigators have provided information on a number of rural **healthcare** and **health status disparities** related to access to care and equity of care:

- While approximately 17% of Americans resided in rural areas at the time of this writing, only 9% of physicians and 16% of nurses choose to practice in rural locations. Inadequate numbers of primary care providers, dental professionals, and mental health practitioners plague rural America.[28]

  - As of December 31, 2019, the U.S. Bureau of Health Workforce identified a total of 7,026 designated **Health Professional Shortage Areas (HPSAs)**. Of these, 4,145 (59.0%) were located in rural areas, while 2,416 (34.39%) were located in nonrural areas. Partially rural areas encompassed 461 HPSAs (6.56%).[29]

  - As of December 31, 2019, the U.S. Bureau of Health Workforce identified a total of 5,833 designated dental HPSAs.[26] Of these, 3,449 (59.13%) were located in rural areas, while 2,042 (35.01%) were located in nonrural areas. Partially rural areas encompassed 337 (5.78%) dental HPSAs.

  - As of December 31, 2019, the U.S. Bureau of Health Workforce identified a total of 5,124 designated mental HPSAs. Of these, 2,721 (53.10%) were located in rural areas, while 1,964 (38.33%) were located in nonrural areas.[29] Partially rural areas encompassed 436 (8.51%) mental HPSAs. Even if mental health services are available, research suggests that in some rural cultures, there may be a substantial stigma associated with the utilization of mental health services.[30]

- Rural residents have less access to public transportation options and may drive older and less reliable vehicles if a personal automobile is available. Thus, the ability to travel to healthcare facilities is reduced in rural areas.[31]

- Since the late 1980s, there has been an alarming trend toward U.S. **rural hospital closures**.[32,33] The number of closures leveled off in the early 2000s, but accelerated again following the Great Recession of 2008. Since 2005, at least 168 rural hospitals have closed, with the majority of closures occurring in the southern United States. Rural hospital closures have been associated with reduced availability of emergency medical services, migration of physicians and other health professionals out of affected communities, and greater difficulty in accessing both primary and specialty care since a hospital is often the gateway to care.[34] While closing a struggling small hospital and subsequently referring patients to a regional institution may be sensible and prudent from a strictly financial standpoint, there are many unexpected consequences and effects of such closures that should be considered. Closure of a rural hospital is devastating economically because the hospital is often one of its community's largest employers.[34] Downstream effects include loss of a substantial percentage of a small community's jobs, shrinkage of the local tax base which may reduce access to other services such as education, reduced per capita income, and increased difficulty attracting potential employers to the affected community.[35] In addition, rural hospitals tend to be centers of community life, which have served local residents for decades during both happy and difficult life events. When such a hospital closes, the ensuing losses are not only economic but emotional, with a community's sense of place, pride, and self-efficacy suffering a severe blow.

- Rural patients are not as likely to have ready access to specialty care clinics such as oncology centers, EDs, or ICUs.[36]

- According to Moy et al., between 1999 and 2014, nonmetropolitan areas experienced higher death rates than metropolitan areas for heart disease, stroke, cancer, accidental injuries, and chronic lung disease.[36] The investigators listed possible causative factors such as reduced access to healthcare and preventive care services, poor access to health insurance, difficulty in accessing high-level emergency care, and reduced emergency response capabilities.

- Emergency service response times have been found to be as much as 50% longer for rural residents than urban residents.[37] Death rates from unintended injury are about 50% higher in rural than urban areas, with longer emergency response times considered a contributing factor.[36] Rural patients are more likely to die from acute myocardial infarctions (heart attacks) than urban patients.[38] One group of investigators who studied data from Nebraska suggested that the larger number of rural deaths from heart attacks could result from (a) discrepancies in the quality of care provided because patients in rural hospitals are less likely to see a cardiologist; (b) lack of equipment and resources in rural hospitals to provide state-of-the-art care; and (c) longer transportation times in accessing care, resulting in delays in the administration of clot-busting medications.

- Rural women are not as likely as urban women to obtain screening mammograms and are more likely than urban women to cite cost and distance as barriers to obtaining screenings.[39]

- Rural residence was associated with a higher incidence of retinopathy in patients diagnosed with diabetes, and the study investigators suggested that distance to care and availability of specialty care could be factors contributing to poor outcomes.[40]

Rural Health Equity and Social Determinants of Health

- Rural residents are less likely to be insured overall, less likely to have private insurance, and often lack access to dental, vision, and mental health benefits.[25,36,41] Many rural health providers, particularly oral health providers, do not accept Medicaid benefits.

- Compared with urban children, rural children are more likely to be poor (23.5% vs. 20.2%). The national average poverty rate at the time of writing is 14.4%; two thirds of America's rural counties have poverty rates equal to or exceeding this benchmark.[2]

- Rural residents' per capita average annual income is $9,242 lower than that of similar urban counterparts, and rural residents' incomes are more likely to fall below the federally designated poverty level.[24]

- While rural areas may have increased needs for infrastructure to support the development and growth of healthy communities, funds to provide vital infrastructure and equitable opportunities are often lacking.[42]

- Lack of availability of equitable educational, economic, and social supports—along with a tendency of young people to migrate to urban areas—have led to high rates of joblessness.[43] Fewer employment opportunities are available in rural areas, leading to higher numbers of uninsured individuals.

- Inability to access resources such as public transportation, broadband Internet services, and affordable housing contributes significantly to rural health disparities.[42]

Thus, access, quality, and equity in healthcare remain serious issues for many rural-dwelling people.

COMMON NUTRITION-IMPACTED HEALTH CONDITIONS ASSOCIATED WITH RURAL SETTINGS

Overall **mortality** rates in the United States have trended downward since this statistic has been measured.[44] Both rural and urban death rates have declined over the decades; however, the declines are consistently smaller for rural as compared to urban populations.[26] For most health measures, micropolitan and noncore areas lag behind more urbanized locations (Figure 8.2).[45]

Mortality and morbidity rates and health disparities for certain racial, ethnic, and regional rural population groups are substantially increased over those of the general rural population.[26] A

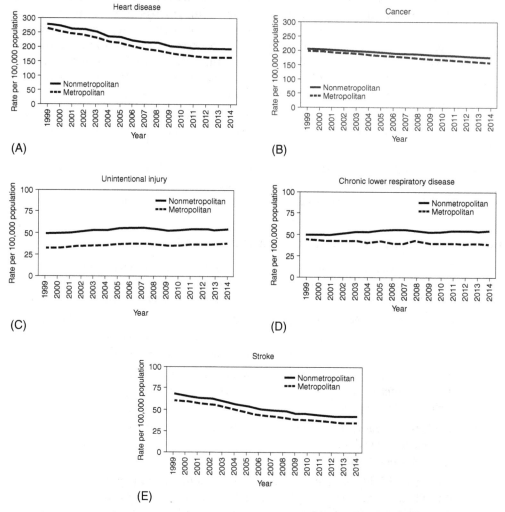

FIGURE 8.2 Age-adjusted death rates among persons of all ages for five leading causes of death in nonmetropolitan and metropolitan areas,* by year.

*Nonmetropolitan and metropolitan areas were identified using the Office of Management and Budget's 2013 county-based classification scheme.

Source: From Moy E, Macarena CG, Bastian B, et al. Leading causes of death in nonmetropolitan and metropolitan areas—United States, 1999–2014. *MMWR Surveill Summ.* 2017;66(6):1–8. https://www.cdc.gov/mmwr/volumes/66/ss/ss6601a1.htm

report prepared by the Centers for Disease Control and Prevention in 2014 found that American Indian and Alaska Native death rates were nearly 50% higher than those of non-Hispanic Whites, with the highest American Indian death rates occurring in the largely rural Northern and Southern Plains.[46] In North Carolina, a state with the highest population of American Indians east of the Mississippi, health outcomes for American Indians are significantly worse than those for Whites.[47] Research indicates that mortality rates for rural African Americans are substantially higher than those for rural Whites.[26] In the Mississippi Delta, a region with many rural counties and a large African American population, the maternal mortality rate is significantly higher than in non-Delta states (18.5/100,000 births vs. 13.6/100,000 births, respectively).[48] Compared to non-Hispanic rural Whites, rural Hispanic populations report higher rates of "fair" or "poor" health.[49] Between 2009 and 2013, the infant mortality rate in Appalachia was 16% higher than the nationwide rate.[50]

Rurality and Mortality

Potentially excess deaths (PEDs) are considered to be those deaths among persons younger than 80 years of age that exceed the number that would be expected for persons of the same ages living in benchmark states, defined as the three states with the lowest death rates for the condition of interest.[36] For each specified condition, the mean death rate in each of the three benchmark states is averaged to determine a single comparison rate for calculating PEDs. Five leading causes of death have been identified based on the *International Classification of Diseases*, 10th Revision (ICD-10), including heart disease, cancer, unintentional injuries, chronic lower respiratory disease, and stroke.[36,51]

When the five leading causes of death in the United States are considered during the years 1999–2014, age-adjusted PED rates are higher in nonmetropolitan areas than in metropolitan areas.[36] While *mortality rate* for heart disease, cancer, and stroke declined for both nonmetropolitan and metropolitan residents during that time period, the decline for heart disease and cancer was slower for nonmetropolitan residents. PEDs from chronic lower respiratory disease increased in nonmetropolitan areas while decreasing in metropolitan areas (54.3% vs. 30.9% PEDs).[36] Unintentional injury PEDs were substantially higher in nonmetropolitan than metropolitan areas during most of the period from 1999 to 2014 (57.5% vs. 39.2%, respectively).[36] PEDs from all of the five leading causes were greater in nonmetropolitan than metropolitan areas. Other causes of death resulting in higher mortality rates for rural areas include diabetes, lung cancer, kidney disease, suicide, influenza, pneumonia, cirrhosis of the liver, Alzheimer's disease, and drug overdose.[36]

Of the five leading causes of death, three—heart disease, cancer, and stroke—are highly associated with nutrition factors that impact both prevention and treatment. Patients suffering from chronic lower respiratory disease—often caused or exacerbated by smoking—may experience significant nutrition difficulties, which require medical nutrition therapy provided by a nutrition professional.[52] Thus, four of the five leading causes of death have strong implications for PHN practitioners.

Substance Abuse in Rural America

Rural residents may be at increased risk for abuse of substances including alcohol, tobacco, and drugs.[53] Remote rural residents admitted to substance abuse treatment facilities were more likely to report their principal drug of abuse as alcohol (49.5%), marijuana (20.9%), and non-heroin opiates, while in large urban areas the primary drugs of abuse were alcohol (36.1%), heroin (21.8%), and marijuana (17.0%).[54] Research comparing rural and urban **substance abuse** statistics is often confounded by which rural/urban definitions are used, as well as other important factors such as race and ethnicity, cultural influences, degree of religiosity, familial relationships and social networks, economic and financial factors, and enforcement of applicable laws and regulations. Data from 2016 indicate that rates of abuse for specific substances vary among nonmetro, small metro, and large metro areas.[89] For example, rates of opioid abuse were 4.0% and 4.5% for nonmetro and large metro areas, respectively.[89] Rural residents typically have less access than urban residents to substance abuse prevention, treatment, and recovery services, thus making substance abuse more problematic even if rates of substance abuse are lower.

Prescription Opioid Abuse

The National Center for Health Statistics (NCHS) reports that the leading cause of death by injury in the United States is poisoning, and that the largest proportion of poison deaths are associated with illegal drugs and pharmaceutical drugs including opioids.[55] States with large rural populations have experienced comparatively greater numbers of deaths and injuries from drug poisoning; examples include the states of West Virginia, Kentucky, New Hampshire, Oklahoma, Utah, Wyoming, New Mexico, Arizona, and Alaska.[56] Public health professionals have indicated that drug poisoning deaths are concentrated in areas with large numbers of rural residents.[56] Higher proportional numbers of drug-related deaths per capita in rural areas may be related to longer first-responder response times, as well as the possibility that continuing education opportunities in regard to drug overdose treatment may be less available in rural settings.[53]

The PHN practitioner should maintain awareness that substance abuse issues can impact the nutrition status of rural populations in a variety of ways. On an individual level, substance abuse may result in a variety of nutrition problems. Macro- and micronutrient deficiencies may become serious and even life-threatening, and are often exacerbated by the secondary effects of drug and alcohol abuse such as drug–nutrient interactions.[57] Overt malnutrition can result from displacement of nutritious foods by substances including drugs and alcohol. Opioid-induced bowel dysfunction, most often manifesting as severe constipation, is a frequent side effect of opioid use even in opioid users supervised by physicians and can have a substantial adverse effect on health and quality of life.[58] On a population level, substance abuse can lead to situations in which appropriate nutrition behaviors are de-emphasized because seeking the substance becomes a primary life priority. Thus, levels of food insecurity for both the affected individual and that person's family may be exacerbated when personal and family resources are used to obtain substances rather than food, with subsequent negative impacts on both individual and family health.[57]

Rural Food Security

The USDA ERS has provided definitions of levels of **food security**.[59] Table 8.2 provides a description of each officially defined category. The USDA ERS reported in 2015 that 84.6% of rural households were food secure compared with 87.8% of metropolitan households, using OMB metropolitan/nonmetropolitan designations.[60] For nonmetropolitan households, 15.4% were food insecure, with 6.1% reporting very low food security. Rates of overall low food security and very low food security for metropolitan residents were 12.2% and 4.9%, respectively. When households with children were considered separately, the overall rates of low food security were 20.5% for nonmetropolitan areas and 15.9% for metropolitan areas.

Poverty is a key indicator of risk for low food security.[61] In rural areas with struggling economies, opportunities for employment sufficient to support an individual's or family's needs may

TABLE 8.2 USDA LEVELS OF FOOD SECURITY

LEVEL	DEFINITION
FOOD SECURITY	
High food security	No reported indications of food-access problems or limitations.
Marginal food security	One or two reported indications—typically of anxiety over food suffi-ciency or shortage of food in the house. Little or no indication of changes in diets or food intake.
FOOD INSECURITY	
Low food security	Reports of reduced quality, variety, or desirability of diet. Little or no indication of reduced food intake.
Very low food security	Reports of multiple indications of disrupted eating patterns and reduced food intake.

USDA, U.S. Department of Agriculture.
Source: From U.S. Department of Agriculture. *Definitions of Food Security.* 2016. https://www.ers.usda.gov/topics/food-nutrition-assistance/food-security-in-the-us/definitions-of-food-security

be scarce or unavailable. Low food security is exacerbated by food-access issues. Availability of adequate, safe, and healthful food may be decreased by the loss of local full-service grocery stores in rural areas; the USDA ERS reported that between 2007 and 2011, nonmetropolitan counties lost an average of 5.77% of their total number of *full-service grocery stores*.[62] Lack of infrastructure for public transportation and/or inability to access private transportation for travel to grocery stores may contribute to higher rates of low food security in rural populations. Food pantries, usually nongovernmental community organizations, which provide emergency food assistance to food-insecure populations, may be less available and accessible to rural residents. In the past two decades, **convenience stores**, including several convenience store chains, have made a concerted effort to locate in rural communities and **food deserts**.[63] Some analysts have expressed concern regarding the impact of convenience stores on existing local businesses. Alongside these concerns, it is acknowledged that convenience stores have brought an expanded selection of foods to rural areas, including some low-fat dairy products, canned and frozen fruits and vegetables, and whole-grain breads and cereals. Few convenience stores offer fresh produce.[63]

Associations Between Low Food Security and Adverse Health Outcomes

Low food security has been linked with higher risk for a number of poor health outcomes.[64,65] Conditions for which low food security is a risk factor include but are not limited to:

- Poor cardiovascular outcomes including hypertension and peripheral arterial disease[64]
- Diabetes[65]
- Chronic kidney disease[66]
- Depression in mothers and behavioral difficulties in preschoolers[67]
- Self-reported fair or poor health, asthma, weight gain, poor academic performance, and social difficulties in children[68]

- Self-reported fair to poor general and mental health, worse academic performance, and compromised dietary intake in university students[69]

- Poor cognitive function, impaired ability to perform activities of daily living (ADLs), increased depressive symptoms, and malnutrition in older adults[70]

Evidence exists to indicate that marginal food security, while not considered low food security, may also be associated with poor outcomes and should be addressed when working with clients.[64]

Because low food security is associated with a plethora of poor health outcomes, the PHN practitioner should assess the food security level of clients and populations and should implement appropriate nutrition education and food-access interventions to improve food security and to link clients/populations with food resources.

CHARACTERISTICS OF HEALTH PROFESSIONALS WHO PRACTICE IN RURAL SETTINGS

Healthcare professionals who choose to build careers in rural settings often report that rural practice is rich in opportunity, fulfilling, and rewarding.[71] Positive aspects of rural health practice include opportunities to get to know patients well over time, to pursue a generalist practice in which one is able to utilize and develop many skills, and to enjoy the feeling of fulfillment that comes from making a positive contribution to the lives of others. Successful rural practice requires autonomy and independence, and persons who enjoy these challenges may thrive. Practitioners also mention quality-of-life advantages: freedom from daily commutes in heavy traffic, less pollution, lower levels of concern regarding crime rates and personal safety, lower costs of living and greater home affordability, a slower pace of life, and perhaps beautiful—even spectacular—natural surroundings.[71] Financial incentives, such as grant monies, state and national funding, and other sources of support are available to some rural providers for repayment of student loans and/or practice start-up costs and maintenance subsidies.[72] Salaries for health providers are not always lower in rural areas: in some locations, the economic law of "supply and demand" may result in sign-on bonuses, generous remuneration, and other incentives such as education benefits and support for practice expenses.

Despite the positive aspects of rural practice, however, recruitment of health professionals to rural settings remains challenging.[73] Financial opportunities in some rural areas may be inadequate for the repayment of the substantial student loans incurred by new practitioners. Amenities, equipment, and facilities to support and enhance practice may be lacking. Employment for an accompanying spouse or partner may be difficult to obtain. Geographic isolation and lack of opportunities to interact with other professionals are challenging. If a practitioner is the only provider in a geographic area, demands for on-call coverage may become problematic. Certain quality-of-life issues can also become barriers to rural practice and may prompt decisions to leave rural settings for relocation to an urban area.[73] Practitioners may be impacted by poor access to cultural, entertainment, and educational opportunities for oneself and one's family, scarcity of important services including quality childcare and excellent schools, lack of adequate shopping resources, and the time and distance required to commute to metropolitan areas to access desired services.

Best Practices for Recruiting Rural Practitioners

A small body of research regarding the recruitment and retention of rural physicians, physician assistants, and nurses provides guidelines for increasing the number of health professionals entering rural practice.[72,74,75] The literature currently provides context and background for interventions designed to augment the workforce of rural practitioners from other specialties such as nutrition and dietetics, public health nutrition, physical therapy, occupational therapy, speech/language therapy, social work, and mental health providers.

Practices such as modifying medical school admission practices by moving from a score-focused admission process to a mission-focused admission process may help to increase the number of rural health practitioners.[74,76] In other words, if a state or region identifies a need to prepare more students to enter rural health practice, careful identification of students who have a strong desire to work in rural areas may be a best practice for achieving desired rural workforce goals. Research findings suggest that rural upbringing and receiving hands-on training in rural health settings are positively associated with physician choice to practice in a rural setting.[77] Best practices for recruiting physicians, and by inference other practitioners including PHN practitioners, to rural areas may include (a) identifying appropriate students, as early as high school age, who want to build their lives and careers in rural settings; (b) keeping those students in-state for their entire education and arranging their practicum experiences in rural health settings; (c) providing seamless support throughout the education process from high school through professional education and credentialing; and (d) providing incentives, including financial incentives, to build practices in rural areas and to remain in those areas.[78-81]

Settings for Rural Practice

Rural nutrition practitioners work in a variety of settings. Settings include but are not limited to rural hospitals and nursing homes; health departments including local/county Special Supplemental Nutrition Program for Women, Infants, and Children (WIC) programs and food assistance programs; nonprofit agencies; public schools; federal, state, and regional administrations; and other organizations.

Two nutrition practice settings of special importance in rural areas are **Rural Health Clinics (RHCs)** or **Federally Qualified Health Centers (FQHCs)**. Both RHCs and FQHCs provide expanded opportunities for underserved and low-income rural residents to access healthcare services.[82] RHCs and FQHCs are important settings for nutrition care, because both types of organizations are able to bill Medicare and Medicaid for diabetes self-management training and medical nutrition therapy.[83] In addition, funding requirements for FQHCs include the provision of **wraparound services** to address social determinants—including nutrition determinants—of health. Table 8.3 provides a side-by-side comparison of RHC and FQHC characteristics.

Distinctives of Rural Practice

Several unique factors may affect rural health practitioners, including rural PHN practitioners. These include privacy concerns, **dual relationships**, the need to attain both generalist and specialist skills, and the need to maintain professional competence and linkages with colleagues.

In sparsely populated rural areas in which extensive kinship networks, long-term friendships and animosities, and shared history result in situations in which many people who live in close proximity know each other well, appropriate legal and personal privacy boundaries can be difficult to maintain.[84] Situations such as well-meant but public sharing of prayer requests at faith-based community organizations and a neighbor recognizing a parked car outside a practitioner office can result in privacy concerns. Attempts to curtail local practices may be viewed by community residents as "outsiders" imposing unwanted control over community customs.[84] Some investigators have found heightened stigma in rural areas surrounding specific health conditions.[30] PHN

TABLE 8.3 DIFFERENCES BETWEEN RHCs AND FQHCs

RHCs	FQHCs
For-profit or nonprofit	Nonprofit or public facility
May be limited to a specific type of primary care practice (e.g., OB/GYN, pediatrics)	Required to provide care for all age groups
Not required to have a board of directors	Required to have a board of directors; at least 51% must be patients of the health center
No minimum service requirements	Minimum service required; maternity and prenatal care, preventive care, behavioral health, dental health, emergency care, and pharmaceutical services
Not required to charge based on a sliding fee scale	Required to treat all residents in their service area with charges based on a sliding fee scale
Not required to provide a minimum of hours or emergency coverage	Required to be open 32.5 hours a week for FTCA coverage of licensed or certified healthcare providers; must provide emergency service after business hours either on-site or by arrangement with another health-care provider
Required to conduct an annual program evaluation regarding quality improvement	Required to have an ongoing quality assurance program
Must be located in a Health Professional Shortage Area, Medically Underserved Area, or governor-designated and secretary-certified shortage area; may retain RHC status if designation of service area changes	Must be located in an area that is underserved or experiencing a shortage of healthcare providers
RHCs must operate in nonurbanized areas	FQHCs may operate in both nonurbanized and urbanized areas
Required to submit an annual cost report; however, auditing of financial reports is not required	Required to submit an annual cost report and audited financial reports

FQHCs, Federally Qualified Health Centers; FTCA, Federal Tort Claims Act; RHCs, Rural Health Clinics.
Source: From Rural Health Information Hub. *Rural Health Clinics (RHCs).* 2019. https://www.ruralhealthinfo.org/topics/rural-health-clinics

practitioners who work in rural areas should be vigilant in regard to maintaining all appropriate legal and ethical privacy boundaries. Examples of situations in which privacy becomes paramount include protecting the privacy of clients seeking nutrition advice or public food assistance.

Dual relationships occur when there is a "blurring" of professional boundaries because of social relationships.[78,84] A PHN practitioner working in a rural setting is very likely to encounter clients in community social settings such as children's school gatherings, local sports events, and community venues such as churches and government agencies. In rural settings, strict prohibition of dual relationships may be counterproductive, since the development of local relationships and a presence in the community are necessary for effective practice. A proactive approach to dual relationships may be helpful.[78] That is, during professional encounters, clients can be told that in a social situation, the practitioner will not refer to any previous professional interaction unless the client initiates the discussion, and even then, the practitioner will not engage in conversation in situations in which privacy cannot be maintained. Practitioners may also find it helpful to develop a pre-prepared answer, or **script**, for occasions when an inappropriate question may be asked in a social setting. For example, if asked to provide information about a particular client, the practitioner may be prepared to reply, "Federal privacy laws prevent me from talking about who does or doesn't visit my facility." A beneficial outcome of such a pre-prepared answer is that trust is built as community residents realize that privacy is respected and taken seriously by the PHN practitioner.

Rural practitioners need both generalist and specialist skills. For example, rural nurses primarily act as generalists, providing care to patients with a variety of common conditions. However, rural nurses also need specialist training in advanced life support skills, needed when preparing severely injured or critically ill patients for transport to higher level facilities. In the same way, rural PHN practitioners need strong generalist knowledge in basic nutrition, nutrition education skills, and nutrition intervention strategies and evaluation, while also acquiring specialist-level knowledge in rural health topics.

Continuing education may be a challenge for rural PHN practitioners. Financial resources may be lacking to provide access to education programs and associated expenses such as tuition and travel. Lack of infrastructure such as broadband Internet access may also impact practitioners' ability to access web-based educational programs. Some rural facilities have been successful in obtaining grant funding, education sponsorships, and other resources to support staff education. Distance education strategies for continuing education for rural practitioners show promise in areas where Internet access is available.[79] Rural facilities may partner with other healthcare organizations and groups to provide continuing education, thus increasing resources for training and continuing education.[90] PHN practitioners should take responsibility for identifying resources and obtaining adequate continuing education to keep knowledge and skills up to date.

CULTURAL COMPETENCE IN RURAL HEALTH SETTINGS IN THE UNITED STATES

There is no one recognized definition of **cultural competence**.[80] According to the National Center for Cultural Competence (NCCC), although there are a number of useful definitions of "cultural competence," the work of Cross et al. in 1989 provided the groundwork for defining the term and has remained the basis for the discipline's fundamental principles since that time. According to Cross et al., cultural competence is

a set of congruent behaviors, attitudes, and policies that come together in a system, agency, or among professionals and enable that system, agency, or those professionals to work effectively in cross-cultural situations.[84]

Cross et al. go on to define "culture" as

the integrated pattern of human behavior that includes thoughts, communications, actions, customs, beliefs, values, and institutions of a racial, ethnic, religious, or social group.[84]

"Competence" is described as

the capacity to function effectively.[84]

Thus, a culturally competent public health nutritionist is one who functions effectively within a diverse variety of professional and community settings to plan, implement, and evaluate respectful, culturally appropriate interventions, which are delivered alongside and in alignment with the target population's distinctive customs, beliefs, and values.

Applications of Cultural Competence Skills in Rural Settings

Respectful care delivery in rural settings requires that the PHN practitioner perform self-assessment of one's **cultural awareness** in regard to populations served. As an example, consider the culture of southern Appalachia, which resulted from the mingling of many groups of people including but not limited to the original American Indian inhabitants, enslaved persons from Africa transported to North America against their will, Scots-Irish settlers who traveled from Europe to the Appalachian mountains before America's War for Independence, and more recent newcomers who have immigrated from an array of nations.[85] Despite this broad diversity, familiar pejoratives such as "hillbillies" and "rednecks" are still used to refer to entire groups of southern Appalachian people.[86] Similar pejoratives have been applied to many other rural population groups around the nation.

Stereotypes are inaccurate and unhelpful because all rural populations are composed of diverse groups of individuals that defy simple categorization and description.[5] The PHN practitioner should not apply cultural generalizations to any particular person. Rather, within a given cultural context, practitioners should respectfully get to know people as individuals.

Stereotypes not only perpetuate harmful myths but impair professionals' ability to provide effective health interventions to rural communities.[87] When initially entering a rural area, it is important for PHN practitioners to take adequate time to observe, listen, and learn about local customs, history, cultural distinctives, and social norms and expectations in all their variety and diversity.[87] PHN practitioners should not underestimate the amount of time needed to develop productive, trusting relationships. A sense of humility and a true willingness to listen carefully to residents will likely be productive in nurturing community connections.

It is essential to gain a thorough understanding of a particular rural culture prior to implementing public health nutrition interventions within that culture. Focusing on the development of relationships with key individuals who can provide consultation and advice regarding specific interventions can be of great help in preventing unintended missteps, especially for entry-level professionals. The PHN practitioner should work to build trust, mutual understanding, and partnerships within the local community. In some rural cultures, people who are "not from around here" will be considered outsiders. Nutrition interventions that are developed in partnership with participatory community members, culturally sensitive, aligned with community values and initiatives, and embedded within existing community frameworks are most likely to be effective.[91]

CULTURALLY COMPETENT PUBLIC HEALTH NUTRITION INTERVENTIONS IN THE RURAL UNITED STATES: AN INTERPROFESSIONAL APPROACH

The Rural Health Nutrition Practice Model

The RHNPM was developed by Gutschall and Thompson as a result of qualitative research involving the coding of in-depth interviews with rural southern Appalachian residents and nutrition practitioners located in the mountainous regions of northwestern North Carolina.[88] The purpose of the RHNPM is to provide an interprofessional framework for developing effective nutrition interventions for specific rural populations. Preliminary findings have suggested that the RHNPM may be applicable to rural populations from areas other than Appalachia.

The RHNPM describes four broad themes, which emerged from coded interviews with rural residents and rural nutrition practitioners in an Appalachian population. Each theme, along with

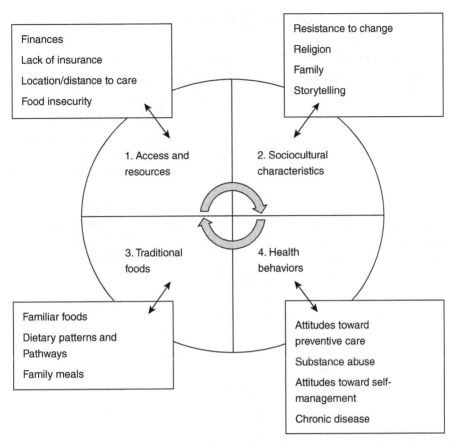

FIGURE 8.3 Rural Health Nutrition Practice Model based on qualitative analysis of interviews with residents and nutrition practitioners from rural Appalachia.

Source: From Gutschall M, Thompson KL. Addressing health disparities in rural nutrition practice: a qualitative model from rural Appalachia. *J Hunger Environ Nutr.* 2017;13(1):84–89.

respective selected subthemes, is represented in Figure 8.3. *Access and resources* refers to the population's ability to access food and nutrition resources as well as the adequacy of available resources. *Sociocultural characteristics* are those culturally related traits, attitudes, beliefs, and practices that may tend to be descriptive of a particular population, although practitioners should always avoid overgeneralizations when working with individuals. *Traditional foods* are particular foods and eating patterns that are important within a particular region and/or population; these may be historical or current foods and eating patterns. *Health behaviors* are common health practices and health beliefs that may impact nutritional well-being and overall health outcomes. Figure 8.4 provides a working example of a PHN intervention implemented within a rural Appalachian context.

PHN practitioners may use the RHNPM to develop culturally appropriate interventions for specific populations. *Within the four broad themes, PHN practitioners should substitute subthemes based on their specific rural populations served.* Identification of population-specific subthemes can be accomplished through a systematic information-gathering and organizing process, as described in the following:

- Conduct focus groups or interviews and/or survey the population served. Structure information-gathering tools and sessions to focus on the four broad areas of access and resources, sociocultural characteristics, traditional foods, and health behaviors.

- Based on the results of information gathering, organize responses within the four broad categories.
- Identify common themes within the responses under each category.
- Summarize and arrange the common themes under each category using the RHNPM worksheet.

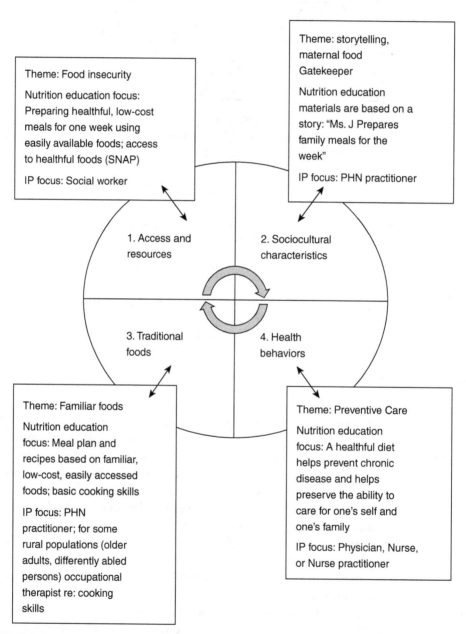

FIGURE 8.4 Intervention example based on Rural Health Nutrition Practice Model, among a rural Appalachian population, with IP suggestions

IP, interprofessional practice; PHN, public health nutrition; SNAP, Supplemental Nutrition Assistance Program.

Source: From Gutschall M, Thompson KL. Addressing health disparities in rural nutrition practice: a qualitative model from rural Appalachia. *J Hunger Environ Nutr.* 2017;13(1):84–89.

Using the RHNPM to Optimize Interprofessional Collaborations

Figure 8.4 provides suggestions for **interprofessional** collaborations within each of the four broad categories of a specific rural public health nutrition intervention. When utilizing the RHNPM, the public health practitioner should recall that interventions may be enhanced through appropriate interprofessional collaborations. Interprofessional involvement in interventions may be through direct participation, or of a consultative nature. Health professionals who are commonly found working in rural health settings include physicians, physician assistants, nurses and nurse practitioners, mental health professionals including school counselors, registered dietitian nutritionists, WIC nutritionists, social workers, public health professionals, physical and occupational therapists, respiratory therapists, and others. The roles of each discipline should be considered carefully, and appropriate collaboration/participation should be considered when planning public health nutrition interventions. Collaboration may not be necessary for every intervention or every step of a particular intervention; however, the process of thinking through the need for interprofessional participation will strengthen the final intervention whether or not other professionals are utilized.

CONTINUING YOUR LEARNING

The rural PHN practitioner should develop a personal plan for continued learning and skill development to support competent practice. Such a plan may include self-assessment of knowledge, skills, and professionalism, along with plans to address identified areas for further development. A number of resources and organizations have focused on rural health, and an abundance of data for study and use is available from federal, state, regional, and local sources. Often the Rural Health Information Hub (the Hub; www.ruralhealthinfo.org) is an excellent place to start when researching rural health topics because the Hub serves as a national clearinghouse for rural health information. In addition to providing both breadth and depth of information, the Hub provides many links to additional information. State offices of rural health can be excellent resources for further learning about rural health. A list of resources for learning more about rural health and rural nutrition practice is provided later in this chapter under Continue Your Learning Resources.

CONCLUSION

Rural health settings offer many strengths and assets that can be leveraged in improving health outcomes for residents as well as specific challenges for the PHN practitioner. A career in rural PHN offers the potential for personal fulfillment while impacting many lives for the better. For PHN practitioners who enjoy practicing with autonomy, developing productive helping relationships with clients over time, cultivating both breadth and depth of professional skills, and enjoying the advantages offered by a rural lifestyle, a career in rural PHN may be an excellent fit.

KEY CONCEPTS

1. There is no one definition of the term "rural." Rural populations and regions are diverse and constantly changing. Three federal definitions of the term are most often used by public health practitioners: the USCB definition, the OMB definition, and the USDA ERS definition of RUCCs and RUCA codes. The federal definitions are

definitions of exclusion: that is, "urban" is defined, and whatever is not urban is rural. The PHN practitioner, when seeking to implement programs and obtain funding for rural programs, should use an appropriate definition for the purpose intended.

2. Rural populations, in regard to health and nutrition care, may face problems and barriers different from those encountered by urban residents.

3a. Rural areas display many strengths and assets that can be leveraged to address community and regional challenges. While rural areas do indeed face health disparities, they can also demonstrate extensive social capital, social networks, close connections among cross-sector partners, and high levels of creativity in addressing challenges.

3b. An understanding of access, quality, and equity issues is central to effective public health nutrition practice in rural areas. The PHN practitioner should seek to identify and define specific access, quality, and equity issues that may create health disparities for the population served.

4a. Rates of potentially excessive deaths from the five leading causes of death in America are higher for rural than for urban populations. The five leading causes of death include heart disease, cancer, unintentional injury, chronic lower respiratory disease, and stroke. Of the five leading causes of death in rural America, three have direct associations with nutrition, and nutrition therapy is important in the treatment of the remaining two causes.

4b. PHN practitioners should be aware that substance abuse is an issue in both rural and urban settings. The PHN practitioner should assess target populations for rates of substance abuse in regard to its impacts on nutrition-related choices and behaviors.

4c. Rural areas tend to have proportionately higher numbers of persons experiencing low food security. Because low food security is associated with a variety of poor health outcomes, the PHN practitioner should assess the food security level of clients and populations and should implement appropriate interventions to improve food security and to link clients/populations with food resources.

5. Rural health practitioners choose to practice in rural areas for a variety of reasons. At the same time, barriers to rural practice are significant and have resulted in a preponderance of HPSAs in nonmetropolitan counties. Persons who were raised in rural areas are more likely to return to rural areas to practice health careers. Barriers to rural practice should be addressed, and PHN practitioners should be provided with training and education specific to common rural issues encountered in practice. Common issues for practitioners may include privacy, dual relationships, the need to develop both generalist and specialist skills, and maintaining competence through continuing education and linkages with colleagues.

6. Cultural competence is necessary when working with rural populations. The PHN practitioner should seek to be culturally competent, defined as a practitioner who functions effectively within a diverse variety of professional and community settings to plan, implement, and evaluate respectful, culturally appropriate interventions, which are delivered alongside and in alignment with the target population's distinctive customs, beliefs, and values. Rural is not homogeneous; rural areas encompass great diversity in terms of race/ethnicity, prominent employment sectors, and regional culture and norms. Culturally competent practitioners approach rural populations with humility and a true desire to learn about their unique community experiences.

7. Effective rural public health nutrition interventions utilize a framework that incorporates the specific target population's available resources and ability to access resources, sociocultural characteristics including sociocultural determinants of health status, traditional foods including cultural and historical dietary patterns, and health beliefs and behaviors including cultural definitions of health, self-management practices, attitudes toward preventive care, and incidence and risk of chronic disease. Sociocultural characteristics and geographic obstacles associated with rurality, reliance on customary food patterns, and adherence to certain culturally based health behaviors may contribute to poor health outcomes. The PHN practitioner should use an appropriate theoretical framework for planning effective nutrition interventions for rural populations.

8. Effective public health nutrition interventions utilize a framework that integrates the skills of the interprofessional healthcare team in order to enhance client outcomes.

9. The PHN practitioner who works in a rural area should develop a personal development plan to maintain and improve both general and setting-focused practice skills.

CASE STUDY: A RURAL FOOD PANTRY CLIENT: HELPING A SINGLE MOTHER INCREASE THE NUTRITIONAL QUALITY OF MEALS PREPARED AT HOME

In a highly rural Midwestern state, an active food pantry *Food for All (FFA)* operates in conjunction with a soup kitchen, homeless shelter, free medical clinic, and free pharmacy. Services are funded by a community nonprofit agency, which is supported by grant funding, donations, a regional food bank, and a number of local volunteers who provide many hours of free labor and services. FFA has worked hard to develop positive, collaborative relationships with local and county religious communities, which provide donations of money, food, and volunteer assistance. The organization's mission, strongly emphasized by its director and governing board, is to (a) provide essential food assistance to county residents, (b) address root causes of hunger, and (c) educate clients and the wider community on hunger-related issues. *FFA* works hard to promote independence and self-efficacy among its client base.

Research has demonstrated that nutrition education promotes self-efficacy and reduces food insecurity scores (measured using the USDA food insecurity scale). *FFA* has partnered with a nutrition and dietetics department in a college in an adjoining county to make individualized basic nutrition education available to its clients. Under the supervision of licensed dietitians, advanced nutrition students are now meeting with selected clients for one-on-one nutrition education appointments. The appointments include training in regard to basic nutrition using materials online (www.choosemyplate.gov), menu planning, optimization of food resources, and cooking skills. Individual nutrition counseling appointments will also include instruction in the use of *FFA's* new food distribution system, the *FFA Fresh Market*. The self-select *Fresh Market* model is arranged to appear as a grocery store so that food pantry clients can browse and self-select available food items. The market is arranged to emphasize fresh fruits and vegetables, whole grains, and other healthful foods. Signage throughout the market is easily readable and provides guidelines for food selections.

Ms. J, a single mother of three children, works full time in her rural county and does not have health insurance. Ms. J and her family qualify for $361.00 in Supplemental Nutrition

Assistance Program (SNAP) benefits monthly, and her children are insured through her state's Children's Health Insurance Program (CHIP). Ms. J's monthly income after deductions is about $1,850, and her housing expenses including utilities consume about 60% of that amount. The remaining funds provide her with less than $200 per week to cover all other expenses. Thus, SNAP benefits are a vital lifeline to nutritious food for Ms. J and her family. Ms. J does have a small kitchen with a stove and refrigerator in good working order, and she enjoys cooking when she has time.

Although Ms. J utilizes the *FFA*, she also takes advantage of a food pantry operated by a local church when emergency expenses cut into the food budget. Ms. J was recently offered a promotion. The offer has placed her in the difficult situation of having to worry if the modest increase in income would result in the loss of some of her SNAP benefits and her children's health insurance, which would ultimately decrease her ability to feed her family. Ms. J is very interested in providing her children with nutritious, healthy meals. She has recently arranged to meet with the *Fresh Market* nutrition student to help her increase the nutritional quality of meals she prepares at home and to provide some healthful, low-cost recipes.

Case Study Questions

For this case study, assume that you are an advanced nutrition student who will be meeting with Ms. J. Answer the following questions:

1. How might you assess Ms. J's current nutrition knowledge?
2. Research indicates that nutrition education can help to reduce food insecurity. What do you think could be the reasons for this?
3. What rural associated factors influence Ms. J's access to food?
4. What barriers do you foresee Ms. J facing in terms of feeding her family?
5. Ms. J has been working at her present job for 4 years and has been asked if she is interested in assuming a management position. Although enticing, she is afraid of losing her SNAP benefits and the children's health insurance if she earns more money. A promotion, she worries, might actually decrease her ability to feed her family once her current benefits are reduced. Which member of the interprofessional team could be most helpful to Ms. J in discussing her options as well as the impact of the promotion on her current SNAP benefits?
6. What nutrition and food resources does Ms. J have available to her at this time?
7. What would be important considerations in selecting appropriate recipes for a rural, low-income client? Select an appropriate recipe and provide it. Why is your chosen recipe appropriate for Ms. J?
8. Which topics (three to five maximum) will you plan to cover during your 45-minute appointment with Ms. J? Why have you chosen each topic?
9. How will you help Ms. J learn to use the new *Fresh Market*?
10. What resources will you recommend to Ms. J for continued learning? Are there any barriers you will need to consider when recommending resources? How will you follow up with Ms. J?

SUGGESTED LEARNING ACTIVITIES

1. Based on the USDA ERS definition of RUCCs, how is your county of residence designated? Now look at RUCCs for your state. Which are your state's most urban counties? Which are the most rural? Do you agree with these designations, and why or why not?

2. For each of the following situations, describe your reasoning regarding the choice of a definition of "rural" to use in applying for grant funding:

   a. Commuting practices of nurses and dietitians who work at a rural county health department providing primary care and WIC services, respectively

   b. Impact of a proposed regional airport on productive farmland in a rural county

   c. Access to food resources such as full-service grocery stores in a metropolitan or micropolitan area

3. Research national, state, or regional databases to find rates for substance abuse, including misuse of alcohol, tobacco, and prescription or recreational drugs in your county or region. How might your findings impact nutrition-related choices and behaviors of residents? Compare rates for an urban and rural county in your region or state. How might you explain your findings?

4. What are rates of food insecurity for your county or region? Visit a rural food pantry to gather information from the pantry director, manager, or another supervisor. How many clients does the pantry serve? How much food is distributed annually? Who are the pantry's typical clients? How is food obtained? Does the pantry offer wraparound services such as job training, stable housing, counseling, nutrition education, or other offerings designed to promote self-efficacy? What are the pantry director's thoughts regarding best practices for approaching rural food insecurity?

5. HPSAs are common in rural regions of the United States. Is there a shortage of health professionals in your county/region? Interview a rural health professional to ask for the practitioner's opinion about advantages/disadvantages of rural practice, as well as the reasons the practitioner thinks some professionals may avoid rural practice.

6. What are some common issues associated with maintenance of patient/client privacy in rural health settings? Develop one or two examples of scripting that could be used in response to inappropriate questions.

7. Develop your own definition of cultural competence. Compare your definition with one or two other colleagues' definitions and revise your definition as appropriate.

8. Use the RHNPM to develop a culturally appropriate nutrition intervention for a chosen rural region. Prepare associated learning materials. Describe members of the interprofessional healthcare team needed for the most effective implementation of your intervention.

9. What are some rural health resources and community assets available in your area/region? What nutrition-specific resources are available? Create a resource list. Implement an Internet search for resources and contact key individuals and organizations as appropriate to complete your list.

10. Create a personal developmental plan to both improve and maintain general and setting-focused skills for rural public health nutrition practice. In your plan, include at least three learning goals, as well as at least three references for appropriate resources for further learning. Justify your choice of each resource.

REFLECTION QUESTIONS

1. What are the strengths and weaknesses of each of the three official government definitions of the word "rural?" If you were asked to choose one of the three definitions as being most representative of the meaning of "rural," which would it be? Justify your answer.

2. What factors should be considered by the PHN practitioner when choosing a definition of "rural" to apply to a particular project?

3. In regard to health and nutrition care, what are some of the problems and barriers rural regions may face compared to urban areas? Provide an example for each of these broad areas of rural issues: (a) access; (b) quality; (c) equity.

4. What leading causes of death in rural areas are nutrition-related? For each of the causes, what are specific associated nutrition concerns?

5. How might substance abuse issues impact the nutrition status of rural individuals and populations?

6. Food insecurity rates tend to be higher in rural areas, compared to urban counterparts. How might the PHN practitioner assess food insecurity levels of individuals residing in rural areas? What are some appropriate interventions?

7. What are some common challenges rural health practitioners face when working in rural areas? What might be some unique challenges for nutrition practice? List and discuss at least three such challenges.

8. What steps would an organization need to take in order to obtain the RHC designation?

9. Why is cultural competence important when working with rural populations?

10. Describe the RHNPM and its application as a theoretical framework for planning effective PHN interventions.

11. Which members of the interprofessional healthcare team might be involved in planning and delivering PHN interventions in rural settings? Describe the role of each profession in intervention delivery.

CONTINUE YOUR LEARNING RESOURCES

The Sheps Center at the University of North Carolina: https://www.shepscenter.unc.edu/programs-projects/rural-health/rural-hospital-closures/
Federal Office of Rural Health Policy: https://www.hrsa.gov/rural-health/index.html
National Rural Health Association: https://www.ruralhealthweb.org
Rural Health Information Hub: https://www.ruralhealthinfo.org/
Rural Health Research Gateway: https://www.ruralhealthresearch.org/centers
Rural Policy Research Institute: http://www.rupri.org
State Offices of Rural Health: https://nosorh.org/

GLOSSARY

Community assets: Any asset, characteristic, or resource (financial, material, human) that has the potential to be used to improve the quality of life in a community (ctb.ku.edu/en/table-of-contents/assessment/assessing-community-needs-and-resources/identify-community-assets/main).

Community strengths: See Community assets.

Convenience stores: Typically, stores with a limited selection of groceries, designed for quick in and out with purchase of only a few items. Convenience stores may provide snack foods, soft drinks, ready-to-eat items such as sandwiches and pizza, and a few staple foods such as milk and bread. Some convenience stores provide a more extensive selection of groceries, but typically lack fresh fruits and vegetables and fresh meats.

Core-based statistical area: The county or counties associated with at least one core (urbanized area or urban cluster of at least 10,000 residents) plus adjacent counties having a significant degree of social and/or economic integration with the core as measured by commuting ties with core-associated counties. The term "core-based statistical area" is used to refer to both metropolitan (population of 50,000 or more) and micropolitan (10,000 to <50,000) designations. Areas with population <10,000 are designated "noncore" (https://www.census.gov/topics/housing/housing-patterns/about/core-based-statistical-areas.html).

Culture: The customary beliefs, social forms, and material traits of a racial, religious, or social group; *also*, the characteristic features of everyday existence (such as diversions or a way of life) shared by people in a place or time (www.merriam-webster.com/dictionary/culture).

Cultural awareness: Acknowledgment of differences, including attitudes, values, and perspectives, between the self and individuals from other backgrounds or parts of the world.

Cultural competence: Cultural competence is a set of congruent behaviors, attitudes, and policies that come together in a system, agency, or among professionals and enable that system, agency, or those professionals to work effectively in cross-cultural situations[84] (nccc.georgetown.edu/curricula/culturalcompetence.html).

Dual relationships: Occur when there is a "blurring" of professional boundaries because of social relationships, as in a situation in which a health practitioner also sees clients socially. Such relationships are often deleterious to professional interactions. Dual relationships are not always inappropriate but should be intentional and carefully monitored by the practitioner.[79]

Federal Office of Rural Health Policy (FORHP): Housed within the Health Resources and Services Administration (HRSA) of the Department of Health and Human Services (DHHS). Designates all nonmetro counties as "rural" and uses an additional designator of rurality, the RUCA codes. The FORHP collaborated with the USDA Economic Research Service to create the RUCAs (www.hrsa.gov/rural-health/index.html).

Federally Qualified Health Center (FQHC): A health center that receives funding from the HRSA and is charged with providing primary care services to underserved populations. FQHCs are mandated to meet a number of requirements, including continuous quality assessment, billing for services on an ability-to-pay sliding scale, and governance by a board that includes at least 51% center patients (www.hrsa.gov/opa/eligibility-and-registration/health-centers/fqhc/index.html).

Food desert: The USDA defines a "food desert" as a neighborhood that lacks healthy food resources; characteristics that contribute to food deserts include income level, distance to supermarkets, and access to vehicles (www.ers.usda.gov/data-products/food-access-research -atlas/documentation).

Food security: Categories are as follows: (a) high food security: no reported food-access problems or limitations; (b) marginal food security: one or two reported indications—typically of anxiety over food sufficiency or shortage of food in the house and little or no indication of changes in diets or food intake; (c) low food security: reports of reduced quality, variety, or desirability of diet and little or no indication of reduced food intake; (d) very low food security: reports of multiple indications of disrupted eating patterns and reduced food intake[59] (https://www.ers.usda.gov/topics/food-nutrition-assistance/food-security-in-the-us/ definitions-of-food-security/).

Full-service grocery store: Typically, a retail store that sells a wide selection of groceries including fresh and frozen fruits and vegetables, meats, dairy products, grains and cereals, and infant foods/formulas. Full-service grocery stores are designed for longer and more extensive shopping trips, in which purchase of all food supplies needed for a period of time can be accomplished (mohealth.uservoice.com/knowledgebase/articles/1849183-what-is-a-full-service -grocery-store).

Healthcare disparities: Differences in access to or availability of facilities and services (www. nlm.nih.gov/hsrinfo/disparities.html).

Health Professional Shortage Area (HPSA): A designation that indicates a specific entity suffers health provider shortages in one or more of three provider types: primary care, dental care, and mental health. HPSAs may be geographically based, population-based (i.e., a shortage of providers for a specific population group), or facility-based (bhw.hrsa.gov/shortage -designation/hpsas).

Health status disparities: Variation in rates of disease occurrence or disabilities among socioeconomic or geographically defined population groups, resulting from health disparities (www.nlm.nih.gov/hsrinfo/disparities.html).

Holler: Geographically, a long, narrow lowland between mountains or hills, often rising in elevation from the entrance to the furthest point along the lowland; often has a creek or river running along the bottom; usually has only one way in and out. In Appalachian parlance, one might say, "I live down in the holler."[85]

Interprofessional: Occurring between or involving two or more professions or professionals. In healthcare, interprofessional collaborations bring together persons who practice two or more healthcare disciplines in order to promote optimized outcomes for patients or clients (www.merriam-webster.com/dictionary/interprofessional).

Metropolitan: A county containing an urbanized area with a population over 50,000; can also include adjacent counties that do not meet the urbanized population requirements for metropolitan status but are linked to the neighboring metropolitan county by commuting and employment patterns. (See Core-based statistical area.)

Micropolitan: A nonmetropolitan county that includes an urbanized area with a population of 10,000 to < 50,000 population.

Mortality: The number of deaths in a given time or place (www.merriam-webster.com/dictionary/mortality).

Non-core rural county: A county that has no urbanized areas with populations in excess of 10,000.

Potentially excess deaths: Deaths among persons <80 years old in excess of the number that would be expected if the group-specific death rates of chosen benchmark states occurred across all states (www.cdc.gov/mmwr/volumes/66/ss/ss6602a1.htm).

Resilience: The ability to adapt successfully to life stressors and adverse events; occurs at both individual and community levels. Resilience is often described as the ability to "bounce back" from negative life occurrences (www.apa.org/helpcenter/road-resilience.aspx).

Rural: According to the USCB, "rural" encompasses any land area that is not urban (https://www.census.gov/programs-surveys/geography/guidance/geo-areas/urban-rural.html).

Rural Health Clinic (RHC): A clinic, designated as such by the Centers for Medicare and Medicaid Services (CMS), providing primary care services to residents of rural, underserved areas. RHCs receive enhanced reimbursement rates from Medicare and Medicaid for approved services. RHCs operate under a different set of requirements than FQHCs (www.cms.gov/Outreach-and-Education/Medicare-Learning-Network-MLN/MLNProducts/downloads/Rural-HlthClinfctsht.pdf).

Rural hospital closures: Rural hospitals have been closing in recent years at rates higher than those of nonrural hospitals. Since 2005, at least 168 rural hospitals have gone out of business, and the trend continues to increase.[32] Closings are usually related to financial challenges. Rural hospitals tend to care for a patient base that is likely to be smaller, and experience difficulties related to physician and caregiver shortages. In addition, rural patients are more likely to be uninsured. The closure of a rural hospital is typically devastating to the communities affected in terms of access to care, consequences to the local economy including direct loss of jobs, and community morale. The populations most affected by rural hospital closures tend to be the poor, minorities, and older adults with chronic conditions (www.hrsa.gov/enews/past-issues/2017/october-19/hospitals-closing-increase.html).

Rurality: A term used to indicate that rural areas are not homogeneous; various degrees of rurality affect the characteristics of a given rural area (www.census.gov/newsroom/blogs/random-samplings/2016/12/rurality_matters.html).

Rural populations: The USCB considers all populations residing outside an urban area, consisting of UAs (50,000+ residents) or UCs (2,500–50,000 residents) to be "rural" populations. The OMB considers all persons residing outside an MSA (>50,000 residents) to be part of the "rural" population; the OMB designation of "rural" includes micropolitan areas. The USDA considers persons living in counties with RUCC designations of 4 to 10 to be "rural" with 10 indicating the highest degree of rurality. In addition, in collaboration with the USDA Economic Research Service, the FORHP considers all census tracts designated 4 to 10 on the RUCA scale to be rural with 10 designating the greatest degree of rurality (www.hrsa.gov/rural-health/about-us/definition/index.html).

Rural–Urban Commuting Area (RUCA) Codes: The FORHP has collaborated with the USDA ERS to develop RUCAs. The system categorizes all census tracts based on population density and work commuting patterns, ranging from 1 for a census tract in a metropolitan area core through 10 for a completely rural tract with no work commuting to an urban area. Typically, RUCAs 1 to 3 are considered urban, with the remainder either micropolitan, small town, or completely dispersed rural. A ZIP code approximation of RUCAs is available for use when census tract information is not available. The use of RUCA codes allows for identification of rural areas within metropolitan counties (RUCCs 1–3); for example, the Grand Canyon is located in an Arizona county designated "metropolitan." In the United States, there are 132 very large area census tracts in which the RUCA code fails to account for long distances to services and low population; therefore, these areas have been designated "rural" although their official RUCA code is 2 or 3 (www.ers.usda.gov/data-products/rural-urban-commuting-area-codes).

Rural–Urban Continuum Codes (RUCCs): The USDA ERS has categorized degrees of rurality by the use of RUCCs, designated from 1 to 9. These codes are assigned by county. Each county in the United States has been assigned an RUCC based on population density, degree of urbanization, and adjacency to metro areas. RUCCs 1 to 3 are designated metropolitan areas; RUCCs 4 to 9 are designated nonmetropolitan areas. An RUCC of 1 indicates a county that has a metropolitan area with a population size of 1 million or more; an RUCC of 9 indicates a county with a population center of <2,500 or completely rural, and nonadjacent to any metropolitan county (www.ers.usda.gov/data-products/rural-urban-continuum-codes.aspx).

Script: Prepared text used for delivering standardized responses in common healthcare situations. Scripts may be useful for greeting clients, answering the telephone, and responding to patient privacy questions. Scripts can be very helpful in enhancing consistency and quality in client interactions as well as reinforcing organizational culture and goals. However, care must be taken when utilizing scripts to remain genuine and authentic and to provide individualized responses to patients (baird-group.com/articles/scripting-for-positive-patient-experience-five-steps-for-success).

Social network: An individual's network of family, friends, and other supportive persons; persons to whom one can go for assistance when needed. Rural persons tend to have larger social networks than urban persons.

Substance abuse: Harmful or hazardous use of psychoactive substances, including alcohol, prescription drugs, and illicit drugs. Substance abuse can lead to psychoactive substance dependency (www.who.int/topics/substance_abuse/en).

U.S. Census Bureau (USCB): Designates "urbanized" and "urban cluster" areas; designates all areas outside urbanized and urban cluster areas as "rural." Definition is based on census tracts, not city or county boundaries (www.hrsa.gov/rural-health/about-us/definition/index.html).

Urban clusters (UCs): Designated by the USCB as areas with a population of 2,500 up to 49,999; UCs do not follow city or county borders (www.hrsa.gov/rural-health/about-us/definition/index.html).

Urbanized areas (UAs): Designated by the USCB as areas with a population of 50,000 or greater; UAs do not follow city or county borders (www.hrsa.gov/rural-health/about-us/definition/index.html).

Wraparound services: At a point of service (such as a county health department), clients may be referred to wraparound services to address social determinants of health with the objective of enhancing clients' self-sufficiency and independence. Typical wraparound services may include federal food assistance programs, physical and mental health and wellness services, skills training opportunities for living wage jobs, and housing assistance.

ACKNOWLEDGMENTS

The authors wish to gratefully acknowledge Michael Meit, MA, MPH, Co-Director, NORC Walsh Center for Rural Health Analysis, and Janice C. Probst, PhD, Former Director, Rural & Minority Health Research Center, Arnold School of Public Health, University of South Carolina. Mr. Meit and Dr. Probst graciously reviewed this chapter, and provided valuable comments and suggestions to the authors.

REFERENCES

1. Federal Office of Rural Health Policy. *Rural Health Information Hub.* 2017. https://www.ruralhealthinfo.org
2. Bolin JN, Bellamy GR, Ferdinand AO, et al. Rural healthy people 2020: new decade, same challenges. *J Rural Health.* 2015;31(3):326–333. doi:10.1111/jrh.12116
3. Singh GK, Siahpush M. Widening rural–urban disparities in all-cause mortality and mortality from major causes of death in the USA, 1969–2009. *J Urban Health.* 2014;91(2):272–292. doi:10.1007/s11524-013-9847-2
4. La Caille John P, Reynnells L. *What Is "Rural"?* 2006. https://www.nal.usda.gov/ric/what-is-rural#INTRO
5. Flora CB, Flora JL, Gasteyer SP. *Rural Communities: Legacy and Change.* Boulder, CO: Westview Press; 2016.
6. Hart LG, Larson EH, Lishner DM. Rural definitions for health policy and research. *Am J Public Health.* 2005;95(7):1149–1155. doi:10.2105/AJPH.2004.042432
7. U.S. General Accounting Office. *Rural Development: Profile of Rural Areas.* Washington, DC: U.S. General Accounting Office; 1993.
8. U.S. Census Bureau. *Urban and Rural.* 2020. https://www.census.gov/programs-surveys/geography/guidance/geo-areas/urban-rural.html
9. Federal Office of Rural Health Policy. *Defining Rural Population.* 2017. https://www.hrsa.gov/ruralhealth/aboutus/definition.html
10. Office of Information and Regulatory Affairs. Office of Management and Budget. 2010 standards for delineating metropolitan and micropolitan statistical areas. *Fed Regist.* 2010;75:37246–37252.
11. U.S. Department of Agriculture Economic Research Service. *Rural-Urban Continuum Codes.* 2013. https://www.ers.usda.gov/data-products/rural-urban-continuum-codes
12. von Reichert C, Greiman L, Myers A, Rural Institute. *The Geography of Disability in America: On Rural-Urban Differences in Impairment Rates.* Missoula, MT: University of Montana; 2014. https://scholarworks.umt.edu/ruralinst_independent_living_community_participation/7
13. Meit M. *Final Report: Exploring Strategies to Improve Health and Equity in Rural Communities.* Bethesda, MD: Walsh Center for Rural Health Analysis; 2018. http://www.norc.org/PDFs/Walsh%20Center/Final%20Reports/Rural%20Assets%20Final%20 Report%20Feb%2018.pdf
14. Crespo R, Shrewsberry M, Cornelius-Averhart D, King HB. Appalachian regional model for organizing and sustaining county-level diabetes coalitions. *Health Promot Pract.* 2011;12(4):544–550.
15. Community-Wealth. *Anchor Institutions.* n.d. https://community-wealth.org/strategies/panel/anchors/index.html
16. Adamy J, Overberg P. Rural America is the new 'inner city'. *Wall Street Journal.* May 27, 2017.
17. Economic Research Service. *Poverty Overview.* Washington, DC: U.S. Department of Agriculture; March 1, 2017.
18. Semeuls A. The graying of rural America. *The Atlantic.* June 2, 2016. https://www.theatlantic.com/business/archive/2016/06/the-graying-of-rural-america/485159
19. U.S. Department of Agriculture, Economic Research Service. *Population and Migration: Overview.* 2017. https://www.ers.usda.gov/topics/rural-economy-population/population-migration.aspx

20. Bailey R. Stuck: A *Reason* writer returns to Appalachia to ask: why don't people who live in places with no opportunity just leave? *Reason*. 2017(January). https://reason.com/2016/12/10/stuck

21. Hing E, Hsiao C. State variability in supply of office-based primary care providers: United States 2012. *NCHS Data Brief*. 2014;151:1–8.

22. Centers for Medicare and Medicaid Services. *Emergency Medical Treatment & Labor Act (EMTALA)*. 2012. https://www.cms.gov/Regulations-and-Guidance/Legislation/EMTALA

23. National Rural Health Association. *About Rural Health Care*. 2017. https://www.ruralhealthweb.org/about-nrha/about-rural-health-care

24. Rural Health Information Hub. *Selected Social Determinants of Health*. 2015. https://www.ruralhealthinfo.org/states/united-states

25. Lu N, Samuels ME, Kletke PR, Whitler ET. Rural-urban differences in health insurance coverage and patterns among working-age adults in Kentucky. *J Rural Health*. 2010;26(2):129–138. doi:10.1111/j.1748-0361.2010.00274.x

26. James W, Cossman JS. Long-term trends in black and white mortality in the rural United States: evidence of a race-specific rural mortality penalty. *J Rural Health*. 2017;33(1):21–31. doi:10.1111/jrh.12181

27. Kozhimannil KB, Hung P, Henning-Smith C, et al. Association between loss of hospital-based obstetric services and birth outcomes in rural counties in the United States. *JAMA*. 2018;319(12):1239–1247. doi:10.1001/jama.2018.1830

28. Council of State Governments. *Capitol Facts and Figures: Health Care Workforce Shortages Critical in Rural America*. April 2011. https://knowledgecenter.csg.org/kc/content/health-care-workforce-shortages-critical-rural-america

29. Bureau of Health Workforce. *Designated Health Professional Shortage Areas Statistics: Third Quarter of Fiscal Year 2019 Designated HPSA Quarterly Summary*. 2019.

30. Stewart H, Jameson JP, Curtin L. The relationship between stigma and self-reported willingness to use mental health services among rural and urban older adults. *Psychol Serv*. 2015;12(2):141–148. doi:10.1037/a0038651

31. Rural Health Information Hub. *Barriers to Transportation in Rural Areas*. 2019. https://www.ruralhealthinfo.org/toolkits/transportation/1/barriers

32. The Cecil G. Sheps Center for Health Services Research. *168 Rural Hospital Closures: January 2005 - Present (126 since 2010)*. 2019. https://www.shepscenter.unc.edu/programs-projects/rural-health/rural-hospital-closures/

33. National Rural Health Association. *NRHA Save Rural Hospitals Action Center. Advocacy*. 2018. https://www.ruralhealthweb.org/advocate/save-rural-hospitals

34. Wishner J, Solleved P, Rudowitz R, et al. *A Look at Rural Hospital Closures and Implications for Access to Care: Three Case Studies. The Kaiser Commission on Medicaid and the Uninsured*. 2016. http://www.kff.org/report-section/a-look-at-rural-hospital-closures-and-implications-for-access-to-care-three-case-studies-issue-brief

35. Holmes GM, Slifkin RT, Randolph RK, Poley S. The effect of rural hospital closures on community economic health. *Health Serv Res*. 2006;41(2):467–485. doi:10.1111/j.1475-6773.2005.00497.x

36. Moy E, Macarena CG, Bastian B, et al. Leading causes of death in nonmetropolitan and metropolitan areas—United States, 1999–2014. *MMWR Surveill Summ*. 2017;66(6):1–8. doi:10.15585/mmwr.ss6601a1

37. Mell HK, Mumma SM, Hiestand B, et al. EMS response times are double in rural vs. urban areas. *JAMA Surg*. 2017;152(10):983–984. doi:10.1001/jamasurg.2017.2230

38. Bhuyan SS, Wang Y, Opoku S, Lin G. Rural–urban differences in acute myocardial infarction mortality: evidence from Nebraska. *J Cardiovasc Dis Res*. 2013;4(4):209–213. doi:10.1016/j.jcdr.2014.01.006

39. Houck K, Wogu AF, Villagra V, et al. National survey of breast cancer screening in rural America. *J Clin Oncol*. 2013;31(26 suppl):13. doi:10.1200/jco.2013.31.26_suppl.13

40. Hale NL, Bennett KJ, Probst JC. Diabetes care and outcomes: disparities across rural America. *J Community Health*. 2010;35(4):365–374. doi:10.1007/s10900-010-9259-0

41. National Center for Health Statistics. *Table 75: Selected measures of access to medical care among adults aged 18–64, by urbanization level and selected characteristics: United States, average annual, 2002–2004 through 2010–2012*. Washington, DC; 2013.

42. Sattelmeyer S. *3 Strategies to Increase Opportunity and Economic Mobility in Rural America. Research and Analysis*. 2016. http://www.pewtrusts.org/en/research-and-analysis/analysis/2016/07/18/3-strategies-to-increase-opportunity-and-economic-mobility-in-rural-america

43. U.S. Census Bureau. *American Community Survey*. 2017. https://www.census.gov/programs-surveys/acs

44. Bastian B, Tejada Vera B, Arias E, et al. Mortality trends in the United States, 1900–2017. *National Center for Health Statistics*; 2019. https://www.cdc.gov/nchs/data-visualization/mortality-trends/index.htm

45. Meit M, Knudson A, Gilbert T, et al. *The 2014 Update of the Rural-Urban Chartbook*. Bethesda, MD: Walsh Center for Rural Health Analysis; 2014.

46. Centers for Disease Control. *CDC Newsroom: American Indian and Alaska Native Death Rates Nearly 50 percent Greater Than Those of Non-Hispanic Whites*. 2014. https://www.cdc.gov/media/releases/2014/p0422-natamerican-deathrate.html

47. North Carolina State Center for Health Statistics and Office of Minority Health and Health Disparities. *North Carolina Minority Health Facts: American Indians*. Raleigh, NC: Department of Health and Human Services; 2010.

48. Smith BL, Sandlin AT, Bird TM, et al. Maternal mortality in the Delta region of the United States. *J Obstet Gynecol Neonatal Nurs*. 2015;44(s1):S66–S67. doi:10.1111/1552-6909.12639

49. Rural Health Information Hub. *Rural Health Disparities*. 2019. https://www.ruralhealthinfo.org/topics/rural-health-disparities#minority-populations

50. Singh GK, Kogan MD, Slifkin RT. Widening disparities in infant mortality and life expectancy between Appalachia and the rest of the United States, 1990–2013. *Health Aff*. 2017;36(8):1423–1432. doi:10.1377/hlthaff.2016.1571

51. World Health Organization. *ICD-10: International Statistical Classification of Diseases and Related Health Problems*. 10th rev ed. Geneva, Switzerland: WHO Press; 2010.

52. Academy of Nutrition and Dietetics Evidence Analysis Library. *Chronic Obstructive Pulmonary Disease Guideline*. 2008. https://www.andeal.org/topic.cfm?menu=5301

53. Rural Health Information Hub. *Substance Abuse in Rural Areas*. 2015. https://www.ruralhealthinfo.org/topics/substance-abuse#drug-abuse

54. Substance Abuse and Mental Health Services Administration. *Treatment Episode Data Set: A Comparison of Rural and Urban Substance Abuse Treatment Admissions*. Washington, DC: U.S. Department of Health and Human Services; 2012.

55. National Center for Health Statistics. NCHS data on drug-poisoning deaths. *NCHS Fact Sheets*. 2017. https://www.cdc.gov/nchs/data/factsheets/factsheet_drug_poisoning.pdf

56. Keyes KM, Cerdá M, Brady JE, et al. Understanding the rural–urban differences in nonmedical prescription opioid use and abuse in the United States. *Am J Public Health*. 2013;104(2):e52–e59. doi:10.2105/ajph.2013.301709

57. Nabipour S, Ayu Said M, Hussain Habil M. Burden and nutritional deficiencies in opiate addiction—systematic review article. *Iran J Public Health*. 2014;43(8):1022–1032.

58. Decher N. Nutritional implications of opioid-induced bowel dysfunction in chronic pain management. *Support Line*. 2009;31(6):19–27.

59. U.S. Department of Agriculture. *Definitions of Food Security*. 2016. https://www.ers.usda.gov/topics/food-nutrition-assistance/food-security-in-the-us/definitions-of-food-security

60. Coleman-Jensen A, Rabbitt MP, Gregory CA, Singh A. *Household Food Security in the United States in 2015*. Washington, DC: U.S. Department of Agriculture Economic Research Service; 2016.

61. Piontak JR, Schulman MD. Food insecurity in rural America. *Contexts: J Am Sociol Assoc*. 2014;13(3):75–77. doi:10.1177/1536504214545766

62. Economic Research Service. *Food Environment Atlas*. Washington, DC: U.S. Department of Agriculture; 2016.

63. Wolfrath J, Ryan B, Nehring P. Dollar Stores in Small Communities—Are They a Good Fit for Your Town? *Downtown Economics*. University of Wisconsin Extension Center for Community and Economic Development, Wisconsin Downtown Action Council; 2018;2019, issue 187.

64. Seligman HK, Laraia BA, Kushel MB. Food insecurity is associated with chronic disease among low-income NHANES participants. *J Nutr*. 2010;140(2):304–310. doi:10.3945/jn.109.112573

65. Seligman HK, Bindman AB, Vittinghoff E, et al. Food insecurity is associated with diabetes mellitus: results from the National Health Examination and Nutrition Examination Survey (NHANES) 1999–2002. *J Gen Intern Med.* 2007;22(7):1018–1023. doi:10.1007/s11606-007-0192-6

66. Suarez JJ, Isakova T, Anderson CA, et al. Food access, chronic kidney disease, and hypertension in the U.S. *Am J Prev Med.* 2015;49(6):912–920. doi:10.1016/j.amepre.2015.07.017

67. Whitaker RC, Phillips SM, Orzol SM. Food insecurity and the risks of depression and anxiety in mothers and behavior problems in their preschool-aged children. *Pediatrics.* 2006;118(3):e859–e868. doi:10.1542/peds.2006-0239

68. Jyoti DF, Frongillo EA, Jones SJ. Food insecurity affects school children's academic performance, weight gain, and social skills. *J Nutr.* 2005;135(12):2831–2839. doi:10.1093/jn/135.12.2831

69. Farahbakhsh J, Hanbazaza M, Ball GDC, et al. Food insecure student clients of a university-based food bank have compromised health, dietary intake and academic quality. *Nutr Diet.* 2017;74(1):67–73. doi:10.1111/1747-0080.12307

70. Frith E, Loprinzi PD. Food insecurity and cognitive function in older adults: brief report. *Clin Nutr.* 2018;37(5):1765–1768. doi:10.1016/j.clnu.2017.07.001

71. Roush D. *Physicians Offer Insights on Practicing Rural Medicine.* 2008. http://www.healthleadersmedia.com/community-rural/physicians-offer-insights-practicing-rural-medicine?page=0%2C1

72. Daniels ZM, VanLeit BJ, Skipper BJ, et al. Factors in recruiting and retaining health professionals for rural practice. *J Rural Health.* 2007;23(1):62–71. doi:10.1111/j.1748-0361.2006.00069.x

73. McGrail MR, Wingrove PM, Petterson SM, Bazemore AW. Mobility of US rural primary care physicians during 2000–2014. *Ann Fam Med.* 2017;15(4):322–328. doi:10.1370/afm.2096

74. Collins C. Challenges of recruitment and retention in rural areas. *N C Med J.* 2016;77(2):99–101. doi:10.18043/ncm.77.2.99

75. South Carolina GME Advisory Group. *Leveraging Graduate Medical Education to Increase Primary Care and Rural Physician Capacity in South Carolina: A report by the South Carolina GME Advisory Group in response to 2013-2014 Appropriations-Bill 3710 Part IB, Proviso 33.34 (E).* Columbia, SC: South Carolina Department of Health and Human Services; 2014.

76. Ballance D, Kornegay D, Evans P. *Factors That Influence Physicians to Practice in Rural Locations: A Review.* Augusta, GA: Medical College of Georgia; 2009.

77. Brooks RG, Walsh M, Mardon RE, et al. The roles of nature and nurture in the recruitment and retention of primary care physicians in rural areas: a review of the literature. *Acad Med.* 2002;77(8):790–798. doi:10.1097/00001888-200208000-00008

78. Rural Health Information Hub. *Rural Health Clinics (RHCs).* 2019. https://www.ruralhealthinfo.org/topics/rural-health-clinics

79. Center for Medicare and Medicaid Services. *Rural Health Clinics (RHCs) and Federally Qualified Health Centers (FQHCs) Billing Guide.* 2016. https://www.cms.gov/Outreach-and-Education/Medicare-Learning-Network-MLN/MLNMattersArticles/Downloads/SE1039.pdf

80. Nelson WA, ed. *Handbook for Rural Health Care Ethics: A Practical Guide for Professionals.* Hanover, NH: Dartmouth College Press: University Press of New England; 2009.

81. Osborn A. Juggling personal life and professionalism: ethical implications for rural school psychologists. *Psychol Sch.* 2012;49(9):876–882. doi:10.1002/pits.21642

82. Berndt A, Murray CM, Kennedy K, et al. Effectiveness of distance learning strategies for continuing professional development (CPD) for rural allied health practitioners: a systematic review. *BMC Med Educ.* 2017;17(1):117. doi:10.1186/s12909-017-0949-5

83. National Center for Cultural Competence. Definitions of Cultural Competence. *Curricula Enhancement Module Series.* 2017. https://nccc.georgetown.edu/curricula/culturalcompetence.html

84. Cross TL, Bazron B, Dennis K, Isaacs M. *Towards a Culturally Competent System of Care.* Vol. 1. Washington, DC: Georgetown University Child Development Center; 1989.

85. Lundy R. *Victuals.* New York, NY: Clarkson/Potter Publishers; 2016.

86. Harkin A. *Hillbilly: A Cultural History of an American Icon.* New York, NY: Oxford University Press; 2004.

87. Veteto JR. Down deep in the holler: chasing seeds and stories in southern Appalachia. *J Ethnobiol Ethnomed.* 2013;9(1):69. doi:10.1186/1746-4269-9-69.

88. Gutschall M, Thompson KL. Addressing health disparities in rural nutrition practice: a qualitative model from rural Appalachia. *J Hunger Environ Nutr.* 2017;13(1):84–89.

89. Substance Abuse and Mental Health Services Administration. Results from the 2016 National Survey on Drug Use and Health: Detailed Tables; 2017, September 27. https://www.samhsa.gov/data/sites/default/files/NSDUH-DetTabs-2016/NSDUH-DetTabs-2016.pdf

90. Holuby RS, Pellegrin KL, Barbato A, Ciarleglio A. Recruitment of rural healthcare professionals for live continuing education. *Med Educ Online*. 2015;20:1–3. doi:10.3402/meo.v20.28958

91. Lengerich EJ, Bohland JR, Brown PK, et al. Images of Appalachia. *Prev Chronic Dis*. 2006;3(4):1–3.

92. United States Department of Agriculture Economic Research Service. Urban Influence Codes. Updated October 24, 2019. Accessed March 13, 2020, at https://www.ers.usda.gov/data-products/urban-influence-codes.aspx

URBAN HEALTH AND URBANIZATION: ACTING ON SOCIAL DETERMINANTS IN URBAN SETTINGS

ARELIS MOORE DE PERALTA, MICHELLE EICHINGER, AND LESLIE HOSSFELD

LEARNING OBJECTIVES

1. Identify social determinants that influence food access and nutritional patterns in urban settings.
2. Understand the role of **urbanization** in food access, availability, and affordability.
3. Explain the components of urban food challenges.
4. Define **gentrification** and understand its role in **food insecurity** and food access.
5. Understand the processes involved with developing a community **food system**.
6. Understand socio-ecological approaches to healthier nutrition in urban settings.
7. Discuss evidence-based practices and protective factors that promote healthier nutritional patterns in urban settings.

INTRODUCTION

The urban environment disproportionately affects vulnerable population groups with poor housing conditions, segregated neighborhoods, and limited access to resources. Maintaining a healthy diet can be challenging in this context. **Food deserts**, gentrification, poverty, and other urban environment processes influence nutritional patterns in these settings. This chapter includes a review of the challenges on access to, affordability of, and availability to food in urban settings. Differences in health are striking in urban communities with poor **social determinants of health (SDOH)** such as unstable housing, low income, unsafe neighborhoods, or substandard education. This chapter presents a description of the Social-Ecological Model (SEM) as well as its application to explore social determinants of nutritional health in urban settings. The chapter portrays the SEM as an integrative framework that shows great promise in improving dietary behaviors and the nutritional status of vulnerable urban populations, including those affected by conditions such as type 2 diabetes. Strategies to improve the urban food environment are reviewed, with a focus on **community gardens** as a promising urban strategy to promote sustainable development.

Two interdisciplinary case studies that utilize an ecological or holistic approach to nutrition and lifestyle improvement are summarized.

Urbanization and Urban Health

Urbanization has been a phenomenon not only in the United States but globally. Urbanization is the population shift from more rural areas to more urban areas, causing expansion of and population growth in cities. Much of this movement is due to economic drivers such as job opportunities and more services.

Urban populations present differing health concerns than populations in rural areas. It is common for children residing in urban settings to experience asthma due to poorer air quality or families having limited access to outdoor recreation space for physical activity. Further, the social and economic determinants of health create disproportionate risk factors that contrast between rural and urban environments. Violent crime rates can be twice as high in urban areas, and sexually transmitted diseases, tuberculosis, infant mortality, and drug and alcohol use are more prevalent in urban areas.[1] The urban environment disproportionately affects vulnerable population groups with poor housing conditions, segregated neighborhoods, and limited access to resources.[2]

In developed countries, diet behavior seems to be associated with cost and convenience. People are working and commuting. Families are struggling with both parents working, which means limited time to prepare, cook, and eat meals, whether it is in the home, at work, or school. In urban areas, convenience stores, fast-food chains, and restaurants line the streetscape. Yet, despite the availability of convenient and inexpensive food, the diet does not necessarily contribute to a healthy lifestyle. Several factors influence diet behavior. When considering the urban environment, these dietary factors often differ from those in nonurban areas, which can influence health outcomes.

Healthy Diet

Urban areas typically have more options for eating. These often include various types of restaurants such as sit-down dining and fast food, but also street food vendors in larger metropolises and different scales of grocery stores. With the variety of food options typically available in urban areas, establishing a healthy diet is possible. According to the U.S. Department of Agriculture (USDA), a healthy diet is a diet rich with whole grains, low-fat or nonfat dairy, a variety of lean proteins, plenty of fresh fruits and vegetables, and food and drinks low in sodium, saturated fat, and added sugars. However, maintaining a healthy diet can be challenging to some population groups, depending on their geographic area and socioeconomic status. Food deserts in urban areas are defined by the USDA as geographic areas with low-income census tracts (i.e., geographically defined areas determined by the U.S. Bureau of the Census, and which are equivalent to neighborhoods) and no supermarket within 1 mile. Low-income census tracts are identified as a census tract with any one of the following:

- At least 20% of the population at or below the federal poverty level (FPL)
- Median household income 80% or less than the state's median household income
- Metropolitan household median income 80% or less than the metropolitan's median household income

Figure 9.1 displays a map of food deserts in Atlanta, Georgia. Residents living in food deserts may rely on the food available in their neighborhood, such as corner stores or dollar stores, or may have to travel distances for more affordable healthy food. Therefore, maintaining a healthy diet may be more challenging for households located in food deserts.

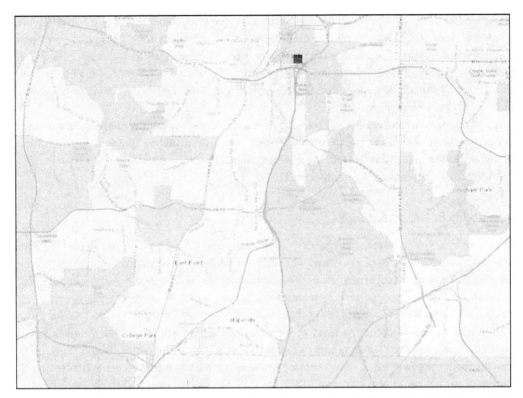

FIGURE 9.1 U.S. Department of Agriculture food desert map of Atlanta, Georgia. The shaded areas are census tracts identified as food deserts. The dark box indicates Atlanta.

Source: From U.S. Department of Agriculture Economic Research Service. *Food Access Research Atlas.* https://www .ers.usda.gov/data-products/food-access-research-atlas/documentation

Urbanization and Gentrification

Urbanization is population movement from rural areas to more urban areas causing an increase in population in cities and the expansion of cities. Urban renewal projects to support economic growth and improve livability in urban areas, and specifically in blighted areas, have attracted new residents and business owners. While this is appealing for cities, it unfortunately can come at a cost to those living in those areas. Gentrification is the change in neighborhood characteristics from low-income communities, often rife with crime, minority populations, and limited resources, to the opposite of high-income households and nonminority population groups. Gentrification results in the displacement of low-income residents following urban renewal or revitalization projects.

Gentrification changes the food retail environment. Urbanization has created a "foodie" culture and has been one of the leading factors of gentrification.[3] High-end supermarkets and food retailers locate in these communities and while these retailers provide an abundance of high-quality food, the costs of the food are too high for long-standing residents.[3] Food prices in urban areas are a contributing influence to food insecurity.[4]

Urban Food Challenges

Food Deserts

In urban areas, we often see "food deserts," or the lack of a supermarket in low-income areas. Supermarkets are not likely to be in cities, but rather in the periphery or suburban areas. There are several reasons for this geographical distribution. Supermarkets often require large square footage of floor space, which requires more land. Cities, with their high density of developed land uses, have a limited amount of open space to meet the needs for supermarkets. Along with limited availability of land to build supermarkets, the cost of land is often high in cities, which contributes to supermarkets locating outside urban areas. Therefore, the availability of healthy foods is limited within cities.

Food retailers located in cities often are smaller with limited availability of healthy foods such as fresh fruits and vegetables and perishable items. Land costs are higher in urban areas resulting in higher leasing and rental costs for storeowners. Consequently, some of these costs are passed on to the consumer through higher food prices.

Availability in Urban Settings

The urban food environment sees a greater variety of food retail and services. Yet, the urban retail food environment may not be associated with increased availability of healthy food options. There are a limited number of supermarkets in urban areas, contributing to food deserts in low-income areas. Instead, small grocers, such as bodegas and corner stores, convenience/gas stores, pharmacies, and dollar stores are often the options available to urban households, especially for those with limited resources. Although small grocers may sell some fresh produce, it is unlikely that nontraditional stores sell whole grains or perishable items, such as fresh fruits and vegetables.[5] Healthy foods are perceived as not profitable by nontraditional food retail owners.[5] Further, as the density of convenience stores increases, as in urban areas, residents are less likely to have a healthy diet.[6] In addition, a new term called **food swamps** describes a geographic location that has a high concentration of businesses that sell "junk food" (high-calorie, low-nutrition food) more so than healthier food outlets.[7] Mobile markets, produce carts, and community gardens and transforming corner stores to include the sale of healthy food can increase opportunities for healthy food in urban settings.[8]

Access to Food in Urban Settings

While healthy food choices may be available, is a healthy diet accessible to everyone? The term "accessible" is broad, but in this section, the term focuses on the ability to get to destinations via transportation. There are transportation disparities related to geographic area, aging, disability, race/ethnicity, and income. As population density increases, vehicle ownership decreases, and about 20% of low-income households do not own a vehicle.[9] In addition, about 40% of those with disabilities, or about 6 million people nationwide, have transportation difficulties such as the inability to drive or no access to other modes of transportation.[10]

Households with no vehicle have limited access to healthy food options and depend on other means to get to supermarkets and healthy food retailers. Households with no vehicle access make fewer shopping trips for groceries than households with sufficient access.[11] In addition, despite access-burdened households and access-sufficient households making comparable trips to unhealthy food retailers (convenience stores, pharmacies, and dollar stores), access-burdened households spend more per capita on food in these retail places.[11] Further, households with no vehicle access are at higher risk of food insecurity, especially among households in public housing.[12] However, a supermarket within walking distance, or within 1,000 meters of home, is associated with lower body mass index and higher consumption of fruits and vegetables, even for disadvantaged population groups.[13,14]

Public transit provides accessibility opportunities, especially for older adults, people with low income, and those with disabilities. As it relates to healthy eating, public transit that connects residential areas to grocery stores and farmers' markets increases access to healthy food. However, transit users have limited choices for supermarkets or grocery stores with limited stops to such food retailers. In addition, travel time is more likely to be longer, including multiple transfers to other routes in order to reach the destination. Transit users also need to factor in travel costs and carrying groceries back to their home.

Affordability in Urban Settings

Cost has been a prohibitive factor in healthy living, especially as it relates to diet choices. In terms of diet, there is a cost disparity between nutrient-rich foods and less healthy food options.[15] This poses an economic challenge, and potential barrier, for those from a lower socioeconomic status. Affordability of healthy foods may have more of an impact on diet patterns than the distance to the nearest supermarket. Grains with added sugars and added fats are less expensive, tasty, and convenient, and have been associated with lower quality diets, lower food costs, and lower socioeconomic status.[16] Further, staple foods such as milk, peanut butter, eggs, legumes, and cereals are up to 50% more expensive in small grocers compared to supermarkets.[17] Lack of affordability of food contributes to food insecurity. Low income and poverty are associated with food insecurity or reduced quality, variety, and desirability of diet with disrupted eating patterns.

Federal programs such as the USDA Supplemental Nutrition Assistance Program (SNAP) and the Special Supplemental Nutrition Program for Women, Infants, and Children (WIC) provide income-eligible households with financial assistance for purchasing foods. Expansion of these programs, including the Senior Farmers' Market Nutrition Program and the WIC Farmers' Market Nutrition Program, increases the purchasing power for healthy foods.[18] The following section conceptualizes SDOH and poor nutritional status as a prevalent SDOH in urban settings.

SDOH: Poor Nutritional Status

Low-resource communities across the country especially face a lack of availability of basic services, which can influence the health of their residents.[19] Research has shown that the health of a community is not determined only by its healthcare system, but it is also determined by access to social and economic opportunities; the resources and supports available in our households, neighborhoods, and communities; the quality of our schooling; the safety of our workplaces; the cleanliness of our water, food, and air; and the nature of our social interactions and relationships.[20] This multitude of factors does not deny that medical care influences health; rather, it indicates that medical care is not the only influence on health and suggests that the effects of medical care may be more limited than commonly thought.[21-24]

The Commission on Social Determinants of Health (CSDH) developed a relevant framework (Figure 9.2) to explain how social, economic, and political mechanisms give rise to a set of socioeconomic positions whereby populations are stratified according to income, education, occupation, gender, race/ethnicity, and other factors. These socioeconomic positions in turn shape specific determinants of health status (intermediary determinants) reflective of people's place within social hierarchies. Based on their respective social status, individuals experience differences in exposure and vulnerability to health-compromising conditions. Together, context, structural mechanisms, and the resultant socioeconomic position of individuals are "structural determinants." The underlying SDOH inequities operate through a set of intermediary determinants of health to shape health outcomes.[25]

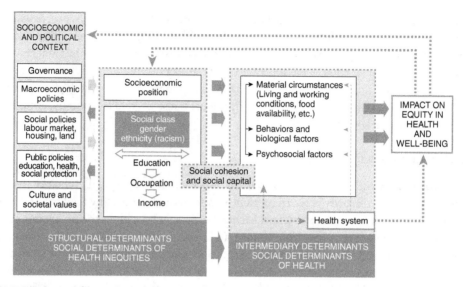

FIGURE 9.2 Final form of the CSDH conceptual framework.

CSDH, Commission on Social Determinants of Health.

Source: From Solar O, Irwin A. A conceptual framework for action on the social determinants of health. *Social Determinants of Health Discussion Paper 2 (Policy and Practice).* Geneva: World Health Organization; 2010.

SDOH are conditions in the environments in which people are born, live, learn, work, play, worship, and age that affect a wide range of health, functioning, and quality-of-life outcomes and risks. Conditions (e.g., social, cultural, political, economic, and environmental) in these various environments and settings (e.g., school, church, workplace, and neighborhood) have been referred to as "place."[20] These place-related factors affect the health of low-resource communities at the varying levels of society, community, and even individuals themselves.[26] For instance, poverty limits access to healthy foods, safe neighborhoods, and strong educational systems. All these factors are predictors of better health. Differences in health are striking in communities with poor SDOH such as unstable housing, low income, unsafe neighborhoods, or substandard education.[27] Education has been identified as one of the relevant SDOH. Figure 9.3 portrays how education affects health, and Figure 9.4 depicts the influence of educational attainment on the perceived health status of individuals among adults aged 25 to 74 years within racial/ethnic groups in the United States, 2008–2010.

Low-resource communities afflicted by a myriad of SDOH are prevalent in urban settings across the globe. The World Health Organization (WHO) has stressed the relevance of the many benefits urban health investments have on individuals and society.[28] However, the WHO warns that there are many inadequacies in the way these health investments are planned and implemented, particularly by focusing mostly on fostering economic growth and better incomes in urban settings. In addition to economic growth and income, the SDOH must be considered.

Fruit and vegetable consumption is declining in the United States, and fat and calorie consumption is increasing. These nutritional status related facts contradict research findings showing that 88% of U.S. household had access, at all times, to enough food for an active, healthy life for all household members.[29] Urbanization and food systems are examples of what WHO labeled as "themes" to consider in addressing SDOH.[28] Regarding food systems, for example, even though urban residents might have more access to, more choices of, and more money for food, they can

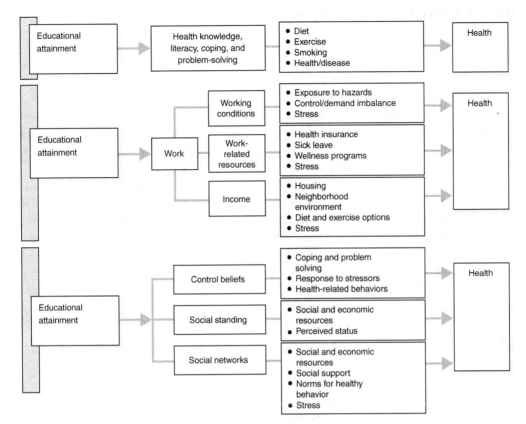

FIGURE 9.3 Pathways through which education can affect health.

Source: From Egerter S, Braveman P, Sadegh-Nobari T, et al. *Education Matters for Health. Exploring the Social Determinants of Health: Issue Brief no. 6.* Princeton, NJ: Robert Wood Johnson Foundation; Copyright 2011. Used with permission from the Robert Wood Johnson Foundation.

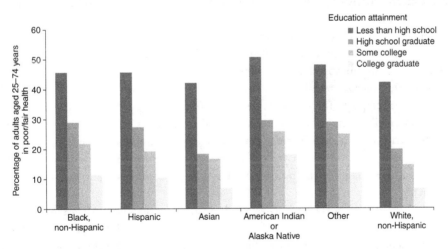

FIGURE 9.4 Socioeconomic gradients in poor/fair health among adults aged 25–74 years within racial/ethnic groups in the United States, 2008–2010.

Note: Age-adjusted. Based on self-report and measured as poor, fair, good, very good, or excellent. "Other" defined as any other or more than one racial or ethnic group, including any group with fewer than 3% of surveyed adults nationally in 2008–2010.

Source: From Braveman P, Egerter S. *Overcoming Obstacles to Health in 2013 and Beyond: Report for the Robert Wood Johnson Foundation Commission to Build a Healthier America.* Princeton, NJ: Robert Wood Johnson Foundation; Copyright 2013. Used with permission from the Robert Wood Johnson Foundation.

be more challenged in nourishment than their rural counterparts. The health and nutritional status of the urban poor may be worse than that of the rural poor.[30] Convenience foods, pricing strategies, agricultural policies, and increases in typical U.S. portion sizes contribute to what has been described as a **toxic environment**.[29] Lower availability of fresh produce, combined with concentrated fast-food outlets and few recreational opportunities, has increased among urban residents, magnifying their opportunities to eat a diet that features higher intakes of fat, sugars, and energy and reducing opportunities to engage in physical activity.[30-32]

Social contexts in urban settings, which include the structure of society or the social relations in society, create social stratification and assign individuals to different social positions. Social stratification in turn engenders differential exposure to health-damaging conditions and differential vulnerability in terms of health conditions and material resource availability. Social stratification likewise determines differential consequences of ill health for more and less advantaged groups (including economic and social consequences) as well as differential health outcomes per se.[25] The following section includes a description of the SEM as well as its application to promote healthier nutritional patterns in urban settings.

SOCIO-ECOLOGICAL APPROACHES TO HEALTHIER NUTRITION IN URBAN SETTINGS

Urie Bronfenbrenner's Ecological Systems Theory (1979) explored influences on behavior as a set of layers, in which each layer had an impact resulting in the next level. The researcher described these layers as being a series of Russian dolls, in which the internal level represents the individual, who is surrounded by different levels of environmental impacts. For example, the social environment of a family, friends, and workplace is embedded within the physical environment of geography and community facilities, which is embedded in policy environments at different levels of government or governing bodies. All levels of the SEM affect the behavior of the individual.[33]

Bronfenbrenner believed that a child's development was affected by everything in his or her surrounding environment. He divided the person's environment into five different levels: the microsystem, the mesosystem, the exosystem, the macrosystem, and the chronosystem (Figure 9.5). The microsystem is the system closest to the person and the one in which he or she has direct contact. This incorporates family/home life, peers (classmates), and school (teachers), and is likely the most influential level of ecological systems. The mesosystem consists of interactions or linkages between different parts of a child's microsystem, for example, the role parents take in the school.[34,35] The interactions can promote or detract from positive developmental outcomes depending on whether the microsystems work together or against one another.

The third level in the model is the exosystem. The exosystem does not involve the child directly, but has an indirect effect nonetheless.[34,35] One example of this would be a parent's employment status. The results of that reality affect the child's environment by affecting his or her parent rather than having a direct influence on him or her. Other examples are neighbors, media, and school administration. The policies implemented by a school change the environment around the child without the child having any direct contact or input in the decisions. The next level of Ecological Systems Theory is the macrosystem. The macrosystem encompasses the attitudes and ideologies of the broader culture surrounding the developing child.[34,35] The final level is the chronosystem. This is the even broader context of sociohistorical setting, the timing of life events, the passing of

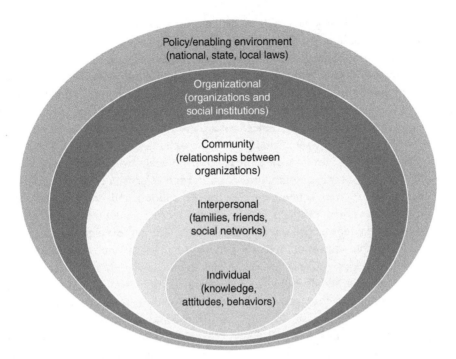

FIGURE 9.5 The Social-Ecological Model.

Source: Adapted from the Centers for Disease Control and Prevention. *The Social Ecological Model: A Framework for Prevention.* https://www.cdc.gov/pcd/issues/2013/12_0204.htm; Bronfenbrenner U. Toward an experimental ecology of human development. *Am Psychol.* 1977;32:513–531.doi:10.1037/0003-066x.32.7.513

time, and transitions.[34,35] This level is important for understanding how the macrosystem became the way it currently exists and can offer perspective on the changing landscape of human development across time and history.

The SEM is usually adapted to suit particular behaviors and population groups. For example, severe mental illness would have various healthcare needs in various environments; therefore, intervention strategies would change for each population. While the components of the SEM would remain the same and can be used in a range of populations, the specific factors within each component will vary depending on the population group. Gardiner emphasized the interactive characteristic of the SEM stating that:

> In short, an individual is seen *not* as a passive, static, and isolated entity on which the environment exerts great influence (much like a *tabula rasa,* or blank slate), but as a dynamic and evolving being that interacts with, and thereby restructures, the many environments with which he or she comes in contact with.[36]

A Socio-Ecological Perspective of Nutritional Patterns

Birch and Anzman posited that within the past three decades, children are developing in an obesity-promoting, or obesogenic, environment. Researchers and practitioners have used socio-ecological perspectives with the purpose of understanding the influence of the environment on the risk of developing health conditions associated with food consumption such as obesity and eating disorders.[37,38] For instance, Fiese and Jones argued that the dynamics of food consumption are linked to socialization practices, individual health, media influences, and contextual factors such as poverty and culture.[39] The authors maintained that food and family connect across different ecologies to result in either poor or optimal outcomes for children under different levels of risk. Neumark-Sztainer used a socio-ecological approach to explore how multiple interacting factors contribute to the etiology of problems within dimensions of weight control in adolescents at the individual, familial, peer, school, community, and societal levels.[38] The author found that families have an important role to play in reinforcing the positive influences at each of these levels and in filtering out the negative influences from the environment. However, the author argued that families could not do it on their own and need support from the more distal environments within which they function.

Fiese and Jones applied the ecological model put forth by Harrison et al., referred to as the Six-Cs Model (cell, child, clan, community, country, and culture), and simplified the model by focusing on the dimensional attributes of the cell, child, clan, community, country, and culture with respect to the food environment (Figure 9.6).[39,40] The authors expanded the model to consider how inadequate sources of food as experienced in food-insecure households may also compromise child development, and focused on how the accumulation of risk across ecologies may account for compromised development. The community sphere focuses on the impact that schools, peers, community factors, and access to food have on the food environment experienced by each child and family. Neighborhoods vary considerably in terms of the types of foods that are offered for purchase, from fast-food outlets and convenience stores to large grocery stores and fruit and vegetable vendors. A family's shopping habits may be directly influenced by their access to food in their neighborhood, which is also affected by socioeconomic resources.[39] Research has shown that there is heightened targeting of energy-dense foods toward African American families, who are also at greater risk for developing obesity.

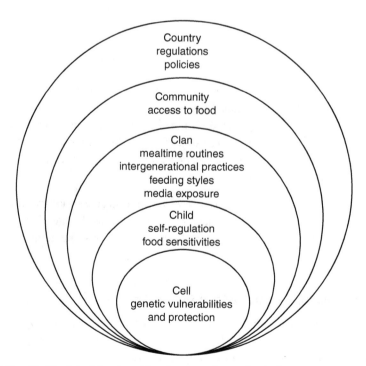

FIGURE 9.6 Five-Cs Model of food and family: A socio-ecological perspective.

Source: From Fiese BH, Jones BL. Food and family: a socio-ecological perspective for child development. *Adv Child Dev Behav.* 2012;42:307–337. doi:10.1016/b978-0-12-394388-0.00009-5

Researchers have used the SEM to explore the role of socioeconomic and cultural factors in determining nutritional patterns in communities. One study explored the role of income and racial–ethnic disparities on fruit and vegetable consumption in urban communities.[41] Other studies had explored determinants of nutritional patterns at school settings. For example, one study explored nutrition-related behavior and food patterns in the school environment, and another study tried to understand the association between factors at different levels of the SEM and pupils' dietary choices.[42,43]

Non-Hispanic Blacks and individuals with lower income are less likely to meet the USDA guidelines for the recommended daily servings of fruits and vegetables. Robinson conducted a literature review to examine dietary behaviors, focusing on fruit and vegetable intake of low-income African Americans from a socio-ecological perspective. Robinson found that dietary behaviors and fruit and vegetable intake among African Americans are the result of a complex interplay of personal, cultural, and environmental factors that can be categorized and described using the five levels of influence conceptualized by the SEM.[41] The author identified factors at the intrapersonal level (taste preferences, habits, and nutritional knowledge and skills); interpersonal level/social environment (processes whereby culture, social traditions, and role expectations impact eating practices; and patterns within peer groups, friends, and family); and at the organizational, community, and public policy levels/physical environment (environmental factors that affect food access and availability).

A study showed that policies at local and school levels reflect the national objectives with respect to nutritional guidelines, but were also influenced by multiple, competing interests at other socio-ecological levels.[42] These competing interests included pupils' food preferences; organizational objectives such as protecting school meal uptake; and the practices of school meal staff. Townsend and Foster used multilevel analysis to study the association of each level of the SEM on student dietary choice while controlling for factors found at other levels in secondary schools in Wales.[43] The authors found that student interpersonal factors, an individual's social environment, had a greater association with the dietary choices students made for lunch than student intrapersonal characteristics, those that reside within the person, which were found to have a greater association with the dietary choices made outside school. School organizational factors, such as rules and policies, had a greater association with whether students ate unhealthy foods, whereas the community nature of the school had a greater association with the choosing of healthy foods. These studies portray that in addition to individual preferences, the ecological systems surrounding the life of these individuals play a key role in shaping dietary behaviors for individuals at the school and community levels.

The multifaceted aspects of the food environment have consequences for child development in several ways including physical health and outcomes associated with nutrition such as obesity and malnutrition.[39] Some of the recommendations, derived from the relevant research reviewed in this chapter, include that school-based interventions can use the SEM to target specific factors and to offer rationale for and guidance on integrating socio-ecological concepts into health promoting programs to improve dietary behaviors. These efforts would change student outcomes in the school setting.[42,43] Moore et al. argued that the reach, effectiveness, adoption, implementation, and maintenance of school food policies and interventions could be maximized by understanding and exploiting the interdependence between levels in the SEM.[44]

The following section includes a discussion on how a variety of factors at different levels of the socio-ecological spectrum in urban settings determine nutritional outcomes for patients affected with type 2 diabetes, with an emphasis on underserved, minority urban populations.

Healthy Food Choice Accessibility, Type 2 Diabetes and Obesity

According to the American Diabetes Association, type 2 diabetes is the most common form of diabetes.[45] Type 2 diabetes is treated with lifestyle changes, oral medications (pills), and insulin. Some people with this illness can control their blood glucose with healthy eating and being active. However, your doctor may need to prescribe oral medications or insulin to help you meet your target blood glucose levels. Type 2 diabetes is more common in African Americans, Latinos, Native Americans, and Asian Americans/Pacific Islanders, as well as the aged population.[45] Medical nutrition therapy is essential in preventing the development of diabetes, and it is recognized as a cornerstone of management in patients who have diabetes.[46] Several factors contribute to unhealthy eating patterns, including lack of knowledge, automatic or habitual choice processes, and preference for convenience. All of these factors can be addressed in the context of the food environment.[47,48] However, high-risk groups including low-income and elderly persons often lack the temporal, spatial, and financial resources needed to obtain and consume a healthy diet.[49]

Over the past 100 years, ethnic minorities and the poor have become increasingly concentrated and isolated in low-income urban neighborhoods.[50] Ensuring adequate medical nutrition therapy is challenging for low-income neighborhood residents, primarily underrepresented minorities. Poor accessibility to healthy and low-cost foods contributes to food insecurity, poor nutrition, and high-calorie consumption among vulnerable groups.[48,49] Ghosh-Dastidar and colleagues posited that a lack of access to healthy foods might explain why residents of low-income neighborhoods, African Americans, and Latinos in the United States have high rates of obesity and type 2 diabetes.[51] The authors added that high prices of healthy foods as well as lack of marketing of these types of foods are also important factors that may explain the increased type 2 diabetes and obesity risk for these minority groups.[51]

The urban poor have limited access to the resources and factors that promote health in the inner city. One of the most health promoting factors in inner cities is food. Food environmental factors shown to be important include the density of restaurants, including fast-food outlets and full-service venues, as well as the density of retail food stores, including supermarkets and convenience stores. However, in the urban context, food choice is often severely constrained.[50] Supermarkets, which offer a wide range of fresh produce, whole-grain products, and unprocessed foods recommended as part of a healthy diet and at less expensive prices than convenience stores, are an important source of affordable and nutritious foods.[49] Changes in urban retailing in cities across the United States include reduction or elimination of urban amenities such as public transportation and large-scale supermarkets, primarily affecting the urban poor.[50] Smoyer-Tomic, Spence, and Amrhein argued that the low point for urban retailing in the United States was in the 1980s, when cities experienced a net loss of supermarkets even as, nationally, store openings exceeded closings.[49] The trend toward fewer, bigger stores located outside cities has continued to the present, leaving urban residents to pay higher prices for a narrower selection of food that often does not include the "nutritious" choices recommended for enhanced health and avoidance of "lifestyle" diseases like type 2 diabetes.[50]

The built environment (e.g., the density of farmers' markets and the presence of farms with direct sales) is associated with the prevalence of obesity and type 2 diabetes, and a strong local food economy may play an important role in prevention.[48] Hence, efforts to prevent obesity and type 2 diabetes at the population level will require changes in the food environment that promote healthy, lower-caloric foods and discourage unhealthy foods.[47,49] Another approach to prevent these conditions is the nutrition labeling on food packages, which addresses knowledge by providing detailed information about the nutritional and caloric content of a food, but many nutrition labels require a high level of literacy and numeracy to interpret.[47]

It may be difficult to change eating behaviors to be more consistent with healthy eating guidelines, particularly in high-risk populations, if affordable and nutritional foods are not readily accessible.[49] Once these nutritional choices are made accessible to the urban poor, nudging strategies that target automatic processes and preferences for convenience can manipulate the food environment to promote healthier choices among them.[47] Salois recommended more research on the influence of the built environment on health, particularly research emphasizing the potential of broad-based community-level interventions.[48] By understanding the ways these problems are rooted in the history of the urban context, local officials, communities, and citizens can begin to creatively address their causes and seek solutions that do not increase dependence on outside forces.[51]

STRATEGIES TO IMPROVE THE URBAN FOOD ENVIRONMENT

The upstream determinants of healthy urbanization include stimulation of job creation, land tenure and land use policy, transportation, sustainable urban development, social protection, settlement policies and strategies, community empowerment, vulnerability reduction, and better security among others.[28] However, the urban food environment has its challenges in offering affordable, accessible healthy foods. Policy-makers and public health practitioners are aware of these challenges and the complexities surrounding urbanization. Considering these issues, there have been strategies to improve the availability, affordability, and accessibility of healthy foods in urban areas.

Urban agriculture initiatives increase the availability of healthy foods. Community gardens and urban farms are growing trends in urban neighborhoods. Community organizations, churches, and even vacant lots have developed space to allow for urban agriculture. Urban park organizations have started garden programs for residents to build gardening skills and provide space to grow their food. Farmers' markets and mobile produce carts can locate themselves in areas with limited healthy food availability. Healthy retail interventions, such as the Healthy Corner Store Initiatives, allow for public–private partnerships to increase the availability of healthy foods in small grocers by providing financial incentives and technical assistance to retail owners to accommodate perishable and healthy foods including grants for refrigeration units and reconfiguring floor design to optimize product placement.[18]

Local policies are sustainable strategies to improve equitable food access and affordability. Land use zoning stipulates land parcels for specified uses. Local municipalities can identify some land uses for urban agriculture. For example, transitional zoning offers a strategy to transform vacant lots to community gardens. Healthy Food Zoning is a land use policy that limits the siting of unhealthy food retailers within proximity to vulnerable population groups, often youth. For example, healthy food zoning may limit dollar stores or fast-food restaurants locating near schools.

Economic policies are often used to incentivize development in blighted areas. For example, Tax Increment Financing (TIF) allows for special tax districts in which a portion of tax revenue is allocated for redevelopment (i.e., rent caps, rent-controlled apartments). As mentioned earlier, this may lead to gentrification, thus exacerbating problems of healthy food access and affordability to low-income and minority population groups. However, thoughtful policies can institute protections toward low-resource or economically disadvantaged neighborhoods. Figure 9.7 depicts SNAP-authorized food retailers in a midsize city. It demonstrates the density of unhealthy food retailers, convenience stores, discount variety stores (e.g., dollar stores), and pharmacies.

Financial institutions combine private funds with federal dollars to support blighted areas with resources and innovative programs. Community Development Financial Institutions (CDFIs) can provide capital financing to support healthy food retail in low-income urban neighborhoods.

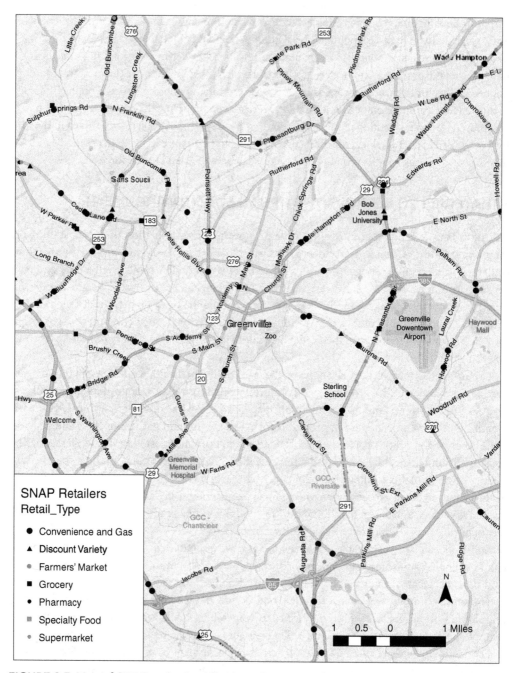

FIGURE 9.7 Map of SNAP-authorized food retailers in a midsize city in the United States.
SNAP, Supplemental Nutrition Assistance Program.
Source: From © OpenStreetMap contributors. Map available by CC BY-SA License (www.openstreetmap.org/copyright).

Healthy Food Financing Initiative is a public–private partnership leveraging public funds to support local food retailers to increase the availability and affordability of healthy foods. This can be through partnerships with SNAP- or WIC-authorized farmers' markets by increasing the value of their public benefits for the purchase of fresh fruits and vegetables.

Urban Agriculture Initiatives

Community agriculture and conservation initiatives have become essential components of sustainable community development strategies, particularly in urban areas and low-income neighborhoods.[52] These initiatives can include community gardens, regional food distribution hubs, zoning for urban agriculture to support food entrepreneurs, food systems in city comprehensive plans, and creation of a healthy retail initiative to promote the availability of healthy, affordable foods in small grocers (i.e., Health Corner Store Initiative). Community gardens are an increasingly popular form of community agriculture, commonly viewed as an effective community development tool in strengthening both individual and community assets.[53] Prior studies indicated the potential of community gardens to revitalize neighborhoods, build social capital and political activism, and foster a sense of belonging and collective efficacy.[54] Furthermore, motivations for participation in community gardening are usually driven by a desire to improve neighborhoods, enjoy nature, increase access to fresh food, and build healthier communities.[55,56] The following is an analysis of the reasons why volunteers participate in community gardens and the environmental, economic, and social benefits of these programs for individual participants and hosting communities.

What Is a Community Garden?

According to Ferris, Norman, and Sempik, community gardens can be described as public enterprises where ownership, access, and democratic control are commonly shared in order to provide local food supplies while offering opportunities for open space, greenery, and leisure and recreational activities.[57] Recent studies have switched from a purely environmental and economic perspective to highlight the importance of community gardens as common places of collective activities that serve a diverse range of social benefits. For example, Sassatelli emphasizes their role as catalysts for creating more sustainable and ethical forms of living as well as community enrichment.[58] Cumbers, Shaw, Crossan, and McMaster gave emphasis to the potential for developing new ways of deriving place-based identity and community, and Wills pinpointed their role as active places bringing diverse groups together to create new and more progressive social relations and diminishing racial tensions.[59,60] A community-based definition described community gardens as a "process for responding to and nurturing neighborhood-based initiative through a nongovernmental intermediary organization where the defining characteristic is the engagement of the program beneficiaries."[61]

Community Gardens and Sustainable Development

Historically, in the United States, community gardens were initially designed to increase local food supplies during the World Wars and Great Depression.[54] In the wake of gross shortages, programs such as the Victory Gardens Program implemented by the USDA produced approximately 40% of the fresh vegetables in the country.[52]

For the past 70 years, community gardens have flourished and declined following the socioeconomic climate of the host communities. In the past few decades, sustainable community development strategies have integrated the use of community gardens as essential components to revitalize and sustain development in communities around the world. Holland studied how community gardens guided the development, evolution, and expansion of local sustainability efforts.[62] The outcomes of Holland's study showed that gardens were all connected through a sense of community participation, and that also provided all three mechanisms to achieve sustainable communities by addressing economic, social, and environmental issues. Today, community activists, public health workers, and planners praise community gardens as a critical urban–rural partnership yielding a myriad of social, economic, environmental, and health benefits.[63]

Citizen Participation and Collective Efficacy in Community Gardens

Citizen participation can be described as the active, voluntary involvement of individuals and groups to modify challenging conditions in their communities and to influence the policies and programs that affect the quality of their lives.[64] For the past few decades, citizen participation has augmented the effectiveness of community-based social work strategies by strengthening individual involvement in democratic processes and building community problem-solving resources and capacities.[65] One of the most frequent challenges for citizen participation is the long-term involvement of individuals. Studies have shown that the majority of community garden programs depend heavily on the participation of their members, not only in terms of physical work and resources, but also in active involvement and time. Therefore, it is imperative that individuals believe they have the capacity to make a difference.

Participation in the planning, development, and maintenance of a community garden can improve individuals' abilities, opportunities, and relationships. An individual's perception regarding his or her ability to work with his or her neighbors to intervene in community issues to solve problems is called collective efficacy.[66] Several studies have shown that community gardens provide the opportunity for place-based social processes that support collective efficacy and, consequently, improve neighborhood conditions, promote health, and sense of belonging.[67,68] Citizen participation in a community garden program can also strengthen the connection among neighbors, commonly referred to as social integration or social capital.[52]

CONCLUSION

Urbanization is a global phenomenon, primarily driven by economic drivers such as job opportunities and more services. However, the urban environment disproportionately affects vulnerable population groups with many SDOH such as poor housing conditions, segregated neighborhoods, and limited access to resources, including those that facilitate achieving a healthy diet. Differences in health are striking in communities with poor SDOH; and low-resource communities afflicted by a myriad of SDOH are prevalent in urban settings across the globe. Living in food deserts, gentrification, poverty, and many other SDOH hinder the capacity of low-income and minority urban residents to access healthy food options. Fortunately, researchers and practitioners are currently using ecological perspectives with the purpose of understanding the influence of the environment on the risk of developing health conditions associated with food consumption such as obesity and eating disorders. These research and related programmatic efforts are helping in identifying community-engaged and holistic strategies to promote healthier eating patterns in urban settings, particularly by demonstrating how the accumulation of risks across ecologies may account for compromised healthy development of children and families. Interventions to address a variety of factors at different levels of the socio-ecological spectrum in urban settings are required. The design of these interventions should incorporate evidence on the influence of the built environment on health, emphasizing the potential of broad-based community-level interventions. By trying to depict how the urban context perpetuates the SDOH that determine poor health outcomes for low-income and minority individuals in urban settings, local officials, communities, and citizens can begin to collaboratively address the factors that perpetuate poor nutritional patterns in urban settings.

KEY CONCEPTS

1. *Urbanization and urban health:* Urbanization is the population shift from more rural areas to more urban areas, causing expansion of and population growth in cities. Much of this movement is due to economic drivers such as job opportunities and more services. Urban populations present differing health concerns than those in rural areas.

2. *Healthy diet:* Maintaining a healthy diet can be challenging to some population groups depending on their geographic area and socioeconomic status.

3. *Urbanization and gentrification:* Urbanization is population movement from rural areas to more urban areas, causing an increase in population in cities and the expansion of cities. Gentrification is the change in neighborhood characteristics from low-income communities, often rife with crime, minority populations, and limited resources to the opposite of high-income households and nonminority population groups. Gentrification results in the displacement of low-income residents following urban renewal or revitalization projects.

4. *Food deserts:* In urban areas, we often see "food deserts," or the lack of a supermarket in low-income areas. Supermarkets are not likely to be in cities, but rather are more often found in the periphery or suburban areas. Food retailers located in cities often are smaller, with limited availability of healthy foods such as fresh fruits and vegetables and perishable items. Land costs are higher in urban areas resulting in higher leasing and rental costs for storeowners. Consequently, some of these costs are passed on to the consumer through higher food prices.

5. *Availability in urban settings:* There are a limited number of supermarkets in urban areas, contributing to food deserts in low-income areas. Instead, small grocers, such as bodegas and corner stores, convenience/gas stores, pharmacies, and dollar stores are often the options available to urban households, especially for those with limited resources.

6. *Access to food in urban settings:* In regard to this topic, accessibility will focus on the ability to get to destinations via transportation. As population density increases, vehicle ownership decreases, and those with disabilities also have transportation difficulties. Public transit provides accessibility opportunities especially for older adults, those with low income, and those with disabilities. However, transit users have limited choices for supermarkets or grocery stores with limited stops to such food retailers. In addition, travel time is more likely to be longer, including multiple transfers to other routes in order to reach the destination. Transit users also need to factor travel costs and carrying groceries back to their home.

7. *Affordability in urban settings:* In terms of diet, there is a cost disparity between nutrient-rich foods and less healthy food options. Lack of affordability of food contributes to food insecurity. Low income and poverty are associated with food insecurity, or reduced quality, variety, and desirability of diet with disrupted eating patterns.

8. *Social determinants of health (SDOH):* Research has shown that the health of a community is not determined only by its healthcare system, but it is also determined by access to social and economic opportunities; the resources and supports available in our households, neighborhoods, and communities; the quality of our schooling; the

safety of our workplaces; the cleanliness of our water, food, and air; and the nature of our social interactions and relationships. SDOH are conditions in the environments in which people are born, live, learn, work, play, worship, and age that affect a wide range of health, functioning, and quality-of-life outcomes and risks.

CASE STUDY 1: LIVEWELL GREENVILLE: MAINTAINING A HEALTHY COMMUNITY IN GREENVILLE COUNTY, SOUTH CAROLINA

LiveWell Greenville is a county-level initiative to create and maintain a healthy community through the promotion and support of policies, systems, and environments that make healthy choices viable to families and communities across Greenville County, South Carolina.[69] Greenville County, South Carolina, has an estimated population of 498,766; 24.2% are younger than 18 years; 76.7% are White; 18.6% are African American; the median household income in 2012–2016 was $52,595; and 15.2% of the population lives below the FPL.[70] Greenville County has one of the highest obesity rates in the nation, with 66% of adults and 41% of youth being overweight or obese. Without providing adequate access to healthy eating and active living, the overall health of this community will continue to decline.[69]

LiveWell Greenville has become the primary vehicle through which partner organizations can successfully promote positive change in the county. A coalition supports schools, neighborhoods, businesses, and other areas of the community through resources, collaboration, and evaluation to promote healthy eating and active living.[69] The healthy eating and active living strategies of the LiveWell Greenville partnership include three overarching initiatives (Figure 9.8), which are active transportation, access to healthy food, and nutrition and physical activity standards in after-school settings.[71] The active transportation improvement initiative aims at increasing bicycle and pedestrian access, including physical changes to streets, construction of trails, installation of wayfinding signage, and development of bike storage stations. The access to healthy food initiative pursues increasing access to affordable and nutritious produce through the implementation of a farmers' market and mobile market in communities with limited access to fresh produce. The nutrition and physical activity initiative aims at increasing policy and environment standards for healthy eating and active living in Out of School Time centers.

LiveWell Greenville is one of 49 community partnerships across the United States that received grants from the Healthy Kids, Healthy Communities (HKHC) national program, funded by the Robert Wood Johnson Foundation (RWJF), with the goal of preventing childhood obesity. The program placed special emphasis on reaching children at highest risk for obesity based on race, ethnicity, income, or geographic location.[71] Efforts to develop the LiveWell Greenville coalition in Greenville county included partnership and capacity-building strategies such as formal retreats and training (over 80 community members and stakeholders), community change agents (the Sterling Land Trust Board, the Nicholtown Neighborhood Association, and Russell Community Church), and community advisory committees (adult and youth planning committees).

LiveWell Greenville's overarching strategy is to influence SDOH in the county including the following: crime, obesity, access to healthy foods, and public transportation.[71] In relation to access to healthy foods, South Carolina has a lower number of healthy food retailers compared to the national average. According to the Nutrition Environment Measures Survey (NEMS), the city

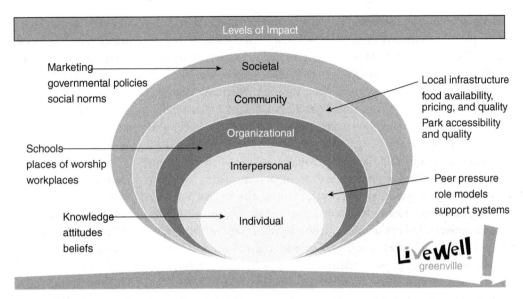

FIGURE 9.8 Levels of impact of LiveWell Greenville in accordance with the socio-ecological framework.

Source: From Powers A. *Live Well Greenville: Making the Healthy Choice the Easy Choice.* Greenville Health System; 2014. http://scholarexchange.furman.edu/records-ghs/3

of Greenville has only six grocery stores, while there are 69 fast casual restaurants, 57 fast-food restaurants, and 97 sit-down restaurants.

Access to healthy food related statistics were generated by the LiveWell Greenville coalition by conducting assessments to better understand access to healthy foods using the NEMS. The NEMS was completed in May 2010 for all food establishments in Greenville County and each municipality to define food desert areas near adult and youth residents. Reports and maps were used within the communities to assist with advocating for changes in the food environment. The County Planning Department developed maps identifying food stores. Additional NEMSs were completed in December 2012. In addition to the surveys, a food policy scan was conducted in fall 2012 by reviewing existing ordinances and codes for various cities in the state of South Carolina. Other assessments included healthy vending assessments and price comparison assessments. A mobile food-vending project was conducted to better understand how Greenville could formulate and implement a policy encouraging the operation of food trucks. A Healthy Eating and Activity Standards in Out of School Time assessment was conducted in 2012 to understand healthy eating and physical activity standards in Out of School Time centers.[71]

Findings from the different assessments conducted by the LiveWell coalition were used to promote population reach and impact related activities including the development of community gardens and mobile markets that were targeted toward residents in three prioritized neighborhoods. In 2012, a 2-acre community garden located in one of these neighborhoods produced approximately 2,000 pounds of food (e.g., collards, okra, asparagus, mustard salad, sweet potatoes, turnip greens), which was distributed free to volunteers, older adults, and residents with disabilities. Some of the challenges identified in one of the community gardens included low participation and lack of community buy-in. Moreover, relationship building was needed owing to distrust among one community and a local faith-based organization. Another relevant strategy implemented as part of the LiveWell Greenville initiative was the Nutrition and Physical Activity Standards in Child Care. As part of this strategy, the City of Greenville instituted a policy change incorporating healthy snacks in all city-sponsored after-school programs in 2012.[71]

Kemper and colleagues conducted a study to determine changes in nutrition and physical activity environments, policies, and practices among 37 after-school programs after their participation in the LiveWell Greenville Afterschool Initiative.[72] The study used a nonexperimental, pre- and postsurvey design. The survey was based on the Nutrition and Physical Activity Self-Assessment for Child Care questionnaire and modified for after-school settings. A 9-month intervention consisted of program staff members completing the preassessment and goal-setting worksheet, receiving technical support and training from LiveWell Greenville staff, attending networking meetings about nutrition and physical activity promotion strategies, and completing a postassessment. Findings of this study showed that the LiveWell Greenville Afterschool Initiative, which involved self-assessment, goal setting, and technical support, is a successful strategy to change nutrition and physical activity environments in after-school settings.[73] Through empirical research and formative and summative evaluations, the LiveWell Greenville initiative has provided evidence of the positive impact on community's health and well-being of implementing holistic and socio-ecological approaches to healthy communities that address SDOH in vulnerable urban communities in the United States.

Case Study Questions

1. Healthier community initiatives require the promotion and support of policies, systems, and environments that make healthy choices viable to families and communities. What could be two examples of policies and two examples of systems and environments you would target for modification and/or development with the purpose of promoting healthier lifestyles at the county level in the United States?

2. Community-based participatory research (CBPR) is a collaborative approach to research that has been useful in working with disadvantaged communities to reduce health disparities. Through CBPR, communities have been directly involved in culturally competent research and interventions. Efforts to develop the LiveWell Greenville coalition in Greenville County incorporated partnership and capacity-building strategies, including formal retreats and training, community change agents, and community advisory committees. Do you believe that the aforementioned partnership and capacity-building strategies and groups were sufficient to foster a CBPR process that accounts for a meaningful participation of most relevant stakeholders in Greenville County? Do you think that Greenville County residents of all ages, race–ethnicity, religion, physical condition, and so on had the same opportunity to have been represented into these programmatic groups? Would you use the same strategies and groups for a similar initiative? If not, what would you do differently?

3. The LiveWell Greenville initiative is framed within the SEM of health and incorporates a holistic and interdisciplinary approach to promote healthier communities through partnerships and collaborations. Identify three elements of this initiative that reflect its socio-ecological perspective, and explain how these three elements reflect this initiative.

CASE STUDY 2: PROGRAMS AND COLLABORATIVES FOR IMPROVING AFFORDABLE HEALTHY FOOD ACCESS IN SAN DIEGO COUNTY, CALIFORNIA

San Diego County in California understood the challenges of healthy living when there are limited healthy food options. With multiple interagency partnerships, there have been a variety of changes to improve affordable, healthy food access. Through the Fresh Food Fund, families and residents participating in SNAP, WIC, and Supplemental Security Income have been able to receive $20 matching funds for every $20 spent at the local farmers' markets for fruits and vegetables. In addition, the San Diego Unified School District implemented a Farm-to-School program for school lunches, which provided fresh, local food to San Diego students, including access to a salad bar. Further, the city of San Diego amended their costly permitting and zoning restrictions to allow for community gardens. The San Diego Food System Alliance is a multisector collaborative aimed at improving food security and healthy food access through a systems-level change strategy by coordinating and collaborating with local partners to address urban agriculture, local food procurement, and food waste recovery.

Case Study Questions

1. The interventions implemented in San Diego required coordination and collaboration from multiple partners from various sectors. Some of these required changes in policy and procurement. In addressing healthy good access through urban agriculture strategies from a socio-ecological perspective, what type of sectors, agencies, and organizations would be part of such collaborative efforts?

2. San Diego's Fresh Food Fund allowed eligible families to increase their purchasing power for healthy, fresh foods. What are the challenges to this program and how would you address those challenges?

3. The San Diego Unified School District implemented a Farm-to-School program. Encouraging children to eat fresh fruits and vegetables as part of a regular diet may be quite the feat. What are some strategies to motivate and introduce children to eating fresh fruits and vegetables, especially with respect to what may be available in a salad bar?

4. San Diego County has a climate that affords a year-round growing season. How might cities in other climates address and support urban agriculture?

SUGGESTED LEARNING ACTIVITIES

1. Visit USDA MyPlate site for interactive engagement of dietary guidelines for specific dietary restrictions or medical conditions (i.e., type 2 diabetes, vegan diet): www.choosemyplate.gov/dietary-guidelines.

2. Visit the USDA Food Access Research Atlas to engage in an interactive map: www.ers.usda.gov/data-products/food-access-research-atlas.

REFLECTION QUESTIONS

1. What is the role of urbanization in shaping nutritional patterns among low-income minority populations?

2. In what ways do food deserts and/or food swamps influence the nutritional status of low-income minority populations in urban settings?

3. What are some of the most relevant social determinants of nutritional health in urban settings?

4. You have been assigned to identify ways to improve the nutritional status of children and adolescents at a school setting by using a socio-ecological approach. Please describe the policies and programs you would recommend for achieving this goal. Which factors, and at which levels of the SEM, are you going to target to achieve your proposed goals?

CONTINUE YOUR LEARNING RESOURCES

- **U.S. Department of Agriculture (USDA)** is responsible for providing a safety net for millions of Americans who are food-insecure and for developing and promoting dietary guidance based on scientific evidence. The USDA works to increase food security and reduce hunger by providing children and low-income people access to food, a healthful diet, and nutrition education in a way that supports American agriculture and inspires public confidence. The Center for Nutrition Policy and Promotion (CNPP) is responsible for developing and promoting dietary guidance that links the best evidence-based scientific research to the nutrition needs of Americans (USDA Child Nutrition Programs: www.usda.gov/topics/food-and-nutrition).

- **Centers for Disease Control and Prevention (CDC) Division of Nutrition, Physical Activity, and Obesity** protects the health of Americans at every stage of life by encouraging regular physical activity, good nutrition, and healthy weight. Through its support of state and community partners, it provides data, programs that work, and practical tools so that Americans have the best possible chance to achieve healthier lives and avoid chronic diseases (Center for Chronic Disease Prevention and Health Promotion, Division of Nutrition, Physical Activity, and Obesity at a Glance: www.cdc.gov/chronicdisease/resources/publications/aag/dnpao.htm).

- **The National Alliance for Nutrition and Activity (NANA)** advocates national policies and programs to promote healthy eating and physical activity to help reduce the illnesses, diseases, disabilities, premature deaths, and costs associated with diet and inactivity. Its efforts include advocating for strong public policy and program funding, supporting effective education programs, and promoting environmental approaches to help the public eat better and be more active (Center for Science in the Public Interest, National Alliance for Nutrition and Activity: cspinet.org/protecting-our-health/nutrition/national-alliance-nutrition-and-activity).

- **The Food Tank:** To counteract unhealthy nutritional messaging, many organizations around the globe are working to instill healthy eating habits, foster food literacy, teach culinary skills, and educate children about the environmental, social, and health consequences of their food choices. Food Tank has selected 35 particularly noteworthy programs (Food Tank, 35 Food Education Organizations: foodtank.com/news/2016/09/thirty-five-food-education-organizations).

- **The Agatston Urban Nutrition Initiative (AUNI)** was developed from an ABCS course taught by Francis Johnston, Professor of Anthropology, in 1991. It was created to help build and sustain healthy communities by promoting nutrition education, food access and sovereignty, and physical fitness in West Philadelphia (The Barbara and Edward Netter Center for Community Partnerships, Agatston Urban Nutrition Initiative: www.nettercenter.upenn.edu/what-we-do/programs/university-assisted-community-schools/agatston-urban-nutrition-initiative).

GLOSSARY

Community garden: Any piece of land gardened by a group of people, utilizing either individual or shared plots on private or public land.

Food desert: Geographic areas with low-income census tracts (i.e., geographically defined areas determined by the U.S. Bureau of the Census and which are equivalent to neighborhoods) and no supermarket within 1 mile.

Food insecurity: The state of being without reliable access to a sufficient quantity of affordable, nutritious food.

Food swamp: Describes a geographic location that has a high concentration of businesses that sell "junk food" (high-calorie, low-nutrition food) more so than healthier food outlets.

Food system: A complex web of activities involving production, processing, transport, and consumption. Issues concerning the food system include the governance and economics of food production, its sustainability, the degree to which we waste food, how food production affects the natural environment, and the impact of food on individual and population health.

Gentrification: The change in neighborhood characteristics from low-income communities, often rife with crime, minority populations, and limited resources, to the opposite of high-income households and nonminority population groups.

Social determinants of health (SDOH): Conditions in the environments in which people are born, live, learn, work, play, worship, and age that affect a wide range of health, functioning, and quality-of-life outcomes and risks.

Socio-ecological perspectives: Contribute with the understanding about the influence of the environment on the risk of developing health conditions.

Toxic environment: A multidisciplinary field of science concerned with the study of the harmful effects of various chemical, biological, and physical agents on living organisms.

Urban agriculture: The growing of plants and the raising of animals within and around cities.

Urbanization: The population shift from more rural areas to more urban areas, causing expansion of and population growth in cities. Much of this movement is due to economic drivers such as job opportunities and more services.

REFERENCES

1. Leviton LC, Snell E, McGinnis M. Urban issues in health promotion strategies. *Am J Public Health.* 2000;90:863–866. doi:10.2105/AJPH.90.6.863
2. Corburn J. Urban place and health equity: critical issues and practices. *Int J Environ Res Public Health.* 2017;14:E117. doi:10.3390/ijerph14020117
3. Cohen N. *Feeding or Starving Gentrification: The Role of Food Policy.* New York, NY: CUNY Urban Food Policy Institute. 2018. https://www.cunyurbanfoodpolicy.org/news/2018/3/27/feeding-or-starving-gentrification-the-role-of-food-policy
4. Cohen MJ, Garrett JL. The food price crisis and urban food (in) security. *Environ Urban.* 2010;22:467–482. doi:10.1177/0956247810380375
5. Caspi CE, Pelletier JE, Harnack L, et al. Differences in healthy food supply and stocking practices between small grocery stores, gas-marts, pharmacies and dollar stores. *Public Health Nutr.* 2016;19(3):540–547. doi:10.1017/S1368980015002724
6. Lind PL, Jensen PV, Glumer C, Toft U. The association between accessibility of local convenience stores and unhealthy diet. *Eur J Public Health.* 2016;26:634–639. doi:10.1093/eurpub/ckv242
7. Cooksey-Stowers K, Schwartz M, Brownell K. Food swamps predict obesity rates better than food deserts in the United States. *Int J Environ Res Public Health.* 2017;11:1366. doi:10.3390/ijerph14111366
8. Khan LK, Sobush K, Keener D, et al. Recommended community strategies and measurements to prevent obesity in the United States. *MMWR Recomm Rep.* 2009;58(RR-7):1–26.
9. Blumenberg E, Pierce G. Automobile ownership and travel by the poor: evidence from the 2009 National Household Travel Survey. *Transp Res Rec.* 2012;2320:28–36. doi:10.3141/2320-04
10. Durant S. *Transportation Difficulties Keep Over Half a Million Disabled at Home.* Washington, DC: Bureau of Transportation Statistics; 2003.
11. Ver Ploeg M, Larimore E, Wilde PE. *The Influence of Food Store Access on Grocery Shopping and Food Spending.* 2017. https://www.ers.usda.gov/webdocs/publications/85442/eib-180.pdf
12. Martinez JC, Clark JM, Gudzune KA. Association of personal vehicle access with lifestyle habits and food insecurity among public housing residents. *Prev Med Rep.* 2019;13:341–345. doi:10.1016/j.pmedr.2019.01.001
13. Murphy M, Koohsari MJ, Badland H, Giles-Corti B. Supermarket access, transport mode and BMI: the potential for urban design and planning policy across socio-economic areas. *Public Health Nutr.* 2017;20:3304–3315. doi:10.1017/S1368980017002336
14. Hossfeld L, Kelly B, Waity J, eds. (2018). *Food and Poverty: Food Insecurity and Food Sovereignty Among America's Poor.* Nashville, TN: Vanderbilt University; 2018.
15. Monsivais P, Mclain J, Drewnowski A. The rising disparity in the price of healthful foods: 2004–2008. *Food Policy.* 2010;35:514–520. doi:10.1016/j.foodpol.2010.06.004
16. Drewnowski A, Rolls BJ. *Obesity Treatment and Prevention: New Directions.* Basel, Switzerland: Karger Medical and Scientific Publishers; 2012.
17. Caspi CE, Pelletier JE, Harnack LJ, et al. Pricing of staple foods at supermarkets versus small food stores. *Int J Environ Res Public Health.* 2017;14:E915. doi:10.3390/ijerph14080915
18. Hossfeld L, Kelly B, Waity J. Solutions to the social problem of food insecurity in the United States. In: Muschert G, Klocke B, Perucci R, Shefner J, eds. *Agenda for Social Justice: Solutions for 2016.* Bristol, UK: Policy Press; 2016.
19. McGinnis JM, Williams-Russo P, Knickman JR. The case for more active policy attention to health promotion. *Health Aff (Millwood).* 2002;21:78–93. doi:10.1377/hlthaff.21.2.78
20. Institute of Medicine. *Disparities in Health Care: Methods for Studying the Effects of Race, Ethnicity, and SES on Access, Use, and Quality of Health Care.* Washington, DC: National Academies Press; 2002.
21. Mackenbach JP. The contribution of medical care to mortality decline: McKeown revisited. *J Clin Epidemiol.* 1996;49:1207–1213. doi:10.1016/S0895-4356(96)00200-4
22. McGinnis JM, Foege WH. Actual causes of death in the United States. *JAMA.* 1993;270:2207–2212. doi:10.1001/jama.1993.03510180077038
23. Mackenbach JP, Stronks K, Kunst AE. The contribution of medical care to inequalities in health: differences between socio-economic groups in decline of mortality from conditions amenable to medical intervention. *Soc Sci Med.* 1989;29:369–376. doi:10.1016/0277-9536(89)90285-2

24. Braveman P, Gottlieb L. The social determinants of health: it's time to consider the causes of the causes. *Public Health Rep.* 2014;129(suppl 2):19–31. doi:10.1177/00333549141291S206

25. Solar O, Irwin A. A conceptual framework for action on the social determinants of health. *Social Determinants of Health Discussion Paper 2 (Policy and Practice)*. Geneva, Switzerland: World Health Organization; 2010.

26. Lovell N, Bibby J. *What Makes Us Healthy? An Introduction to the Social Determinants of Health.* London, UK: Health Foundation; 2018:1–61.

27. Centers for Disease Control and Prevention. *Social Determinants of Health: Know what affects health.* 2018. Retrieved from https://www.cdc.gov/socialdeterminants/index.htm

28. Commission on Social Determinants of Health. *Closing the Gap in a Generation: Health Equity Through Action on the Social Determinants of Health.* Geneva, Switzerland: World Health Organization; 2008. https://www.who.int/social_determinants/en

29. Anderson ES, Winett RA, Wojcik JR. Self-regulation, self-efficacy, outcome expectations, and social support: social cognitive theory and nutrition behavior. *Ann Behav Med.* 2007;34(3):304–312. doi:10.1007/BF02874555

30. World Health Organization. *Our Cities, Our Health, Our Future: Toward Action on Social Determinants of Health in Urban Settings.* A synopsis of the report of the knowledge network on urban settings to the WHO Commission on Social Determinants of Health. Kobe, Japan: WHO Centre for Health Development; 2008.

31. Gordon-Larsen P, Nelson MC, Page P, Popkin BM. Inequality in the built environment underlies key health disparities in physical activity and obesity. *Pediatrics.* 2006;117:417–424. doi:10.1542/peds.2005-0058

32. Cummins S, Macintyre S. Food environments and obesity—neighborhood or nation? *Int J Epidemiol.* 2006;35:100–104. doi:10.1093/ije/dyi276

33. Asfour L, Huang S, Ocasio MA, et al. Association between socio-ecological risk factor clustering and mental, emotional, and behavioral problems in Hispanic adolescents. *J Child Fam Stud.* 2017;26:1266–1273. doi:10.1007/s10826-016-0641-0

34. Bronfenbrenner, U. (1977). Toward an experimental ecology of human development. *Am Psychol.* 1977;32:513–531.doi:10.1037/0003-066x.32.7.513

35. Bronfenbrenner U. Ecological systems theory. In: Bronfenbrenner U, ed. *Making Human Beings Human: Bioecological Perspectives on Human Development.* Thousand Oaks, CA: Sage Publications; 2005:106–173.

36. Gardiner HW. *Lives Across Cultures: Cross-Cultural Human Development.* New York, NY: Pearson; 2018:14.

37. Birch LL, Anzman SL. Learning to eat in an obesogenic environment: a developmental systems perspective on childhood obesity. *Child Dev Perspect.* 2010;4:138–143. doi:10.1111/j.1750-8606.2010.00132.x

38. Neumark-Sztainer D. Preventing the broad spectrum of weight-related problems: working with parents to help teens achieve a healthy weight and positive body image. *J Nutr Educ Behav.* 2005;37:S133–S139. doi:10.1016/S1499-4046(06)60214-5

39. Fiese BH, Jones BL. Food and family: a socio-ecological perspective for child development. *Adv Child Dev Behav.* 2012;42:307–337. doi:10.1016/b978-0-12-394388-0.00009-5

40. Harrison K, Bost KK, McBride BA, et al. Toward a developmental conceptualization of contributors to overweight and obesity in childhood: the Six-C's model. *Child Dev Perspect.* 2011;5:50–58. doi:10.1111/j.1750-8606.2010.00150.x

41. Robinson T. Applying the Socio-ecological Model to improving fruit and vegetable intake among low-income African Americans. *J Community Health.* 2008;33:395–406. doi:10.1007/s10900-008-9109-5

42. Moore SN, Murphy S, Moore L. Health improvement, nutrition-related behaviour and the role of school meals: the usefulness of a socio-ecological perspective to inform policy design, implementation and evaluation. *Crit Public Health.* 2011;21:441–454. doi:10.1080/09581596.2011.620604

43. Townsend N, Foster C. Developing and applying a socio-ecological model to the promotion of healthy eating in the school. *Public Health Nutr.* 2011;16:1101–1108. doi:10.1017/S1368980011002655

44. Moore L, de Silva-Sanigorski A, Moore SN. A socio-ecological perspective on behavioural interventions to influence food choice in schools: alternative, complementary or synergistic? *Public Health Nutr.* 2013;16:1000–1005. doi:10.1017/S1368980012005605

45. American Diabetes Association. *Facts About Type 2 Diabetes*. 2015. http://www.diabetes.org/diabetes -basics/type-2/facts-about-type-2.html?loc=db-slabnav

46. Ziemer DC, Berkowitz KJ, Panayioto RM, et al. A simple meal plan emphasizing healthy food choices is as effective as an exchange-based meal plan for urban African Americans with type 2 diabetes. *Diabetes Care*. 2003;26:1719–1724. doi:10.2337/diacare.26.6.1719

47. Thorndike AN, Riis J, Sonnenberg LM, Levy DE. Traffic-light labels and choice architecture: promoting healthy food choices. *Am J Prev Med*. 2014;46:143–149. doi:10.1016/j.amepre.2013.10.002

48. Salois MJ. Obesity and diabetes, the built environment, and the 'local' food economy in the United States. *Econ Hum Biol*. 2012;10:35–42. doi:10.1016/j.ehb.2011.04.001

49. Smoyer-Tomic KE, Spence JC, Amrhein C. Food deserts in the prairies? Supermarket accessibility and neighborhood need in Edmonton, Canada. *Prof Geogr*. 2006;58:307–326. doi:10.1111/j.1467 -9272.2006.00570.x

50. Eisenhauer E. In poor health: supermarket redlining and urban nutrition. *E Geo J*. 2001;53:125–133. doi:10.1023/A:1015772503007

51. Ghosh-Dastidar B, Cohen D, Hunter G, et al. Distance to store, food prices, and obesity in urban food deserts. *Am J Prev Med*. 2014;47:587–595. doi:10.1016/j.amepre.2014.07.005

52. Ohmer ML, Meadowcroft P, Freed K, Lewis E. Community gardening and community development: individual, social and community benefits of a community conservation program. *J Community Pract*. 2009;17:377–399. doi:10.1080/10705420903299961

53. Jones L. Improving health, building community: exploring the asset building potential of community gardens. *Evans Sch Rev*. 2012;2:66–84. doi:10.7152/esr.v2i1.13732

54. Saldivar-Tanaka L, Krasny ME. Culturing community development, neighborhood open space, and civic agriculture: the case of Latino community gardens in New York City. *Agr Hum Values*. 2004;21:399–412.

55. Schumacher JR, Lanier JA, Calvert K. Fostering community health through community gardens. *J Acad Nutr Diet*. 2014;114:A88. doi:10.1016/j.jand.2014.06.296

56. Andersson E, Barthel S, Ahrné K. Measuring social–ecological dynamics behind the generation of ecosystem services. *Ecol Appl*. 2007;17:1267–1278. doi:10.1890/06-1116.1

57. Ferris J, Norman C, Sempik J. People, land and sustainability: community gardens and the social dimension of sustainable development. *Soc Policy Adm*. 2001;35:559–568. doi:10.1111/1467-9515.t01- 1-00253

58. Sassatelli R. Consumer culture, sustainability and a new vision of consumer sovereignty. *Sociol Ruralis*. 2015;55:483–496. doi:10.1111/soru.12081

59. Cumbers A, Shaw D, Crossan J, McMaster R. The work of community gardens: reclaiming place for community in the City. *Work Employ Soc*. 2018;32:133–149. doi:10.1177/0950017017695042

60. Wills J. Place and politics. In Featherstone D, Painter J, eds. *Spatial Politics: Essays for Doreen Massey*. Chichester, UK: Wiley-Blackwell; 2013:133–145.

61. Tranel M, Handlin LB Jr. Metromorphosis: documenting change. *J Urban Aff*, 2006;28:151–167. doi:10.1111/j.0735-2166.2006.00265.x

62. Holland L. Diversity and connections in community gardens: a contribution to local sustainability. *Local Environ*. 2004;9:285–305. doi:10.1080/1354983042000219388

63. Kearney SC. *The Community Garden as a Tool for Community Empowerment: A Study of Community Gardens in Hampden County* (master's thesis). Amherst, MA: University of Massachusetts; 2009:361.

64. Gamble DN, Weil MO. Citizen participation. *Encycl Soc Work*. 1995;1:483–494.

65. Ohmer M, Beck E. Citizen participation in neighborhood organizations in poor communities and its relationship to neighborhood and organizational collective efficacy. *J Sociol Soc Welfare*. 2006;33:179.

66. Wandersman A, Florin P. Citizen participation and community organizations. In: Rappaport J, Seidman E, eds. *Handbook of Community Psychology*. Boston, MA: Springer; 2000:247–272.

67. Alaimo K, Reischl TM, Allen JO. Community gardening, neighborhood meetings, and social capital. *J Community Psychol*. 2010;38:497–514. doi:10.1002/jcop.20378

68. Teig E, Amulya J, Bardwell L, et al. Collective efficacy in Denver, Colorado: strengthening neighborhoods and health through community gardens. *Health Place*. 2009;15:1115–1122. doi:10.1016/ j.healthplace.2009.06.003

69. Powers A. *Live Well Greenville: Making the Healthy Choice the Easy Choice*. 2014. http://scholarexchange. furman.edu/records-ghs/3

70. U.S. Census Bureau. *QuickFacts*. Greenville County, South Carolina. 2018. https://census.gov/quickfacts/fact/table/greenvillecountysouthcarolina/RHI725216

71. Mazdra B, Behlmann, T, Brennan LK. *LiveWell Greenville Case Report*. St. Louis, MO: Transtria; 2014. http://www.transtria.com/hkhc

72. Kemper KA, Pate SP, Powers AR, Fair M. Promoting healthy environments in afterschool settings: the LiveWell Greenville afterschool initiative. *Prev Chronic Dis*. 2018;15:1–10. doi:10.5888/pcd15.180164

73. LiveWell Greenville. *Making the Healthy Choice the Easy Choice*. 2019. https://livewellgreenville.org

GLOBAL HEALTH: IMPORTANCE OF INTERPROFESSIONAL APPROACH

LAUREN R. SASTRE, JIGNA M. DHAROD, AND DANIELLE L. NUNNERY

LEARNING OBJECTIVES

1. Describe global **nutrition security (NS)** and associated, complex socioenvironmental factors.

2. Identify major organizations working on nutrition issues worldwide.

3. Identify key nutrition and health issues that the public health practitioner should consider when working with a global population.

4. Understand the importance of food insecurity in predicting health and productivity of the population.

5. Examine the role of water in sustaining food security and ensuring optimal nutritional status at the global level.

6. Explain various mechanisms for migration and the unique nutrition and health risks that individuals face pre-, peri-, and postmigration.

7. Define cultural competence and describe ways in which public health practitioners can effectively meet the social, cultural, and linguistic needs of the communities they serve.

INTRODUCTION

This chapter outlines key health and nutrition considerations for public health nutrition (PHN) practitioners when they work with individuals in the global setting, be it abroad or in the United States. Specific topics include food and **water security**, immigration status and access to services, the role of **resettlement**, and best practices for working with diverse populations, including evidence-based resources and cultural competency.

GLOBAL NUTRITION AND NUTRITION SECURITY

Major Global Nutrition Issues and Defining NS

The concept of NS is one lens through which we can examine nutrition risks, nutrition concerns, and the status of nutrition in individuals and communities globally. It is defined in a position paper on NS by the Academy of Nutrition and Dietetics:

> Nutrition security requires that all people have access to a variety of nutritious foods and potable drinking water; knowledge, resources, and skills for healthy living; prevention, treatment, and care for diseases affecting nutrition status; and safety-net systems during crisis situations, such as natural disasters or deleterious social and political systems.[1]

NS is complex and includes interrelated contextual (e.g., social–environmental) and behavioral determinants of nutritional status and security. Food insecurity is a more familiar nutrition measure and it is included within the concept of NS, for without food security one cannot have NS. However, NS expands to include health services, environmental conditions, and health and nutritional status. NS moves beyond food to encompass optimal nutritional status and the conditions necessary to support it. A conceptual framework and definitions were developed by Gross et al. (see Figure 6 on page 7 of "The Four Dimensions of Food and Nutrition Security: Definitions and Concepts," www.fao.org/elearning/course/fa/en/pdf/p-01_rg_concept.pdf).[2]

Nutrition insecurity (NIS) includes both deficiencies and excesses, which are demonstrated by inadequate nutrient intake, underweight, and overweight status.[1] NIS is a global problem; however, because of the complex factors that influence NIS, it is not easy to address because of such a wide range of interrelated determinants. These determinants include food insecurity; poverty; poor nutritional intake and status (e.g., micronutrient deficiencies, macronutrient excesses); water, hygiene, and sanitation; agricultural systems that do not ensure diverse nutrients or sustainability; infectious diseases, which increase needs and impact absorption, as well as **noncommunicable diseases (NCDs)**; lack of gender equality (inequality for use of household resources as well as educational opportunities, most commonly manifested as a risk for women) and education (lack of financial resources to attend school or lack of school access), limited investment and capacity for economic stability; and an overall aging global population.[1] Within poor nutrition intake and micronutrient deficiencies, there are five common global nutrient deficiencies, which are the primary focus of PHN and clinicians globally. They include iron, folate, vitamin A, zinc, and iodine.[1]

The Socioeconomic Context

In order to address micronutrient deficiencies and NIS, it is critical to understand the complex socioeconomic factors that affect low- and lower-income countries, arguably the countries most burdened by NIS.[1] Low-income countries (previously labeled as "developing countries") are now classified by the World Bank into four economic classifications based on **gross national income (GNI)**: low-, lower middle, upper middle, and high-income countries.[3] Recent discussions have focused on the limitations of using groupings based on income such as "developing" country as there is no consensus on the meaning of this definition and often it only reflects national wealth and industry. More appropriate and inclusive classification definitions have been developed in order to aid in setting nutrition and health priorities and goals.[3] A newer more inclusive and comprehensive category has been developed by the United Nations (UN) and is called the **Human Development Index (HDI)**, which goes beyond income classifications to include more factors of

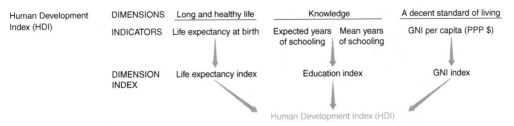

FIGURE 10.1 Human Development Index developed by the United Nations includes three key indicators that reflect the health and economic and status of a country: life expectancy at birth, education, and GNI per capita.

GNI, gross national income.

Source: From Human Development Index. *United Nations Development Programme: Human Development Reports.* 2019. http://hdr.undp.org/en/content/human-development-index-hdi

capacity: a life expectancy index (life expectancy at birth), education index (expected and mean years of schooling), and a GNI index (**GNI per capita**);[4] see Figure 10.1. The HDI overlaps with economic capacity and the **social determinants of health** (**SDOH**), making it a more useful tool for nutrition public health workers and researchers to classify countries when prioritizing programming, funding, and resources.

Major Global Organizations Addressing NIS

Within the UN, four organizations were formed to address NIS. Most were established after World War II; they are World Health Organization (WHO), United Nations Children's Fund (UNICEF), Food and Agriculture Organization of the UN (FAO), and the World Food Programme (WFP). Table 10.1 provides an overview of each of these on the global scale.[5-11]

Each of these organizations plays a crucial role in addressing short-term and long-term nutrition risks and needs for vulnerable communities worldwide. In Busoro, Rwanda, UNICEF provided children with a meal during a community nutrition event (www.unicef.org/nutrition/index_action.html). The children were then weighed and measured as part of growth and nutrition monitoring.

The WFP provides "food baskets" for crisis situations and/or refugee camps. Basic WFP rations include a grain staple (e.g., flour, rice), legumes (lentils, chickpeas, pulses, or beans), vegetable oil fortified with vitamins A and D, sugar, and iodized salt. Food rations per individual include 2,100 kcal, 10% to 12% from protein and 17% from fat, and micronutrients vitamin A, iron, iodine, and zinc. Although these rations are intended to reduce common nutritional deficiencies and provide basic nutrition support, they may be the staple diet for populations that have experienced conflict and/or for refugees for longer term crises. For example, several conflicts and refugee crises in the regions have been occurring for decades. Long-term lack of produce or fresh produce further puts these individuals and groups at risk for long-term adverse health outcomes.

The previously described organizations are large-scale players striving to address global nutrition risks with a primary focus on malnutrition/undernutrition. Organizations such as UNICEF and WHO provide a wide coverage of surveillance and programming, but there are smaller **nongovernmental organizations** (**NGOs**) working toward addressing nutrition risks at the community level. Of these, successful approaches include programmatic elements that build capacity by addressing primary risk factors associated with poor nutrition, including but not limited to

TABLE 10.1 MAJOR GLOBAL ORGANIZATIONS THAT PROVIDE NUTRITION AND HEALTH SERVICES

ORGANIZATION	FOUNDED (YEAR)	OVERVIEW/MISSION	LOCATIONS
World Health Organization (WHO)[5]	1948	The primary global organization addressing nutrition is WHO. WHO's mission includes a focus on health systems, health through the life span, communicable and noncommunicable diseases, emergency preparedness, surveillance, response, and corporate services around the globe. WHO also coordinates efforts with governments and NGO partners to coordinate national health priorities and policies to meet global health goals.	150 countries
United Nations Children's Fund (UNICEF)[6]	1946	Priority areas include child protection and inclusion, child survival (nutrition), education, emergency response, gender inequality, as well as research. UNICEF nutrition-specific initiatives focus on the following: baby-friendly hospital initiatives, breastfeeding/complementary foods, micronutrients, SAM, HIV, and nutrition as well as integration of nutrition into other areas, including health, water, and sanitation.	90 countries
Food and Agriculture Organization of the UN (FAO)[7,8]		The FAO specifically focuses on addressing and eradicating hunger. The FAO's primary focus is on five key areas: (a) elimination of hunger, food insecurity, and malnutrition; (b) increase sustainability and productivity of agriculture, forestry, and fisheries; (c) reduce rural poverty; (d) enable inclusive and efficient agricultural/food systems; and (e) increase the resilience of livelihoods (work/careers) to threats and crises. The FAO's priorities fit well within the 2015–2030 SDGs set by the UN, which include multiple areas associated with food insecurity and environmental goals to increase health equity. (See Continue Your Learning Resources for link to interactive SDGs.)	130 countries

(continued)

TABLE 10.1 MAJOR GLOBAL ORGANIZATIONS THAT PROVIDE NUTRITION AND HEALTH SERVICES (continued)

ORGANIZATION	FOUNDED (YEAR)	OVERVIEW/MISSION	LOCATIONS
World Food Programme (WFP)[9]	1961	The WFP's primary function is as a crisis and relief organization that directly provides emergency food, although they do also work on longer term initiatives within communities to improve nutrition. One in nine individuals still do not have enough to eat and while emergency food assistance is still vital to addressing nutrition insecurity in the short term, other areas of capacity and community building are needed to break cycles of hunger and poverty that create long-term food insecurity. The WFP is not only committed to addressing hunger but also nutrition, and they offer many resources to help assess communities to identify barriers to accessing and consuming healthy and nutritious foods such as the Fill the Nutrient Gap tool. The WFP also works along with other organizations and initiatives such as SUN. SUN was established in 2010 and is a collaborative effort including individuals, the UN, businesses, and researchers to address nutrition, especially malnutrition, and works toward achieving all of the **SDGs**.	80+ countries
International Rescue Committee (IRC)[10]	1933	The IRC works primarily within humanitarian crises and responds during conflict and disasters cities with a focus on the provision of clean water, shelter, healthcare, education, and empowerment. The IRC in particular has a focus on addressing child malnutrition in particularly remote areas. The IRC conducts research to ensure the use of evidence-based practices in addressing malnutrition and infant and child feeding initiatives. They also train lay health workers in their own communities, also known as the **Community Health Worker Model**, to address nutrition, particularly SAM.[11]	40+ countries and 26 U.S. cities

NGO, nongovernmental organization; SAM, severe acute malnutrition; SDGs, Sustainable Development Goals; SUN, Scaling up for Nutrition; UN, United Nations.

poverty, gender and education inequalities, limited healthcare access, and low nutrition and health literacy (knowledge) as well as sustainability.

One approach that has demonstrated success in regions throughout the world is goat herding programs whereby farmers are given goats or **microloans** to purchase a herd. Many of the world's most at-risk populations are in rural, poor areas working on small-scale farms. These "goat projects" provide a source of protein, nutrient-rich milk, and manure for compositing and enriching soil. Additionally, goat's milk may be used as soap, which supports hygiene or additional opportunities for income and goats are relatively small, inexpensive, easy animals to raise and provide additional income when they or their products are sold. Research has shown that agriculture projects, including animal husbandry, are most effective when they include educational and empowerment opportunities that address gender inequality, nutrition and health literacy, and budgeting/financial literacy.[12] Furthermore, research evaluating agricultural and animal husbandry projects on NIS is limited but warranted to drive efforts by NGOs and other organizations to ensure the best use of limited resources to maximize the capacity within communities. Necessary business and related math skills (e.g., pricing, budgeting) should also be addressed.

GLOBAL NUTRITION RISKS TO HEALTH STATUS ACROSS THE LIFE SPAN

In this section, we expand on global nutrition security and insecurity through discussion of specific risks throughout the life span as well as the socioenvironmental contextual factors that influence these globally.

The Dual Burden of Malnutrition

Malnutrition represents an imbalance in an individual's intake of nutrients and covers the two major ends of the spectrum of nutritional status, including both undernutrition and overnutrition. As the name suggests, undernutrition refers to a deficiency of **macronutrients** and/or **micronutrients** caused by starvation and characterized by low body weight, **wasting**, and **stunting**. Globally, anemia related to iron deficiency is one of the most common issues of undernutrition (Figure 10.2). Iron, vitamin A, iodine, and zinc are the most prevalent vitamin and mineral deficiencies in the world. When one considers which foods are rich in these nutrients and the tendency toward a grain-heavy (processed grain) diet, it is not surprising that these are the most common deficiencies globally.

In contrast, overnutrition represents the condition of excess in which an individual is chronically exceeding the daily requirements for macronutrients (excess calories), leading often to obesity but possibly getting limited amounts of critical quality micronutrients. In mapping the prevalence of these two nutrition imbalances, in general, overnutrition is mainly a problem of high-income countries like the United States, China, and Canada, while undernutrition is mainly seen in middle- and low-income countries. For instance, according to the Global Obesity Observatory, approximately 38% of adult men in the United States are obese, while in Kenya (a lower middle income country), the obesity rate among adult men is about 4%.[13] Similarly, undernutrition among children (for example, stunting, wasting, and being underweight) is a major problem in middle- to low-income countries. However, owing to the increase in urbanization, economic growth, and technological advancement, the issue of malnutrition has become more complex and multinomial in recent years. Around 45% of deaths among young children are linked to undernutrition in low- and middle-income countries. At the same time, in these same

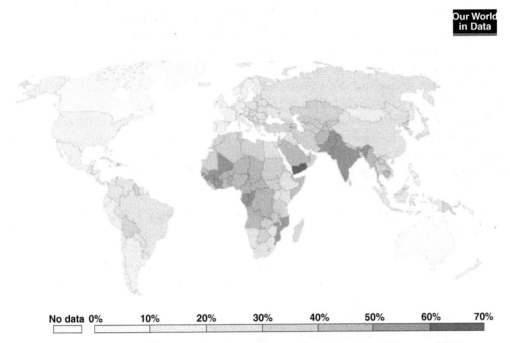

FIGURE 10.2 Prevalence of anemia in women of reproductive age (15–29 years; 2016), measured as the percentage of women with a hemoglobin level less than 110 grams per liter at sea level.

Source: Adapted from Ritchie H, Roser M. *Micronutrient Deficiency.* 2019. https://ourworldindata.org/micronutrient -deficiency

countries, rates of childhood overweight and obesity are rising.[14] This coexistence of under- and overnutrition, which is seen at the individual, household, or population level, is referred as "the double burden of malnutrition." According to Perez Escamilla, this double burden of malnutrition is an effect of economic disparities and food insecurity.[15] Especially, it is noted that the double burden of malnutrition is common among food-insecure households in which access to safe and nutritious food is a problem.

Food Insecurity

At the 1996 UN World Food Summit, the importance of **food security** was highlighted, and its definition was established to include three key components: food availability, food access, and food utilization and stability. Food security is also a critical component of NS—one cannot achieve nutrition security without food security. Food security was defined as occurring "When all people, at all times, have physical, social and economic access to sufficient, safe and nutritious food which meets their dietary needs and food preferences for an active and healthy life."[16] In contrast, food insecurity occurs when people do not have consistent access to a sufficient amount of safe and nutritious food due to issues in food availability, access, and/or its utilization. According to the FAO report on the global state of food insecurity, in 2017, approximately 770 million people, or 10% of the world's population, were experiencing hunger.[17] By continents, the rate of hunger ranges from about 1.4% in Northern America and Europe to 30% in sub-Saharan Africa. Hunger represents the most severe level of food insecurity, in which individuals cut portion sizes or skip meals due to lack of food. In food insecurity, coping strategies often include reliance on calorie-dense but nutrient-poor staple foods, which has been a significant cause of the double burden of malnutrition resulting in high rates of overweight and obesity among both children and adults.[18,19] This phenomenon has now become well documented as the **food insecurity–obesity paradox**.[20,21] In a nutritional assessment of 4,299 pairs of 15- to 49-year-old mothers and their children in Brazil, it was found that overweight mothers were significantly likely to have a stunted child and the odds of this combination were significantly higher among food-insecure house-holds.[22] In a similar cross-sectional survey in Indonesia, 24% of households in the study had a combination of a within-household stunted child and an overweight/obese mother. In examining the predictors, again it was found that the odds of this combination were about two times higher among food-insecure households.[23]

EFFECTS OF FOOD INSECURITY DURING THE FIRST 1,000 DAYS OF LIFE

In order to understand this coexistence of over- and undernutrition within families, it is criti-cal to examine food insecurity in the context of the **life-course approach or perspective**.[24] The life-course perspective recognizes that experiences of food shortage or food insecurity during childhood affect how an individual manages and views food in adulthood. Additionally, and per-haps most critically, the life-course approach recognizes that food insecurity affects nutritional status and health right from the beginning of life. The **first 1,000 days of life**, representing the period between conception and one's second birthday, is a critical period of opportunity to estab-lish foundations for optimal health, growth, and neurodevelopment for the lifetime. Hence, food insecurity or limited access to nutritious foods (including critical vitamins and minerals) during this period can have serious detrimental effects on potential growth and development, which can ultimately affect long-term health in childhood and beyond into adulthood.

Research studies have shown that food insecurity is associated with obesity among women in the United States and other countries.[25] Additionally, it is noted that food insecurity is significantly associated with stress and depression, which in turn, also influence food choice and dietary pat-tern.[26,27] Specifically, stress hormones and neuropeptides alter metabolism to favor and increase cravings for highly palatable foods. Chronic stress, common among food-insecure women, acti-vates the hypothalamic–pituitary–adrenal axis, which is associated with a high preference for high-sugar, high-fat foods to dampen the stress response.[28] Increased release of stress-related hormones in chronic stress is also associated with shifting metabolism favoring deposition of visceral (fat around the organs) or central abdominal fat. Studies have shown that higher levels of perceived stress are associated with uncontrolled eating and emotional eating among low-income women.[29] Considering the stress of poverty, limited educational and economic opportunities, and gender inequality, one can easily see the excessive burden on the world's most vulnerable populations.

Further, studies in the United States show that, low-income, minority women, who are at a higher risk of experiencing food insecurity, tend to gain excess weight during pregnancy and are more likely to retain excess weight post partum.[30-32] As a result, in the subsequent pregnancy, women are entering pregnancy with excess weight and are likely to repeat the cycle of excess gestational weight gain and postpartum weight retention. Research examining the life-course perspective indicates that prepregnancy overweight or obesity and excess weight gain during pregnancy are both significant predictors of high body fat and weight among infants and chil-dren later in their lives. Further, food insecurity can compound its effect on the next generation because it is associated with restricted feeding and high-fat and high-sugar complementary feeding. Qualitative research indicates that food-insecure mothers are often stressed and worried that they might not have the "capacity" to produce enough milk for their babies.[33]

Food insecurity not only poses a risk of overweight and obesity during the first 1,000 days of life, but it is also likely to affect growth and development through micronutrient deficiencies and lack of variety in the diet. Brain development occurs at the most rapid rate in the last trimester of pregnancy and the first two years of life. The first 1,000 days are characterized by rapid proliferation of neural cells, myelination, and development of connectivity in the brain, and hence, represent a window of greatest vulnerability to any nutrient deficiency. For optimal development, the brain requires a range of micronutrients including protein and polyunsaturated fatty acids. Additionally, minerals such as iron, zinc, copper, and iodine are particularly important. Iron deficiency is the most common nutrient deficiency in the world, and it is often associated with lack of variety in the diet due to food insecurity.[34] Worldwide, approximately 47% (293 million) of all young children and 42% (56 million) of all pregnant women are anemic, and in about half of them iron deficiency is the cause. A recent report from UNICEF indicates that prevention of iron deficiency during the first 1,000 days of life is very important to prevent lower mental development and poor productivity in adulthood.[35] Addressing food insecurity and promoting optimal nutrition during this critical phase of the first 1,000 days of life is needed to break the cycle of poverty and promote health equity around the world.

Addressing Food Insecurity: Moving Forward

Three main pillars of our food system must be strengthened in order to address global food insecurity: food availability, food access, and food utilization. Food availability is generally measured at the country level referring to agricultural input and output, national trade practices, and import and export policies that allow the country to have enough food to feed and nourish its population. This is a critical piece in predicting food security of the country or vulnerability to food insecurity at the national level. In measuring food availability, the estimate of daily dietary energy supply per capita is used, which is measured by adding net food production and imports and deducting food exports and food lost, stored, or used for animal feed or industry. Recently, the food availability or daily dietary supply per capita has worsened in parts of sub-Saharan African, Southeast Asia, and Western Asia. This deterioration has been attributed mainly to regional conflicts and conflicts combined with natural disasters of droughts or floods.[17] For instance, civil conflicts, which began in 2012 in the Central African Republic, have led to a 57% reduction in cultivated crop areas and a decrease in food production by 54%. In addition to crop reduction, conflicts have also led to livestock-related loss, with 46% for cattle and 57% for small ruminants (goats, sheep), forcing one fourth of rural farmers to shift to other sources for livelihoods.[17]

In 2010, the UN recognized access to clean water as a basic human right, yet a majority of the world's population in low-income countries experience moderate to severe water scarcity. Approximately, 1.8 billion people lack access to safe drinking water, and this situation is predicted to get worse by the year 2025.[36] It is important to realize that clean water is an essential nutrient and meeting its daily requirement is critical to ensure optimal absorption and utilization of nutrients at the physiological level. Additionally, clean water is needed to ensure food safety and hygiene and is critical in prevention of infectious diseases that lead to diarrhea. In low-income countries, 50% of all undernutrition cases in children are related to repeated diarrhea and intestinal parasite related infections.[37] As indicated in Figure 10.3, research indicates that water security or consistent access to a safe and sufficient of amount of clean water is a critical component in

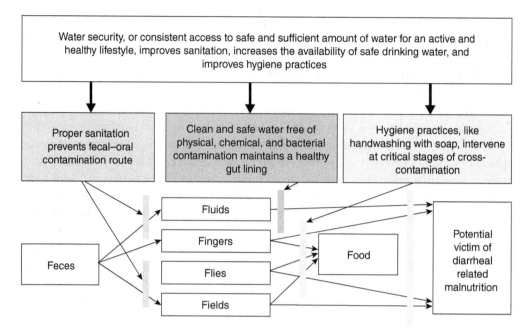

FIGURE 10.3 Interrelationship among water, diarrhea, and food utilization (third pillar of food security). Feces are the main vehicle of transmission for diarrhea, causing bacterial and parasitic infections. Transmission and contamination of food occur when feces gets into "fluids" (water supplies), when there is poor handwashing or inability to wash after defecation ("fingers"), when feces-contaminated water covers food crops ("fields"), and when "flies" alight on bacteria-laden feces and then land on foods to be consumed.

Source: From Nounkeu DC. *Assessment of the Relationship Between Water Insecurity, Hygiene Practices, and the Incidence of Diarrhea Among Children from Rural Households of the Menoua Division - West Cameroon.* 2017. http://libres.uncg.edu/ir/uncg/listing.aspx?styp=ti&id=22592

preventing diarrhea and poor food utilization—a leading cause of malnutrition among children in low-income countries (Figure 10.3).[38]

The UN Water Report established the definition of water security:

the capacity of a population to safeguard sustainable access to adequate quantities of and acceptable quality water for sustaining livelihoods, human well-being, and socio-economic development, for ensuring protection against water-borne pollution and water-related disasters, and for preserving ecosystems in a climate of peace and political stability.[39]

Further, to promote water security, one of the goals of 2015–2030 Sustainable Development Goals is to "Ensure availability and sustainable management of water and sanitation for all."[17,40] Additionally, key water access related indicators were established to monitor and evaluate the success in achieving the Sustainable Development Goals (SDGs).[40] According to the UN, water access is considered poor when (a) per capita water use is less than 50 liters per day, (b) total water collection time is more than 30 minutes, (c) water source is not within 1,000 meters of home, and (d) water cost is more than 3% of the household income. Establishment of these standards has been very critical in monitoring and planning specific water-related issues. However, it is very much interrelated to food security and the progress we make in improving maternal and child nutrition in developing or low-income countries.

An understanding of global nutrition issues and interrelated risk factors (e.g., food security, water security, SDOH) and their effect particularly on maternal and child nutrition (e.g., first

1,000 days) is not only critical for the PHN practitioner working globally, but also for the PHN practitioner working domestically with foreign-born individuals and communities. Thus far, we have provided an overview of global nutritional issues and now we transition to include an introduction to U.S. migration as well as related postarrival nutritional risk factors. When working domestically, the PHN practitioner must not only be familiar with prearrival or premigration global nutrition risks but also postarrival or postmigration risks. We begin the next section with an overview of **migration** (e.g., Who comes? Why and to where? What are the different immigration categories and how do they impact nutrition resources in the United States?) and then expand to focus on specific risks and key considerations when working with diverse, foreign-born populations in the United States.

U.S. MIGRATION: GARNERING AN UNDERSTANDING OF THE EXPERIENCES, CONTEXT, ACCULTURATION PROCESS, AND RISKS ASSOCIATED WITH MIGRATION

Introduction to U.S. Migration–Immigration and Refugee Resettlement

By 2044 it is expected that, for the first time, the United States will switch to a "minority-majority" nation.[41] By 2060, the foreign-born population of the United States is expected to increase by 85%, which will lead to dramatic demographic shifts in the United States.[41] The estimated percentage of individuals with Hispanic or Latino origin is expected to increase by 114.8% from 2014 to 2060, and they are the third fastest growing population, with the "two or more races" identification category projected to be the fastest and the Asian population to be the second fastest growing.[41] In order to address nutrition and related health needs of an increasingly diverse U.S. population, PHN practitioners should have a foundational knowledge of the categories and causes for migration to the United States as well as the socioenvironmental premigration context. In the next section, we provide an overview of the following: (a) definition of terms related to migration, (b) primary geographic regions globally where the United States receives high numbers of foreign-born individuals, and (c) an overview of the acculturation process and risks associated as demonstrated by the model proposed by Schwartz and colleagues.

The U.S. immigration policy is guided by the Immigration and Nationality Act (INA, 1952) and current reasons for migration to the United States primarily include family reunification, U.S. labor market contribution, origin-country diversity, and humanitarian assistance.[42] The INA sets a ceiling on permanent immigration admissions at 675,000 total individuals per year. However, this number does not represent refugee resettlement numbers, which are determined by the U.S. president and Congress annually.[42] Limits are also set by the INA, which include a 7% cap for any category of entrance to the United States per nationality called a "per-country limit" or "cap." Table 10.2 summarizes U.S. INA defined migration categories.

Reasons for Migration

Individuals migrate for a variety of reasons, and it is valuable to the PHN practitioner to understand the differences and categories for new arrivals to the United States as each has its own nutrition-related prearrival risks and unique SDOH. For example, refugees are a unique category. Refugees are identified as fleeing because of persecution or fear of persecution for "race, religion, nationality, membership in a particular social group, or political opinion." These individuals are identified by the United Nations High Commissioner for Refugees (UNHCR) and currently

TABLE 10.2 SUMMARY OF U.S. INA MIGRATION CATEGORY DEFINITIONS

TERM	DEFINITIONS AS PER THE U.S. PRIMER ON U.S. IMMIGRATION POLICY
Aliens*	"people who are not U.S. citizens, including those legally and not legally present"
Unauthorized aliens	"foreign nationals who reside unlawfully in the United States and who either entered the United States illegally ('without inspection') or entered lawfully and temporarily ('with inspection') but subsequently violated the terms of their admission, typically by 'overstaying' their visa duration"
Immigrants†	"foreign nationals lawfully admitted to the United States for permanent residence"
Nonimmigrants	"foreign nationals temporarily and lawfully admitted to the United States for a specific purpose and period of time, including tourists, diplomats, students, temporary workers, and exchange visitors, among others"
Noncitizens	"persons who have not naturalized and may include immigrants as well as nonimmigrants"
Naturalized citizens	"LPRs who become U.S. citizens through a process known as naturalization, generally after residing in the United States continuously for at least five years"
Refugees and asylees‡	"persons fleeing their countries because of persecution, or a well-founded fear of persecution, on account of race, religion, nationality, membership in a particular social group, or political opinion"

*The terms "alien," "foreign national," and "noncitizen" are synonymous.
†The terms "immigrant," "lawful permanent resident" (LPR), and "green-card holder" are synonymous.
‡Refugees and asylees are not classified as immigrants under the INA, but once admitted, they may adjust their status to LPR.
INA Immigration and Nationality Act.
Source: Data from Kandel WA. A Primer on U.S. Immigration Policy. 2018. https://digitalcommons.ilr.cornell.edu/key_workplace/2119

57% of all refugees come from five countries: Syria, Afghanistan, South Sudan, Myanmar, and Somalia.[43] Some individuals flee and enter another country before they can be recognized as refugees and they are called **asylum seekers** or **asylees** and they may petition their host country for refugee status.[44] Individuals who flee persecution or violence but who do not leave their home country are known as **internally displaced people (IDPs)**. IDPs are not protected by international law or eligible to receive aid as refugees.[44] For more information about refugee resettlement in the United States, visit www.unrefugees.org/refugee-facts/usa.

Many U.S. foreign-born individuals may have lived decades in a refugee camp setting with limited access to healthcare and education as well as water and food insecurity, all of which after fleeing persecution and violence. Some refugee camps do not even have adequate lighting.[68] This prearrival socioenvironmental context and related health and nutrition risks are important to keep in mind when working with groups after their arrival to the United States (see Box 10.1).

Although the United States receives very diverse groups annually, there are some countries from which the United States has received larger numbers of immigrants and/or refugees and asylees. However, these trends shift over time and would have looked very different 10 or 20 years ago. From 2015 to 2017, the bulk of immigrants entering and obtaining permanent legal status in the United States were from Mexico, China, India, Philippines, and Cuba (15.1%, 7.1%, 6.1%, 5.4%, and 5.2%, respectively).[45]

BOX 10.1

PRACTITIONER NOTES: IMMIGRATION STATUS DETERMINES ACCESS TO SOCIAL SERVICES

Different classifications for foreign-born individuals (e.g., refugee vs. immigrant vs. unauthorized aliens) result in different access to health and social services:

- **Refugees**, for example, enter the United States through a formal resettlement program, are provided a Social Security number and have access to healthcare (Medicaid), SNAP assistance, and WIC as well as other resources (e.g., employment assistance, ESL classes) for a few months (up to 1 year) after arrival. It is important to highlight that although refugees may receive initial government benefits, they are also a vulnerable group with many having experienced recent active war and trauma in combination with the stress of being new in a foreign country.

- **Immigrants** vary based usually on their legal status. Unauthorized aliens or "undocumented" individuals will not be able to receive benefits like SNAP or Medicaid, whereas documented immigrants are able to connect with and receive social service benefits. (Important note: Undocumented families may be eligible for WIC.) Undocumented immigrants are at great risk for food insecurity, poor healthcare access, and adverse health outcomes.

ESL, English as a second language; SNAP, Supplemental Nutrition Assistance Program; WIC, Special Supplemental Nutrition Program for Women, Infants, and Children.

The states receiving the highest numbers for persons obtaining permanent residence from 2015 to 2017 were California, New York, and Florida (19.9%, 12.4%, and 11.3%, respectively).[45] In contrast to general immigration, refugees have arrived over the past decade primarily from Southeast Asia (Burma, Bhutan), the Middle East (Iraq), and Africa (Somalia, Democratic Republic of Congo).[46] Texas, California, and New York were the top three states in the United States receiving immigrants and refugees (10.7%, 8.2%, 5.8%, respectively).[46]

Acculturation

During and after the complex migration process, foreign-born individuals experience some degree of **acculturation**. Acculturation is a process by which individuals adopt behaviors and beliefs of the host culture. This process has also been associated with the **immigrant paradox** in which an individual's health declines over time particularly when he or she migrates to Eurocentric Westernized countries.[47] Typically, this decline in health is related to lack of activity and an increase in consumption of a more Westernized diet (fast foods, processed and packaged foods) results in the development and/or exacerbation of chronic disease like diabetes, hypertension, and heart disease.

Acculturation has traditionally been defined as a linear progression where the individual becomes more and more like his or her receiving culture in terms of language, food practices, and behaviors. Theoretically, this linear progression would mean that they would be more successful economically (stable job, access to education) and socially (acquire language, customs) as they assimilate or become more like the host country. However, Schwartz and colleagues proposed that this linear progression is inaccurate and proposed the "Multidimensionality of Acculturation" model, which suggests that individuals retain their own culture in certain areas and adopt the host culture in others, sometimes moving back and forth along the continuum for different practices, values, and identifications (self). Schwartz et al. propose that they are more resilient and successful because of this variable adoption of practices. Their model explores the complexity of the process and associated factors, and they identified two primary areas of variance based on (a) culture and ethnicity and (b) socioenvironmental context of reception.[47]

PUTTING IT ALL TOGETHER: BEST PRACTICES FOR PHN PROFESSIONALS WORKING WITH DIVERSE AUDIENCES

Understand the Context

Individuals live in complex social, political, economic, and cultural (religion, ethnicity/race) contexts that shape their physical and mental health. As a PHN professional, it is critical to consider all of the elements that intersect in this context or "bigger picture" when you work with clients either locally or abroad. Within this context, there are several key issues for consideration: education/literacy, prior job training/skills, mental and physical health, previous food shortage, and gender inequality. These factors ultimately impact the individual's ability to adapt, grow, and succeed both pre- and postmigration. A model summarizing these factors is presented in Figure 10.4, and further description follows.

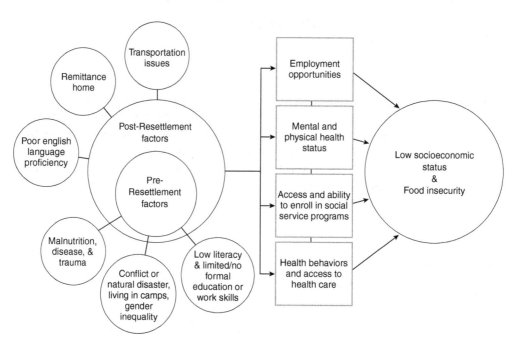

FIGURE 10.4 Pre- and postmigration factors that impact health and socioeconomic status. Refugees and immigrants bring with them previous experiences of limited opportunities and unstable living conditions in resettlement. On top of that, they experience issues such as language barriers and responsibility of supporting families or friends living in camps or other countries. This combination of embedded pre- and postresettlement factors affect the individual's ability to seek employment, health status, ability to access social services and programs, and ultimately increase risk for food insecurity.

Source: Adapted from Nunnery DL, Dharod JM. Potential determinants of food security among refugees in the U.S.: an examination of pre- and post-resettlement factors. *Food Secur.* 2017;9(1):163–179. doi:10.1007/s12571-016-0637-z

Education and Literacy

Public education in grades K–12 is available and compulsory (up to a certain age) in most middle-income and higher income countries like the United States, Canada, China, and Mexico. However, in some countries, education is not always compulsory and is often only accessible if families can afford to pay for private education and/or ensure transportation and safety. Generally, these countries may be considered lower income and most have suffered severe prolonged conflict or natural disasters that have destroyed government, financial, and community infrastructure. However, educational attainment and literacy cannot be assumed based on the country of origin; much is dependent on resources and location for schooling. In a study examining food insecurity among Liberian refugees ($n = 33$) resettled in the United States, it was observed that some women had education as high as bachelor's and master's degrees while others could not read or write even in their native language.[48]

Literacy, or the ability to read and write in one's native language, is critical to navigating a majority of positions in the workforce and successfully providing a stable income for one's family. Additionally, literacy can be critical to the development and self-actualization of the individual. Even within the United States, a higher income country, approximately 50% of adults read below an eighth-grade reading level and roughly 30 million Americans read below very basic prose literacy (reading for very minor, most basic skills).[49] Literacy has been posited as a direct correlate to poverty and food insecurity as it greatly impacts earning potential throughout the lifetime of the individual.[50] Moreover, literacy in one's native language can be critical to learning reading and writing skills in a new language, especially for those who are migrating and need to procure work and support services in the receiving country. We may take it for granted, however, even basic literacy and proficiency in English are critical for tasks such as driving and even navigating public transportation. Low literacy coupled with the inaccessibility of transportation can directly impact employment and access to support services. See Figure 10.5 for estimated literacy rates around the world.

Educational attainment and literacy directly affect individuals' prospects for jobs/careers and their potential to develop work and trade skills that could ensure a stable income whether they are in their home country or have migrated. Literacy is also important for PHN practitioners to consider as they would with any individual and community they work with to appropriately target and tailor resources and programming.

Prior Job Training and Skills

For immigrants and refugees, one of the first assessments conducted upon arrival examines prior employment and any job or trade skills. For individuals who have lived in countries with prolonged conflict or loss of infrastructure, much of the general work and even schooling has been halted and people are often placed into refugee or IDP camps. Refugee and IDP camps are meant to be temporary living shelters, with housing made of plastic or canvas tents, limited or no electricity, and no formal infrastructure (police/safety, education, sanitation, etc.).[51] Unfortunately, these temporary shelters may become permanent housing for long periods of time, up to decades, depending on the severity of conflict and upheaval in the region. People living in camps may have access to education and employment opportunities, but this is not guaranteed, and may be sporadically offered only when funds or resources are available. This means that upon arrival, many refugees may lack applicable training or job skills that could secure employment.

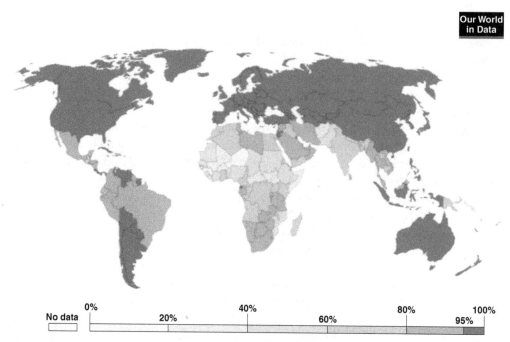

0%   40%   80%   100%

No data   20%   60%   95%

FIGURE 10.5 Global literacy rate, 2015. Estimates correspond to the share of the population older than 14 years that is able to read and write. Specific definitions and measurement methodologies vary across countries and time.

Source: From *Our World in Data: CIA World Factbook.* https://ourworldindata.org/literacy#note-1

Mental and Physical Health: Trauma Pre- and Postconflict/Migration

People tend to migrate to improve their circumstances. Refugees, asylees, and those in various immigrant categories (particularly undocumented immigrants) flee their home country because of fear of persecution or even death in the face of whatever conflict (civil, political, etc.) or natural disaster has gripped their country. Social and political unrest has led to many bitter and violent conflicts in parts of the world where families are often separated and loss of life is high. In the course of migration out of this conflict, people and their families may have faced long periods of travel in harsh weather with little support or resources along the way. They may have relinquished all of their financial means toward escape, and these losses, coupled with any physical and mental trauma experienced premigration, conspire to deteriorate mental health. Refugees, asylees, and undocumented migrants are at significantly increased risk for posttraumatic stress disorder (PTSD), severe anxiety, and depression.[52,53] In addition to mental health conditions, refugees and immigrants may also have physical health conditions (chronic diseases, infectious diseases like HIV/AIDS) that become exacerbated perimigration when medical care/medication is inaccessible or sporadic.

PRIOR FOOD DEPRIVATION, FOOD INSECURITY, AND REMITTANCE

Prior food deprivation experiences are common among individuals who have lived through civil conflict, especially if they have spent time in refugee camps. Periods of food deprivation may exacerbate food insecurity postmigration. Studies examining food insecurity among resettled refugees in the United States have shown rates ranging from 30% to as high as 85% compared to roughly 12% food insecurity nationally.[54–56] In a sample of Cambodian refugees, it was found that those who experienced prior food deprivation were significantly more likely to resort to unhealthy behaviors and coping strategies such as overeating high-fat foods when available. These refugees were subsequently more likely to also be overweight and obese, mirroring the phenomenon seen in the food insecurity–obesity paradox described earlier.[57] For many refugees and migrants, the issue of food insecurity is further complicated due to **remittance**, or the act of sending portions of their income back to family still in their home country. Remittance can account for a significant amount of an individual's income. In 2017, the World Bank estimated around $466 billion dollars in remittances to low- and middle-income countries.[58]

Gender Inequality

It is critical to understand the intersection between global health, migration, and gender. Gender inequality in and of itself may be the impetus for migration. In patriarchal societies that experience civil conflict/disasters and extreme poverty, women, girls, intersex people, and individuals of the LGBTQ community often receive the least resources and experience high rates of violence and discrimination.[59] Education of women and girls is not typically prioritized and males receive preference in schooling and other educational resources. Gender-based violence can lead to deterioration of mental health that further compromises the success and well-being of individuals as they resettle in new countries. Women, especially those who act as caregivers and meal preparers of the family, experience higher rates of food insecurity and anxiety around food acquisition both pre- and postmigration.[60-62]

Evidence-Based Practice for Education, Services, and Resources

Validated Resources

In order to gain valuable insight on the community or group of individuals you are working with, the first step is to research and critically evaluate existing evidence-based practice resources. The WHO e-Library of Evidence for Nutrition Actions (eLENA) is a great starting resource to learn about specific and effective nutrition and health interventions for the population of interest. These resources are divided by specific period in the life course with WHO recommendations, reports, and research defining the interventions. The Nutrition Landscape Information System (NLiS), also created by WHO, is a major repository of data on the nutrition and health profiles of particular countries and regions. The NLiS provides online tools that include downloadable data from a wide range of global sources.[63] The NLiS helps public health professionals and researchers to quickly identify nutrition risks and priorities globally.

WHO also provides critical health warnings (infectious disease outbreaks) and information about vaccinations and/or sociopolitical issues for professionals who might be traveling to unfamiliar parts of the world. For additional resources, see Continue Your Learning Resources.

Educational Materials and Assessments

Many existing educational resources are culturally relevant and linguistically appropriate for the needs of diverse audiences. Do not reinvent the wheel, especially if a good wheel already exists. The U.S. Committee for Refugees has done extensive research and pooled resources to develop the Healthy Living Toolkit and additional nutrition resource handouts. The toolkit and nutrition handouts are designed to educate not only refugees and immigrants, but also the resettlement agencies, clinics, and community-based organizations that serve them. The toolkit and nutrition resources come in over 15 different languages (including English). The toolkit covers topics such

---

BOX 10.2

PRACTITIONER'S INSIGHT: INTERPRETATION AND TRANSLATION

The terms interpretation and translation are often used interchangeably; however, translation is used in the context of written materials (direct word for word or phrase for phrase). Interpretation is typically done orally in person or over a language line and involves some actual interpretation of the context and possibly meaning of what the individual is saying, especially if the concepts being interpreted are not similar between the cultures/languages.

It is the practitioner's duty to attempt to find a professional interpreter or translator when possible. Having children or family members interpret/translate is highly problematic because it violates the privacy of the individual and may put children and family members in situations that they do not understand or that cause undue stress. Most agencies, organizations, or health facilities will have access to a **language line (phone network for interpreter services)** if they do not have professional interpreters on staff. If there is no other option, *you must be sure that your client or patient consents to proceed with family interpretation.*

---

as navigating medical services and dental care and the nutrition resource covers topics such as food safety, breastfeeding, reading nutrition labels, and increasing foods with adequate calcium and iron.

The Centers for Disease Control and Prevention (CDC) has created a resource page for Refugee Health Guidelines that defines all the guidelines for predeparture and postarrival medical screening and treatment of U.S.-bound refugees. From this main page, you can also find a link to U.S.-Mexico Public Health resources including health and education communication tools. See Box 10.2 for helpful tips about using interpreters and translators with clients and patients.

Build Bridges: Interprofessional Collaboration and the Community Health Worker Model

As PHN professionals, much of our work is interprofessional including collaborations with social workers, medical providers, school, and other governmental (state health departments, Supplemental Nutrition Assistance Program [SNAP], Special Supplemental Nutrition Program for Women, Infants, and Children [WIC], Medicaid/Medicare) and nongovernmental (resettlement agencies, legal counsel) organizations. It is important to reach out and build a resource network of individuals who care about and understand the complex health and nutrition needs of a diverse audience.

Further, to provide culturally appropriate care and education, the professional must go beyond their evidence-based practice resources and strive to assess and meet the community where they are. One of the most effective, well-documented ways to do this is by working with community health workers (**CHWs**). CHWs are individuals from the community of interest who are trained to provide medical and nutritional care or at the very least to act as liaisons and educators on these services for their community. They typically share ethnicity/race, language, and cultural background with their community and are most effective when they are viewed as a trusted member of their community. CHWs can act as a gatekeeper and bridge to the community. The use of the CHW model has been integral in conducting nutrition needs assessments and research with refugee and migrant groups who may feel hesitancy and fear in working with outsiders.[64] The CDC offers a *CHW Toolkit* and the Rural Health Information Hub offers descriptive educational modules on Training CHWs and sustainability for nutrition interventions using this framework.

Develop Your Cultural Competence

Cultural competence is defined as the ability of providers and organizations to effectively deliver healthcare services (education, counseling, treatment) that meet the social, cultural, and linguistic needs of their patients/clients and the community they serve. In order to work with diverse populations, be it locally or globally, it is necessary to take a holistic approach and cultivate four key areas of your development as public health professionals: awareness, attitude, knowledge, and skills.[65,66]

- Awareness: Build self-awareness by reflecting on your own cultural identity and potential biases toward other identities.

- Attitude: Cultivate an attitude of open-mindedness, compassion, and genuine interest in learning about those different from yourself. Strive for genuine empathy and never make assumptions despite how much you think you know or have researched. People will always surprise you.

- Knowledge: Strive to learn more about the different cultural practices, ideas, and concepts that are important to your patients or clientele. Learn about the specific cultural, political, and economic environments that might have influenced their migration.

- Skills: Practice cross-cultural skills and put yourself out there by trying new cultural foods/restaurants, visiting new places (even in your own town), and attending different cultural events and celebrations. Speak with and learn directly from individuals of different backgrounds. Learn a new language.

It is important to understand that developing your cultural competence can be uncomfortable and challenging. However, developing cultural competence is an ongoing (lifelong) growth process that we commit to in order to provide the best care for our clients/patients. **Cultural humility** is an additional key trait of the culturally competent PHN practitioner, and it is within the context of cultural competency. Cultural humility includes a self-awareness of one's limitations regarding the depth of understanding of another culture's beliefs, attitudes, values, and practices. Cultural humility is a cautious, yet open approach to working with individuals and/or groups that vary from one's own culture and practices.[67]

CONCLUSION

In this chapter, we began by introducing the concept of NS, then expanded to discuss specific nutritional risks throughout the life span, introduced organizations addressing nutritional issues globally, and provided an overview of the immigration process and considerations and risks for diverse foreign-born individuals and groups peri- and postarrival to the United States. Whether working globally or domestically as a PHN practitioner, an understanding of the socioenvironmental context and SDOH that groups experience is critical. Moreover, foundational knowledge and understanding of the target community (cultural competence) is necessary to cultivate best practices for any area of public health programming. It is impossible to offer appropriate or tailored efforts to a global or foreign-born U.S. community without knowledge of current global issues and their complexity. While we offer a foundation for PHN practitioners to expand their knowledge of global nutrition issues, this alone is not adequate. We urge you to utilize the resources provided at the end of this chapter to further develop your cultural competence. We have provided a wide range of tools and resources to expand your knowledge, understanding, and skills for working with populations internationally and/or domestically including a reflection activity, toolkits with nutrition and health education resources in many languages, online global nutrition databases, additional primary literature articles, case studies, best practices and guidelines for public health/healthcare workers, books, and other media. In addition to these, we highly recommend volunteering with organizations that serve diverse populations domestically or internationally to further develop your skills as a global minded, culturally competent PHN practitioner.

KEY CONCEPTS

Community Health Worker (CHW) Model: A model whereby public health and social service workers are trained to provide health services and education to the communities they are close to. CHWs often share ethnicity, language, socioeconomic status, values, and life experiences with the community members they serve. CHWs are and should be chosen by the community and aid as a bridge to critical health services.

Cultural Competence: The ability of providers and organizations to effectively deliver healthcare services (education, counseling, treatment) that meet the social, cultural, and linguistic needs of patients/clients and the community they serve.

Food insecurity–obesity paradox: The concept that those who experience food insecurity are paradoxically more likely to also be overweight or obese, particularly in middle-income and higher income countries. This association is best-documented in adult women. Findings are mixed among men and children. This paradox is often attributed to relying on cheap, calorie-dense, but nutrient-poor foods when the individual is food-insecure.

Immigrant paradox: The concept that individuals immigrating often experience health declines over time and especially associated with acculturation processes in Eurocentric Westernized countries.

Life-course approach (perspective): A framework that examines how individual health trajectories vary and asserts that patterns can be predicted for populations and communities based on social, economic, and environmental exposures and experiences. Life is viewed as a continuum of exposures, experiences, and interactions that intersect to influence the overall health (genetic, biological, and behavioral) of individuals and future generations.

CASE STUDY: HEALTH LITERACY AND RESETTLED REFUGEES: DR. LAUREN SASTRE ON HER RESEARCH WITH BURMESE REFUGEES

It is important not to make any assumptions regarding health literacy. I worked on a project that explored hypertension knowledge and related behavioral risk factors (e.g., diet, lack of physical activity, excess adiposity) with a local refugee group. I was invited to work with a group of resettled adult Burmese refugees, mostly of Chin ethnicity, by a nurse who worked at a local community free clinic. She told me the medical staff had been noticing consistent high blood pressure, and she was very concerned. I began the project by providing digital cameras to the group to document their food for 2 weeks. While we waited for the pictures, we provided health screenings and had small group discussions about the clinical measurements and health concerns the group had.

Prior to working with the group I immersed myself in any literature I could find as well as cultural information online (e.g., CDC provides profiles of refugee groups). Burmese refugees are a unique group—having fled ethnic, political, and religious persecution over 30 years ago with many having lived in either rural refugee camps along the Thai border (rural) or in urban settings within Malaysia where they are treated like undocumented immigrants. Being stateless for 30+ years dramatically influenced education and healthcare access. Moreover, pre-U.S. socioenvironmental contexts varied drastically between Malaysia and Thailand. This is one of the largest refugee groups resettled in the United States in the past 10 years and there are distinct ethnic groups within the overall "Burmese" group as well as individual languages, food practices, and so on. Although I had prepared myself with background cultural and socioenvironmental information, I was not prepared for how limited the group I worked with would be in regard to health literacy.

During our small group facilitated discussions (scheduled by the nurse through an interpreter they worked with who was part of the Chin Burmese community and held on Saturdays for a month), I quickly realized there was no understanding of blood pressure and while they had been told several times their blood pressure was high they did not understand what this meant or what the risk was. I explained the relationship between blood pressure and the heart and how high blood pressure is risky for the heart. I then (using the digital photographs of the food as well as info from a grocery store trip we took together to learn more about what they were eating) discussed diet and lifestyle changes that could help with blood pressure, focusing on the basics: (a) less salt; (b) more fruits and vegetables following the DASH diet, with examples from their traditional foods based on the photographs; (c) portion control, hopefully leading to some weight loss; and (d) increased physical activity.

At the last Saturday session we held together, several in the group were very emotional—they expressed they did not know their high blood pressure could impact their heart and that it was so risky for their health. They told me they were so happy they had learned what was going on with them and how to change it. I was incredibly humbled.

Case Study Questions

1. Taking time to "do your homework" and learn about a group you are not familiar with is an important first step to providing culturally competent services and care; however, it is possible such preparation could lead to the development of inaccurate assumptions or even biases or stereotyping. What information might you focus on obtaining during your preparation? How might you avoid pitfalls previously highlighted when you develop materials or begin to interact with groups?

2. Educational opportunities may be limited or fully interrupted for some groups, especially refugees if they fled active war or were in camps for extended time periods or immigrants in low-income countries. This may impact general literacy as well as nutrition and health literacy. How might you cautiously assess and address general as well as nutrition and health literacy? What creative approaches might you use to modify your materials or approach? Describe three example approaches you might take for a group or individual with low literacy in which you are teaching general nutrition education topics (e.g. food label, portion sizes, MyPlate).

3. During my experience with the Chin Burmese, I attempted to use motivational interviewing techniques (an evidence-based practice with Western-Eurocentric groups), which support the individual to drive the focus of the conversation. This did not go over well with the Chin Burmese. At one point, one of the women actually said to me (as I pushed for the group to guide the topics for our sessions), "I don't know. You are the expert . . . you tell us!", which brought a round of laughter from the group.

   Groups might vary not only in their food habits, health beliefs, perceptions of gender roles, and religion . . . but also in their perceptions of the role of healthcare providers (as well as the expectations of the healthcare process and services). How might I have avoided this situation? Find specific evidence to support modifications to how you would have approached the facilitated group discussions with the Chin Burmese. Outline a different, more culturally appropriate approach using your sources (be sure to cite your sources).

Source: Smith EB, Sastre LR. "We didn't know": An examination of health and nutrition knowledge, behaviors and clinical risk factors to guide a pilot health education intervention for refugees from Burma. *J Refugee Global Health.* 2019;2(2):article 2. doi:10.18297/rgh/vol2/iss2/2

SUGGESTED LEARNING ACTIVITIES

Journaling about experiences is one way to critically think about and analyze your feelings and thoughts on working with others different from yourself.

Building Self-Awareness and Empathy

Think about a time when you were the only one of your race/ethnicity, religious group, age, or gender (or any other aspect of your identity that you feel strongly defines you) in a social situation. Write a 1-page journal style entry describing the social situation, why you were there, and how you felt to be the only one of your particular identity.

If you have never had this experience: Consider what it would feel like to move to a new country very different from your own, where you do not speak the language very well, do not know many people, and are unfamiliar with the cultural practices. Write a 1-page journal style entry describing what this might feel like for you (any frustrations, stress, excitement). How would you adapt or learn about your new receiving country? What would you have to consider to gain employment, find housing, and navigate your new city? What would you do if you had to bring aging parents and/or children with you to this new country (think about the potential issues with enrolling into programs/school, for example)?

REFLECTION QUESTIONS

1. List at least four reasons people migrate and describe how these reasons might affect their migration status (refugee, asylee, undocumented, etc.) and access to resources.

2. Define cultural competence and describe three strategies that a public health practitioner can use to effectively meet the social, cultural, and linguistic needs of the communities they serve.

3. Identify four key nutrition and health issues that the public health practitioner should consider when working with a global population. Identify and describe resources you

could use to educate your clients on these nutrition and health issues (i.e., what materials would you use?).

4. Describe the role that water plays in sustaining food security and ensuring optimal nutritional status at the global level.

CONTINUE YOUR LEARNING RESOURCES

Evidence-Based Practice for Nutrition Care in the Global Setting

World Health Organization: e-Library of Evidence for Nutrition Actions (eLENA). https://www.who.int/elena/en

World Health Organization: Selected Guidelines and Reports on Nutrition Recommendations. https://www.who.int/publications/guidelines/nutrition/en

World Health Organization. Regional Offices (important health and nutrition resources grouped by region of the globe). https://www.who.int/about/who-we-are/regional-offices

Centers for Disease Control and Prevention. Nutrition: Micronutrient Malnutrition. Global Health and Nutrition Resources. https://www.cdc.gov/nutrition/micronutrient-malnutrition/resources/index.html

Rural Health Information Hub. Evidence-based toolkits: Community health worker toolkit. https://www.ruralhealthinfo.org/toolkits/community-health-workers/1

Academy of Nutrition and Dietetics: Evidence Analysis Library (must be a member of the Academy of Nutrition and Dietetics to access this resource). https://www.andeal.org/projects.cfm

Develop Cultural Competence

Georgetown University Center for Child and Human Development: National Center for Cultural Competence. https://nccc.georgetown.edu

U.S. Department of Health and Human Services: National Standards for Culturally and Linguistically Appropriate Services (CLAS) in Health and Health Care. https://www.thinkculturalhealth.hhs.gov/clas

Expert Panel on Cultural Competence Education for Students in Medicine and Public Health (2012). *Cultural competence education for students in medicine and public health: Report of an expert panel.* Washington, DC: Association of American Medical Colleges and Association of Schools of Public Health. https://pcpcc.org/sites/default/files/resources/Cultural%20Competence%20Education%20for%20Students%20in%20Medicine%20%26%20Public%20Health.pdf

Increase Knowledge About Nutrition and Health Disparities

National Collaborative for Health Equity. http://www.nationalcollaborative.org

U.S. Department of Health and Human Services. National Institute on Minority Health and Health Disparities. https://www.nimhd.nih.gov

World Health Organization. Nutrition Landscape Information System (NLiS provides snapshot on nutrition and health status of different countries). https://www.who.int/nutrition/nlis/en

U.S. Department of Agriculture, Economic Research Service. Food Security in the United States (definitions, statistics, and tools used to measure food security in the United States). https://www.ers.usda.gov/topics/food-nutrition-assistance/food-security-in-the-us

UN 2015–2030 Sustainable Development Goals. https://www.un.org/sustainabledevelopment/blog/2015/12/sustainable-development-goals-kick-off-with-start-of-new-year

Educational and Support Resources for a Diverse Audience

U.S. Committee for Refugees and Immigrants. Research and Reports, Library of Materials: Health and Nutrition (educational resources available in multiple languages). https://refugees.org/research-reports

U.S. Department of Health and Human Services. Office of Refugee Resettlement: Refugee Health. https://www.acf.hhs.gov/orr/programs/refugee-health

Centers for Disease Control and Prevention. Immigrant and Refugee Health. https://www.cdc.gov/immigrantrefugeehealth

Centers for Disease Control and Prevention. United States-Mexico Public Health. https://www.cdc.gov/usmexicohealth/index.html

Examples of the Migration Experience From Film and Literature

Fadiman A. *The Spirit Catches You and You Fall Down: A Hmong Child, Her American Doctors, and the Collision of Two Cultures.* New York, NY: Farrar, Straus & Giroux; 1998.

Pipher M. *The Middle of Everywhere: Helping Refugees Enter the American Community.* New York, NY: Harcourt; 2002.

Martínez R. *Crossing Over: A Mexican Family on the Migrant Trail.* New York, NY: Metropolitan Books; 2001.

Nazario S. *Enrique's Journey: The True Story of a Boy Determined to Reunite With His Mother.* New York, NY: Ember; 2014.

Eggers D. *What Is the What : The Autobiography of Valentino Achak Deng: A Novel.* San Francisco, CA: McSweeney's; 2006.

Falardeau P, director. *The Good Lie.* United States: Warner Bros., Summit Entertainment; 2014.

Schweitzer RD, Vromans L, Ranke G, Griffin J. Narratives of healing: A case study of a young Liberian refugee settled in Australia. *Arts in Psychother.* 2014;41(1):98–106.

GLOSSARY

Acculturation: The degree of assimilation to a different culture (most commonly the dominant or receiving culture).

Asylee: A person who is seeking or has been granted political asylum or protection by the receiving nation or a nation outside his or her home country.

Community Health Worker (CHW) Model: A model whereby public health and social service workers are trained to provide health services and education to the communities they are close to. CHWs often share ethnicity, language, socioeconomic status, values, and life experiences with the community members they serve. CHWs are and should be chosen by the community and aid as a bridge to critical health services.

Cultural competence: The ability of providers and organizations to effectively deliver health-care services (education, counseling, treatment) that meet the social, cultural, and linguistic needs of patients/clients and the community they serve.

Cultural humility: Self-awareness of one's limitations regarding the depth of understanding of another culture's beliefs, attitudes, values, and practices.

First 1,000 days of life: The period between conception and a child's second birthday. This period is considered a critical window of development and growth.

Food insecurity–obesity paradox: The concept that those who experience food insecurity are paradoxically more likely to also be overweight or obese, particularly in middle and higher income countries. This association is best-documented in adult women. Findings are mixed among men and children. This paradox is often attributed to relying on cheap, calorie-dense, but nutrient-poor foods when the individual is food-insecure.

Food security: "When all people, at all times, have physical, social, and economic access to sufficient, safe and nutritious food which meets their dietary needs and food preferences for an active and healthy life."[16] Food insecurity is the opposite term and is characterized by anxiety related to acquiring food, compromising quality and compromising quantity of food.

Gross national income (GNI): A measurement of a country's income that includes all the income earned by a country's residents and businesses, including any income earned abroad. Income is defined as all employee compensation plus investment profits and includes earnings from foreign sources. Typically measured per person (GNI per capita).

Human Development Index (HDI): A more comprehensive assessment of a country beyond economic growth alone and includes quality of life, education, and standard of living (GNI per capita).

Immigrant paradox: Assimilation or acculturation is associated with adverse health outcomes, while more recent immigrants are at reduced risk despite higher overall social and economic vulnerability.

Internally displaced people: Individuals who flee persecution or violence but who do not leave their home country.

Life-course approach (perspective): Framework that examines how individual health trajectories vary and asserts that patterns can be predicted for populations and communities based on social, economic, and environmental exposures and experiences. Life is viewed as a continuum of exposures, experiences, and interactions that intersect to influence the overall health (genetic, biological, and behavioral) of individuals and future generations.

Macronutrients: A class of nutrients that provide calories and therefore energy to the body. Carbohydrates, protein, and fat are the three macronutrients.

Malnutrition: The condition of having poor nutrition, caused by not having enough to eat, not having adequate intake of quality macronutrients that provide energy (carbohydrates, protein, fat) and micronutrients such as vitamins, minerals, and fiber.

Microloan: A small sum of money lent at low interest to businesses and individuals. Providing microloans to small businesses and farms is under examination as one way to reduce poverty, empower the community, and improve the economy in low- and middle-income countries.

Micronutrients: A class of nutrients that do not provide calories but are necessary in small quantities for the optimal function of metabolism and growth in the body. Vitamins and minerals are the two types of micronutrients.

Migration: Movement of people from one place to another, whether it be inside their own country or to another country, with the intentions of settling there either temporarily or permanently.

Noncommunicable diseases (NCDs): Health conditions that cannot be transmitted to another person and which are most commonly associated with diet and lifestyle (e.g., diabetes, cardiovascular disease) but may also include others (e.g., Alzheimer's disease).

Nongovernmental organizations (NGOs): Nonprofit organizations not affiliated with a government entity.

Nutrition insecurity (NIS): A situation in which one or more of the qualities of nutrition security are absent. This is the opposite condition to NS.

Nutrition security (NS): "Nutrition security requires that all people have access to a variety of nutritious foods and potable drinking water; knowledge, resources, and skills for healthy living; prevention, treatment, and care for diseases affecting nutrition status; and safety-net systems during crisis situations, such as natural disasters or deleterious social and political systems."[1]

Remittance: Sending resources and money to family members back in their home country.

Resettlement: Transfer of refugees from one country (often the asylum country and/or neighboring country from the one they have fled) to another country that has agreed to admit them and grant them permanent settlement.

Social determinants of health (SDOH): Conditions in the environments in which people are born, live, learn, work, play, worship, and age that affect a wide range of health, functioning, and quality-of-life outcomes and risks (CDC definition).

Stunting: A low height for age caused in relation to chronic starvation of both macro- and micronutrients that ultimately has affected growth and development of the individual.

Wasting: A reduction in overall body muscle mass in relation to acute starvation of protein and calories characterized by a low weight for height.

Water security: The capacity of a population to safeguard sustainable access to adequate quantities of and acceptable quality water for sustaining livelihoods, human well-being, and socioeconomic development for ensuring protection against waterborne pollution and water-related disasters and for preserving ecosystems in a climate of peace and political stability.[39]

REFERENCES

1. Nordin SM, Boyle M, Kemmer TM. Position of the Academy of Nutrition and Dietetics: nutrition security in developing nations: sustainable food, water, and health. *J Acad Nutr Diet.* 2013;113(4):581–595. doi:10.1016/j.jand.2013.01.025
2. Gross R, Schoeneberger H, Pfeifer H, Preuss H-JA. The four dimensions of food and nutrition security: definitions and concepts. *Nutr Food Secur.* 2000:1–17. http://www.ieham.org/html/docs/The_Four_Dimensions_FNS_Definitions_and_Concepts.pdf
3. The World Bank: Data. *How Does the World Bank Classify Countries?* 2019. https://datahelpdesk.worldbank.org/knowledgebase/articles/378834-how-does-the-world-bank-classify-countries
4. Human Development Index (HDI). *United Nations Development Programme: Human Development Reports.* 2019. http://hdr.undp.org/en/content/human-development-index-hdi
5. World Health Organization. *Who We Are: History.* 2019. https://www.who.int/about/who-we-are/history
6. UNICEF. Nutrition: What we do. https://www.unicef.org/nutrition/index_action.html. Updated December 24, 2015.
7. Food and Agriculture Organization of the United Nations. *About FAO: What We Do.* 2019. http://www.fao.org/about/what-we-do/en
8. Food and Agriculture Organization of the United Nations (FAO). *About FAO.* 2019. http://www.fao.org/about/en
9. World Food Programme. *Overview.* 2019. https://www1.wfp.org/overview
10. International Rescue Committee. *Who We Are: The IRC's Impact at a Glance.* 2019. https://www.rescue.org/page/ircs-impact-glance
11. International Rescue Committee. *Nutrition at the International Rescue Committee.* 2019. https://www.rescue.org/resource/nutrition-international-rescue-committee?edme=true
12. Girard AW, Self JL, McAuliffe C, Olude O. The effects of household food production strategies on the health and nutrition outcomes of women and young children: a systematic review. *Paediatr Perinat Epidemiol.* 2012;26:205–222. doi:10.1111/j.1365-3016.2012.01282.x
13. World Obesity Federation. *Global Obesity Observatory: Obesity Prevalence Worldwide.* World Obesity; 2018. https://www.worldobesitydata.org/map/overview-adults
14. World Health Organization. *Report of the Commission on Ending Childhood Obesity Implementation Plan: Executive Summary.* Geneva, Switzerland: World Health Organizaton; 2017. https://apps.who.int/iris/bitstream/handle/10665/259349/WHO-NMH-PND-ECHO-17.1-eng.pdf

15. Perez-Escamilla R, Bermudez O, Buccini GS, et al. Nutrition disparities and the global burden of malnutrition. *BMJ*. 2018;361:k2252. doi:10.1136/bmj.k2252

16. Hamilton WL, Cook JT, Thompson WW, et al. *Household Food Security in the United States in 1995: Technical Report of the Food Security Measurement Project*. Cambridge, MA: Abt Associates; 1997:95. https://fns-prod.azureedge.net/sites/default/files/TECH_RPT.PDF

17. FAO, IFAD, UNICEF, WFP, and WHO. *The State of Food Security and Nutrition in the World 2017. Building Resilience for Peace and Food Security*. Rome, Italy: Food and Agriculture Organization; 2017:S129.

18. Marriott BP, Olsho L, Hadden L, Connor P. Intake of added sugars and selected nutrients in the United States, National Health and Nutrition Examination Survey (NHANES) 2003-2006. *Crit Rev Food Sci Nutr*. 2010;50:228–258. doi:10.1080/10408391003626223

19. Wallace TC, McBurney M, Fulgoni VL. Multivitamin/mineral supplement contribution to micronutrient intakes in the United States, 2007-2010. *J Am Coll Nutr*. 2014;33(2):94-102. doi:10.1080/07315724.2013.846806

20. Alaimo K, Olson CM, Frongillo EA Jr. Low family income and food insufficiency in relation to overweight in US children: is there a paradox? *Arch Pediatr Adolesc Med*. 2001;155(10):1161–1167. doi:10.1001/archpedi.155.10.1161

21. Dinour LM, Bergen D, Yeh MC. The food insecurity-obesity paradox: a review of the literature and the role food stamps may play. *J Am Diet Assoc*. 2007;107(11):1952–1961. doi:10.1016/j.jada.2007.08.006

22. Gubert MB, Spaniol AM, Bortolini GA, Pérez-Escamilla R. Household food insecurity, nutritional status and morbidity in Brazilian children. *Public Health Nutr*. 2016;19:2240–2245. doi:10.1017/S1368980016000239

23. Mahmudiono T, Nindya TS, Andrias DR, et al. Household food insecurity as a predictor of stunted children and overweight/obese mothers (SCOWT) in urban Indonesia. *Nutrients*. 2018;10:535. doi:10.3390/nu10050535

24. Pérez-Escamilla R, Kac G. Childhood obesity prevention: a life-course framework. *Int J Obes Suppl*. 2013;3(suppl 1):S3–S5. doi:10.1038/ijosup.2013.2

25. Hernandez DC, Reesor LM, Murillo R. Food insecurity and adult overweight/obesity: gender and race/ethnic disparities. *Appetite*. 2017;117:373–378. doi:10.1016/j.appet.2017.07.010

26. Laraia BA, Leak TM, Tester JM, Leung CW. Biobehavioral factors that shape nutrition in low-income populations: a narrative review. *Am J Prev Med*. 2017;52(2):S118–S126. doi:10.1016/j.amepre.2016.08.003

27. Flórez KR, Dubowitz T, Ghosh-Dastidar M (Bonnie), et al. Associations between depressive symptomatology, diet, and body mass index among participants in the supplemental nutrition assistance program. *J Acad Nutr Diet*. 2015;115(7):1102–1108. doi:10.1016/j.jand.2015.01.001

28. Scott KA, Melhorn SJ, Sakai RR. Effects of chronic social stress on obesity. *Curr Obes Rep*. 2012;1(1):16–25. doi:10.1007/s13679-011-0006-3

29. Richardson AS, Arsenault JE, Cates SC, Muth MK. Perceived stress, unhealthy eating behaviors, and severe obesity in low-income women. *Nutr J*. 2015;14:122. doi:10.1186/s12937-015-0110-4

30. Laraia B, Epel E, Siega-Riz AM. Food insecurity with past experience of restrained eating is a recipe for increased gestational weight gain. *Appetite*. 2013;65:178–184. doi:10.1016/j.appet.2013.01.018

31. Metallinos-Katsaras E, Siu E, Colchamiro R. Food insecurity's association with gestational weight gain varies by pre-pregnancy weight and parity. *FASEB J*. 2016;30(1_suppl):149.7. http://www.fasebj.org/cgi/content/long/30/1_Supplement/149.7

32. Larson NI, Story MT. Food insecurity and weight status among U.S. children and families: a review of the literature. *Am J Prev Med*. 2011;40(2):166–173. doi:10.1016/j.amepre.2010.10.028

33. Gross RS, Mendelsohn AL, Arana MM, Messito MJ. Food insecurity during pregnancy and breastfeeding by low-income Hispanic mothers. *Pediatrics*. 2019;143:e20184113. doi:10.1542/peds.2018-4113

34. World Health Organization. Global Nutrition Targets 2025: Policy Brief Series. *(WHO/NMH/NHD/142)*. 2014. https://www.who.int/nutrition/publications/globaltargets2025_policybrief_overview/en

35. Unicef Office of Research-Innocenti. *The First 1,000 Days of Life: The Brain's Window of Opportunity*. 2018. https://www.unicef-irc.org/article/958-the-first-1000-days-of-life-the-brains-window-of-opportunity.html

36. WHO/UNICEF. *Progress on Drinking Water, Sanitation and Hygiene: 2017 Update and SDG Baseline*. 2017. https://www.unicef.org/publications/index_96611.html

37. Prüss-Üstün A, Bos R, Gore F, Bartram J. *Safer Water, Better Health: Costs, Benefits and Sustainability of Interventions to Protect and Promote Health.* Geneva, Switzerland: World Health Organization; 2008.

38. Nounkeu DC. *Assessment of the Relationship Between Water Insecurity, Hygiene Practices, and the Incidence of Diarrhea Among Children from Rural Households of the Menoua Division - West Cameroon.* 2017. http://libres.uncg.edu/ir/uncg/f/Nounkeu_uncg_0154M_12349.pdf

39. United Nations. *UNESCO World Water Assessment Programme. 2019.* The United Nations World Water Development Report 2019: Leaving No One Behind. 2019. http://www.unesco.org/new/en/natural-sciences/environment/water/wwap

40. United Nations. *Sustainable Development Goals: About the Sustainable Development Goals.* 2015. https://www.un.org/sustainabledevelopment/sustainable-development-goals

41. Colby BSL, Ortman JM. *Projections of the Size and Composition of the U.S. Population: 2014 to 2060.* Population Estimates and Predictions. 2015.

42. Kandel WA. *Congressional Research Service Report: A Primer on U.S. Immigration Policy.* 2018.

43. Refugee Facts. *USA for UNHCR: The UN Refugee Agency.* 2019. https://www.unrefugees.org/refugee-facts/usa

44. USA for UNHCR: The UN Refugee Agency. *Refugee Facts: What Is a refugee?* 2019. https://www.unrefugees.org/refugee-facts/what-is-a-refugee

45. Witsman K. *Annual Flow Report: Lawful Permanent Residents August 2018.* 2018. https://www.dhs.gov/sites/default/files/publications/Lawful_Permanent_Residents_2017.pdf

46. Mossaad N. *Annual Flow Report Refugees and Asylees: 2017.* 2019. https://www.dhs.gov/sites/default/files/publications/Refugees_Asylees_2017.pdf

47. Schwartz SJ, Unger JB, Zamboanga BL, Szapocznik J. Rethinking the concept of acculturation: implications for theory and research. *Am Psychol.* 2010;65(4):237–251. doi:10.1037/a0019330

48. Nunnery DL, Dharod JM. Potential determinants of food security among refugees in the U.S.: an examination of pre- and post- resettlement factors. *Food Secur.* 2017;9(1):163–179. doi:10.1007/s12571-016-0637-z

49. Baer J, Kutner M, Sabatini J, White S. *Basic Reading Skills and the Literacy of America's Least Literate Adults: Results From the 2003 National Assessment of Adult Literacy (NAAL).* Washington, DC: National Center for Education Statistics; 2009:1–66. https://nces.ed.gov/ pubsearch/pubsinfo.asp?pubid=2009481

50. De Muro P, Burchi F. *Education for Rural People and Food Security: A Cross Country Analysis.* Rome: Food and Agriculture Organization of the United Nations; 2007. https://ftp://ftp.fao.org/docrep/fao/010/a1434e/a1434e.pdf

51. Dharod JM, Croom J, Sady CG, Morrell D. Dietary intake, food security, and acculturation among Somali refugees in the United States: results of a pilot study. *J Immigr Refug Stud.* 2011;9(1):82–97. doi:10.1080/15562948.2011.547827

52. Davidson G, Murray KE, Schweitzer R. Review of refugee mental health and wellbeing: Australian perspectives. *Aust Psychol.* 2008;43(January):160–174. doi:10.1080/00050060802163041

53. Garcini LM, Murray KE, Zhou A, et al. Mental health of undocumented immigrant adults in the United States: a systematic review of methodology and findings. *J Immigr Refug Stud.* 2016;14(1):1–25. doi:10.1080/15562948.2014.998849

54. Coleman-Jensen A, Rabbitt MP, Gregory C, Singh A. *Household Food Security in the United States in 2017, ERR-256.* Washington, DC: U.S. Department of Agriculture, Economic Research Service; 2018.

55. Piwowarczyk L, Keane TM, Lincoln A. Hunger: the silent epidemic among asylum seekers and resettled refugees. *Int Migr.* 2008;46(1):59–77. doi:10.1111/j.1468-2435.2008.00436.x

56. Hadley C, Zodhiates A, Sellen DW. Acculturation, economics and food insecurity among refugees resettled in the USA: a case study of West African refugees. *Public Health Nutr.* 2007;10(4):405–412. doi:10.1017/S1368980007222943

57. Peterman JN, Wilde PE, Liang S, et al. Relationship between past food deprivation and current dietary practices and weight status among Cambodian refugee women in Lowell, MA. *Am J Public Health.* 2010;100(10):1930–1937. doi:10.2105/AJPH.2009.175869

58. The World Bank: Press Release. *Record high remittances to low- and middle-income countries in 2017.* 2018. https://www.worldbank.org/en/news/press-release/2018/04/23/record-high-remittances-to-low-and-middle-income-countries-in-2017

59. IASC. *Guidelines for Integrating Gender-Based Violence Interventions in Humanitarian Action.* 2015. https://interagencystandingcommittee.org/working-group/documents-public/iasc-guidelines-integrating-gender-based-violence-interventions

60. Gottingen G, Stuttgart M, Weingarter L. *Achieving Food and Nutrition Security: Actions to Meet the Global Challenge: A Training Course Reader.* Feldafing; 2005.

61. Patil CL, Hadley C, Nahayo PD. Unpacking dietary acculturation among New Americans: results from formative research with African refugees. *J Immigr Minor Health.* 2009;11(5):342–358. doi:10.1007/s10903-008-9120-z

62. Dharod JM, Croom J, Sady CG, Morrell D. Dietary intake, food security, and acculturation among Somali refugees in the United States: results of a pilot study. *J Immigr Refug Stud.* 2011;9(1):82–97. doi:10.1080/15562948.2011.547827

63. World Health Organization. *Nutrition: Nutrition Landscape Information System (NLiS).* 2019. https://www.who.int/nutrition/nlis/en

64. Nunnery D, Dharod J. Community health worker model: its implementation and importance in reaching refugee populations in the U.S. *Int J Migr Health Soc Care.* 2015;11(3):169–178. doi:10.1108/IJMHSC-04-2014-0014

65. Black CM. A handbook for developing multicultural awareness. *NASSP Bull.* 1988;72(511):115–116. doi:10.1177/019263658807251131

66. Pedersen P. *A Handbook for Developing Multicultural Awareness.* Alexandria, VA: American Association for Counseling; 1988.

67. Foronda C, Baptiste D, Reinholdt MM, Ousman K. Cultural humility: a concept analysis. *J Transcult Nurs.* 2015;27(3):210–217. doi:10.1177/1043659615592677

68. UNHCR. IOC Launches Campaign to Bring Light to Refugee Camps. 2017.https://www.unhcr.org/news/latest/2017/11/5a1307884/ioc-launches-campaign-bring-light-refugee-camps.html

III

COMMUNITY ASSESSMENT, PLANNING, IMPLEMENTING, AND EVALUATION

COMMUNITY ASSESSMENTS IN PUBLIC HEALTH NUTRITION

BECKY ADAMS AND KAREN L. PROBERT

LEARNING OBJECTIVES

1. Understand the basics and the complexities of conducting a community assessment.

2. Identify the most common models and tools to guide the community assessment process.

3. Describe the four categories of information to collect and analyze in conducting a community assessment oriented toward nutrition and physical activity needs.

4. Describe the value of collaboration and **community engagement** in conducting a community assessment and explain the difference between the two.

5. List at least two key points on the use of social media and innovative technology in conducting a community assessment.

INTRODUCTION

Community assessment is not a public health philosophy or theory. Community assessment is something a health practitioner does. In simple terms, when conducting a community assessment, one studies information about a community in order to identify strengths, opportunities, needs, wants, and concerns related to the health of people in the community.

For years, professionals in public health departments conducted community assessments; now, hospitals and clinics are also performing community assessments. This chapter begins by describing various terms and definitions for community assessment. Several national public health and healthcare organizations have developed community health assessment models and tools. Some of these models and tools are reviewed in this chapter. The reasons for conducting assessments and approaches to conducting community assessment are discussed in this chapter. Types of data, data sources, data collection methods, and challenges along with steps for developing a plan to assess the target population with key stakeholders are also described. Important skills needed by public health professionals and emerging technologies that may be used in community assessment and programs are reviewed.

CONDUCTING COMMUNITY-BASED NEEDS ASSESSMENTS AND ENVIRONMENTAL SCANS

This section includes terms used for community assessment, definitions of community assessment, reasons for conducting a community assessment, and approaches to community assessment.

Terminology

Community assessment, community health assessment, community needs assessment, environmental scan, population-level needs assessment, community-based health needs assessment, population-based needs assessment, and so on are all "community assessment" terms with similar meaning. These terms have slightly different definitions, but the key points include gathering and studying information about a community in order to identify strengths, opportunities, needs, wants, and concerns related to the health of people in the community. Practitioners should know that these terms essentially mean the same thing while also understanding that some terms are specific to a particular model of community health assessment. Going forward, this text will use these terms interchangeably.

Definitions

There are many definitions of community assessment, but the two provided here are used widely by public health and healthcare sectors. The Centers for Disease Control and Prevention (CDC) describes **community health assessment (CHA) and community health needs assessment (CHNA)** broadly as

> the process of community engagement; collection, analysis, and interpretation of data on health outcomes and health correlates/determinants (. . . health determinates); identification of health disparities; and identification of resources that can be used to address priority needs.[1]

The Public Health Accreditation Board (PHAB) defines community health assessment as

> a systematic examination of the health status indicators for a given population that is used to identify key problems and assets in a community. The ultimate goal of a community health assessment is to develop strategies to address the community's health needs and identified issues.[2]

Another term related to collecting information about a community is "environmental scan." In the public health field, the term is not clearly defined, nor has it been evaluated. It is used to describe an approach to community assessment that involves reviewing stakeholders, health data, **focus group** findings, and key informant interview results. The phrase has also been used to describe an audit of the types of food available in retail stores. In the business field, where environmental scan has been well-defined, environmental scanning is a process used to assess internal strengths and challenges and external opportunities and threats. Decision-makers use environmental scans to collect, organize, and analyze data on their assets and shortcomings in external and internal environments to guide strategic planning and decision-making. Environmental scanning integrates multiple strategies for information collection. The purpose of an environmental scan is to understand context; collect information; and identify resources, links, and gaps.[3] Given this description, the increasing popularity of this concept in public health practice is understandable.

Justification

There are two overarching reasons for conducting a community health assessment: it is good practice and/or it is required. Successful programs address the needs and wants of the community, and the best way to find out what a community needs and wants is to conduct a community assessment.[4] Community health assessments are used to identify unmet needs; prioritize the use of resources; guide activities of coalitions, organizations, or agencies; and guide advocacy efforts or policy change. For example, United Way conducts periodic community health needs assessments to help direct funding and resources toward identified priority needs.[5]

The second reason for conducting a community health needs assessment is that it may be a required activity for a public health or healthcare entity. The following is a list of four institutions that require community assessment.

Nonprofit community hospitals. Through the Patient Protection and Affordable Care Act of 2010, all nonprofit hospitals are now required to conduct a community health needs assessment every 3 years. If this assessment is not conducted, the hospital will be assigned a tax of $50,000 per year because the hospital is not compliant. Hospitals are to consult public health and other community partners with information relevant to the health needs of the community served by the hospital.[6] Neither the law nor the subsequent regulations have provided much detail on what is included in the community health needs assessment.

Public health agency accreditation. A community health assessment is a prerequisite of public health accreditation under PHAB standards, and the standards address data collection, data analysis, and health assessment results.[7]

Community health center (CHC). According to amendments of the Public Health Services Act, CHCs conduct a community health assessment in order to be eligible for formal designation and federal funding. And CHC assessments must include the numbers and types of health professionals to aid in designation as Medically Underserved Areas or Health Professional Shortage Areas.[5]

Maternal and Child Health (MCH) Block Grant Program. The Title V Maternal and Child Health legislation requires states to complete a statewide, comprehensive needs assessment every 5 years. The Title V legislation (Section 505(a)(1)) requires the state, as part of the application, to prepare and

> transmit a comprehensive statewide Needs Assessment every five years that identifies (consistent with the health status goals and national health objectives) the need for: (1) Preventive and primary care services for pregnant women, mothers and infants up to age one; (2) Preventive and primary care services for children; and (3) Services for children with special healthcare needs. Findings from the Five-Year Needs Assessment serve as the cornerstone for the development of a five-year Action Plan for the State MCH Block Grant.[8]

Some states rely on community health assessments completed by local agencies to develop the statewide needs assessment.

Funding institutions. And less specific, but still a requirement, conducting a community needs assessment is a prerequisite to a grant application or a requirement after grant funding is obtained.

At the community level, many of these required community assessments will overlap. To avoid burnout by community members and health practitioners, reduce duplication of efforts, maximize limited resources, and obtain comprehensive data and information about the community, it is worthwhile for public health and healthcare agencies to work together when conducting community assessments. In fact, the CDC developed the Community Health Improvement Logic

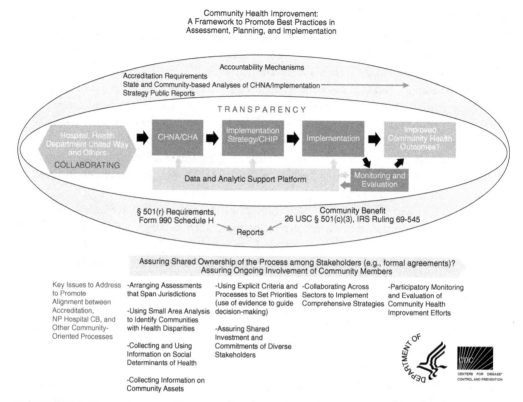

FIGURE 11.1 Community Health Improvement Logic Model.

CHA, community health assessment; CHIP, Children's Health Insurance Program; CHNA, community health needs assessment.

Source: From Barnett K. *Best Practices for Community Health Needs Assessment and Implementation Strategy Development: A Review of Scientific Methods, Current Practices, and Future Potential Report Proceedings from a Public Health Forum and Interview of Experts.* Oakland, CA: Public Health Institute; 2012. http://www.phi.org/uploads/application/files/dz9vh55o3bb2x56lcrzyel83fwfu3mvu24oqqvn5z6qaeiw2u4.pdf

Model (Figure 11.1), which depicts the alignment between the processes and expectations of tax-exempt hospitals, public health agencies, and other community-based organizations.[5]

A 2017 resource developed by the Association of State and Territorial Health Officials and the National Organization of State Offices of Rural Health reviews the potential for nonprofit hospitals and public health agencies to collaborate on community health assessments. This resource also includes models of collaboration from several states.[9,10] The next section includes details for some of the most common community health assessment models. In general, however, there are two approaches to the process of conducting a community health assessment. A community health assessment may examine a broad spectrum of issues important to the health of the population within the community, and the results identify top health concerns. For example, following a comprehensive community health assessment, adult obesity and infant mortality could emerge as top health concerns of the community. The other approach to a community health assessment is to orient toward a particular disease, the needs of a particular population, or specific risk factors, such as poor nutrition and physical inactivity. For example, a community-based health needs assessment may be conducted in a specific neighborhood to identify the barriers to and opportunities for healthy eating among adolescents.

COMMUNITY HEALTH ASSESSMENT MODELS

National public health organizations and national healthcare organizations have developed tools to help professionals conduct a community assessment. The different tools, or models, reflect different priorities. Each model varies in the number of steps involved, the people to engage in the process, the types of data to collect, and the approach to the task. There are also community health assessment tools that provide guidance and resources but do not prescribe a specific model. In addition, because assessment is the base for planning programs and services, some of the community assessment tools also include the steps that come after assessment including prioritizing, program design, implementation, and evaluation.

Key components of each model include building an assessment team, defining the community, deciding the purpose, engaging the community, collecting and analyzing information, and reporting findings. If program planning is part of the model, then prioritizing findings, developing goals and objectives, designing interventions, and evaluating actions are also included. In the following, we review two models used primarily by public health entities, one model designed for nonprofit hospitals, a website with tools for anyone conducting a community-based needs assessment, and a model used when the only interest is population-based nutrition and physical activity.

Mobilizing for Action Through Planning and Partnership (MAPP)

MAPP is a community assessment tool developed by the National Association of County and City Health Officials (NACCHO), which is a national nonprofit organization representing city and county public health departments. This model (Figure 11.2) is not exclusively about community assessment, and in fact, the resource is described as helping with community health assessment and community health improvement planning. There is a PDF document, but the resource is also available online (www.naccho.org/programs/public-health-infrastructure/performance-improvement/community-health-assessment/mapp) with modifiable documents and worksheets, webinars, presentation slides, and success stories. Two unique features of this community assessment model are that (a) one of the assessment steps is focused entirely on the capacity of the local public health system and (b) the approach permits a focus on health equity, and NACCHO has supplementary resources to help a community address health inequity.[11]

Community Health Assessment and Group Evaluation (CHANGE)

The CHANGE tool was developed by the CDC, which is the nation's federal agency focused on health promotion and disease prevention. There are multiple PDF documents, Excel spreadsheets, and success stories that are accessible on CDC's website (www.cdc.gov/nccdphp/dnpao/state-local-programs/change-tool/index.html). Three unique features to this community assessment model are that (a) it is data-intensive with several specific questions to ask of major institutions in the community plus formatted Excel spreadsheets to help gather and organize data and information; (b) it focuses on the key factors that affect chronic disease including tobacco exposure, healthy eating, physical activity, and disease management; and (c) it allows tracking of community-level systems changes, for example, food and beverage choices for school students, worksite promotion of using stairwells, or healthy food options at meetings or events.[12]

CHANGE describes five phases to community assessment and then provides instruction and resources for eight action steps. The five phases of this process are commitment, assessment, planning, implementation, and evaluation (Figure 11.3).[12] The eight action steps are (a) assemble the

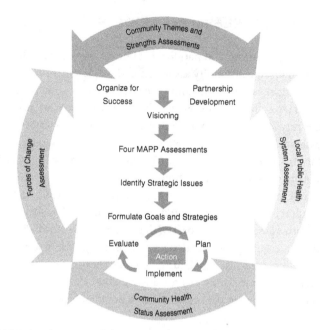

FIGURE 11.2 MAPP Academic Model. The six phases of MAPP are: (1) organize for success/ partnership development, (2) visioning, (3) four MAPP assessments, (4) identify strategic issues, (5) formulate goals and strategies, and (6) action cycle.

MAPP, Mobilizing for Action through Planning and Partnership.

Source: From National Association of County and City Health Officials. *Mobilizing for Action through Planning and Partnerships (MAPP).* https://www.naccho.org/programs/public-health-infrastructure/performance-improvement/ community-health-assessment/mapp/phase-1-organize-for-success-partnership-development

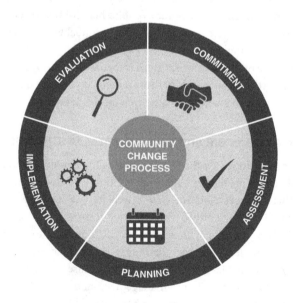

FIGURE 11.3 CHANGE Model for community assessment and action.

CHANGE, Community Health Assessment and Group Evaluation.

Source: From Centers for Disease Control and Prevention. *Community Change Process and the CHANGE Tool.* 2018. https://www.cdc.gov/nccdphp/dnpao/state-local-programs/change-tool/community-change-process.html

community team, (b) develop team strategy, (c) review all five CHANGE sectors, (d) gather data, (e) review data gathered, (f) enter data, (g) review consolidated data (includes four substeps and worksheets), and (h) build the community action plan.[13]

Community Health Assessment Toolkit

The Association for Community Health Improvement (ACHI) is an affiliate of the American Hospital Association and the Health Research & Educational Trust. With funding from CDC, ACHI produced the Community Health Assessment Toolkit, which can help a nonprofit hospital meet the Internal Revenue Service (IRS) requirement of conducting a community health needs assessment every 3 years. The toolkit includes nine steps starting with "Reflect and Strategize" and ending with "Evaluate Progress." Steps three and four are "Define the Community" and "Collect and Analyze Data," respectively. This is *not* a stand-alone tool; instead, the toolkit provides a framework for the community assessment process and includes links to other resources for each of the nine steps.[14]

Community Tool Box

Maintained by the Center for Community Health and Development at the University of Kansas, the Community Tool Box is used around the world by people working to build healthier communities. It includes information, checklists, templates, examples, and PowerPoint presentations summarizing information in each section. The Community Tool Box covers topics such as partnerships, assessing community needs and resources, building leadership, and sustaining the work.[15] The information in this resource can be used to complement a community health needs assessment process being conducted using another model, or it can be used to provide step-by-step guidance to conducting an assessment and building an intervention in a community.

Moving to the Future: Nutrition and Physical Activity Program Planning

Moving to the Future is a resource produced by the Association of State Public Health Nutritionists, which is a nonprofit membership organization of public health nutrition professionals. Moving to the Future is a program planning resource that emphasizes community assessment. It is exclusively focused on helping practitioners develop community-based nutrition and physical activity programs. This model is an online resource (movingtothefuture.org) with information, worksheets, and tip sheets in PDF and Word format.[16] General or broad community health needs assessments typically do not address the community-based food, nutrition, and physical activity needs or opportunities. An assessment with an area of interest needs to be done as a stand-alone or supplemental assessment.

METHODS FOR DATA COLLECTION AND CHALLENGES

Primary and secondary data are used in a community health assessment. **Primary data** is data that is collected by the practitioners involved in the community health needs assessment process. **Secondary data** is collected by someone else, typically a government agency such as the U.S. Census Bureau or a state health department. Methods for data collection depend on the category of data collected. For example, if the category of data to be collected is community opinion, then the method will likely be primary data collection and the practitioner might be administering community opinion surveys or organizing a **photovoice** project. If the data being collected is on the demographics or health status of the population, then the method will be secondary data collection.

As noted previously, each community assessment model calls for different types of information to be gathered. All models do, however, direct users to gather demographics and health status data. But the collection of information to describe community opinions and the community environment varies substantially across the models. Thinking broadly about community health needs and assets, the categories of information to gather and analyze can be organized into four buckets: (a) population data, (b) opinion and perception information, (c) community environment, and (d) public policy environment.[17]

Categories

Population data includes sociodemographic descriptors and indicators of the health and nutritional status of the selected population. There are many population data points to consider; examples include poverty rates, education levels, race, ethnicity, infant mortality, adult obesity, physical inactivity, diabetes monitoring, breastfeeding rates, and so on. The CDC, the Council of State and Territorial Epidemiologists, and the National Association of Chronic Disease Directors developed 124 chronic disease indicators that uniformly define and provide reliable datasets for chronic diseases and associated risk factors. There are 38 nutrition, physical activity, and weight status indicators, such as prepregnancy overweight or obesity, infants breastfeeding at 6 months, and no leisure-time physical activity among adults aged over 18 years.[18]

Opinion and perception information includes perceived needs, priorities, norms, and values of the priority population and other constituencies and stakeholders. Some examples of ways to collect this information include conducting a media survey, photovoice project, community opinion/concern survey, key informant interviews, and listening sessions.[17]

Community environment includes programs, services, and resources available in a community and their quality attributes, plus community influencers and social networks. One can gather this information using checklists, audits, surveys, or interviews. A few specific examples include asset mapping, walkability audit, Nutrition Environment Measures Survey (NEMS), and Physical Activity Resource Assessment (PARA).[17]

The *public policy environment* involves identifying relevant public policy issues and their status, including related legislation, regulation, ordinances, and so on at local, state, and national levels as well as national standards and guidelines from government agencies.[17] This is the point at which a practitioner can gather information on the social determinants of health by considering "incidental" laws and policies that affect income, education, housing, or other factors that have an indirect impact on health outcomes. Two other types of policy to consider include (a) "infrastructural" laws and policies that authorize development and financing of institutions and programs meant to improve the public's health (e.g., Healthy, Hunger-Free Kids Act) and facilitate the uptake of social services and (b) "interventional" approaches meant to limit exposure to potentially harmful materials (e.g., banning soda on children's menus), discourage unhealthy behaviors (e.g., junk food tax), encourage healthy behaviors (e.g., calorie labeling on restaurant menus), or engage in a combination of such approaches.

The community and public policy environments, described earlier, and their effect on the food and physical activity habits of people have generated a lot of interest among researchers and practitioners. As a result, there are several tools to assess the environment as it affects the foods we eat and level of physical activity in our daily life. There is not, yet, however, consensus on the single way to approach the "environment" categories of community nutrition and physical activity needs assessment. Several tools exist to assess the physical activity environment and the food and nutrition environment, and some are reviewed in the following.

The Built Environment Assessment Tool measures the core features and qualities of the built environment that affect health, especially walking, biking, and other types of physical activity. An example finding from this assessment could be that a community has several public parks, but they are located in remote, out-of-the-way areas of the community.[19]

To determine the quantity and quality of physical activity resources in a community one can complete the PARA instrument. The PARA is a brief, 1-page, check-box instrument used to assess the type, features, amenities, quality, and incivilities of a variety of physical activity resources (e.g., parks, churches, schools, sports facilities, fitness centers, community centers, and trails).

The **food environment** has been defined to include the physical, social, and person-centered environments that all play a role in what people choose to eat.[20] Measuring the physical food environment considers location and quality of food available and example tools to use include geographic information systems (GISs) and observational scans or audits. Measuring social environment assesses social support; policies, practices and rules; and parent practices as related to food. An example survey is the School Health Policy and Practice Survey, a CDC-conducted survey. Measuring person-centered environment assesses perceptions of availability, access, social norms, and social support; phone interviews and questionnaires are example tools for gathering this information.[20]

The nutrition environment is any place where people buy or eat food and is almost a subcategory of physical food environment described in the previous paragraph. The Center for Health Behavior, University of Pennsylvania, developed and/or inspired NEMS (https://nems-upenn.org/) for several places—restaurants, stores, corner stores, vending machines, grab-and-go food outlets, farmers' markets, hospitals, and national parks, plus a survey for perceived nutrition environment.[21]

Challenges

There are challenges in conducting community health assessments. The three that almost always come up for practitioners are (a) gathering too much or not enough information, (b) the limitations of health indicator data at the local level, and (c) the conflict between community opinion/perception findings and objective findings.

Regarding the quantity of information to gather, a practitioner can either get bogged down in gathering too much data and information or decide the whole process is too much and only gather a small amount of information. To answer the question "How much information does one need to gather?", use common sense. Collect as much information as possible, given the time frame and capacity. At a minimum, gather some information from each of the following categories: population data, opinions, community environment, and public policy environment. In general, the more information one has, the better. However, this must be balanced with making this step manageable and with getting the work done in a reasonable amount of time. To avoid not gathering enough information, remember that the point of community assessment is to learn about the community; so be sure to gather and analyze information in an area that is unfamiliar. Gathering more data and information during the next community assessment in the future is always a possibility.

In a perfect world, local-level health status and nutrition and physical activity behavior data would be available to practitioners conducting a community-based health needs assessment.

However, this type of data is typically only available at the state level and at county or city level for large population centers. For example, state-level data are available on the percentage of people who consume fruits and vegetables daily and the percentage of people who do not consume any vegetables or fruits, but this information is less likely to be available for a small area like a neighborhood or a small county/parish/borough. There is recognition of the need to have data at smaller units of analysis (e.g., zip code, census tract) in order to identify where there may be high prevalence for particular health conditions or to help identify pockets of risk in a larger population center.[5] Until such community-specific health, nutrition, and physical activity data are available, there are options. The following is a list of tips if data are not available for the specific community one is working with.

- Use a subcategory of data that the state does tabulate and that is similar. For example, the state may break down the data into these categories: rural, urban, or suburban, or by geographic region.

- Ask the state health agency and/or an academic institution for help in calculating data for a specific community or region. State health agencies may have access to local-level data and may help generate data that will meet the practitioners' needs.

- Use data from a community that is similar in demographics and geography.

- Use program data. Be sure everyone understands the limits of the data. For example, the Special Supplemental Nutrition Program for Women, Infants, and Children (WIC) program collects body mass index (BMI) data on children in the program. A community health assessment team could use this data to assess childhood overweight in a specific community. However, everyone needs to be clear that the data are for children 5 years old and younger from low-income families.

- Use state or even national data, but this choice should be a last resort.[22]

Another common challenge in conducting a community health needs assessment occurs when community perception findings differ from results of objective findings.[23,24] An example would be if the community perception reports indicate no access to healthy foods in neighborhoods, but through census tract data, practitioners discover several retailers with healthier food choices. Knowing that the community perceives things differently than what the objective data show is essential to developing community-based programs and services. Exactly how to address this conflict will vary depending on many factors.

- Health professionals can ignore the findings from the community with the risk of alienating the community and seeing failed programs and services over time.

- At the other extreme, health practitioners could develop programs and services that directly and solely address the community perceptions. For example, based on community opinion, the top adolescent health concern is teen substance abuse; yet, recent data show a steady decline in use of illegal substances over the past 5 years and an alarming increase in percentage of teens not doing any leisure-time physical activity. The community's health planning team that is conducting the community needs assessment could decide to work with the community and address teen substance abuse. Then over time the team might develop interventions to help increase levels of physical activity among school-age children.

- The third option to dealing with the situation of community perception conflicting with objective assessment results is to engage the community and work together to identify solutions that address the different findings. This solution will be the most successful in both the short and the long term.

BASIC NEEDS ASSESSMENT: DEVELOPING A PLAN FOR THE TARGET POPULATION

Using the tools and principles identified throughout this chapter, it is important to plan your assessment. Community assessment provides an opportunity to engage many stakeholders in the community. Engaging diverse community members during the planning phase of assessment can facilitate more robust engagement and identification of a broader range of resources.

Once the target population has been identified, develop a planning group that represents the community. The role of this group may be to oversee, coordinate, and/or conduct parts of the assessment. It is important to determine the goals of the assessment and how much or what kind of data are needed to answer questions in order to achieve the goals of the assessment. It is necessary to identify resources such as human resources, capacity/skills in various aspects of community assessment, existing data sources or previous/concurrent assessments, and funding available for primary data collection. Develop a plan that includes methods for gathering information, how to reach community members for input, how the data will be analyzed, who will collect and analyze the data, and a realistic timeline. Decide on a method of documentation and presentation of the results of the assessment and assign tasks. Present the plan to the planning committee, make adjustments as needed, and implement the plan.[25]

SKILLS IN ASSESSMENT OF COMMUNITIES

The previous sections have defined and described community health needs assessment. This section reviews the skills and principles necessary to successfully conduct a community health assessment. According to the Council on Linkages Between Academia and Public Health Practice,[26] there are eight skill areas for public health professionals:

- Analytical/assessment skills
- Policy development/program planning skills
- Communication skills
- Cultural competency skills
- Community dimensions of practice skills
- Public health sciences skills
- Financial planning and management skills
- Leadership and systems thinking skills

Obviously, in conducting a community-based health assessment, a practitioner needs all the abilities under the analytical/assessment skills area, which include identifying and understanding data, turning data into information for action, assessing needs and assets to address community health needs, developing community health assessments, and using evidence for decision-making.[26] Many of the abilities under the areas of communication, cultural competency, community dimensions of practice, and leadership and systems thinking are also needed for a practitioner to successfully conduct a community needs assessment. For example, an ability under communication skills is "soliciting and using community input," which would help a practitioner collect perceptions and opinions of community members; and an ability under leadership and systems thinking is "creating opportunities for collaboration among public health, healthcare, and other organizations," which is an essential skill when working with other health organizations also conducting a community health assessment.[26]

In addition to practitioners having the necessary skills to conduct a community health needs assessment, in 2013 a set of basic principles for approaching the work to improve community health were written to help implement the Affordable Care Act's requirement for not-for-profit hospitals to conduct a community health needs assessment every 3 years. Considering the public health literature, seven basic principles were proposed:

- Multisector collaborations that support shared ownership of all phases of community health improvement, including assessment, planning, investment, implementation, and evaluation

- Proactive, broad, and diverse community engagement to improve results

- A definition of community that encompasses both a significant enough area to allow for population-wide interventions and measurable results, and includes a targeted focus to address disparities among subpopulations

- Maximum transparency to improve community engagement and accountability

- Use of evidence-based interventions and encouragement of innovative practices with thorough evaluation

- Evaluation to inform a continuous improvement process

- Use of the highest quality data pooled from, and shared among, diverse public and private sources[27]

BUILDING SUSTAINED STAKEHOLDER RELATIONSHIPS AND ENGAGEMENT

Collaboration is fundamental to community assessment. Four of the seven principles to implementing a community needs assessment, listed earlier, had the theme of collaboration and/or engagement. Also, as noted previously in this chapter, there is likely to be more than one community organization conducting a community health assessment, and a collaborative relationship is inevitable. And, in the models for conducting a community-based health assessment (covered previously in this chapter), a team or committee is assumed and integral, or forming a team is a stand-alone step in the community assessment process. Plus cross-sectoral collaboration is a built-in component of Public Health 3.0, a model for governmental public health defined in 2017 and that goes beyond the traditional public health department functions and programs.[28]

There are several benefits to working with partner organizations when conducting a community health needs assessment. Other organizations that have either conducted or plan to conduct an assessment can share information and findings. With a diverse coalition, there is a greater chance of successfully addressing health inequities. Collaboration among organizations conducting community health assessments can help reduce fatigue among community members asked to participate. And collaboration during the assessment phase will likely increase partner and community member engagement in the intervention and evaluation phases of community health improvement.

Who needs to be involved? Multiple agencies should be involved in this work, and many factors affect the final roster of partners.

1. Expertise. Include someone who has experience collecting and analyzing community data and information. If this expertise is not available, seek locally to involve someone from a university, college, or state health agency who is knowledgeable about data collection. Also, state offices of rural health have a history of helping rural communities

with needs assessment and are a good place to find such expertise. Involvement of experts could be limited, as an advisor to provide technical assistance; the person would not have to fully engage in the community health needs assessment process.

2. Topic. The content focus of the community assessment will also influence who is part of the team. A food security coalition will have different people than a local hospital's community health assessment committee.

3. Committee structure. The community needs assessment team may require people to engage at different levels. For example, there might be a working committee of seven to 10 people from multiple agencies that meets monthly to review and analyze information and then every 4 months holds an open meeting to update anyone who is interested in the progress and to solicit comments.

4. Community size. A rural community may have four agencies, total, that work on nutrition and physical activity related issues, whereas an urban or suburban community could have hundreds of agencies offering nutrition and physical activity programs and services. So, in a rural community, everyone is involved, but in an urban or suburban community not everyone can be involved. A state-level community assessment, in which the community is the whole state, may also struggle to get all relevant agencies involved.

5. Interest. Not everyone is interested in the work to be done in conducting a community assessment. Some people are uncomfortable with data or are uninterested in assessing the community perspective or environment, and some only want to work on implementation. A person's interest in the community assessment work should be considered.

6. Grant funding. A funder may recommend agencies or disciplines that should be involved.

7. Philosophy. A group's philosophy may be to continually invite new people to participate, whereas another committee might draw up the list of agencies to involve with community assessment and not open up participation until they move to a new phase, such as implementation.[4]

8. Health equity. By engaging specific stakeholders, a community health needs assessment team can assess a community's health disparities and engage the right people to develop strategies to achieve health equity. The types of stakeholders to include are as follows:

   ○ Population groups that are affected by health disparities due to racism, gender inequity, socioeconomic status, and other structural inequities

   ○ Individuals with decision-making ability and the knowledge and power to influence policies, investments, and laws that have caused (or can prevent) health inequity

   ○ Individuals with expertise in data analysis and measurement of social, economic, and health inequity indicators

   ○ Groups that can communicate the causes of health inequities in a way that inspires people to work on achieving health equity

   ○ Facilitators that can create an environment that leads to productive discussions about health inequities and possible solutions or collaborative action[10]

Many resources exist to guide a community health needs assessment team in their work together. The community health assessment models reviewed previously in this chapter (MAPP, CHANGE, and Community Tool Box) have guidance, worksheets, videos, sample materials, and similar materials for use by practitioners. There is a relatively new trend in community health assessment to use the principles from **community-based participatory research (CBPR)**. A nationally developed toolkit using CBPR as a model does not exist, but journal articles describing the process used in specific communities do exist.[29-31]

Different from collaboration and partnering, but similar in that the practice involves working with others, is engagement. Engaging people from the community when conducting a needs assessment will greatly increase community support of the findings and next steps, plus it is an effective strategy to reduce health inequalities.[32] Community engagement involves members of the public in agenda-setting, decision-making, and program- and policy-forming activities. Without community engagement, the work of conducting a community health needs assessment is completed solely by professionals. This was the practice for many years; now, however, community members are involved in the community needs assessment process. The level of engagement ranges from professionals simply sharing information with community members to freely supporting independently made community decisions.[32] Generally, a high level of authentic community engagement yields more accurate community assessment findings and greater success in the programs and services developed as a result of the community assessment.

Social Media, Innovative Technologies, and Communication Strategies

Community health needs assessment has a long history of being conducted by governmental public health agencies, which means the work has been poorly funded; plus the scrutiny and accountability of public funds decreases the opportunities to try new, untested approaches, which can hinder innovation. As a result, newer technology is slow to be adapted. Public health leaders have called upon the field to develop new technology tools to help practitioners conduct community health assessments.[28,33] The models and tools for conducting community-based health needs assessments do not address using social media or innovative technologies in collecting community information, nor do these models provide guidance on using new or unique strategies to communicate assessment findings.

Despite this lack of guidance in existing community assessment tools and minimal information in the peer-reviewed literature, there are obvious potential uses and clear benefits. According to anecdotal reports and case studies, professionals use social media and innovative technologies to engage people in tasks such as collecting community opinion, assessing the community environment, and reporting information out to team members and community members. Here is an example from a regional planning advisory council in Central Arkansas, and the group of local governments is called Metroplan.

A collaborative effort brought "health" to the table with Metroplan's 2030 strategic plan, Imagine Central Arkansas. Because community input was deemed critical in shaping the mission of Imagine Central Arkansas, Metroplan used a mixture of low- and high-tech methods to engage citizens and other stakeholders across an urban area and several rural counties in a dialogue about the future.[34] Imagine Central Arkansas used:

- A "Kickoff Event"
- A series of mobile workshops throughout the region. The workshops were held at places that people visit daily such as malls, parks, shopping centers, schools, and so on.
- "Hometown Visits" to festivals, community events, shopping centers, campuses and other places across the region

- A speaker's bureau where representatives of the project would speak to organizations
- Email updates and posts on Twitter and Facebook
- Virtual opportunities to "imagine" Central Arkansas:
  - What do you love about Central Arkansas? Identify and vote for Treasured Places.
  - Have a killer idea? Share it and vote for others on IdeaScale.
  - Think you know Central Arkansas? Take our interactive quiz at Know Your Region.
  - Want to learn more about Imagine Central Arkansas?
- A web-based platform/game where individuals could select their top five priorities for the future by dragging icons depicting priorities such as faster commute, no tax increase, more transportation options, parks and natural areas, convenience (shopping, services, work nearby), and protecting the environment into empty slots on the page. Then they were asked several more questions about specific options or decisions by the decision-makers as a graphic on the page showed how each decision or set of decisions impacted the individual's priorities
- **Crowdsourcing** with online and mobile idea generation tools including IdeaScale and MindMixer;[34] see Figure 11.4

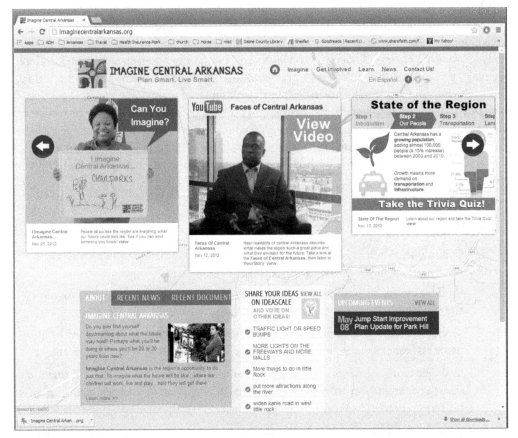

FIGURE 11.4 Imagine Central Arkansas homepage.
Source: From Metroplan. *Imagine Central Arkansas Plan Smart. Live Smart.*

Being innovative and using new technologies when conducting a community health assessment require special expertise and rigor. For example, if a needs assessment team plans to use GISs to evaluate the accessibility and availability of foods in a geographic area, there must be someone who knows how to access the data and use the related software.[20] Or, if a team proposed using the community-based participatory action research method, photovoice, to obtain the perspective of a marginalized group of people in the community, it is necessary to secure expertise on this assessment method to ensure the method is conducted accurately and the results are valid.

CONCLUSION

Community health assessment is of interest because assessment is the foundational first step to developing successful programs and services that improve health. The models described in this chapter help guide community assessment and some also include steps in program planning. There are key components across models and some differences that reflect different priorities. One component that suggests an important skill for the public health nutrition professional and carries through assessment, program planning, and implementation is community engagement. Community engagement and relationships are essential for a successful community assessment and for the success of programs and services that are developed as a result of the assessment. Collaboration with other organizations interested in community assessment within the community can contribute to a more complete assessment, reduce burden (assessment fatigue) on the community, and conserve scarce resources. The Woodruff County case described in Case Study 1: Woodruff County, Arkansas, Case Study on Community Assessment is a good example of engaging key community members and organizations in the assessment phase who formalized to develop and implement a plan for their community, brought resources, and continued to conduct follow-up assessments and planning. This case also describes the use of secondary and primary data, and tools for assessment of nutrition and physical activity using the MAPP tool to guide community assessment. This model is also used for program planning and implementation. Program planning will be discussed in Chapter 12, Public Health Nutrition Program Planning.

KEY CONCEPTS

1. Community health assessment is an activity facilitated by health professionals and includes other stakeholders.

2. Community health assessment is the foundational step to planning health programs and services.

3. Several terms are used to mean community assessment including community health needs assessment, environmental scan, and community-based needs assessment.

4. In simple terms, when conducting a community assessment, one studies information about a community in order to identify strengths, opportunities, needs, wants, and concerns related to the health of people in the community.

5. The CDC defines community health assessment as "a process of community engagement; collection, analysis, and interpretation of data on health outcomes and health

correlates/determinants (. . . health determinates); identification of health disparities; and identification of resources that can be used to address priority needs".[1]

6. Many community organizations conduct community assessment, including public health agencies, nonprofit hospitals, clinics, and other nonprofit organizations.

7. Two overarching reasons for conducting community assessment are that it is good practice and it may be required.

8. Community assessment can be broad in scope to yield top health concerns or narrow and prescriptive to identify barriers to and opportunities for a specific health issue.

9. There are several models and tools to help practitioners conduct a community health needs assessment.

10. Special tools and models are needed to conduct a community assessment that is oriented toward needs and opportunities related to nutrition and physical activity.

11. Primary data are collected by practitioners, and an example of primary data is information collected via a community opinion survey.

12. Secondary data are collected by someone else, typically a government agency, and examples include demographics or population health status data.

13. There are four categories of information to collect in a community-based health needs assessment focused on nutrition and physical activity: (a) population data, (b) opinion and perception information, (c) community environment, and (d) public policy environment.

14. From population data, one learns about the demographics of the population of interest, about the health status of the population as a whole, and about the food and physical activity habits of the population.

15. In gathering opinion and perception information, health practitioners learn about the viewpoints and perspectives of the community of interest.

16. Assessing the community environment identifies community assets, barriers, and gaps to achieving good health. This part of the assessment can identify inequities.

17. The public policy environment includes legislation, regulations, and ordinances at the local, state, and national levels that impact community health.

18. There are several tools and surveys to assess the community environment and public policy environment related to physical activity and food and nutrition.

19. The three challenges that almost always come up when conducting a community health needs assessment are (a) gathering too much or not enough information, (b) the limitations of health indicator data at the local level, and (c) the conflict between community opinion/perception findings and objective findings.

20. To overcome the challenge regarding how much information to gather, a practitioner needs to use common sense. Collect as much information as possible, given the time frame and capacity of the team, and gather some information from each of the four categories.

21. One way to overcome the challenge of not having local-level health, nutrition, and physical activity data is to use a subcategory of data that is similar and available.

22. If community assessment findings from objective measures conflict with findings collected via community opinion surveys, a good solution is to increase engagement with community members to better understand community perceptions and involve community members in developing solutions.

23. A practitioner uses several skills and abilities in the work of conducting a community assessment including understanding data, assessing needs and assets, soliciting and using community input, and creating opportunities for collaboration among public health, healthcare, and other organizations.

24. Collaboration with other organizations to collect and share data, information, perspectives, and findings is integral to the work of conducting a community assessment.

25. Consider several factors when deciding who should be on the community assessment team such as expertise, community assessment topic, community size, requirements, and population of focus.

26. Community engagement is a process by which people (typically not health professionals) from the community of interest give their opinions, set the agenda regarding community health concerns, and make decisions about how to create a health promoting community.

27. There are several opportunities for new technologies to be used in the work of conducting a community assessment. For example, online or social media based surveys can be used to gather community opinion, online environment surveys/checklists may be conducted to assess the physical environment, or social media posts may be used to report progress and/or findings.

CASE STUDY 1: WOODRUFF COUNTY, ARKANSAS, CASE STUDY ON COMMUNITY ASSESSMENT[35–37]

The catalyst for this community assessment was a funding opportunity, the CDC High Obesity Program. Land grant universities were funded to implement evidence-based interventions in counties with adult obesity rates greater than 40%. The University of Arkansas System Division of Agriculture Research and Extension—Cooperative Extension Service obtained the funding. Several counties in Arkansas met the criteria of greater than 40% adult obesity rate. In order for a county to be selected for intervention, the County Family and Consumer Science Agent was required to opt in and express an interest in built environment and food access.

Woodruff County was selected to participate. This county has four municipalities, Cotton Plant, Augusta, Patterson, and McCrory. At the first stakeholder meeting, all communities were represented and for the purpose of this community plan assessment and strategic action plan, the community was defined as the entire county. Community Coalition Action Theory was employed to guide the development and sustainability of the coalition and strategic plan. The MAPP tool was used to guide the community needs and assets assessment.

The grant administrator and interventionists were from the State Extension Office in Little Rock. They had a prior relationship with the county extension agent, who was a 30-year resident of Woodruff County. The county extension agent knew many of the people in the communities who contributed to the success of the project.

Secondary data collection:

▨ Data from the U.S. Census Bureau was used to describe the sociodemographic profile of the population. As per the 2010 U.S. Census, Woodruff County had a population of 7,260. White/Caucasian made up 69.9%, Black or African American 27.5%, American Indian and Alaska Native 0.2%, Native Hawaiian and Other Pacific Islander 0.1%, Two or More Races 1.4%, and Hispanic or Latino 1.2%. The number of households recorded from 2011 to 2015 was 2,911. The median household income (in 2015 dollars) from 2011 to 2015 was $28,933. The poverty rate was 25.8%.

▨ Arkansas Department of Health County Health Fact Sheets provided county numbers and percentages; state percentages and county rank within the state for demographics (e.g., total population, race, and ethnicity); economic indicators (e.g., income, poverty rates among children and all ages, single-parent homes, uninsured, and no transportation); injury; health indicators and major health risk factors (e.g., adult and youth smoking rates, low birth weight babies, life expectancy, natural teeth, water fluoridation, infant mortality and teen births, food insecurity, physical inactivity, obesity and overweight for adults and youth, low literacy, and youth substance abuse); and Department of Health services/programs, such as WIC, and participation rates. Woodruff County ranks 71st of 75 counties in life expectancy, with an average life expectancy of 72.6 years. The obesity rates in Woodruff County were 41.1% for adults and 30.8% for children. Food insecurity in Woodruff County was 24.1%. Physical inactivity in Woodruff County was 30.9%.

▨ The Robert Wood Johnson Foundation's County Health Rankings were used to compare relevant indicators with other similar counties, the State of Arkansas, and the United States. The County Health Rankings were used to obtain state-level data such as the "food environment index" (U.S. Department of Agriculture [USDA] Food Environment Atlas, Feeding America Map the Meal Gap), "access to exercise opportunities" (Business Analyst, Delorme Map Data, ESRI, and U.S. Census Files), and long commutes (American Community Survey).

▨ The Healthy Food Access Portal, USDA Food Desert Map, and Feeding America data were used to help describe access to foods and food insecurity in the county.

▨ Behavioral Risk Factor Surveillance System (BRFSS) data obtained from the Arkansas Department of Health provided county estimates for hypertension, diabetes, and overweight/obesity rates.

Primary data collection:

▨ A focus group was conducted by trained staff including a moderator and assistant moderator who kept notes. The sessions were also digitally audiorecorded. A moderator guide that included semistructured questions was used. The location was determined by the local county extension agent with input from community members. A large cross section of people were invited including elected county and city officials, faith-based leadership, business owners, civic organization leaders, community volunteers, school personnel, and library staff. The focus group revealed a perception of lower quality produce in local grocery stores. The focus group also revealed that those who were able drove 20 minutes from the cities in Woodruff County to shop for food in neighboring counties because of better selection, price, and quality. Many residents have no or very limited transportation to get to the grocery store. Major challenges identified were transportation, distance to grocery stores, and financial constraints (food insecurity). Cotton Plant had no grocery stores but did have a food pantry. The times and day of the week of operation limited participation. Standard methods of qualitative analysis were used to examine the focus group data. A panel of experts and community members provided feedback for selected data collection tools, instruments, surveys, and focus group questions. The panel assisted with interpretation and validation of qualitative data coding (i.e., grounded theory) and qualitative analyses.

- In order to obtain data more specific to the county and food access, the Nutrition Environment Measures Survey in Stores (NEMS-S) was completed in Woodruff County by an intern housed in Pulaski County. The same survey was completed in Pulaski County, which identified disparity in access to grocery stores between the two counties. There was a small disparity in variety, a large disparity in price, and no disparity in quality of foods according to the NEMS-S.

- Two physical activity assessments were conducted by the intern: the PARA and two of three parts of the Rural Active Living Assessment (RALA). The walkability assessment portion was deferred until it could be conducted with community members. The time and resources of the community were initially directed to the nutrition objectives.

During the first stakeholder meeting, the quantitative and qualitative data were presented in a variety of ways. For example, one way the focus group discussion was presented was in a word cloud.

The major stakeholders were the county and local governments, mayors, schools, church pastors, ARcare (Federally Qualified Health Centers [FQHCs]), State and County Extension Service, and community volunteers including a very active retired couple. A wide variety of people were involved from the beginning. It was important that the right person ask specific individuals to participate in order to ensure participation of appropriate and representative stakeholders.

The group formed the Woodruff County Health Improvement Coalition. The emphasis of the coalition turned to access to healthy foods as the need for emergency food distribution in McCrory was identified by the group. Community members willing to walk 3 miles for food assistance and other results of the focus groups and the NEMS-S confirmed the need for food access.

A facilitated planning process was conducted. See Case Study 2: McCrory Local Foods, Local Places Assessment.

CASE STUDY 2: MCCRORY LOCAL FOODS, LOCAL PLACES ASSESSMENT

The city of McCrory obtained a Local Foods, Local Places grant funded through the USDA, the U.S. Environmental Protection Agency, the CDC, and the Delta Regional Authority. A second community assessment was conducted in the city of McCrory that built on the Woodruff County assessment.

- The Environmental Protection Agency's EJSCREEN: Environmental Justice Screening and Mapping Tool (www.epa.gov/ejscreen) provides demographic and environmental data. The reports from EJSCREEN were generated on the city and the county. A second set of reports from the Healthy Food Access Portal, Research Your Community web portal (www.healthyfoodaccess.org/access-101/research-your-community) provided demographic, workforce, food environment, and health indicator data for the city and county.

- The final report was generated from the Ag Census, which only includes data at the county level.
- Through focus groups, the coalition identified additional projects.

Lauren Morris[36] provided these important takeaways:

1. Went in with grand plans from what had been seen in other places. Let plans/ideas be generated from community—good to share ideas from others, but don't want them to adopt something just because someone else did.

2. It is sometimes important who asked specific people to participate in the process.

3. Eating healthy and physical activity is personal and not something most want to talk about and must be tied to another priority more important to the stakeholders.

4. Don't push too fast. Plan is a living document. The Coalition would not have had the Warehouse but would have probably only had the community gardens if the organizers had pushed the community too fast. The Coalition needed an early win.

5. Make sure to ask what they love about their community, what makes it unique, special, a place you want to live.

6. The process helps to create a pathway and hope.

Case Study Questions

1. What were some of the factors motivating this rural community to conduct an assessment?

2. What community assessment model was used?

3. What tools were used to assess the community environment?

4. What category of information was collected by community assessment team members?

5. Who were the stakeholders involved in the community assessment?

6. How were community members engaged?

7. What were some of the key learnings/findings?

SUGGESTED LEARNING ACTIVITIES

1. An essay: Answer the following questions. Consider the Woodruff County case study and our class discussions about the community assessment models and methods.
   - How was community defined?
   - What was the impetus for the assessment?
   - Where might they have obtained data for the assessment?
   - Write three of the goals/objectives as specific, measurable, achievable, realistic, and, timely (SMART) objectives.

2. Team assignment: Teams will consist of three to four students per team randomly grouped by the instructor. May be assigned community member roles.
   - Group work during class:
     - Determine your target population and your target problem.

- ○ Determine how/who will find demographic and background information about your target population. Arrange a deadline to have this information to the group.
- ○ Exchange phone numbers and discuss possible group meeting times.
- ○ Review and make sure you all understand the overall assignment.
- ○ Divide up workload and assign responsibilities.

- ▦ Written plan: Plan should be double-spaced, typed, and without grammatical errors. All components listed in the following must be included and written in correct format. The following components must be included:
  - ○ Title of program
  - ○ Names of team members
  - ○ Mini "Community Assessment"
    - – Description of the community and/or demographic profile
    - – Perceived needs and assets (results from the opinion survey and/or other sources). One important part of the assessment involves surveying the perceived needs of community members. As a group, decide what segment of the population you might like to target for your assessment. Each student should survey at least five members of your targeted community.
    - – Health and/or nutrition status of the target population
    - – Available resources (assets)
  - ○ Write a needs statement
  - ○ Write one or two goals
  - ○ Write two objectives per goal

3. Oral presentation:
   - ▦ Presentation: 5 to 10 minutes.
   - ▦ It is the team's choice as to whether or not all group members should be present; however, all team members must come to the front of the classroom.
   - ▦ Audiovisual aids are recommended but not required.
   - ▦ The presentation should involve a broad overview of the goals and implementation plan.
   - ▦ Any necessary audiovisual equipment should be prearranged with the instructor.

REFLECTION QUESTIONS

1. What is the simple definition of community assessment and the basic components of the task?

2. What are the complexities of conducting a community assessment?

3. What are the most common models and tools used to conduct a community assessment among public health agencies, nonprofit hospitals, and other community-based nonprofit organizations?

4. When conducting a community health assessment with an orientation toward nutrition and physical activity, what are the categories of information to collect and analyze and what kind of information is learned in each category?

5. Why is collaboration among stakeholders important when conducting a community assessment?

6. What is community engagement and how is it different from collaboration?

7. What are the considerations to using social media and innovative technologies when conducting a community assessment?

CONTINUE YOUR LEARNING RESOURCES

- Moving to the future is an online tool for guiding nutrition assessment. https://movingtothefuture.org/chapter-1-community-assessment/

- There are two free online courses offered related to the BEAT Institute (http://www.med.upenn.edu/beat/online-courses.html):
  - Assessing the Built Environment for Physical Activity
  - Assessing the Nutrition Environment

- The Built Environment Assessment Tool is located at https://www.cdc.gov/nccdphp/dnpao/state-local-programs/built-environment-assessment/index.htm

- CDC's Center for State, Tribal, Local and Territorial Support Public Health Professionals Gateway at https://www.cdc.gov/stltpublichealth provides tools, information, and resources related to health department accreditation, community health assessment and planning, national health initiatives, strategies and action plans, funding opportunities, training, and other resources. Community Health Assessment & Health Improvement Planning resources are available at https://www.cdc.gov/stltpublichealth/cha

GLOSSARY

Community-based participatory research (CBPR): A process for conducting research that involves partnership between community members and researchers in which the community is valued and involved in every phase of the project.

Community engagement: A process whereby people (typically not health professionals) from the community of interest give their opinions, set the agenda regarding community health concerns, and make decisions about how to create a health promoting community.

Community health assessment (CHA) and community health needs assessment (CHNA): Defined broadly as "a process of community engagement; collection, analysis, and interpretation of data on health outcomes and health correlates/determinants (. . . health determinates); identification of health disparities; and identification of resources that can be used to address priority needs."[1]

Crowdsourcing: A process for obtaining ideas, input, and sometimes services, goods or funding from a large group of people, often through technology.

Focus group: A guided, small-group interview that uses group interaction to elicit information from group members.

Food environment: Includes the physical, social, and person-centered environments that all play a role in what people choose to eat.

Photovoice: A community opinion data collection method whereby community members take photographs of various aspects of their community and tell stories about the photographs. Examples could include foods available in vending machines, grocery or corner stores, or cafeterias, or other aspects of the environment such as walkability of an area.

Primary data: Data collected by the practitioners involved in the community health needs assessment process.

Secondary data: Data collected by someone else, typically with a government agency such as the U.S. Census Bureau or a state health department.

REFERENCES

1. U.S. Centers for Disease Control and Prevention. *Community Health Assessment for Population Health Improvement: Resource of Most Frequently Recommended Health Outcomes and Determinants.* Atlanta, GA: Office of Surveillance, Epidemiology, and Laboratory Services; 2013. https://cdn.ymaws.com/www.cste .org/resource/resmgr/CrossCuttingI/FinalCHAforPHI508.pdf
2. Public Health Accreditation Board. *Acronyms and Glossary of Terms.* Version 1.0. http://www.phaboard .org/wp-content/uploads/PHAB-Acronyms-and-Glossary-of-Terms-Version-1.02.pdf. Published September 2011.
3. Wilburn A, Vanderpool RC, Knight JR. Environmental scanning as a public health tool: Kentucky's human papillomavirus vaccination project 160165. *Prev Chronic Dis.* 2016;13:E109. doi:10.5888/ pcd13.160165
4. Probert KL. *Moving to the Future: Conduct a Community Assessment—Chapter Overview.* https:// movingtothefuture.org/chapter-1-community-assessment/
5. Barnett K. *Best Practices for Community Health Needs Assessment and Implementation Strategy Development: A Review of Scientific Methods, Current Practices, and Future Potential Report Proceedings from a Public Health Forum and Interview of Experts.* Oakland, CA: Public Health Institute; 2012. http:// www.phi.org/uploads/application/files/dz9vh55o3bb2x56lcrzyel83fwfu3mvu24oqqvn5z6qaeiw2u4.pdf
6. The Network for Public Health Law. *Issue Brief: New Requirements for Nonprofit Hospitals Provide Opportunities for Health Department Collaboration.* 2011. http://www.networkforphl.org/_asset/ fqmqxr/CHNAFINAL.pdf
7. Public Health Accreditation Board. *Public Health Accreditation Board Acronyms and Glossary of Terms Version 1.0.* Alexandria, VA: Public Health Accreditation Board; 2012. http://www.phaboard.org/ wp-content/uploads/PHAB-Acronyms-and-Glossary-of-Terms-Version-1.02.pdf
8. Health Resources and Services Administration. *Title V Maternal and Child Health Services Block Grant to States Program: Guidance and Forms for the Title V Application/Annual Report.* (Application Guidance No. OMB # 0915-0172.) Rockville, MD: U.S. Department of Health and Human Services; 2019:17–18. https://mchb.tvisdata.hrsa.gov/uploadedfiles/Documents/blockgrantguidance.pdf
9. National Organization of State Offices of Rural Health. *Community-Based Health Needs Assessment Activities: Opportunities for Collaboration Between Public Health Departments and Rural Hospitals.* (Issue Brief). Arlington, VA: Association of State Health Officers; 2017. http://www.astho.org/uploadedFiles/ Programs/Access/Primary_Care/Scan%20of%20Community-Based%20Health%20Needs%20 Assessment%20Activities.pdf
10. National Association of County and City Health Officials. *MAPP User's Handbook: Health Equity Supplement 2014.* 2014. http://eweb.naccho.org/eweb/DynamicPage.aspx?WebCode=proddetailadd&ivd_ qty=1&ivd_prc_prd_key=044bc66e-8d1f-4c1d-a85d-33976a21a6a6&Action=Add&site=naccho& ObjectKeyFrom=1A83491A-9853-4C87-86A4-F7D95601C2E2&DoNotSave=yes&ParentObject= CentralizedOrderEntry&ParentDataObject=Invoice%20Detail

11. National Association of County and City Health Officials. *Mobilizing for Action Through Planning and Partnerships (MAPP).* https://www.naccho.org/programs/public-health-infrastructure/performance-improvement/community-health-assessment/mapp/phase-1-organize-for-success-partnership-development

12. Centers for Disease Control and Prevention. *Community Health Assessment and Group Evaluation (CHANGE) Action Guide: Building a Foundation of Knowledge to Prioritize Community Needs.* 2019. https://www.cdc.gov/nccdphp/dnpao/state-local-programs/change-tool/index.html

13. Centers for Disease Control and Prevention. *Community Health Assessment and Group Evaluation (CHANGE) Tool Action Steps.* 2019. https://www.cdc.gov/nccdphp/dnpao/state-local-programs/change-tool/action-steps.html

14. Association for Community Health Improvement. *Community Health Assessment Toolkit.* 2017. https://www.healthycommunities.org/assesstoolkit

15. University of Kansas Center for Community Health and Development. *Community Tool Box: Table of Contents.* 2018. https://ctb.ku.edu/en/table-of-contents

16. Probert KL. *Moving to the Future: Tools for Planning Nutrition and Physical Activity Programs.* http://movingtothefuture.org

17. Splett P, Probert KL. *Assessment Terms for Community Nutrition Needs Assessment.* Unpublished manuscript; 2019.

18. Centers for Disease Control and Prevention. *Chronic Disease iIdicators.* 2015. https://www.cdc.gov/cdi

19. Centers for Disease Control and Prevention. *Built Environment Assessment Tool Manual.* 2019. https://www.cdc.gov/nccdphp/dnpao/state-local-programs/built-environment-assessment/index.htm

20. Lytle L, Myers A. *Measures Registry User Guide: Food Environment.* Washington, DC: National Collaborative on Childhood Obesity Research; 2017. http://www.nccor.org/downloads/NCCOR_MR_User_Guide-Food_Environment-FINAL.pdf

21. Glanz K. *Nutrition Environment Measures Survey.* https://www.med.upenn.edu/nems

22. Probert KL. *Moving to the Future, Conduct a Community Assessment. "No Data Tip Sheet."* https://movingtothefuture.org/wp-content/uploads/2017/05/No_Data_Tip_Sheet.pdf

23. Florian J, Roy NM, Quintiliani LM, et al. Using photovoice and asset mapping to inform a community-based diabetes intervention, Boston, Massachusetts, 2015. *Prev Chronic Dis.* 2016;13:E107. doi:10.5888/pcd13.160160

24. Ko LK, Enzler C, Rodriguez E, et al. Food availability and food access in rural agricultural communities: use of mixed methods. *BMC Public Health.* 2018;18(1):634. doi:10.1186/s12889-018-5547-x

25. University of Kansas Center for Community Health and Development. *Community Tool Box: Chapter 3 Developing a Plan for Assessing Local Needs and Resources.* 2018. https://ctb.ku.edu/en/table-of-contents/assessment/assessing-community-needs-and-resources/develop-a-plan/main

26. Council on Linkages Between Academia and Public Health Practice. *Core Competencies for Public Health Professionals.* http://www.phf.org/programs/corecompetencies/Pages/Core_Competencies_Domains.aspx

27. Rosenbaum S. *Principles to Consider for the Implementation of a Community Health Needs Assessment Process.* Washington, DC: George Washington University School of Public Health and Health Services, Department of Health Policy; 2013. http://nnphi.org/wp-content/uploads/2015/08/PrinciplesToConsiderForTheImplementationOfACHNAProcess_GWU_20130604.pdf

28. DeSalvo KB, Wang YC, Harris A, et al. Public health 3.0: a call to action for public health to meet the challenges of the 21st century. *Prev Chronic Dis.* 2017;14:E78. doi:10.5888/pcd14.170017

29. Akintobi TH, Lockamy E, Goodin L, et al. Processes and outcomes of a community-based participatory research-driven health needs assessment: a tool for moving health disparity reporting to evidence-based action. *Prog Community Health Partnersh.* 2018;12(1S):139–147. doi:10.1353/cpr.2018.0029

30. Kirk CM, Johnson-Hakim S, Anglin A, Connelly C. Putting the community back into community health needs assessments: maximizing Partnerships via community-based participatory research. *Prog Community Health Partnersh.* 2017;11(2):167–173. doi:10.1353/cpr.2017.0021

31. Williams KJ, Bray PG, Shapiro-Mendoza CK, et al. Modeling the principles of community-based participatory research in a community health assessment conducted by a health foundation. *Health Promot Pract.* 2016;10(1):67–75. doi:10.1177/1524839906294419

32. O'Mara-Eves A, Brunton G, Oliver S, et al. The effectiveness of community engagement in public health interventions for disadvantaged groups: a meta-analysis. *BMC Public Health.* 2015;15:159. doi:10.1186/s12889-015-1352-y

33. King AC, Glanz K, Patrick K. Technologies to measure and modify physical activity and eating environments. *Am J Prev Med.* 2015;48(5):630–638. doi:10.1016/j.amepre.2014.10.005
34. Metroplan. *Imagine Central Arkansas plan smart live smart.*
35. Bullington LA. In: Adams BA, ed. *Personal communication between Leigh Ann Bullington and Becky Adams on September 18 and October 19 2018 regarding the Woodruff County community assessment and planning process.* 2018.
36. Morris L. In: Adams BA, ed. *Personal communication between Lauren Morris and Becky Adams on August 30, 2018 regarding the Woodruff County community assessment and planning process.* 2018.
37. Washburn L, Freasier L, Morris L, Conner J. *Collaborations to activate local communities [PowerPoint].* (No. 1). Association of State Public Health Nutritionists; 2017. https://asphn.org/cdc-dnpao-conference -call-november-9-2017-collaborations-activate-local-communities

PUBLIC HEALTH NUTRITION PROGRAM PLANNING

KAREN L. PROBERT AND BECKY ADAMS

LEARNING OBJECTIVES

- Describe the steps to program planning.
- Tell why it is important to review community assessment results as the first step to developing a program plan.
- Understand the difference between health goals and objectives.
- Describe the criteria for SMART objectives.
- Understand the difference between evidence-based programs and practice-based evidence.
- Understand levels of evidence of public health programs.
- Describe how to find evidence-informed programs.
- Tell why selecting and implementing programs are described as a science and an art.
- List the common components to a program plan.
- List three other plans that accompany a program plan.
- Describe the different types of community resources and collaborations.
- Describe the difference between a centralized and decentralized model of managing implementation of the plan.

INTRODUCTION

The previous chapter covered the process of conducting a community health assessment. The natural next step following assessment is to develop programs and services to improve the health of people in the community. This chapter includes a description of the steps to program planning and reviews essential elements to developing a successful public health nutrition program plan. In this chapter, the words "program" or "intervention" are used broadly and could encompass any group of activities including projects, services, programs, and policy, system, or environmental changes.

FUNDAMENTALS OF PUBLIC HEALTH NUTRITION PROGRAM DESIGN, PLANNING, AND MANAGEMENT

Program planning is like vacation planning. The decision to go on vacation is based on some kind of assessment that includes a list of needs and wants from a vacation. The first big decision in vacation planning is setting the destination and defining some key parameters of the vacation (mode of transportation, length of time away, and approximate amount of money to spend). Next, the details are figured out such as a place to stay, things to do, planning for meals, and deciding what to pack. And many of these decisions are based on research including reviews, recommendations, reports, etc. Then you go on vacation! And while on vacation, you are monitoring your experiences and making tweaks to the plan to optimize the vacation. Public health nutrition program planning is a similar process. Based on findings from the community health needs assessment, a community health goal, or destination, is set (e.g., healthy weight among families with children); in addition, some key factors are defined that provide guidance to achieving the health goal (e.g., increase healthy eating and active living habits among families with children). Next, based on available evidence, the specific project ideas are selected (e.g., worksite programs to improve diet and physical activity, healthy corner stores, and safe routes to schools). Details about how to implement the projects are written down in an action plan. Then the work on these projects begins! Throughout implementation of the projects, people are assessing how things are going and deciding what modifications to make to ensure success and improve health. Again, public health nutrition program planning is a process and is similar to planning other significant events.

This chapter reviews seven program planning steps starting with listing community assessment findings and ending with implementing the intervention and monitoring for effectiveness. If public health practitioners want to create a successful intervention, all steps are important and the order of the steps is important. For example, it is tempting to decide the public health nutrition intervention, or program, before the goals and outcome objectives have been determined, but using the vacation-planning analogy, this is equivalent to packing a down parka and snow shoes before the family ultimately decides to vacation in the Bahamas.

REVIEW OF COMMUNITY ASSESSMENT RESULTS

Obviously, reviewing community assessment results is not a difficult step, but it can only be done if a community health needs assessment has been conducted. This step is essential to planning programs that improve health because it reminds practitioners to plan programs based on the needs and wants of a community, which are learned from conducting a community health assessment. Key public health documents plus all of the community assessment tools reviewed in Chapter 11, Community Assessments in Public Health Nutrition, direct a public health practitioner to list, identify, review, and/or report primary health issues based on community health assessment findings.

For this step of reviewing community assessment results, a practitioner compiles all the community health concerns and community assets identified from analyzing the four categories of data identified in Chapter 11, Community Assessments in Public Health Nutrition: **population data**, **opinion and perception information**, **community environment**, and **public policy environment**. It is tempting to compile the list of findings based on one's own opinions or beliefs, but at this point, it is best to simply list all findings. Reviewing the list of findings is then used in the next step of defining goals and objectives.

Along with listing or reviewing community health needs assessment results, some resources emphasize the task of creating a community assessment report.[1,2] By writing an assessment report, details of the community needs assessment work are not lost, and all the information from the assessment process is located in one place, making it easy to pull facts as needed to fulfill requests for information from the community health needs assessment process. For example, information from the report can be used to create social media postings that keep community members and partners informed of the work, or the information can be used in a grant application to secure funding for next steps. Although the specific categories of information to include vary among resources, in general, the community health assessment report includes a community profile or a description of the community served and assessed, a listing of community assessment team members involved in the assessment, a description of the process and methods used to conducting the community health needs assessment, findings, and next steps.[1,2]

Define Program Goals and Objectives With Community Stakeholders

After generating and reviewing a list of health concerns based on the community assessment, the next step is to focus the team's efforts. This is accomplished by determining priorities, and writing goals and objectives related to the priorities. The other value to defining goals and objectives is realized later after implementing the program when practitioners are monitoring progress and evaluating whether the program made a difference in the community.

The assumption here is that defining goals and objectives is done with others from a team or coalition. As noted in Chapter 11, Community Assessments in Public Health Nutrition, collaboration is fundamental to community assessment and it is essential to program planning.[3,4] It would be impossible to do this work alone, and without stakeholders involved, the program will fail. With input on goals and objectives from people living in the community and from stakeholders, there is built-in support for the efforts to improve health, increasing the likelihood of success.

If the community needs assessment was broad in scope, there may be a long list of issues or concerns that the community could address. It is best to prioritize by choosing one or two health issues to focus on. There are materials and techniques available to facilitate a committee's effort to identify priorities. Among them are resources from the University of Kansas[5] and the National Association of County and City Health Officials.[6]

If the community health needs assessment was specifically assessing needs related to nutrition and physical activity, the coalition may already have a priority health issue, such as "child and adolescent healthy weight," or "food security," or "heart disease prevention," or some other nutrition-related priority. If so, this step of prioritizing is not necessary now.

Once one or two health priorities are set, the program planning team can write health goals and objectives. Begin by writing a health goal. There is no single, standard definition of health goal, and agencies and organizations define it differently. Considering the many ways that health goal is defined, a general description for health goal is a statement about a long-term desired state of health, clarifying what you want to achieve. Goals are often positive statements, such as everyone has healthy food to eat, promote daily physical activity, and promote healthy weight, rather than reduce hunger, decrease inactivity, or prevent cancer, respectively. Specific measurements and time frames are not generally included in goals, and goals are broad-based. A community health goal is derived from a health priority or health concern.[7] For example, if obesity is identified as a top community health concern, then "Promote healthy weight in the community" could be the health goal. A simple worksheet like the one provided in Exhibit 12.1 helps practitioners

EXHIBIT 12.1

MOVING TO THE FUTURE: WRITING GOALS WORKSHEET

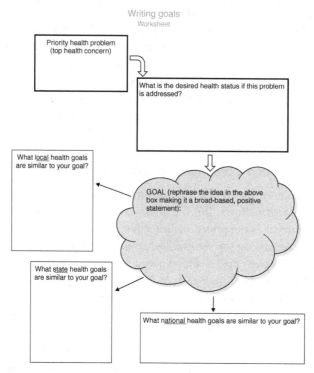

Source: From Probert KL. *Moving to the Future: Nutrition and Physical Activity Program Planning, Chapter 2: Identify Priorities, Goals and Objectives, Section: Writing Goals – Overview.* Tucson, AZ: Association of State Public Health Nutritionists; 2006. https://movingtothefuture.org/chapter-2-determine-goals/writing-goals-overview

write community health goals connected to top health concerns of the community. As noted in the worksheet, it may also be helpful to record existing health goals in the community or at the state and national levels. Knowing this information can give guidance on wording and/or help the community connect to larger efforts.

Specific ways of achieving the goal belong in the objectives, strategies, and action steps. Once the team has finalized its health goal, then it is time to write objectives. Objectives are the pathways to achieving a goal. An objective is a specific, measurable, intended result of your committee's work.[8] Objectives need to relate logically to a goal, and they should include specific measurements and time frames. Most resources identify two or three levels of objectives. The different levels or types consider (a) length of time to achieve and (b) whether the end point has to do with setting up and implementing the program or has to do with changing behaviors or health status. The terminology for and categorization of objectives varies. For example, an objective having to do with the proportion of adolescents eating the recommended intake of fruits and vegetables could be defined as an outcome objective, intermediate objective, or health behavior objective, depending on the resource. Or, an objective directing the establishment of a school employee wellness program might be considered a process objective, a policy objective, or even a strategy for an objective focused on improving the school health environment, depending on the resource. The exact term for an objective is not important. It is important that goals, objectives, and strategies are logically related and that objectives are well written. A logical relationship among goals, objectives, and strategies helps make sure that your work will impact what you are striving to achieve.

After writing a health goal, the types of objectives to define are generally called outcome or intermediate, or behavioral and/or community-level. Again, the objective name is dependent on the resource used as a guide. This text will use "outcome" to describe this type or level of objective. Generally, it will take a community at least 3 years to achieve outcome objectives. Here are examples of two outcome objectives:

- Over the next 3 years and by December 31, 20xx, convert downtown [City Name] to a pedestrian-friendly design that complies with the state Department of Transportation's Pedestrian and Streetscape Design Guidelines.

- In 5 years by June 30, 20xx, increase from 30% to 35% the percentage of people in [County Name] who have a healthy weight. (Baseline data source: 20xx Behavioral Risk Factor Surveillance System [BRFSS] data with data from [County Name] and 10 peer counties. The state chronic disease **epidemiologist** generated this regional data. Goal source: the upper 95% CI from this same regional data.)

Exhibit 12.2 presents another worksheet that can help public health nutrition practitioners write objectives that are related to the health goal.

Healthy People is a national effort that sets goals and objectives to improve the health and well-being of all people in the United States. The Healthy People Initiative has been going since 1979 with a Healthy People report issued every decade (1990, 2000, 2010, 2020, and 2030).[9] The goals and objectives are evidence-based and have input from several federal agencies, public health experts, and the public. Healthy People addresses those aspects of health that are the most critical to overall health and well-being. One of the greatest benefits of Healthy People objectives is that any community health team can adopt the goals and objectives, and they can be used as is or altered to meet a community's needs. It is smart to take advantage of the expertise required to set these health goals and objectives, and use Healthy People goals and objectives to guide the writing of community health goals and objectives.

Most resources use the term "process objectives" for the type of objectives having to do with setting up and implementing a program. The length of time to achieve a process objective is short, usually about a year. Process objectives are more relevant later when discussing the program plan.

The last point about objectives is that they must be SMART. A SMART objective is one that meets these criteria:

- Specific: It tells how much of what is to be achieved or who will change and by how much.
- Measurable: The information can be collected, detected, or obtained.
- Achievable: The intended result is realistic.
- Relevant: The result fits with the mission of the group.
- Time bound: A timeline is included.[8]

EVIDENCE-BASED PROGRAMS IN PROGRAM PLANNING

With direction provided by the health goal and outcome objectives, the next move is to decide what programs to pursue. The choice cannot be random or based on a practitioner's preference;

EXHIBIT 12.2

MOVING TO THE FUTURE: WRITING OBJECTIVES OUTCOMES WORKSHEET

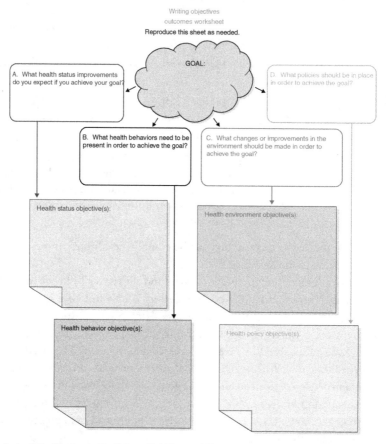

Writing objectives
outcomes worksheet
Reproduce this sheet as needed.

GOAL:

A. What health status improvements do you expect if you achieve your goal?

D. What policies should be in place in order to achieve the goal?

B. What health behaviors need to be present in order to achieve the goal?

C. What changes or improvements in the environment should be made in order to achieve the goal?

Health status objective(s):

Health environment objective(s):

Health behavior objective(s):

Health policy objective(s):

Source: From Probert KL. *Moving to the Future: Nutrition and Physical Activity Program Planning, Chapter 2: Identify Priorities, Goals and Objectives, Section: Writing Objectives.* Tucson, AZ: Association of State Public Health Nutritionists; 2006. https://movingtothefuture.org/chapter-2-determine-goals/writing-objectives-overview

instead, the programs selected need evidence of a positive effect on the defined health goal and/ or outcome objectives. For example, if "achieving healthy weight among working-age adults" is the health goal, then one evidence-based program to consider would be worksite nutrition and physical activity program(s) that have strong evidence of effectiveness for reducing weight among employees.[10] Another option to consider would be to increase healthy options in vending machines at work places.[11] There are many program ideas that community members and stakeholders will want to do, but the program will not have evidence of effectiveness. Continuing with the example above, some community members may have lost weight recently by following the ketogenic diet and want to do a program that includes this diet. Teaching people how to follow the ketogenic diet, however, does not have evidence that it is an effective community-based intervention in obesity prevention and control; hence ketogenic diet classes should not be considered as a program to improve public health. There are many community-based programs with evidence that supports nutrition-related health goals and many program ideas without evidence of effectiveness. Public health nutritionists who understand, advocate for, and implement evidence-based programs will help improve the health of the community they serve. This chapter reviews history and clarifies terminology related to evidence-based programs, reviews definitions for programs with varying levels of evidence, and addresses the concern of using evidence-based programs.

TERMINOLOGY

Public health practitioners, managers, and leaders use the term "evidence-based" frequently and perhaps without knowing the intricacies of the term. Put simply, "evidence-based" means that you use evidence to decide what to do. Regarding evidence-based programs, this simple meaning gets complicated because (a) evidence has varying levels of strength or proof, (b) community stakeholders have varying levels of trust in the different types of evidence, (c) there are always other community factors not accounted for in the evidence that affect the program outcomes in actual communities, and (d) not all possible solutions to health concerns have been researched or evaluated so the science does not always exist to say whether an idea will work or not.

Adding more complexity to the adjective "evidence-based" is the fact that it is used to describe the practice of public health, that is, evidence-based public health, and the term is used in a general way to identify preferred public health programs, that is, evidence-based programs or evidence-based interventions. Plus, "evidence-based" is a specific category of interventions in the classification of interventions by level of evidence. Because of this specific meaning for "evidence-based," the adjective "evidence-informed" has emerged as a descriptor of programs that are based on some level of evidence that will have a positive effect on health. This chapter uses "evidence-informed" as a general description of programs that have some level of evidence of effectiveness and uses "evidence-based" when the specific, narrow meaning is intended.

HISTORY AND EVOLUTION OF TERMS AND DEFINITIONS

The notion of evidence-based or evidence-informed programs has not always been part of public health programming. Before the evidence-based public health (EBPH) movement that started in the late 1990s,[12] public health practitioners often selected programs that "sounded good."[13] Although programs that "sounded good" were the only option and may have occasionally resulted in population-wide health improvements, we now know that using evidence-informed programs will yield steady improvements in community health and demonstrate responsible use of program funding.[14]

EVIDENCE-BASED PUBLIC HEALTH

The concept of EBPH is young and started, formally, in the late 1990s.[14] The newness of EBPH means that there is not a settled-on definition for the phrase. The definition is evolving as more research is published and as practitioners use evidence-based programs and report their findings and experience.[14] Proof that there is not yet agreement on the definition of EBPH, provided here are three descriptions from reputable sources. An article in the *Annual Review of Public Health* entitled, "Evidence-Based Public Health: A Fundamental Concept for Public Health Practice," whose authors are leading experts on the topic, listed key characteristics of EBPH, which some consider a definition:

> making decisions using the best available peer-reviewed evidence (both quantitative and qualitative research); using data and information systems systematically; applying program-planning frameworks (that often have a foundation in behavioral science theory); engaging the community in assessment and decision making; conducting sound evaluation; and disseminating what is learned to key stakeholders and decision makers.[14]

The Rural Health Information Hub defines EBPH as "Development, implementation, and evaluation of effective programs and policies in public health. It employs scientific reasoning to systematically use data and information systems, and appropriately use behavioral science theory and program planning models."[15] In a paper published in 2017, the international public health community defined EBPH as "a process of integrating evidence from scientific research and practice to improve the health of the target population."[16] There are many other definitions circulating in published materials. Generally, however, EBPH can be described as a combination of scientific evidence and values, resources, and context.[14]

EBPH is not the same as evidence-based programs, but the terms are related. Evidence-based programs are a significant component of EBPH, but community assessment is also a component of EBPH. At times, the two phrases, EBPH and evidence-based programs, are conflated. Their meanings did evolve together with several key events happening at roughly the same time. In the early 1990s, evidence-based medicine (EBM) was coined and practitioners were encouraged to follow the newest research findings to improve patient health outcomes instead of practitioners relying solely on intuition and experience.[12] When EBM was introduced, it provided excitement and a new focus on how to improve health across many health disciplines. Public health science was close behind in identifying approaches to improve population health. EBPH was first proposed in 1997.[12] The connection between EBM and EBPH is strong, and in fact, a simple description of EBPH is that it applies the principles of EBM to the field of public health.[17] The next key point on the EBPH timeline was the development of the Healthy People 2020 objectives. The Secretary's Advisory Committee on National Health Promotion and Disease Prevention Objectives for 2020 was asked to suggest actions for achieving the Healthy People 2020 objectives because "just setting the targets" was not adequate.[13]

Since then, EBPH has experienced substantial attention and growth. The collective effort of many researchers and practitioners to develop a cross-cutting definition and methodology of evidence-based practice to guide medicine, nursing, psychology, social work, and public health is a sign of the permanence and value of evidence-based work.[12] "Evidence-based practice" is the term used to describe an approach to how a health professional ought to conduct business in his or her discipline. Figure 12.1 is a model of "evidence-based practice" that all health disciplines could use, that is, a transdisciplinary model of evidence-based practice. The model incorporates the strengths of each discipline's model and tries to address the deficiency of each independent model.

EVIDENCE-INFORMED PROGRAMS

From here forward in this chapter, the focus is on evidence-informed and evidence-based programs. According to the strictest definition of evidence-based, an evidence-based program follows research protocols in design and implementation to determine whether the program made a difference. Evidence-based programs are typically highly controlled and well resourced with trained staff and adequate funding. The flip side of this coin is practice-based evidence, which describes when a

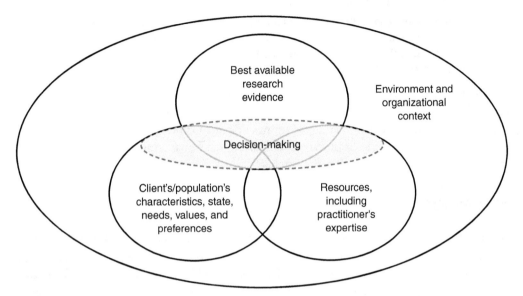

FIGURE 12.1 Revised evidence-based practice model.

Source: From Satterfield JM, Spring B, Brownson RC, et al. Toward a transdisciplinary model of evidence-based practice. *Milbank Q.* 2009;87(2):368–390. doi:10.1111/j.1468-0009.2009.00561

public health program is launched in a community, and the process and results are documented and measured; that is, the researcher observes and records what happens when a public health program is operating in the real-world environment, which has several imperfections from a research perspective. The impact of the public health program is then measured and reported out.[18]

As noted previously, "evidence" has varying levels of strength or proof, which some refer to as a continuum of evidence. Fortunately, a typology for classifying interventions or programs was developed in 2009 and is mostly used by public health researchers and practitioners. The typology includes evidence-based interventions, effective interventions, promising interventions, and emerging interventions.[14]

Although some of the category terms may be used interchangeably or imprecisely by practitioners, the typology is well adhered to in publications. Some organizations have written definitions for each category based on the typology. For example, the Rural Health Information Hub defines evidence-based, effective, promising, and emerging programs as follows, which is very close to the classification described in 2009:

- Evidence-based programs: Published in systematic reviews, syntheses, or meta-analyses whose authors have conducted a structured review of published high-quality, peer-reviewed studies and evaluation reports. Evidence-based strategies produce significant, positive health or behavioral outcomes and/or intermediate policy, environmental, or economic impacts.

- Effective programs: Published in high-quality, peer-reviewed studies and have produced significant positive health or behavioral outcomes, and policy, environment, or economic impacts.

- Promising programs: Based on exploratory evaluations that show potentially meaningful health or behavioral outcomes, and policy, environment, or economic impacts. They have strong qualitative or quantitative data supporting positive outcomes, but are not yet generalizable to public health outcomes.

■ Emerging programs: Based on guidelines, protocols, or standards that may be in the process of being evaluated by researchers to measure their positive impact on public health. Emerging practices are new and there is not enough information to make a decision about effectiveness.[15]

A footnote about these classifications of interventions by level of evidence: The classification is recognized and followed by most public health researchers and most governmental public health agencies, but entities that have developed ratings systems for program/intervention databases may veer from these specific classifications and create their own terms and levels. The ratings classifications are, however, based on the typology.

BEST PRACTICE

One new level of evidence has emerged since the typology was proposed, and it is called "best practice." Best practices are rooted in the practice-based evidence idea mentioned earlier. There is no consensus on a definition nor on the characteristics of best practices. In 2015, a working definition was proposed: "practices that have shown evidence of effectiveness in improving population health when implemented in a specific real-life setting and are likely to be replicable in other settings."[19] A best practice would be an evidence-informed program. Unfortunately, the term "best practice" is overused and misused and, at times, has little meaning. Public health practitioners who understand the term use it correctly and help implement best practices, which will help advance this emerging area of evidence-informed programs and improve population health.

VALUE OF EVIDENCE-INFORMED PROGRAMS

Although not stated explicitly so far, it is assumed is that there is value in using evidence-informed public health programs in communities. The value can be summarized in two words: cost and respect. By implementing evidence-informed public health programs, a practitioner saves resources including money, community members' time, and stakeholder time.[20] There is also an opportunity cost when an ineffective program is developed and used in a community. Somewhat related, but a value by itself, is the respect shown to stakeholders, funders, and community members when public health practitioners develop programs that have evidence of making a difference and helping achieve the community's health goals.

CONCERN REGARDING FOCUS ON EVIDENCE

Although there are many clear advantages to using evidence-informed programs to improve population health, some public health practitioners are cautious about the heavy emphasis on programs with evidence. The concern is the potential loss of innovation if "everyone" is only using evidence-based programs. It is true that the field would go stale and practitioners would feel like they were working with a straitjacket on if only evidence-based programs were used. However, this concern is not warranted. The typology for classifying interventions by level of evidence includes an "emerging" category. An emerging program could easily be innovative as long as it is based on some evidence, including word of mouth or personal experience and that it will be evaluated. The practice-based evidence approach is also applicable here. Hence, even with much focus on evidence, innovation is permitted. The burden of innovation does, however, fall on practitioners who must conduct program evaluation and publish their findings or connect with researchers who will publish findings. Finally, philanthropy tends to nurture the innovative side of practice, making their role in the field much more critical than simply providing funding for interventions.

Identifying Evidence-Informed Programs in Public Health Nutrition

This is the step in program planning that many practitioners enjoy the most—finding programs to implement. This step involves (a) making a list of potential programs that have evidence to meet the health goal and outcome objectives and (b) narrowing down the options with community health team members. The information in this section describes how to accomplish these two steps.

Because of the focus and attention on evidence-based public health, there are several websites to support public health practitioners in finding and implementing evidence-informed programs that positively affect public health. The key feature of these websites is a database of evidence-informed programs. At the time this text was published, there were 16 websites that included evidence-informed programs to improve diet and exercise behaviors of communities (see Appendix at the end of the book). Most of the 16 websites are domestic ones, with .gov or .org attached to their URLs, but two are international websites from the Public Health Agency of Canada and the United Kingdom's National Institute for Health Care Excellence. Most websites have a database that dynamically generates a list of programs based on criteria selected. The websites include information either posted directly on the website and/or program information that is available via a link to another website. There are some similarities and several differences across these websites. Here are some website traits with a general comment on how they vary.

- Each website fills a specific niche. For example, one website is oriented toward non-profit hospital staff, another includes programs and resources for the Title V Maternal and Child Health Services Block Grant Program, and another website is oriented toward local leaders wanting to create sustainable community change.

- Available programs in each website are only as good as what has been added to the database. Most of the websites add programs as evidence is available to justify inclusion in the website database. Hence, effective programs in practice but without evidence in the published literature will not be in many of the website databases.

- Each website is costly to maintain. Some websites lost funding a few years after they were created. It seems, however, that if financial support is cut, the website developer keeps the web-based database available, but no new content is added after the funding ended.

- The programs included in each website database vary in their level of evidence or form of evidence. For example, a couple of the websites only include evidence-based programs while other websites include programs across the continuum of evidence.

- The source of the programs in each database and how programs are added vary. Some websites include programs submitted by practitioners and others include only programs selected by experts.

- Most websites have programs and some resources that help implement, but two websites are a list of resources only.

- Most websites with programs have a rating system, and although the rating systems vary across websites, rating systems are clearly explained on each site.

- Each agency and organization with a website uses their own process to identify what is evidence-based, but often a systematic review or a meta-analysis is used to evaluate the body of evidence in a given field.

- All websites have a frequently asked questions (FAQ) section or include a clear explanation of the information on the website.

For many reasons, a detailed explanation of each website is not feasible. One reason, for example, is that the programs in the database and the sorting features constantly change, so detailed explanations would quickly be outdated. Some information is needed, however, to understand these new and much-needed tools for public health practitioners implementing evidence-informed programs. Three websites with evidence-informed programs are reviewed here and Table 12.1 describes the intended user of the website, the methodology of selecting interventions to review, and the ratings used.

- The *What Works for Health* program database is sponsored by Robert Wood Johnson Foundation. This full-service website includes "a menu of evidence-informed policies and programs that can make a difference locally."[11] The intervention database is one component of the County Health Rankings & Roadmaps website that also includes information and resources on assessment, prioritization, evaluation, and collaboration.[11]

- The *Community Guide* is sponsored by the Community Preventive Services Task Force. The Guide to Community Preventive Services (The Community Guide) includes evidence-based programs that consider health outcomes and cost-effectiveness. The findings are based on systematic reviews of peer-reviewed literature.[21]

- The *SNAP-Ed Toolkit* is sponsored by the Regional Nutrition Education Centers of Excellence, National Coordination Center at the University of Kentucky with funding from the U.S. Department of Agriculture. This intervention database is a collection of evidence-informed obesity prevention and policy, system, and environmental change interventions. The interventions in the toolkit are only a partial list of interventions that are used in SNAP-Ed (Supplemental Nutrition Assistance Program Education). All the interventions are intended to achieve the goal of helping SNAP-eligible households make healthy eating and physical activity choices on a limited budget.[22]

Independent of the website's focus or intent, they all have information for practitioners looking for evidence-informed programs. A public health nutritionist working for a local health department could find possible program ideas in the website oriented toward nonprofit hospital staff. A practitioner could review many websites to generate a list of evidence-informed program ideas. Users should find programs that will address the community health goal and outcome objectives and should be smart and creative in using the website databases. For example, a program with evidence of effectiveness in community-based obesity control and prevention can be considered by a cancer prevention program even if the program is not in Research-Tested Intervention Programs (RTIPs), a database of evidence-based cancer control interventions, because obesity is a risk factor for some forms of cancer.

Armed with definitions, an understanding of the nuances of evidence-informed work, and several websites with evidence-informed programs, a practitioner is ready to find, choose, and implement evidence-informed programs. Practitioners and researchers note that these actual tasks of selecting and implementing programs are a science and an art. The science part is selecting programs based on epidemiological, behavioral, and policy research showing which interventions are likely to be effective in addressing the problems.[14] The art is in the application so that the

TABLE 12.1 WEBSITES THAT REVIEW EVIDENCE-INFORMED PROGRAMS: COMPARISON OF INTENDED USER, METHODOLOGY OF SELECTING INTERVENTIONS FOR REVIEW, AND RATINGS USED

	WHAT WORKS FOR HEALTH	COMMUNITY GUIDE	SNAP-ED TOOLKIT
Intended User	Not specific, but language does call out local leaders wanting to create sustainable community change.	Not specific, but lists possible users as public health and healthcare practitioners, employers, researchers, and other decision-makers.	SNAP-Ed administrators and implementing agencies.
Summary of Methodology	To assess evidence, this resource combines information from science and observations of unbiased experts. Programs are included based on information from systematic review resources, other rating organizations, and published and grey literature.	A team of experts considers the results of systematic review of interventions. The team includes topic experts, an economist, research fellows, a federal agency representative, a member of the Community Preventive Services Task Force, and a CDC coordinating scientist.	Through a peer-review process, the interventions are reviewed by USDA Food and Nutrition Service, Association of SNAP Nutrition Education Administrators, National Collaborative on Childhood Obesity Research, and Center for Training and Research Translation. Practitioners can submit interventions for review.
Ratings	Each program receives an evidence rating and a disparity rating. The evidence ratings are: • Scientifically supported • Some evidence • Expert opinion • Insufficient evidence • Mixed evidence • Evidence of ineffectiveness The disparity ratings are: • Likely to decrease disparities • No impact on disparities likely • Likely to increase disparities	Each intervention receives a finding: • Recommended with strong evidence • Recommended with sufficient evidence • Recommended against • Insufficient evidence	Each intervention is classified as • Research-tested • Practice-tested • Emerging

CDC, Centers for Disease Control and Prevention; SNAP-Ed, Supplemental Nutrition Assistance Program Education; USDA, United States Department of Agriculture.

programs selected have the greatest likelihood of success. And success will come from identifying the programs with the strongest evidence of effect balanced with partner and community member buy-in for specific programs.[14]

This science and art idea has a catchphrase—evidence-informed decision-making (EIDM). The description of EIDM conveys perfectly how a practitioner selects and implements public health programs. EIDM involves "using research findings plus public health expertise and resources, and knowledge about community health issues, local context, and political climate to make policy and programming decisions."[20] Below are five fictional vignettes that translate the theoretical EIDM process into a real case story:

- Several commercial business districts in a region have tried point-of-decision prompts for physical activity, specifically motivational signs near stairwells and elevators, but they just are not making a difference with workers in these neighboring business districts. Understand that motivational signs near stairwells may not be a good program to try in the specific community despite the strong scientific evidence of increasing physical activity levels. Or, consider an assessment of workers in the area to determine why the point-of-decision prompts are not working.

- A team of practitioners are working to find and use evidence-informed programs to increase healthy eating and active living in a Native American community. Several program ideas are highly recommended by The Community Guide, which is sponsored by the Centers for Disease Control and Prevention. Understand that the possible programs from this government publication may have to be put aside because of the distrust of the U.S. government by many people in the specific Native American community. Other evidence-informed programs are available and need to be considered.

- A mildly effective intervention (making water easily available in childcare settings) has anecdotal evidence from some local childcare providers to reduce the amount of "sweet drinks" that kids are drinking. Understand that despite the weaker level of evidence for the "water availability" intervention, it should be considered for implementation in more childcare settings. With time, after childcare providers have confidence in their ability to improve the nutritional health of children in their care, a different evidence-informed program can probably be considered that has greater evidence of effectiveness. Also, consider connecting with a researcher who could help gather evaluation information on the program in childcare settings, which would contribute to the evidence base for "water availability" programs.

- The child of a community health team member was hit by a vehicle while walking to school. Understand that despite the extremely strong evidence of increasing the numbers of students walking and biking to school, and the fact that the purpose of the program is to make walking and biking safer, the **Safe Routes to Schools** program may not be a feasible option right away.

- A new medical doctor just moved to the community and wants to be involved with the community-based health improvement efforts. In her previous community, the physician was an advisor to the community health team that was experimenting with a program that did not have any level of evidence of effectiveness other than expert opinion. The doctor is pushing to do the same experimental program in the new community. Consider whether the value of having the new doctor engaged in the community work to improve health may be more important than whether this low-level evidence program is done. Perhaps there are some research-based modifications to the program design that can be done to improve its level of evidence, and consider working with the other community to see whether with evaluation data the program could become a best practice. Also, remember that the experimental program does not have to be the only program selected to address the community health goal.

Prepare Program Plan and Management System

Before launching evidence-informed programs in a community, it is important to make a plan. A program plan describes step-by-step how to get started and how to stay on track. Based on what was learned through the community health assessment, what was envisioned in the writing of health goals and outcome objectives, and what was discovered while researching evidence-informed interventions, a public health program plan translates the program ideas into action. A plan should clearly describe the who, what, when, and where of implementing the program(s).

Many public health program planning "how to" tools exist. All the tools reviewed in Chapter 11, Community Assessments in Public Health Nutrition, on community assessment include guidance on how to develop a program plan. There is also an online software strategic planning resource, called OnStrategy, used by some public health agencies to guide practitioners through the process of developing a program plan.[23]

The information that "should" be included in the program plan and the terminology vary with every resource. For example, some resources use the term "action plan" instead of "program plan," or resources will refer to a coordinator versus a lead contact to describe the person who is responsible for a specific step or activity. There are several terms used to describe the objectives included in a program plan, such as "process objective" versus "annual objective." In general, however, the plan will include a health goal, outcome objectives, intervention descriptions, process objectives, and details such as strategies, activities or action steps, partners, lead contact, and timeline. By developing a plan, practitioners can verify that health goals, outcome objectives, and intervention plans are logically related so that the interventions will contribute positively to the health goal. The plan template provided in Exhibit 12.3[24] is a good demonstration of this.

Several resources exist to help practitioners develop a plan. There are program planning resources that provide specific guidance with forms that continue a process which started with community assessment. For example, in the Mobilizing for Action through Planning and Partnerships (MAPP) tool, phases four, five, and six take the user from community assessment findings to an action plan. The six phases of MAPP are: (a) organize for success/partnership development, (b) visioning, (c) four MAPP assessments, (d) identify strategic issues, (e) formulate goals and strategies, and (f) action cycle.[25] The action plan templates available on the MAPP website are examples from community teams that have used the MAPP planning process: www.naccho.org/programs/public-health-infrastructure/performance-improvement/community-health-assessment/mapp.

Another program planning resource reviewed in the community assessment chapter, Community Health Assessment and Group Evaluation (CHANGE) Tool,[26] walks the user through two steps to generate a detailed action plan. In Action Step 7, CHANGE instructs a user to complete a planning template, which calls for minimal but essential information to launch and maintain an intervention. The planning template (Exhibit 12.4)[27] calls for the change strategy (e.g., healthy food choices at corner stores and convenience stores), the "next steps" related to the change strategy (e.g., generate a list of stores, meet with store owners to discuss vision and success stories, assess interest of store owners, form a work group of interested store owners, provide training and technical assistance to interested store owners), the lead contact, and the timeline. Then in Step 8 (Build the Community Action Plan), CHANGE calls for much more detail with 1-year and multiyear objectives, activities, number of people reached, etc. See the template in Exhibit 12.5.[28]

EXHIBIT 12.3

MOVING TO THE FUTURE: PROGRAM WORK PLAN WORKSHEET

Program work plan

GOAL:

Outcome objective:

Process objective: _____

_____

Strategy: _____

Action steps	Due date	Agency responsible	Resources required

How would you monitor and evaluate the strategy and/or action steps?

Source: From Probert KL. *Moving to the Future: Nutrition and Physical Activity Program Planning, Chapter 3: Develop a Plan – Chapter Overview.* Tucson, AZ: Association of State Public Health Nutritionists; 2006. https://movingtothefuture.org/chapter-3-develop-a-plan/develop-a-plan-chapter-overview

EXHIBIT 12.4

COMMUNITY HEALTH IMPROVEMENT PLANNING TEMPLATE

SECTOR: POLICY/ENVIRONMENTAL CHANGE STRATEGY	NEXT STEPS	LEAD/ PRIMARY CONTACT	TIMELINE
1.			
2.			

Source: From Centers for Disease Control and Prevention, Division of Nutrition, Physical Activity and Obesity. *Community Health Assessment and Group Evaluation (CHANGE) Tool: Action Step 7d: Complete the Community Health Improvement Planning Template.* 2019. https://www.cdc.gov/nccdphp/dnpao/state-local-programs/change-tool/actionstep7.html

EXHIBIT 12.5

EXAMPLE OF A COMMUNITY ACTION PLAN

Project Period Objective	Description of the Objective	Priority Area
Annual Objective	Description of the Objective	Sector
		Number of People Reached
Activities	Activity Title	Description

Source: From Centers for Disease Control and Prevention, Division of Nutrition, Physical Activity and Obesity. *Community Health Assessment and Group Evaluation (CHANGE) Tool: Action Step 8.* 2019. https://www.cdc.gov/nccdphp/dnpao/state-local-programs/change-tool/actionstep8.html

If the plan is part of grant-funded work, there is almost certainly a plan template provided, requesting applicants to provide the information that the funder has deemed relevant and useful. There are also generic templates available that are not tied to a specific program planning process. An example generic plan template from the Community Tool Box is provided in Exhibit 12.6.

The Rural Health Information Hub and Community Tool Box includes resources that provide step-by-step guidance for planning specific community programs. The Rural Health Information Hub includes a toolkit for community health program planning in rural communities plus toolkits for addressing specific community health concerns, such as chronic obstructive pulmonary disease, food access, obesity prevention, and many more.[15] And the Community Tool Box includes links to action planning guides for specific community issues, such as improving access and eliminating disparities in community health, promoting child well-being, and preventing chronic disease.[29]

There is even a tool that helps practitioners plan interventions in the context of other interventions. The Matrix Assisting Practitioner's Intervention Planning Tool (MAP-IT) does not guide

EXHIBIT 12.6

COMMUNITY TOOL BOX ACTION PLAN TEMPLATE

Action Plan for [Community or Initiative Name]

Community Focus Area: _____

Community Change to Be Sought: _____

Collaborating Organization(s) Group(s): _____ Community Sector: _____

ACTION STEPS

ACTION STEPS	BY WHOM	BY WHEN	RESOURCES AND SUPPORT AVAILABLE/NEEDED		POTENTIAL BARRIERS OR RESISTANCE	COMMUNICATION PLAN FOR IMPLEMENTATION
What needs to be done?	Who will take actions?	By what date will the action be done?	Resources available	Resources needed (financial, human, political, and other)	What individuals and organizations might resist? How?	What individuals and organizations should be informed about/involved with these actions?
Step 1: By _____						
Step 2: By _____						
Step 3: By _____						
Step 4: By _____						

Source: From KU Center for Community Health and Development. *Chapter 3, Section 1: Developing a Plan for Assessing Local Needs and Resources.* Lawrence, KS: University of Kansas; 2019. http://ctb.ku.edu/en/table-of-contents/assessment/assessing-community-needs-and-resources/develop-a-plan/main

a user through the steps of planning a specific intervention, but instead forces practitioners to think through all the types of interventions needed to support behavior change—the needs of the individual and the needs for the environment.[30] The assumption with public health nutrition is that programs will focus on changes to the environment or systems rather than changes to individual behavior, for example, helping hospitals achieve the Baby-Friendly designation rather than individual counseling to pregnant women about the benefits of breastfeeding. This focus on the environment or system does not suggest that the individual behavior change strategies are not important. Clearly, the individual makes the change that leads to improved health and quality of life. There needs to be a focus on environmental change *and* individual change, and MAP-IT helps practitioners see the need for all interventions.

In addition to developing a program plan for evidence-informed intervention(s), a community health team may also develop a sustainability plan, a communication plan, and/or an evaluation plan that accompanies the program plan. Some community health teams might, instead, incorporate sustainability, communication, and evaluation objectives and related activities into the program plan.

Sustainability planning considers ways to sustain funding, activities, success, partners, outcomes, system changes, and community commitment to good health and wellness.[31-33] Several public health resources include additional information on sustainability plans.

According to the Centers for Disease Control and Prevention, "an evaluation plan is a written document that describes how you will monitor and evaluate your program, so that you will be able to describe the 'What,' the 'How,' and the 'Why It Matters' for your program and use evaluation results for program improvement and decision making."[34] An evaluation plan is designed to answer questions that partners, the community, the funder, and the practitioners most involved in implementation have about the program. Two example evaluation questions would be: What were the effects of the **Farm to Preschool** programs on children's fruit and vegetable consumption? Or Did the Farm to Preschool programs benefit local farms? The evaluation plan will yield a report with results on how successful the program was and recommendations on how to improve the intervention(s).

A communication plan describes who will receive information, when to send the information, and how the information will be shared. Regarding the public health nutrition program planning process, a communication plan can help the community and partners understand community health concerns, possible solutions, progress with program implementation, and program results.[35]

Planning is critical to implementing successful evidence-informed programs and interventions, and several tools are available to help public health nutrition practitioners develop plans. The challenge, however, is to not become paralyzed in the planning step. Not all of these plans have to be done perfectly every year.

Identification of Resources and Collaborations

Public health nutritionists always need to partner with others to do their work. Evidence-informed public health nutrition programs call for changes to a system that is owned or controlled by others, and that is the primary reason for identifying partners and resources when planning programs. Each intervention presented here could be led by a public health nutrition professional and would require collaboration with other people and organizations: increasing the healthy food choices in vending machines; training home visiting staff to deliver simple, healthy eating messages to clients; encouraging obstetricians to screen for excessive weight gain and refer to a qualified professional for additional weight management counseling; implementing school wellness policies; launching a school garden and school salad bar project; increasing the number of breastfeeding-friendly childcare centers; increasing fruit and vegetable choices in the Child and Adult Care Food Program; and the list goes on.

Collaboration is also required to sustain the effect of successful, evidence-informed public health nutrition programs. Bringing together different organizations with similar goals plus organizations with different goals, but that benefit from the system and health changes and improvements, will significantly increase the long-term effects of one's work.[36]

Every community will have different types of assets that can help to implement and sustain public health interventions or outcomes. Through the process of conducting a community health assessment and the process of developing a program plan, a list of community resources and partners will emerge. A list of potential partners and other resources helpful to implementing and sustaining programs that improve access to healthy, affordable foods and safe places for physical activity in communities is provided here:

- Community members—look for people with time, expertise, and connections. Be open and inclusive of people who are not typically invited to transform their community, but who have knowledge about the community, such as a stay-at-home parent or local librarian or volunteer firefighter. Also, consider individuals with expertise in specific areas related to your goals, such as a master gardener, or with skills in services you need like a social media expert. Everyone in the community has abilities and talents to contribute.

- Formal community leaders—these people are commonly thought of as partners, but they are often very busy: elected persons, government agency heads, local business owners, and board members of local nonprofit organizations.

- Community groups—associations, local foundations, civic groups, faith-based organizations, local government agencies and businesses, economic development corporations, service clubs, etc.

- Community services—public transportation, community sports facilities, early care and education centers and homes, community recycling facilities, cooperative extension, public health agencies, other government agencies, municipal parks and recreation centers, senior activity centers, cultural organizations, community colleges or universities, community centers, etc.

- Food-related groups—food service organizations, food vendors, local food policy council, farmers, farm bureaus, grocers, food pantries and food banks, regional dietetic associations, state or regional checkoff organizations (beef, dairy, almond, mushroom, etc.), SNAP-Ed providers, Child and Adult Care Food Program (CACFP) providers, Women, Infants, and Children (WIC) clinics, etc.

- Health groups—doctors, dentists, physician practices, hospitals, health clinics, nonprofit voluntary health agencies (e.g., American Heart Association, American Cancer Society), home health agencies, etc.

- State and federal experts—food, nutrition, agriculture, and health expert staff in government agencies or state-level organizations.

- Physical structures or places—land and buildings, such as schools, hospitals, churches, libraries, recreation centers, social clubs, unused buildings, empty lots, parks, wetlands, or other open spaces.

- Financial resources—local foundations, Foundation Center; grants.gov; state health department website; state council, society, or association of foundations; The Grantsmanship Center; Rural Health Information Hub.

This list was generated based on information from the Community Tool Box about partnerships and community assets and resources[37,38] and a manual written by faculty at the Asset-Based Community Development Institute.[39]

This planning phase is the opportune time to coordinate and combine resources with partners to build successful public health nutrition programs.

Implementation and Monitoring of Program Effectiveness

Finally, it is time to carry out the planned activities. The program plan will include steps to get started, and when to the point of actually implementing the specific program (e.g., healthy food initiatives in food banks) a practitioner can return to the websites with evidence-informed programs for how-to guidance.

The scope of the program plan and the capacity of the team leading implementation of the plan will dictate how the work will be managed. The approach to plan management may be centralized or decentralized. With a centralized model of managing implementation, there is one person or a small group managing and directing the work. The centralized model of implementation would more likely be used if the program plan has only a few interventions. For example, a few practitioners would manage a program plan with the health goal of improving children's eating habits that has two activities focused on early care and education settings—farm to preschool and breastfeeding-friendly child care centers.

With a decentralized model, there are several people or organizations leading major portions of the plan. The decentralized model of implementation would be used if the program plan was comprehensive and involved the work of many organizations and included several activities. An example would be a countywide health plan focused on healthy eating and active living with interventions in multiple settings (early care and education centers, hospitals, schools, community facilities, small grocers, and local government buildings), where different organizations would be leaders for the activities in a setting or two.

Whether management is centralized or decentralized, monitoring progress using the program plan should be done as often as determined by the lead workers. Basic checks on whether activities are being accomplished according to the timeline is a good place to start.

CONCLUSION

Program planning falls between community health needs assessment and interventions. This, of course, makes sense because practitioners must get organized after learning what the community wants and needs to improve community health and before launching new programs. In public health nutrition practice, much of the information in this chapter will be used and referred to throughout one's career. For practitioners who enjoy getting organized, the challenge will be to not spend too much time planning and get everything perfect before starting programs. For practitioners who race through the steps of getting organized, it will be essential to spend time at each step addressed in this chapter to increase the chance of implementing a successful public health nutrition program.

KEY CONCEPTS

- The seven steps to planning programs are (1) review community assessment results, (2) define health goals and objectives, (3) understand evidence-informed programs, (4) find evidence-informed programs, (5) write a plan, (6) identify partners and other resources, and (7) implement and monitor.

- Compile community health concerns and community assets based on community health assessment results. Do not judge or modify the list based on personal opinion.

- Health goals are written based on community health concerns and provide long-term vision for the program plan. Goals are positive, broad-based, and without time frames.

- Objectives are pathways to achieving the goal. Outcome objectives logically related to a health goal, take at least 3 years to achieve, and address changes in health behaviors or in health status.

- SMART objectives are specific, measurable, achievable, relevant, and time bound. All objectives should meet these SMART criteria.

- Practitioners need to choose programs or interventions with evidence of a positive effect on the health goal and/or outcome objectives.

- Evidence-based public health, evidence-based program, effective program, promising program, emerging program, best practice, and practice-based evidence are all terms that are imprecisely used by many practitioners, but these terms do have specific, precise definitions.

- An evidence-based program follows research protocols in design and implementation. Evidence-informed programs are based on some level of evidence that shows they will have a positive effect on health. Evidence-informed programs include evidence-based programs plus effective, promising, and emerging programs, and best practices.

- Several websites exist with evidence-informed programs and most websites have a database that dynamically generates a list of programs based on criteria selected. The websites differ in many ways including, but not limited to, who the intended user of the website is and what rating system is used.

- The value of using evidence-informed public health programs can be summarized in two words: cost and respect.

- Selecting and implementing programs are a science and an art, and can best be described by the term evidence-informed decision-making (EIDM), which involves using research findings plus public health expertise and resources, and knowledge about community health issues, local context, and political climate to make policy and programming decisions.

- A program plan clearly describes the who, what, when, and where of implementing programs. Generally, a plan includes a health goal, outcome objectives, intervention description(s), process objectives, and details such as strategies, action steps, partners, lead contact, and timeline. Several plan templates exist to use as designed or to modify as needed.

- Plans that address sustainability, evaluation, and communication can accompany the program plan.

- Planning is critical; however, do not become paralyzed by only planning.

- Public health nutritionists always need to partner with others to do their work. Evidence-informed, public health nutrition programs call for changes to a system that is owned or controlled by others. Every community has resources including people, organizations, and physical structures to help implement public health nutrition programs.

- With a centralized model of managing implementation, there is one person or a small group managing and directing the work. The centralized model of implementation would likely be used if the program plan has only a few interventions.

- With a decentralized model, there are several people or organizations leading major portions of the plan. The decentralized model of implementation would be used if the program plan was comprehensive and involved the work of many organizations and included several activities.

CASE STUDY: THE HOWARD COUNTY HOMETOWN HEALTH IMPROVEMENT COALITION: IMPROVING NUTRITION AND INCREASING ACCESS TO HEALTHY FOODS IN HOWARD COUNTY, ARKANSAS

The population of Howard County was approximately 15,000 in 2003. The county seat is Nashville, Arkansas, which had a population of 4,782.[40] The county is designated medically underserved by the Health Resources and Services Administration (HRSA).[40]

The Howard County Hometown Health Improvement (HHI) Coalition began in 2003. The HHI Coalition serves all of Howard County, although most activities were concentrated in Nashville, Arkansas.[40] According to the 2003 BRFSS, 80% of adults in the county reported not eating the recommended amount of vegetables, 42% of adults reported no leisure time physical activity, and 70% to 80% did not get the recommended physical activity. The adult obesity rate was 68%, and 58% of adults reported a diagnosis of hypertension. The active members identified the need for a change in culture and attitudes regarding health. Education and engagement in the larger community was needed. The Coalition wanted to do something like a community garden.

The 2005 Committee goals[40] were to:

- Improve the nutrition of low-income county residents
- Provide healthy foods to needy county residents
- Expand availability of affordable fresh produce and healthy foods
- Partner with existing community programs to access target populations
- Generate community support for program sustainability

Committee Projects[40]

1. **Veggie Swap Shop:** A weekly Veggie Swap Shop was implemented at New Light CME Church. The produce was coupled with existing food pantry items for senior adults. The Veggie Swap Shop Program expanded to include the local Senior Citizen Center and the Senior Outreach Program. Produce not distributed through the church was taken to the Senior Citizen Center for distribution during the week or delivered to homebound senior adults through the Senior Outreach Program. The Veggie Swap idea began from a conversation at a Coalition meeting (2005).

2. **Plant an Extra Row (2006):** A media campaign began in February to encourage gardeners to plant extra produce for donation to the Veggie Swap Shop. Local seed retailers donated seed to support the project.

3. **Program Garden (2006):** The Veggie Swap Committee hosted a Community Coffee to gain support for a Program Garden. The City of Nashville, Arkansas, donated land adjacent to the Senior Citizen Center for the community garden. Community volunteers and 4-H students started the garden, but there was not sufficient infrastructure to coordinate and maintain the garden. The local Master Gardener club took over the garden as a teaching garden. Harvest was donated to Veggie Swap targeting area senior adults. In 2007, there was so much community support for the idea that three locations committed to provide space, supplies, and volunteers for gardens in the county. The three locations were the Senior Citizen Center, Stepping Stones Day Care, and Dierks

Nursing and Rehab Center. Local 4-H groups were utilized as volunteers to plant the gardens. Other local children joined them just for fun. The students in the summer and after-school programs worked in the garden. It was a great educational opportunity for the youth. Senior adults were provided nutrition education sessions by the Cooperative Extension Office with help from the 4-H youth.

4. **Demonstration Organic Garden (2008):** Crops grown in the demonstration garden were donated through the Veggie Swap Committee. Raised beds, an irrigation system, and fencing were built.

Outcomes noted were free, healthy produce for those in need: an outlet for local gardeners to donate produce, and public workshops focusing on organic, low-maintenance gardening.[40]

As the Veggie Swap and Demonstration Garden projects matured, the HHI Coalition began an effort to identify the perceived needs and interest of the community for additional projects. The HHI Coalition members presented at community and civic club meetings. They held focus group and key informant interviews. The Coalition engaged decision-makers such as mayors and city council members. They decided to establish a Farmers' Market with nutrition education.[41] The key stakeholders were behind it. The goals of the program were to provide a means for area residents to acquire fresh locally grown produce and a centralized location for local farmers and gardeners to sell produce. It was also designed as a location for workshops, health fairs, public social activities, and other events.[40]

Partners:[40]

- Red Dirt Master Gardeners
- Howard County Health Improvement
- Howard County
- City of Nashville, Arkansas
- Howard County Health Department
- Senior Outreach Program
- Howard County Cooperative Extension Service and 4H
- Howard County Sheriff's Office
- Area businesses
- Individuals

Funding and resources:

- Grant funds: $29,750 construction costs
- Howard County: land, grading, and dirt work; maintenance of pavilion and parking areas
- City of Nashville, Arkansas: grass mowing
- Chamber of Commerce: administrative costs
- Howard County Health Improvement Coalition/Red Dirt Master Gardeners: raised beds, demonstration garden, and activities held there
- Red Dirt Master Gardeners: on-site management during hours market is open
- Vendor rental fees: operational funds for the Farmers' Market (utilities, advertising, etc.)

Growing Healthy Communities (GHC) Immersion Training is a project of the Arkansas Coalition for Obesity Prevention (ArCOP) to build capacity within communities to reduce obesity by increasing physical activity and access to healthy foods, and implementing environmental and policy changes that support healthy living. Attendance by the community chief executive officer (e.g., mayor, county judge, university president) along with two additional decision-makers and five community implementers (e.g., city planner, members of chamber of commerce, school board, local public health administrator) is required. The training included networking with and presentations by national, state, and local leaders on evidence-informed interventions to address access to healthy foods and physical activity, community assessment, and coalition building/community engagement. Facilitated strategic planning for each community began at the training with instruction for completion back home. An initial community needs assessment was required for GHC application. Following the GHC training, the communities were required to complete a comprehensive assessment, implement strategies, and ensure that the strategies are sustained. Howard County successfully applied for GHC Immersion Training and funding.

Following the ArCOP GHC Immersion Training, the Howard County HHI Coalition's Veggie Swap Committee formalized the GHC Committee to develop and implement Nashville, Arkansas's plan. In April, the Committee submitted their plan to ArCOP, who approved the plan following some minor modifications. Nashville, Arkansas's 2011 "4G" (Get Informed, Get Active, Get Involved, and Get Healthy) Initiative was broad in scope and included a number of strategies/activities to promote physical activity and improve access to healthy nutrition.[42] These strategies/activities were:

1. Develop a website to coordinate Growing Healthy Communities' activities with other community activities and events—"One Place to Go to Find Out What Is Happening!"

2. Develop a series of 12 "NFD TV" programs for local television each composed of three 10-minute modules dealing with healthy nutrition and physical activity. While the programs were developed for local television and were televised during 2012, the modules were also used for community workshops, educational activities, and media promotions.

3. Develop a series of 12-weekly, 30-minute radio talk programs to promote healthy nutrition and physical activity, and to highlight upcoming and on-going events related to healthy lifestyles.

4. Develop a volunteer engagement strategy.

5. Create a partnership with Nashville, Arkansas School District. Quarterly meetings between the Coalition and school nurses were initiated and the Coalition funded the SPARK curriculum for the junior high school.

6. Develop community gardens.

7. Integrate organic farming methods in the local agriculture industry.

8. Complete the certified kitchen at the farmers' market (for cooking demonstrations and nutrition workshops, and for growers to process locally grown produce for sale at market).

9. Increase the number of growers participating at the farmers' market. Ten new growers participated.

10. Offer a series of health screenings, workshops, and cooking demonstrations encouraging healthy nutrition. Five healthy cooking demonstrations were given by the Howard County Extension Agent.

11. Initiate policy that encourages/supports physical activity and healthy nutrition. Initial plans were for each GHC participant to look for policy changes within their organizations to encourage healthy nutrition and physical activity, and implement any desired changes possible. Nashville, Arkansas Parks and Recreation immediately made improvement in selections at park concession stands; Howard County Farmers' Market continued to enforce its policy that unhealthy choices will not be served in market-sponsored events; and Howard County Memorial Hospital added a baked or broiled meat selection to their cafeteria line and expanded salad bar items. Evaluating existing policy and looking for areas of improvement have become a strategy that is planned to continue in the future.

12. Complete a walkability, bikeability, rollability assessment. Three routes were evaluated (City Park to schools, City Park to Downtown, and Downtown to Farmers' Market) over four high-traffic periods.

13. Improve Hispanic participation through the following activities: (1) identify leaders and others in the Hispanic community and get at least one representative on the GHC Committee, (2) translate farmers' market informational brochures, registration forms, and other items into Spanish, and (3) identify potential Hispanic growers and encourage participation at the market.

In 2014, another assessment and strategic planning process was conducted as part of GHC grant funding. This included a Photovoice assessment and presentation.[41] The resulting initiative was called "Eating Fresher in Howard County 2017." The goal of "Eating Fresher in Howard County 2017" is linking community resources to improve nutrition behaviors while increasing consumption of and access to locally grown fresh produce.

The primary strategy is to promote self-efficacy regarding health behaviors, utilizing community health awareness campaigns and traditional focused training. Other strategies were the establishment of individual and community sustainable gardens, amplified grower participation, local farmers' markets, and continued education to increase consumption of fresh produce. The funded activities enhanced and expanded previous efforts in promoting healthy lifestyles through partnerships. The GHC projects included direct education that affects primary and secondary targets, but also leaning heavily on media campaigns to raise awareness for all county residents and the surrounding area.[43]

The 2017 "Eating Fresher in Howard County" project has directly reached more than 2,967 people, including adults and children.[43]

Activity 1—Program Promotion: The "Getting the Word Out" program promotion includes project notices in each local newspaper, two radio stations, email notices, Facebook, and various local websites.[43]

Activity 2—"You Can Do It Gardens" has directly reached a total of 342 individuals through the Square Foot Garden Class, Square Foot Garden Club activities at local community gardens, and the Farm to Table Summit for 6th graders.[43]

Activity 3—"Community & Universally Accessible (UA) Garden" project reached more than 3,300 people at gardening, beekeeping, and drip irrigation workshops and activities.[43]

Activity 4—Physical Activity & Nutrition Programs. In 2017, more than 392 individuals participated in the cooking demonstrations and tastings at Howard County Farmers' Market. The Farm to Table School Summit had 240 participants. Desk cyclers purchased for sixth-grade students. Approximately 61 Extension Homemakers received training on food preservation.[43]

Activity 5—Regional Grower Training in 2016 targeted all 17 counties in southwest Arkansas. In 2017, the GHC Committee organized training with 298 participants.[43]

Activity 6—Healthy Living Libraries includes the "Master Gardener Special Collection" of gardening, recipe, and nutrition books and the existing "Beekeeping Special Collection" located at the public library.[43]

More information is available at the Nashville Arkansas Growing Healthy Communities website at nashvilleghc.com/fullscreen-slider.[44]

In December 2017, the Howard County HHI Coalition conducted a strategic planning day to revise the Committee work plans. The facilitated planning process asked the coalition members to determine what is being done now that needs to be sustained and how to sustain or do the activity better in the coming year. This included determination of all resources needed and available (funding, volunteers, training needs, etc.). Specific Action Steps for each project were developed. These include:

- Specific dates/schedules where possible
- Specific resources needed and how they will be secured
- Assigned volunteers, volunteer recruitment plan (included training needs)

Note: Community gardens, farmers' markets, and fruit and vegetable tasting all have evidence ratings of "Some Evidence" according to "What Works For Health," a Robert Wood Johnson Foundation database of strategies with ratings of effectiveness. Urban agriculture, food hubs, and fruit and vegetable gleaning programs are all rated as "expert opinion." School gardens and fruit and vegetable incentive programs, such as "Double up bucks" for SNAP participants are rated as "scientifically supported." Through the years and iterations of committee and action plans, the Howard County community has used these or adaptations of these strategies among others.[11]

Case Study Questions

1. What were some of the community assessment findings reviewed by the HHI Coalition?

2. Are the health goals related to the health assessment findings? Explain why or why not?

3. Outcome objectives are not included in the case study, but can you write one or two outcome objectives that meet SMART criteria that could be feasible for this case study?

4. Explain whether the initial committee projects were evidence-informed programs? And what about the activities done later?

5. Given the initial list of committee projects and later added activities, what partners and other resources were essential? Were there other community partners and resources that could have been included?

6. With information in the case study, create a program plan using any of the sample plan templates included in this chapter.

7. Would this plan be managed using a centralized or decentralized model? Explain.

8. This community was very successful! What were some of their successes? What might be some of the reasons for their success?

9. What projects and activities seemed interesting to you and why?

SUGGESTED LEARNING ACTIVITIES

1. An essay: Answer the following questions. Consider the Howard County case study and our class discussions about program planning models and methods.

    ▪ What Health Goals were identified in 2003?

    ▪ What are some examples of where the community might have used concepts of evidence-informed decision-making?

    ▪ How did the community increase the likelihood of sustainability?

    ▪ Where might they have obtained ideas for evidence-informed strategies/ programs?

    ▪ What assets/resources did the committee identify for implementation and sustainability?

    ▪ Choose one activity from the 2011 4G initiative and one activity from the 2017 Eat Fresher in Howard County initiative and write one SMART objective for each initiative with the information provided in the case study.

2. Team assignment (continued from Chapter 11, Community Assessments in Public Health Nutrition): Teams will consist of three to four students per team randomly grouped by the instructor. They may be assigned community member roles.

    ▪ Group work during class:

      ○ Review the community assessment

      ○ Determine one health goal

      ○ Determine a model for use in developing your community action plan

      ○ Exchange phone numbers, discuss possible group meeting times

      ○ Review and make sure you all understand the overall assignment

      ○ Divide up workload, assign responsibilities

    ▪ Written plan:

      ○ Plan should be double-spaced, typed, and without grammatical errors. All components listed below must be included and written in correct format. The following components must be included:

      ○ Title of program

      ○ Names of team members

      ○ Mini "community action plan"

        – Complete each step in a planning model resulting in a mini community action plan addressing the health goal

        – Brief assessment report from the Chapter 11, Community Assessments in Public Health Nutrition, community assessment assignment

        – Health and/or nutrition status of the target population

        – Available resources (assets)

        – Two to three SMART objectives

        – Evidence-informed strategies

      – Method of monitoring (how will you measure success)

      – Sustainability plan

3. Oral presentation:

- Presentation: 5–10 minutes
- It is the team's choice as to whether or not all group members will be present; however, all team members must come to the front of the classroom.
- Audiovisual aids are recommended but not required.
- The presentation should involve a broad overview of your goals and implementation plan.
- Any necessary audiovisual equipment should be prearranged with the instructor.

REFLECTION QUESTIONS

- What is evidence-informed decision-making?
- What is the difference between evidence-based, effective, promising, emerging, and best practice programs?
- What are four components of the Evidence-Based Practice Model?
- What are the seven steps to program planning?
- Why is it important to review community assessment results as the first step to developing a program plan?
- What is the difference between goals and objectives?
- What are SMART objectives?
- What is the difference between evidence-based and practice-based evidence?
- What is the difference between evidence-based public health and evidence-based programs?
- What are the levels of evidence of public health programs?
- How can a practitioner find evidence-informed programs? List four sources.
- Why is selecting and implementing programs described as a science and an art?
- In general, what are the components included in a program plan?
- What are the other three plans that might accompany a program plan or be incorporated into the program plan?
- What are some types of community resources and who are some potential partners?
- What is the difference between a centralized and decentralized model of managing implementation of the plan?

CONTINUE YOUR LEARNING RESOURCES

Assessment Planning Models

The CDC has several assessment planning models that can be found at https://www.cdc.gov/stlt publichealth/cha/index.html and https://www.cdc.gov/stltpublichealth/cha/assessment.html#four. Organization(s): Centers for Disease Prevention and Control

Global Childhood Obesity Recommendations

The National Collaborative on Childhood Obesity Research (NCCOR) has resources and recommendations for research and for communities to help reduce childhood obesity around the word at https://www.nccor.org/projects/globallessons. You can also learn more about evidence and key concepts for Health, Behavioral Design, and the Built Environment at https://www.nccor.org/projects/health-built-environment.

Organization(s): National Collaborative on Childhood Obesity Research (NCCOR)

The Community Guide

The Community Guide is a repository of evidence-based and promising policies, programs, or strategies on a wide range of topics related to health and disease prevention in communities, including asthma, physical activity, and tobacco.

Organization(s): Centers for Disease Control and Prevention

Evidence-Based Practice

Website

Resources on child well-being and use of rigorously evaluated programs that target the needs of children and helping them have healthy development: https://www.aecf.org/work/evidence-based-practice and https://www.aecf.org/work/evidence-based-practice/evidence2success.

Organization(s): Annie E. Casey Foundation

Promising Practices from the WICHE Project Archive

Video/Multimedia

The webinar is a technical assistance guide for communities running promising practices in rural America to understand what qualifies their work as a "promising practice." The guide also provides information about the strategies, methodologies, and resources necessary to become evidenced-based practices: https://www.wiche.edu/archive/mh/promisingPractices.

Organization(s): Western Interstate Commission for Higher Education

Date: 10/2010

Evidence-Based Public Health

Tutorial/Training

This online book is a tutorial in evidence-based public health. It introduces readers to the main themes associated with the topic and provides useful resources for further learning. In particular, it describes analytical strategies and literature review methods that can help practitioners integrate the concepts in their own work: https://www.ruralhealthinfo.org/toolkits/rural-toolkit/2/evidence-base.

Organization(s): Rural Health Information Hub[45]

Mobilizing Action through Planning and Partnerships (MAPP)

Webinars/Handbook

To learn more about using MAPP you can access a free MAPP Handbook and webinars.

Free MAPP Handbook: http://eweb.naccho.org/eweb/DynamicPage.aspx?WebCode=proddetail
add&ivd_qty=1&ivd_prc_prd_key=8cb05f83-904e-471b-b588-8c51e9628c8b&Action=Add
&site=naccho&ObjectKeyFrom=1A83491A-9853-4C87-86A4-F7D95601C2E2&DoNotSave
=yes&ParentObject=CentralizedOrderEntry&ParentDataObject=Invoice%20Detail.
MAPP webinars and resources: https://www.naccho.org/programs/public-health-infrastructure/
performance-improvement/community-health-assessment/mapp.
Organization(s): National Association of County and City Health Officials (NACCHO)

GLOSSARY

Community environment: Programs, services, and resources available in a community and
their quality attributes, plus community influencers, and social networks.

Epidemiologist: A scientist who studies the incidence, prevalence, spread, and distribution
patterns of disease conditions and risk factors in populations.

Farm to Preschool: Encompasses efforts to serve local or regionally produced foods in early
childcare and education settings; provides hands-on learning activities, such as gardening,
farm visits, and culinary activities; and integrates food-related education into the curriculum
(from a USDA factsheet).

Opinion and perception information: Perceived needs, priorities, norms, and values of the
priority population and other constituencies and stakeholders.

Population data: Sociodemographic descriptors and indicators of the health and nutritional
status of the selected population.

Public policy environment: Relevant public policy issues and their status, including related
legislation, regulation, ordinances, etc. at local, state, and national levels as well as national
standards and guidelines from government agencies.

Safe Routes to Schools: "[A]n approach that promotes walking and bicycling to school through
infrastructure improvements, enforcement, tools, safety education, and incentives to encourage walking and bicycling to school.[46]

REFERENCES

1. Association for Community Health Improvement. *Community Health Assessment Toolkit: Step 6: Document and Communicate Results.* 2017. https://www.healthycommunities.org/resources/toolkit/files/step6-document-community-results
2. Probert K. *Moving to the Future: Nutrition and Physical Activity Program Planning, Chapter 1: Community Assessment, Summarize and Report Information.* Tucson, AZ: Association of State Public Health Nutritionists; 2006. https://movingtothefuture.org/chapter-1-community-assessment/summarizing-and-reporting-information
3. Association for Community Health Improvement. *Community Health Assessment Toolkit: Step 7: Plan Implementation Strategies.* 2017. https://www.healthycommunities.org/resources/toolkit/files/step7-plan-implementation
4. University of Kansas, Center for Community Health and Development. *Community Tool Box: Chapter 8, Section 5: Developing an Action Plan.* 2019. https://ctb.ku.edu/en/table-of-contents/structure/strategic-planning/develop-action-plans/main
5. University of Kansas, Center for Community Health and Development. *Community Tool Box: Chapter 3, Section 23: Developing and Using Criteria and Processes to Set Priorities.* 2019. https://ctb.ku.edu/en/table-of-contents/assessment/assessing-community-needs-and-resources/criteria-and-processes-to-set-priorities/main

6. National Association of County and City Health Officials. *Mobilizing for Action Through Planning and Partnerships (MAPP): Phase 4: Identifying and Prioritizing Strategic Issues.* 2019. https://www.naccho.org/programs/public-health-infrastructure/performance-improvement/community-health-assessment/mapp/phase-4-identify-strategic-issues

7. Probert K. *Moving to the Future: Nutrition and Physical Activity Program Planning, Chapter 2: Identify Priorities, Goals and Objectives, Writing Goals—Overview.* Tucson, AZ: Association of State Public Health Nutritionists; 2006. https://movingtothefuture.org/chapter-2-determine-goals/writing-goals-overview

8. Centers for Disease Control and Prevention, National Center for Chronic Disease Prevention and Health Promotion, Division for Heart Disease and Stroke Prevention, State Heart Disease and Stroke Prevention Program. *Evaluation Guide Writing SMART Objectives.* 2017:3–4. https://www.cdc.gov/dhdsp/evaluation_resources/guides/writing-smart-objectives.htm

9. U.S. Department of Health and Human Services, Office of Disease Prevention and Health Promotion. *Healthy People 2020.* 2019. https://www.healthypeople.gov/2020/About-Healthy-People/Development-Healthy-People-2030/Framework

10. Community Preventive Services Task Force. *Guide to Community Preventive Services. Obesity: Worksite Programs.* 2019. https://www.thecommunityguide.org/findings/obesity-worksite-programs

11. Robert Wood Johnson Foundation. *County Health Rankings and Roadmaps What Works for Health: Increase Access to Healthy Food Options.* 2019. https://www.countyhealthrankings.org/take-action-to-improve-health/what-works-for-health/policies?f%5B0%5D=field_program_health_factors%3A12058&f%5B1%5D=field_program_topics%3A24736

12. Satterfield JM, Spring B, Brownson RC, et al. Toward a transdisciplinary model of evidence-based practice. *Milbank Q.* 2009;87(2):368–390. doi:10.1111/j.1468-0009.2009.00561

13. U.S. Department of Health & Human Services. *Evidence-Based Clinical and Public Health: Generating and Applying the Evidence.* Secretary's advisory committee on national health promotion and disease prevention objectives for 2020; 2010. https://www.healthypeople.gov/sites/default/files/EvidenceBasedClinicalPH2010.pdf

14. Brownson RC, Fielding JE, Maylahn CM. Evidence-based public health: a fundamental concept for public health practice. *Annu Rev Public Health.* 2009;30:175–201. doi:10.1146/annurev.publhealth.031308.100134

15. Rural Health Information Hub. *Rural Health Information Hub Evidence-Based Toolkits for Rural Community Health.* 2018. https://www.ruralhealthinfo.org/toolkits

16. Vanagas G, Bala M, Lhachimi K. Evidence-based public health 2017. *Biomed Res Int.* 2017;2017:2607397. doi:10.1155/2017/2607397

17. Lhachimi SK, Bala MM, Vanagas G. Evidence-based public health. *Biomed Res Int.* 2016;2016:5681409. doi:10.1155/2016/5681409

18. Ammerman A, Smith TW, Larissa C. Practice-based evidence in public health: improving reach, relevance, and results. *Annu Rev Public Health.* 2014;35(1):47–63. doi:10.1146/annurev-publhealth-032013-182458

19. Ng E, de Colombani P. Framework for selecting best practices in public health: a systematic literature review. *J Public Health Res.* 2015;4(3):577. doi:10.4081/jphr.2015.577

20. Yost J, Dobbins M, Traynor R, et al. Tools to support evidence-informed public health decision making. *BMC Public Health.* 2014;14:728. doi:10.1186/1471-2458-14-728

21. Community Preventative Services Task Force. *Guide to Community Preventive Services.* 2019. https://www.thecommunityguide.org

22. U.S. Department of Agriculture. *SNAP-ed Toolkit.* 2018. https://wicworks.fns.usda.gov

23. OnStrategy. *OnStrategy.* 2019. https://onstrategyhq.com

24. Probert K. *Moving to the Future: Nutrition and Physical Activity Program Planning, Chapter 3: Develop a Plan—Chapter Overview.* Tucson, AZ: Association of State Public Health Nutritionists; 2006. https://movingtothefuture.org/chapter-3-develop-a-plan/develop-a-plan-chapter-overview

25. National Association of County and City Health Officials. *Mobilizing for Action Through Planning and Partnerships (MAPP).* https://www.naccho.org/programs/public-health-infrastructure/performance-improvement/community-health-assessment/mapp/phase-1-organize-for-success-partnership-development

26. Centers for Disease Control and Prevention. *Community Health Assessment and Group Evaluation (CHANGE) Tool Action Steps.* 2019. https://www.cdc.gov/nccdphp/dnpao/state-local-programs/change-tool/action-steps.html

27. Centers for Disease Control and Prevention, Division of Nutrition, Physical Activity and Obesity. *Community Health Assessment and Group Evaluation (CHANGE) Tool: Action Step 7d: Complete the Community Health Improvement Planning Template.* 2019. https://www.cdc.gov/nccdphp/dnpao/state -local-programs/change-tool/actionstep7.html

28. Centers for Disease Control and Prevention, Division of Nutrition, Physical Activity and Obesity. *Community Health Assessment and Group Evaluation (CHANGE) Tool: Action Step 8.* 2019. https://www .cdc.gov/nccdphp/dnpao/state-local-programs/change-tool/actionstep8.html

29. University of Kansas, Center for Community Health and Development. *Community Tool Box: Chapter 3 Developing a Plan for Assessing Local Needs and Resources.* 2018. https://ctb.ku.edu/en/table-of-contents/ assessment/assessing-community-needs-and-resources/develop-a-plan/main

30. Hansen S, Kanning M, Lauer R, et al. MAP-IT: A practical tool for planning complex behavior modification interventions. *Health Promot Pract.* 2017;18(5):696–705. doi:10.1177/1524839917710454

31. Aldridge WA, Boothroyd RI, Fleming WO, et al. Transforming community prevention systems for sustained impact: embedding active implementation and scaling functions. *Transl Behav Med.* 2016;6(1):135–144. doi:10.1007/s13142-015-0351-y

32. Rural Health Information Hub, University of North Dakota. *Rural Community Health Toolkit, Module 5: Planning for Sustainability.* 2019. https://www.ruralhealthinfo.org/toolkits/rural-toolkit/5/sustainability -planning

33. University of Kansas, Center for Community Health and Development. *Community Tool Box: Chapter 46, Section 1: Strategies for the Long-Term Sustainability of an Initiative: An Overview.* 2019. https://ctb .ku.edu/en/table-of-contents/sustain/long-term-sustainability/overview/main

34. Centers for Disease Control and Prevention, National Center for Chronic Disease Prevention and Health Promotion, Office on Smoking and Health, & Division of Nutrition, Physical Activity and Obesity. *Developing an Effective Evaluation Plan: Setting the Course for Effective Program Evaluation.* Atlanta, GA: Centers for Disease Control and Prevention; 2011:1.

35. University of Kansas, Center for Community Health and Development. *Community Tool Box: Chapter 6, Section 1: Developing a Plan for Communication.* 2019. https://ctb.ku.edu/en/table-of-contents/ participation/promoting-interest

36. NORC at the University of Chicago. *Developing a Conceptual Framework to Assess the Sustainability of Community Coalitions Post-Federal Funding.* (Literature Review). Washington DC: U.S. Department of Health and Human Services, Assistant Secretary for Planning and Evaluation; 2011. https://aspe.hhs .gov/system/files/pdf/76066/report.pdf

37. University of Kansas, Center for Community Health and Development. *Community Tool Box: Chapter 3, Section 8: Identifying Community Assets and Resources.* 2019. https://ctb.ku.edu/en/table-of-contents/ assessment/assessing-community-needs-and-resources/identify-community-assets/main

38. University of Kansas, Center for Community Health and Development. *Community Tool Box: Toolkit 1: Creating and Maintaining Partnerships.* 2019. https://ctb.ku.edu/en/creating-and-maintaining-partnerships

39. Kretzmann JP, McKnight JL. *Building Communities from the Inside Out: A Path Toward Finding and Mobilizing a Community's Assets.* Evanston, IL: Institute for Policy Research; 1993:1–11.

40. Bolding D. *Growing healthy communities, Howard county [PowerPoint slides] 2010.* Unpublished manuscript; 2010.

41. Powell S, Adams B. Personal communication. September 2018.

42. Bolding D. *City of Nashville Arkansas Growing Healthy Communities Final Report December, 2011.* Unpublished manuscript; 2011.

43. Howard County Health Improvement Coalition. *Eating Fresher in Howard County, Community First Wellness Grant Report January 1, 2017–December 31, 2017.* Unpublished manuscript; 2018.

44. Nashville Growing Healthy Communities Committee. *Nashville Growing Healthy Communities.* 2019. http://nashvilleghc.com/about

45. Rural Health Information Hub. *Review of the Evidence Base.* 2018. https://www.ruralhealthinfo.org/ toolkits/rural-toolkit/2/evidence-base

46. U.S. Department of Transportation. *Safe routes to school programs.* https://www.transportation.gov/ mission/health/Safe-Routes-to-School-Programs. Updated August 24, 2015.

PUBLIC HEALTH NUTRITION INTERVENTIONS AND EVALUATION

JESSICA SOLDAVINI, CAITLIN HILDEBRAND, AND ALICE AMMERMAN

LEARNING OBJECTIVES

1. Understand the critical role of evaluation in both the design and assessing the impact of interventions.

2. Recognize the importance of planning evaluation strategies early in the process of intervention design that fit the appropriate stage: formative, process, outcome, and impact.

3. Be aware of the potential for logic models to identify appropriate inputs and outcomes and to evaluate process and impact.

4. Understand the wide variety of current and emerging evaluation strategies for interventions as diverse as policy and social media.

5. Appreciate the importance of interprofessional approaches to intervention implementation and evaluation.

INTRODUCTION

Program evaluation is a critical component of public health nutrition **interventions**. Without program evaluation, it is difficult to know whether interventions are having the intended effects. Program evaluation can also be used to help improve public health nutrition interventions. This chapter describes strategies for evaluating public health nutrition interventions. A variety of types of evaluation (formative, process, outcome, and impact) and methods for collecting both qualitative and quantitative data are discussed. Evaluation frameworks are useful when evaluating public health nutrition interventions. This chapter provides an overview of two evaluation frameworks commonly used in public health nutrition: the Centers for Disease Control and Prevention (CDC) Framework for Program Evaluation and the **RE-AIM framework**. Program evaluation is important for all types of public health nutrition interventions, and this chapter describes methods that can be used for a variety of approaches.

IMPLEMENTATION AND EVALUATION OF FOOD AND NUTRITION INTERVENTIONS

This chapter complements earlier chapters regarding program and policy interventions by describing strategies for program evaluation. In this chapter, we define **intervention** as any activity taken to improve public health nutrition. Evaluation can help determine whether nutrition interventions and programs are effective and to identify areas in need of improvement.[1]

There is increasing focus on the science of implementation and dissemination as mechanisms to ensure that interventions are effective and efficient and that those programs and interventions achieving these goals are scaled up to benefit the greatest number of people. Implementation research is a form of evaluating the degree to which an intervention fits within the context and can be very helpful in informing program or policy redesign to achieve greater impact. An example would be a public health department offering nutrition education for low-income individuals with diabetes. To be effective, such a program would need to be accessible to and affordable for the target population, be culturally relevant, create an effective referral process, and ideally be part of reimbursable clinical service delivery.

The Difference Between Evaluation and Research

Before further discussing the specifics of evaluation methods, it is important to consider the differences and similarities between evaluation and research in public health nutrition. It can sometimes be difficult to distinguish whether something should be considered research or evaluation, and it is possible for a project to include both. One of the major differences between research and evaluation is the primary goal. In general, research aims to gain new information and produce generalizable knowledge through answering a question in a controlled environment while evaluation seeks to assess the effectiveness of an intervention in a real-world setting. Research and evaluation projects often use similar methods and strategies. Some community organizations and funders are more comfortable with the term "evaluation" as it implies, perhaps, a more practical and applied effort. At the same time, community partners should be reassured that evaluation is designed to improve programs and not to judge their implementers.

Types of Evaluation

There are a variety of different types of evaluations. Common types of evaluations used in public health nutrition program evaluation are described in the following.

Formative evaluation typically occurs during the development of a new intervention, modification of an existing intervention, or adaptation of an intervention to a new setting or population. Needs assessments, which were discussed in Chapter 11, Community Assessments in Public Health Nutrition, are an example of formative evaluation. Formative evaluation helps to ensure that the intervention is appropriate and feasible before it is fully implemented. It is important to conduct a formative evaluation prior to implementing an intervention so that you can develop and implement an intervention that is likely to be successful and meet the needs of the population served.

Process evaluation determines if an intervention was implemented as intended. It can help you understand why and for whom an intervention did or did not have the intended outcomes. Key process evaluation components include reach, dose delivered, dose received, **fidelity**, implementation, recruitment, and context.[2] Reach is typically measured as the proportion of the target audience participating in an intervention or intervention component. An attendance sheet from a nutrition class is an example of a commonly used way to measure reach. Dose delivered refers to how much of an intended intervention is actually delivered. An example is the number of lessons from a curriculum that were actually taught. Dose received refers to the extent to which participants receive and engage with intervention materials or components. Examples of ways to assess this include questionnaires or interviews with intervention participants. Fidelity refers to whether the intervention was implemented as planned. Common ways of assessing fidelity include fidelity checklists and observations. Implementation aims to understand the extent that the intervention was implemented and received by the target audience and is a composite score of reach, dose delivered, dose received, and fidelity. Assessing recruitment involves documenting the approaches used to recruit participants into the intervention. This component of process evaluation can be helpful for understanding things such as whether and why certain types of individuals or organizations were more or less likely to participate. Context focuses on assessing aspects of the larger environment (social, political, and environmental) that may influence the intervention.

Outcome and impact evaluations help to understand whether an intervention was effective at creating change. **Outcome evaluation** measures the effects of the intervention on achieving a program's outcome objectives. **Impact evaluation** assesses how effective the intervention is in achieving its ultimate goals.

Logic Models

Logic models are a useful tool for program planning and evaluation. They can be helpful for depicting what your intervention will do and the expected results. They illustrate the sequential relationships between your intervention activities and intended effects.[1] There are several variations of logic models; however, common elements include the following:

- **Inputs** are the resources invested into the program. Examples of inputs include funding, staff time, materials, and partners.

- **Activities** are what the intervention does with the inputs. Examples of activities include developing resources, conducting workshops, providing training, and establishing partnerships.

- **Outputs** are the direct results of the activities that are intended to lead to the intervention's outcomes. Examples of outputs include resources developed, number of workshops held, number of participants trained, and number of partnerships established.

- **Outcomes** are the changes that your intervention expects to achieve. Outcomes may correspond to one or more levels of the Social-Ecological Model. Outcomes are often divided into short-term, medium-term, and long-term outcomes. Short-term outcomes are the more immediate outcomes of an intervention, such as changes in knowledge, skills, or attitudes. Examples of medium-term outcomes include behavioral changes and policy, systems, and environmental (PSE) changes. Long-term outcomes are the more distal outcomes of an intervention, an example being changes in health conditions or status.[1]

Logic models can help you determine what indicators to measure in your evaluation. The different sections of a logic model correspond to the different types of evaluation. Information gathered during formative evaluation can be used to refine the activities indicated in the program logic model. Process evaluation focuses on tracking the outputs of the program logic model. Outcome evaluation focuses on assessing the short- and intermediate-term outcomes section of the program logic model. Impact evaluation assesses the long-term outcomes of the logic model.

Evaluating Multiple Levels of the Social-Ecological Model

Intervention implementation can happen at many different levels of the Social-Ecological Model. Traditionally, the focus of nutrition education programing has been targeted at the individual or group level. Increasingly, however, interventions are aimed at PSE change, moving upstream to create environments that make the "healthy choice the easy choice." This could include community-level organizational change in schools or worksites or move further upstream to changes in the built environment (urban gardens, increased availability of healthy foods in parks and recreation areas) or policy (Supplemental Nutrition Assistance Program [SNAP], Special Supplemental Nutrition Program for Women, Infants, and Children [WIC], and Child Nutrition Programs).

Evaluation strategies vary by level of the Social-Ecological model. Most people are familiar with **individual-level strategies**. Generally, data are collected before and after an intervention to determine if there has been a change. Ideally, this would involve a control or comparison group so that any conclusion about impact could rule out the potential for change due to chance or to "secular trend." For example, if an evaluation study is addressing an intervention to increase the intake of folic acid and the Food and Drug Administration (FDA) announces the need to include folic acid levels on nutrition labels, this could influence dietary change above and beyond any impact of the intervention. Individual-level measures could be clinically focused (body mass index [BMI], blood pressure, hemoglobin A1c, etc.) or address diet-related behaviors. Other individual-level evaluation involves assessment of knowledge, attitudes, and beliefs. The constructs from the behavior theories your intervention is based on can help to select what to measure in your evaluation. This can involve both qualitative and quantitative assessment using structured/semistructured interviews, focus groups, or surveys. Qualitative measures are more commonly used for formative assessment prior to intervention implementation or after it is complete, in order to better understand how to design and conduct an intervention, based on the population served. To quantify intervention impact, surveys and structured observation are more appropriate, recognizing that any sort of self-report measure involves subjectivity. Care must be taken to ensure respondents that there are no "right answers" and their responses are most helpful to improving nutrition for all if candid and accurate.

At other levels of the Social-Ecological Model, evaluation can involve a wide variety of measurement strategies, from tracking changes in monitoring data to media coverage and policy processes. A helpful tool to identify both variables and measurement instruments is the SNAP-Ed Evaluation Framework.[3] This framework divides the Social-Ecological Model into individual, environmental settings, and sectors of influence, which parallel the Social-Ecological model, and is organized in a logic model format. The interactive framework offers specific variables to be measured and, in many cases, validated measurement instruments. With the increasing interest in "food systems" change as an approach to public health nutrition, this framework can be a helpful guide in evaluating, for example, the impact of community gardens from the individual level (taste preferences for vegetables, knowledge about cooking, etc.) to sectors of influence (food policy council formation and impact, zoning policies regarding community gardens, "brown field" regulations, and funding to address contaminated soil for urban gardens, etc.). In the case of policy, short-term outcomes might include forming a coalition, medium-term outcomes could be achieving the legislative action of passing a bill or regulation, and long-term outcomes would include whether the bill was implemented as planned and its impact on the original concern. An example would be forming a coalition around creating a walking trail to increase physical activity, influencing the city council to designate land for the trail, documenting if the trail is built as specified, and assessing whether it results in increased physical activity of individuals in the community.

Data Collection Methods

As previously discussed, both quantitative and qualitative data collection methods can be used. It is common to use a mixed methods approach that collects both quantitative and qualitative data.

Triangulation of data refers to using multiple data sources to evaluate an outcome,[4] which helps to verify the results of the different methods and provide more credibility to the results.

Questionnaires are commonly used to assess outcomes and can assess quantitative and/or qualitative outcomes as they may contain closed and/or open-ended questions. They can be used to collect data on a variety of topics including outcomes such as dietary intake, physical activity, and feedback on an intervention. New questionnaires do not need to be developed for every intervention. It can be helpful to select tools that have been shown to be valid and reliable in similar populations. A pretest–posttest design is often used where questionnaires are administered before and after an intervention in order to assess change. Some interventions only administer questionnaires at the end of an intervention. A useful tool for evaluating change over time when you are only administering a questionnaire at the end of an intervention is a retrospective pre–post survey, which collects information on outcomes before and after an intervention at the same time. This method can be useful when it is not feasible to administer both pre- and postsurveys, such as when giving a one-session nutrition lesson. Questionnaires may be administered through a variety of modes including pencil and paper (in person or by mail), telephone, or online.

Focus groups and structured interviews are commonly used methods to collect qualitative data. Similar information can be collected through these methods, and the choice of which to use depends on a variety of factors. Focus groups allow you to collect information from more individuals at one time; however, if individuals are not all able to participate in the same place at the same time, interviews may be a better option. Focus groups are helpful when interactions among the participants can be helpful. If you are discussing a sensitive topic that participants may not be comfortable discussing with others, have respondents with different characteristics, or have a large amount of materials for participants to review, interviews may be a more appropriate option for data collection.

Photovoice is a type of participatory action research in which participants use photographs to capture and reflect on different issues.[5,6] Participants help to identify themes for the project to focus on and take pictures related to those themes using a prompt selected by the group, like "What helps me be healthy and what gets in the way?" They then gather for group discussions to reflect on those images and the issues they represent. Discussions are often guided by the **SHOWeD method**, which guides participants through a series of questions to help them reflect on the photos.[6] The questions include:

- What do you **S**ee here?
- What is really **H**appening here?
- How does this relate to **O**ur lives?
- **W**hy does this situation, concern, or strength exist?
- What can we **D**o about it?

One of the potential goals of photovoice is to reach policy-makers or others who can influence change.[5,6] Photos and stories resulting from the project can be shared with community leaders and policy-makers through a variety of ways, including community forums or presentations, exhibits, and community locations, such as libraries, schools, parks and recreation facilities, or town halls. They can also be shared online through websites or social media as well as through traditional media coverage or publications.

Not all data used in program evaluation need to be new data collected specifically for this purpose. For example, administrative data can be used, such as data collected by school meals programs on the number of meals served to assess the effect of an intervention on increasing participation in school meals programs. Depending on the target population of your intervention, you may be able to use national, state, or local data from surveillance systems to help assess change in outcomes such as dietary behaviors or physical activity over time. This is useful when your intervention is focused on community-level change. The Behavioral Risk Factor Surveillance System is an example of a survey developed and administered by the CDC that collects data across the United States and is able to provide state-level estimates as well as local-level estimates in some cases.[7]

A variety of observational methods can be used to collect quantitative or qualitative data. Examples of observational methods in process evaluation include observers completing fidelity checklists while observing intervention activities to determine whether the planned components occurred. Observers can also assess participant engagement. Additionally, observational methods can be used as part of outcome and impact evaluation. Many public health nutrition interventions are interested in assessing changes in dietary behaviors. While many evaluations rely on self-reported information, observational methods also exist. Observational methods of collecting dietary intake are often used with interventions in school or childcare settings to assess changes in what children eat in meals served in these settings. Young children often have difficulty accurately recalling what they ate, limiting the value of self-reported methods for this population. Observational methods for collecting dietary data typically involve observing meal trays and/or children eating and subtracting how much food was left at the end from how much they were served.[8,9] Observers may also watch the children while they eat to determine if they dropped, spilled, traded, or were provided with extra portions. As an alternative to estimating the amount consumed through observation, the food items served can be weighed before and after a meal (plate waste monitoring) to determine how much was wasted and how much was eaten.[10,11] Limitations of these methods include being time-consuming and only being able to observe specific meals where it is possible to make observations as opposed to overall dietary intake. Observational methods are also used in PSE change interventions and can be used to determine if changes are being implemented. An intervention to increase the amount of fruits and vegetables sold in corner stores may have observers report information such as the type, amount, price, and quality of fruits and vegetables sold in the store, for example. Sometimes this is referred to as "disappearance data" when the amount of food remaining on the shelf is subtracted from what is originally stocked.

EVALUATION METHODS AND BEST PRACTICES

Given that evaluation can serve various purposes, the process can take many forms. Approaching evaluation through a systematic and methodical approach allows for both comprehensive learning and focused efforts, depending on the needs of the evaluation participants and audience.[1]

Guiding Frameworks for Evaluation

The product of an evaluation has the potential for considerable utility for programs and stakeholders. In addition, conducting an evaluation requires valuable time and resources. Thus, approaching an evaluation through the lens of a comprehensive framework allows for greater efficiency while securing useful results. Several frameworks have been developed as a guide for public health practitioners. This section provides an overview of the general approach to program evaluation using the CDC Framework for Program Evaluation in Public Health[1] and RE-AIM framework.[12]

The CDC Framework for Program Evaluation in Public Health

The CDC Framework for Program Evaluation in Public Health outlines steps and standards to guide the performance of an evaluation.[1] It is designed as a practical tool that can be used not only for looking at program outcomes but also for incorporating evaluative processes into everyday organizational practices. The framework considers contextual factors of a program to allow for more tailored and thus impactful evaluation strategies from the start. The framework's design allows for its use in a variety of applications and settings, from specific program operations and public health research to policy-level changes. Remember that planning your evaluation should be a focus of activity from the very beginning of program or policy implementation. The steps outlined in the CDC evaluation framework[1] are as follows:

STEP 1: ENGAGE STAKEHOLDERS

Stakeholders, which are individuals and organizations with an interest in what will be learned from the evaluation, are important to engage from the beginning in order to ensure the evaluation meets their needs. Stakeholders may include the individuals who are involved with implementing the intervention, served by the intervention, or identified as primary users of the evaluation.

STEP 2: DESCRIBE THE PROGRAM

The program description is a critical step in the evaluation process as it provides a framework to guide decision-making in future steps of the evaluation process. Items to include in the program description are need, expected effects, activities, resources, stage of development, and context. A logic model can help illustrate the interrelationship of these components.

STEP 3: FOCUS THE EVALUATION DESIGN

It is important to focus the evaluation design to ensure that the issues that are most important to the stakeholders are being addressed and that time and resources are being used efficiently. To focus the evaluation design, start by determining the purpose of the evaluation, which may include gaining insight, changing practices, assessing effects, or impacting participants. The users of your evaluation findings and how they will use them should be defined. These components will then help you to select your evaluation questions and the methods you will use to gather the information needed. Agreements may be developed related to the evaluation plan that addresses areas such as how it will be implemented, who will implement it, and how ethical standards will be maintained.

STEP 4: GATHER CREDIBLE EVIDENCE

Information gathered during the evaluation needs to be credible. It is helpful to use the logic model to select which indicators to measure. The sources of data you use and the quality and quantity of data influence how credible your findings will be. Logistics are important to keep in mind when gathering evidence, as the most appropriate techniques can vary based on factors such as timing, physical infrastructure, and techniques used. It is also important to take the cultural norms of individuals and organizations into consideration when determining methods of gathering data.

STEP 5: JUSTIFY CONCLUSIONS

Justifying conclusions is an important step because it promotes increased stakeholder trust in the outcomes of the evaluation, thus enhancing the potential utility of the evaluation results for stakeholders. Stakeholder values guide the standards for justifying conclusions from an evaluation and provide a measure for judging program efficacy. Analysis and synthesis of evidence have the potential to reveal patterns from evaluation results that may be helpful for drawing conclusions. Results gained through evaluation require further interpretation to gain meaningful conclusions, ideally through incorporating stakeholder input. Within an evaluation, judgments reflect the merit or significance of the program and require assessing how results compare to specifically chosen standards, such as program objectives or participant needs. Finally, the resulting recommendations from an evaluation should consider not only the evidence gathered and resulting conclusions but also stakeholder input and context. Presenting recommendations with multiple options to consider may prove more useful for stakeholders.

STEP 6: ENSURE USE AND SHARE LESSONS LEARNED

The final component of the CDC Evaluation Framework entails strategies to improve implementation and dissemination of evaluation results. Factors such as the design of the evaluation, preparation of stakeholders for using the findings, and obtainment of continuous feedback are important. Engaging in follow-up after the conclusion of an evaluation is a way to provide programs with support and promote appropriate application of findings. Finally, evaluators should work with stakeholders to consider how best to disseminate the results of the evaluation as well as "lessons learned."

The RE-AIM Framework

The growing field of implementation science examines how to best put knowledge from evidence-based studies into practice.[13] Several factors may impact implementation of evidence-based studies.[13] For example, barriers to implementation may include cost or lack of population representativeness.[13,14] Potential strategies to improve implementation of evidence-based studies include greater attention given to external validity and increased involvement of stakeholders;[2] taking these measures may help make the intervention more relevant for users.[13]

The RE-AIM framework is an example of a framework used in dissemination and implementation science and is an attempt to shift the focus of evaluation away from simply the effect or outcome and capture other important elements of program and policy impact. For example, if the target population is not *reached* (commonly interventions end up "preaching to the choir" rather than reaching those in greatest need), even a very effective intervention will not have the impact desired. Similarly, if the intervention effect only occurs during the brief period of evaluation and is not *maintained* over time, it offers little value in the long run. RE-AIM consists of five dimensions to consider in evaluation: reach, efficacy, adoption, implementation, and maintenance.[12] These five dimensions are also considered the "five steps to translate research into action" and are defined as follows:[15]

1. Reach refers to the absolute number or proportion of the target audience and the representativeness of participants in an intervention compared with the target audience.

2. Effectiveness/efficacy considers the outcomes of an intervention and should take into account both positive and negative effects.

3. Adoption refers to the absolute number of settings or staff who are willing to implement a program as well as the proportion and representativeness.

4. Implementation looks at whether an intervention was carried out as planned and resources expended to deliver the intervention.

5. Maintenance occurs at both the individual and organizational levels. Maintenance at the individual level refers to the long-term outcomes 6 months or longer after an intervention. Maintenance at the organizational level looks at the degree of uptake of a policy or program.

HEALTHY FOOD ENVIRONMENTS (HFE) PRICING INITIATIVE INTERVENTION EXAMPLE

The HFE Initiative, implemented by the organization NC Prevention Partners, was an intervention targeting both the policy and environmental levels to promote healthy eating behaviors in the hospital setting throughout North Carolina with later expansion to South Carolina.[16] The intervention aimed to encourage healthier eating behaviors by hospital visitors, staff, and volunteers by making healthy food options more accessible and visible. Specifically, the initiative used a pricing model to incentivize healthier eating through price discounts on healthy foods while simultaneously charging more for unhealthy foods. In addition, the intervention incorporated strategies to educate consumers at the point of purchase with healthy food labels. HFE included changes not only in cafeterias but also in vending machines and catering. The five underlying principles of the HFE Initiative are:

- Provide access to healthy foods: achieved through actions such as incorporation of dietary guidelines and working with vendors to procure healthier foods.

- Use pricing to promote healthy foods: achieved through pricing incentives that encourage the purchase of healthier foods and discourage the purchase of less health-promoting foods.

- Use marketing techniques to promote healthy foods: achieved through point-of-sale strategies such as healthy food icon labels and product placement to encourage purchasing healthier items.

- Use benefit design and incentives to encourage behavior change: achieved through implementing programs such as those targeting hospital employee wellness.

- Educate staff and visitors about healthy foods: achieved through initiatives such as healthy food choice education and training and hosting cooking demonstrations.[16]

The evaluation for the program was based on the RE-AIM framework. Figure 13.1 shows the logic model for the intervention and Exhibit 13.1 shows the evaluation plan as depicted on the website for the Center for Training and Research Translation (Center TRT).[16] Center TRT developed a framework for evaluating PSE change interventions and identifies, reviews, translates, and disseminates evidence-based interventions that promote healthy eating and physical activity.[17-19]

INVENTION AND REINVENTION OF APPROACHES BASED ON HEALTH OUTCOMES

Although evaluation is often seen as the final step in the intervention process, it is much more productive (and fun/useful) to see it as a process of invention and reinvention. Any good innovator/entrepreneur knows that "failure" is part of the learning process and is expected to happen

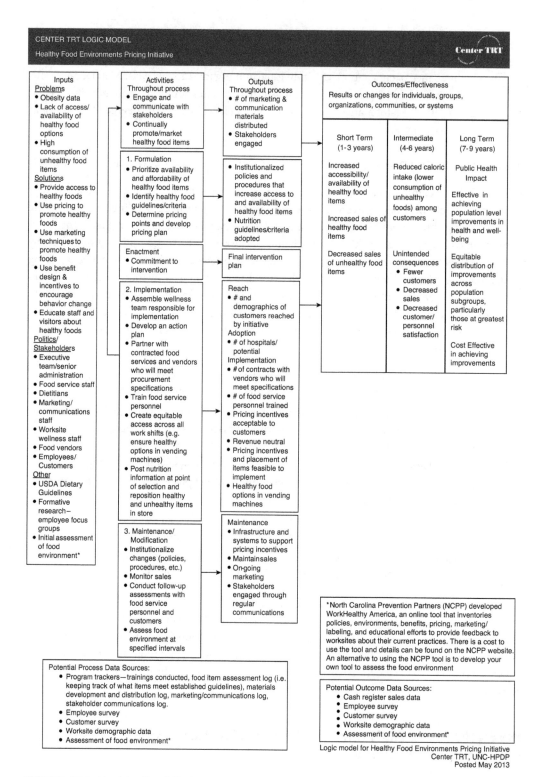

FIGURE 13.1 Healthy Food Environments Pricing Initiative logic model.

Center TRT, Center for Training and Research Translation.

Source: Center for Training and Research Translation. From Healthy Food Environments Pricing Initiative. http://www.centertrt.org/?p=intervention&id=1099

EXHIBIT 13.1

HEALTHY FOOD ENVIRONMENTS PRICING INITIATIVE EVALUATION MODEL

CENTER TRT EVALUATION PLAN
Healthy Food Environments Pricing Initiative

Purpose: The purpose of this evaluation plan is to determine the extent of implementation, acceptability, and effectiveness of a Healthy Food Environments (HFE) Pricing Initiative similar to the North Carolina Prevention Partner's HFE Pricing Initiative. This evaluation plan provides a **menu of options** for evaluation questions covering several dimensions commonly included in program evaluations, including: reach, adoption, extent of program implementation, and effectiveness in addressing targeted outcomes. Please note that this suggested evaluation plan focuses on program implementation; a list of other relevant evaluation questions is available in the Evaluation section of the Center TRT website.

Evaluation questions: This evaluation plan likely includes many more evaluation questions than will be feasible to answer. Similarly, it may include questions that are less important for your particular context or lack questions that should be prioritized for your context. Center TRT recommends working with your stakeholder group to prioritize the evaluation questions you will seek to answer.

Design: The evaluation is a pre- and post-test design with no comparison group.

Data collection: A variety of data collection tools are referenced throughout the evaluation plan. These data collection tools will need to be created to apply to your context. These same tools also appear in the lower section of the Center TRT Logic Model.

Process evaluation tools:
- Program trackers – These are logs used to monitor various aspects of program reach, adoption, and implementation. The wellness team and food service personnel would probably maintain such logs. The program trackers we suggest keeping are: trainings conducted, food item assessment log (i.e. keeping track of what items meet established guidelines), materials development and distribution log, marketing/communications log, stakeholder communications log, etc.
- Cash register sales data
- Employee survey
- Customer survey
- Worksite demographic data
- Assessment of food environment* *(either the NCPP tool or tool created for your context)*

Short-term (1-3 year) outcome evaluation tools:
- Cash register sales data
- Assessment of food environment* *(either the NCPP tool or tool created for your context)*

*North Carolina Prevention Partners developed WorkHealthy America, an online tool that inventories policies, environments, benefits, pricing, marketing/labeling, and educational efforts to provide feedback to worksites about their current practices. **There is a cost to use the tool and details can be found on the NCPP website.** *An alternative to using the NCPP tool is to develop your own tool to assess the food environment.* All other tools will need to be developed to apply to your context.

Contact information for the developers is available on the Center TRT website within the HFE Pricing Initiative intervention package. Please contact the intervention developers for questions about the intervention itself.

(continued)

EXHIBIT 13.1

HEALTHY FOOD ENVIRONMENTS PRICING INITIATIVE EVALUATION MODEL (*CONTINUED*)

PROCESS EVALUATION		
This section should address the *reach* of the intervention into the intended population; the *adoption* or uptake of the intervention by setting; and the fidelity of *implementation* of the intervention components and core elements.		
Evaluation Questions	**Data to Be Collected**	**Data Collection Method**
Reach How many people were exposed to the pricing initiative? What were the demographics of customers purchasing food from the hospitals?	Number of customers per day Demographics (age, gender, etc.) of customers at hospitals	• Cash register sales data • Customer demographic data and/or customer survey
Adoption What proportion of hospitals adopted the pricing initiative? What are the characteristics of the hospitals adopting the pricing initiative?	Percentage of hospitals that adopt the pricing initiative out of the total number that could adopt Size (number of beds), public/private, specialties, setting (urban/rural)	• Program tracker—hospital adoption log • Program tracker—hospital adoption log
Implementation What nutrition guidelines/criteria were identified? What pricing points were developed? Who was on the wellness team assembled? How many and what type of contracts were established with vendors who will meet specifications? How many food service personnel were trained and what was the content of the training? Were pricing incentives acceptable to customers? Were pricing initiatives feasible for personnel to implement? Was the program revenue neutral? Did hospitals fully implement the pricing initiative, including: • Labeling healthy food items • Posting nutrition information at point of selection • Place less healthy food items in lower traffic areas and healthy food items in higher traffic areas • Adjust pricing points to encourage consumption of healthier food items and discourage consumption of less healthy food items	Nutrition guidelines/criteria Pricing points Existence and composition of wellness team Number and what type of contracts Number of food service personnel trained Training content Acceptability of incentives Feasibility of implementation Budget records (purchases and sales) Number of hospitals that fully implemented the pricing initiative, including: • Labeling healthy food items • Posting nutrition information at point of selection • Place less healthy food items in lower traffic areas and healthy food items in higher traffic areas • Adjust pricing points to encourage consumption of healthier food items and discourage consumption of less healthy food items	• Program tracker—Materials development log • Program tracker—Planning log or Materials development log • Program tracker—Planning log • Cash register sales data • Program tracker—training log • Training curriculum and agenda • Customer survey • Employee survey • Cash register sales data • Program tracker—implementation log or hospital adoption log

(continued)

EXHIBIT 13.1

HEALTHY FOOD ENVIRONMENTS PRICING INITIATIVE EVALUATION MODEL (*CONTINUED*)

OUTCOME EVALUATION		
This section should address the <u>effect</u> of the intervention on the intended short-term outcomes (those you can measure at the end of a 1–3-year project period).		
Evaluation Questions	**Data to Be Collected**	**Data Collection Method**
Short-Term Outcomes		
Outcome 1: Increased accessibility/availability of healthy food items		
Did access to healthy food items at hospitals increase?	Number of "healthy" (use identified nutrition guidelines/criteria) food items available at each hospital: • Baseline • Follow-up	• Cash register sales data • Assessment of food environment (*either NCPP tool or tool created for your context*)
Outcome 2: Increased sales of healthy food items		
Did sales of healthy food items increase?	"Healthy" (use identified nutrition guidelines/criteria) food item sales: • Baseline • Follow-up	• Cash register sales data
Outcome 3: Decreased sales of unhealthy food items		
Did sales of unhealthy food items decrease?	"Unhealthy" (use identified nutrition guidelines/criteria) food item sales: • Baseline • Follow-up	• Cash register sales data

Center TRT, Center for Training and Research Translation.

Source: From Center for Training and Research Translation. *Healthy Food Environments Pricing Initiative.* http://www.centertrt.org/?p=intervention&id=1099

some if not much of the time. Continuing with this theme, often product testing results in "pivoting" to a different approach that is more likely to be satisfactory to the customer. This same approach can apply to public health nutrition interventions. Despite careful formative evaluation work, there is always the potential that an intervention may fail to have the desired impact. Collecting good process data using implementation theory frameworks, such as RE-AIM or the Consolidated Framework for Implementation Science,[20] will help enormously in understanding what might have gone wrong and what might be corrected or "reinvented."

For example, we have plenty of evidence that a healthier diet for children (more whole grains, more fruits and vegetables, higher quality fats and oils, and fewer simple carbohydrates) is associated with better long-term outcomes. It seems obvious that school lunches should implement these guidelines given the large potential for impact nationally. However, implementation of the policy has been rocky due to unexpected resistance from school lunch program leaders and staff, in part because they felt they were not adequately consulted regarding the implementation process. There were also logistical challenges, such as the unappealing consistency of whole-grain pasta products kept hot on the lunch line and limited knowledge about vegetable preparation among school cafeteria staff. However, rather than "ditching" the idea of the cafeteria guidelines in the Healthy Hunger-Free Kids Act, various evaluations have demonstrated that serving practices can be modified and that staff/children adjust to the new foods and preparation strategies over time.

COMMUNICATION STRATEGIES

As you have seen in other chapters, health communications can play an important role in improving health outcomes, and evaluation is key to identifying the most effective and efficient approaches. Health communication strategies can be used to reach a variety of audiences including community members, health professionals, and policy-makers.

Examples of Communication Channels

A variety of communication channels can be used to disseminate health messages. The specific channels you use depend on a variety of factors, including who is the intended audience you are trying to reach and what is the message you are trying to deliver. Interpersonal channels, such as a healthcare provider sharing information with a patient, are often used to convey health messages. Telehealth strategies, such as videoconferencing, can be used to share health messages over long distances. Print materials, such as posters, brochures, and newsletters, are commonly used to distribute health information. Promotional items with health messages can also be distributed. Water bottles with a message about drinking water are a great way to promote drinking water instead of sugary drinks, for example. Mass media, such as radio, television, newspapers, billboards, bus advertisements, and direct mailings are also often used. In addition, online channels, such as websites and social media, are very popular. The wide variety of communication channels requires a diverse set of evaluation strategies.

Development and Evaluation of Health Communication Programs

Successful health communication programs involve thoughtful planning and evaluation. The four stages of developing a health communication program are planning and strategy development; developing and pretesting concepts, messages, and materials; implementing the program; and assessing effectiveness and making refinements.[21] This is a circular process, and evaluation plays an important role in each stage.

Stage 1: Planning and Strategy Development

Approaches to evaluation should be considered and implemented throughout the planning process. During the first stage, you will conduct formative evaluation. Begin by assessing the health issue/problem and identifying all components of a possible solution. Data should be gathered and reviewed on the health issue/problem, who is affected, and possible causes and solutions. In this step, it is important to evaluate all possible components of a solution and whether health communication is an appropriate strategy alone or in combination with other approaches. During this stage, you will also develop communication objectives. Communication objectives should be SMART (specific, measurable, achievable, relevant, and time-bound), which helps in building in an evaluation component. This stage also involves defining and learning about the intended audience(s) of the communication program; thinking about the settings, channels, and activities that the communication program will use to reach the intended audience; and identifying potential partners to work with on the communication program. The final step of stage 1 is to develop a communication strategy and draft communication and evaluation plans.

Stage 2: Developing and Pretesting Concepts, Messages, and Materials

Before beginning to develop new materials, it is important to identify and evaluate existing materials to see whether there is a need to create something new. Using or adapting existing materials can help to save time and money and prevent you from having to "reinvent the wheel."

Next, you will develop message concepts, which are rough forms of how you will present the information, and test them with the intended audience. Concept testing is important because it can help to assess reactions to your proposed messages and materials and to identify which messages will work best for the intended audiences. The information gathered can be used to help refine your messages and materials prior to producing them. Focus groups and in-depth interviews are common strategies for testing concepts. Cognitive response testing is another method that can be used and allows you to understand how members of your target audience interpret and comprehend your messages. Individuals are shown the messages and complete a semistructured interview answering questions related to areas such as how they interpret or perceive certain words or phrases.[22] They are also able to provide suggestions on different ways of wording messages to make them easier to understand and to increase the relevance of the information.[22]

After testing message concepts, you will decide what materials to develop. Materials should be pretested with the intended audience to ensure they understand the message, are relevant, and are doing what you want them to do. A variety of strategies are used to pretest materials, such as questionnaires, theater testing of large groups of individuals who respond to messages, and observational studies in which materials are put out and the behaviors of individuals are observed.

Stage 3: Implementing the Program

Process evaluation is an important component of implementing a health communication program and helps to assess whether the program was implemented as intended. Areas assessed during process evaluation include who was reached; what was done; when, where, and how activities were carried out; and audience satisfaction. Examples of methods to collect process data include activity tracking sheets, website or social media metrics, and status reports and/or meetings with staff and partners. Surveys can be conducted with your audience to help assess areas such as audience satisfaction, how well the characteristics of those reached match those of your intended audience, and how the materials were used. Intercept surveys are commonly used in evaluating communication campaigns. With this method, interviewers go to a public location or business to recruit, screen, and interview individuals who are at that location. These interviews are typically short as individuals are interviewed as they are recruited and will not have planned to be participating in advance. Intercept surveys have the benefits of being able to quickly collect data at a low cost; however, there are limitations, such as not having a representative sample as only individuals at the location and time of data collection are able to participate. Intercept surveys can also be conducted online, such as a brief survey popping up when someone visits a website. The data collected through process evaluation should be reviewed regularly to determine whether adjustments should be made.

Stage 4: Assessing Effectiveness and Making Refinements

In developing an outcome evaluation, determine what information you need to obtain from the evaluation and the type of data you will need to collect. There are a variety of types of outcomes you may want to consider, including changes in knowledge, attitudes, or behaviors; awareness of the health communication program; or whether policies or institutional actions were taken. Next, you will determine which type of evaluation design you will use. The data collection instruments will then be developed and pretested. Both quantitative and qualitative methods can be used. Data collection will then take place. Ideally, data collection takes place both before and after the program so that you can assess change. Analyze your data and use it to develop an evaluation report that can be shared with key stakeholders. The results of the evaluation can be used to refine the health communication program.

Social Media

Much of what was discussed before applies to evaluating social media campaigns as well. In this section, we discuss metrics relevant to social media. As with the evaluation of most other types of public health nutrition programs, reach is often an important process measure to consider. In the context of social media, reach typically refers to the number of unique individuals who had the opportunity to see your content.[23] This differs from impressions, which is the number of times a piece of content has been viewed. Many social media platforms provide metrics for reach and/or impressions.[23] They may also provide information on the demographics of the individuals you reached. Depending on the platform, other ways of assessing these include number of likes, followers, views, subscribers, or visitors. Engagement refers to taking some type of action beyond exposure.[23] Examples of ways to measure this include number of likes, comments, retweets, content embeds, replies, shares, hashtag use, and votes. Posts, comments, or other pieces of content can also be qualitatively analyzed to assess outcomes, such as whether engagement with your campaign is positive, neutral, or negative in sentiment. You can also survey individuals to assess outcomes of interest through social media platforms.

Telehealth

With telehealth interventions becoming increasingly used, it is important that they are evaluated. As with any public health nutrition intervention, evaluation planning should begin while the intervention is being developed. Formative evaluation is important in telehealth interventions to help ensure that the strategies being used are appropriate and feasible for the providers and participants. Process, outcome, and impact evaluation are also important to conduct throughout the implementation of the intervention to ensure it is being implemented as planned and producing the desired effects. The technology aspects of the intervention should be considered in the evaluation process, such as usability, participant satisfaction, workload, and cost-effectiveness.[24,25] There is currently no "gold standard" evaluation framework or methods surrounding telehealth interventions. A variety of different frameworks have been developed specifically for telehealth interventions, although many nonspecific frameworks including those discussed previously, such as RE-AIM, have been used.[24]

mHEALTH APPLICATIONS AND NUTRITION MONITORING

Cell phone use has been increasing worldwide.[26] In the United States, 96% of adults own a cell phone, with 81% owning a smartphone.[27] Although there are multiple definitions of mHealth, it generally refers to the use of mobile and wireless devices to improve health.[28] Using mobile technologies in health programs and research is an expanding area in both developed and developing countries. A variety of mHealth technologies are used including text messages, mobile apps, global positioning system (GPS), Bluetooth, and wearables and sensors.[26]

mHealth is used in both medical care and community settings. Examples in medical care include text message appointment reminders, mobile apps allowing access to electronic health records, and video consultations with patients.[26] A variety of mHealth applications and interventions have been developed both for general health and for prevention or treatment of specific conditions such as obesity, diabetes, and cardiovascular disease.[29,30] There have even been specific apps developed for individuals participating in certain federal nutrition programs, such as the WIC.[31]

Nutrition programs can use mHealth in a variety of ways. Nutrition messages can be sent via text message and may or may not include links to websites with additional content. A variety of mobile apps have been developed. Examples of app features include nutrition education, social connectivity features such as forums and team participation, encouragement and prompts such as rewards and push notifications, goal setting, game elements, environmental supports such as menu suggestions, and dietary tracking.[29]

There are a variety of ways that mHealth applications can be used in evaluation and nutrition monitoring. Mobile phones can be used to collect survey data from participants. This can be especially helpful when participants live in hard-to-reach areas.[32] Telephone surveys can be used to reach participants. Some public health interventions use text messages to send questions to participants who can then text back their responses. Participants can also complete online surveys on their phones or through mobile apps.

Dietary outcomes are commonly assessed in public health nutrition interventions. There are numerous apps available to track dietary data.[33] These apps allow participants to enter the foods they are eating and can be analyzed to see specific foods, food groups, or nutrients. Physical activity can also be assessed through mobile apps, through self-report methods in which participants record their physical activity, or through objective measurements as captured by activity trackers.[34] Information such as weight or blood glucose levels can also be tracked. These forms of gathering information can be used by individuals to track their own dietary intake and/or can be seen by healthcare providers to help with monitoring their patients.

CONCLUSION

Evaluation plays an important role in public health nutrition interventions. Using a framework to systematically approach an evaluation is a helpful strategy, especially given how varied evaluations can be in purpose and type. Examples of evaluation frameworks include the CDC Framework for Program Evaluation in Public Health and the RE-AIM framework. Common types of evaluation include formative, process, outcome, and impact. When performing an evaluation, a logic model is a useful tool that can provide a schematic representation of program elements such as inputs, activities, and expected outputs and outcomes. Interventions can be implemented at varying levels, ranging from a focus on the individual to broader PSE change; thus, evaluation strategies can differ based on the contextual level. Data collection methods in an evaluation can be quantitative, qualitative, or mixed methods. Planning an evaluation should commence with the start of implementing a program and should include continual engagement of stakeholders to increase utility and acceptability of results. Additionally, evaluations present an opportunity to "reinvent" or improve interventions if needed. Finally, evolving strategies and technology in public health nutrition, such as an increasing use of social media, may necessitate adapting evaluation approaches and also offers new and innovative approaches to effective evaluation.

KEY CONCEPTS

▨ Evaluation can assume varying forms depending on the purpose of the evaluation and the needs of the audience; common types of evaluation include formative, process, outcome, and impact.

▨ The logic model is a useful tool to guide an evaluation and commonly incorporates inputs, activities, outputs, and outcomes.

▨ Methods for collecting data in an evaluation can be quantitative or qualitative; often, evaluations use a mixed methods approach, which includes a combination of quantitative and qualitative methods.

▨ A variety of frameworks are available to provide a systematic guide to evaluation; the CDC Framework for Program Evaluation in Public Health and the RE-AIM framework are examples.

▨ Evaluation can provide opportunities to both invent and reinvent an intervention depending on needs and results from previous interventions.

▨ The process of evaluation must continually adapt as approaches to public health interventions evolve, as seen in the use of PSE change strategies promoting healthy environments, health communication programs engaging audiences through social media, and interventions incorporating mHealth applications.

CASE STUDY: A FARM-TO-SCHOOL PROGRAM IN THE HAPPY VALLEY SCHOOL DISTRICT

Happy Valley School District, which includes 10 schools (five elementary schools, three middle schools, and two high schools), is going to start a farm-to-school program for their district. The school wellness committee for the district will be leading the project. The program includes the following components:

▨ Procurement: The school district plans to increase the amount of local fruits and vegetables purchased, promoted, and served in the school cafeteria.

▨ School gardens: The school district would like to start school gardens where students can participate in hands-on activities.

▨ Education: Nutrition education related to fruits and vegetables, gardening, and how to prepare fruits and vegetables will be provided through classroom lessons and special events. There will also be information shared with parents through methods such as a special section of the school website, social media, and paper handouts sent home with children.

▨ Farm visits: Opportunities will be available for students to visit a farm as part of a class field trip to understand more about agricultural production.

The school district does not currently serve local produce but is looking into partnering with local farmers to provide it. The district also does not currently have school gardens, but the school wellness committee has received a $20,000 grant from a local foundation to support the establishment of school gardens in the district. The principals of the schools must agree to having the garden and provide a location for it. The local health department has nutrition educators who are interested in providing nutrition education to interested classrooms. The School Wellness Committee has also identified a local farm that is willing to provide tours to students.

The school wellness committee would like to evaluate their efforts over the course of the next two school years and has partnered with a local university to assist with the evaluation. They are interested in learning about how the different components of the farm-to-school program are implemented at the schools within their districts and whether participation in the activities is associated with changes in attitudes, preferences, and consumption of fruits and vegetables. They would also like to know what is working well and what can be improved upon.

For this case study, assume that you are a nutrition student from a local university who will be assisting the school wellness committee with the evaluation.

Case Study Questions

1. Who are the stakeholders you would want to engage in the evaluation?

2. What outputs would you assess through your process evaluation?

3. What outcomes would you assess?

4. Thinking about the RE-AIM framework, what would you consider measuring to assess reach, effectiveness, adoption, implementation, and maintenance?

5. Create a logic model for the program that includes the inputs, activities, outputs, and outcomes.

6. What data collection methods would you use?

7. How would you use the data you collect to provide conclusions and recommendations to the school wellness committee?

SUGGESTED LEARNING ACTIVITIES

- Learn more about PSE change interventions. Visit snapedpse.org to browse PSE change examples by setting using the Snap-Ed Interactive Map. If interested in learning more about school gardens, find this setting and explore!

- Expand your evaluation framework "toolbox" by learning more about the SNAP-Ed Evaluation Framework found on the SNAP-Ed Toolkit's website (snapedtoolkit .org).

- Enhance your mHealth knowledge by exploring examples of mHealth interventions such as Text2BHealthy (snapedtoolkit.org/interventions/programs/text2 bhealthy).

- Visit the Center TRT website at www.centertrt.org for more materials developed for the HFE Pricing Initiative Intervention example from this chapter. Check out other interventions on the website!

- Perform a literature search of evaluations using the RE-AIM framework and select a paper to review. A list of publications can be found online (www.re-aim.org/category/ publications).

REFLECTION QUESTIONS

1. What are some challenges you may face if you wait until an intervention is already being implemented to plan the evaluation?

2. What do you think are some of the benefits and challenges of using social media as an avenue for public health interventions?

3. What are some interventions you have encountered that you would like to "reinvent"? How would you do so?

4. Think about a public health nutrition program with which you are familiar. Who are the key stakeholders involved in the intervention?

CONTINUE YOUR LEARNING RESOURCES

CDC Evaluation Framework. https://www.cdc.gov/eval/framework/index.htm.
Center TRT. http://www.centertrt.org.
RE-AIM. http://www.re-aim.org.
SNAP-Ed Evaluation Framework. https://snapedtoolkit.org/framework/index.

GLOSSARY

Activities: What the intervention does with the inputs in order to achieve the desired outcomes.

Fidelity: The degree of exactness with which something is copied or reproduced.

Formative evaluation: Typically occurs during the development or adaptation of an intervention to ensure the intervention is feasible and acceptable.

Impact evaluation: Assesses how effective an intervention is at achieving its ultimate goals.

Individual-level strategies: Intervention approaches that work directly with individuals one-on-one vs. in groups.

Inputs: Resources invested into a program.

Intervention: Any activity taken to improve public health nutrition.

Logic model: A conceptual tool that illustrates the sequential relationships between an intervention's inputs, activities, outputs, and outcomes.

Outcome evaluation: Assesses the effects of an intervention on achieving a program's outcome objectives.

Outcomes: The changes an intervention expects to achieve.

Outputs: The direct results of the intervention's activities that are intended to lead to the desired outcomes.

Photovoice: A type of participatory action research that involves participants using photographs to capture and reflect on different issues.

Process evaluation: Assesses how an intervention was implemented and whether it resulted in particular outputs.

Program evaluation: A systematic method for collecting, analyzing, and using information to answer questions about programs and policies, particularly about their effectiveness and efficiency.

RE-AIM framework: An evaluation framework that consists of five steps (reach, effectiveness, adoption, implementation, and maintenance) and aims to translate research into action.

SHOWeD method: A process that guides participants through a series of questions to help them reflect on photos and the issues they represent.

REFERENCES

1. Centers for Disease Control and Prevention. *Framework for Program Evaluation in Public Health.* Atlanta, GA: Centers for Disease Control and Prevention; 1999.
2. Steckler A, Linnan L. Process evaluation for public health interventions and research: an overview. In: Steckler A, Linnan L, eds. *Process Evaluation for Public Health Interventions and Research.* San Francisco, CA: Jossey-Bass; 2002:1–23.
3. *UNC Center for Health Promotion and Disease Prevention. SNAP-Ed Toolkit: SNAP-Ed Evaluation Framework.* 2016. https://snapedtoolkit.org/framework/index
4. Morse JM. Approaches to qualitative-quantitative methodological triangulation. *Nurs Res.* 1991;40(2):120–123.
5. Wang C, Burris MA. Photovoice: concept, methodology, and use for participatory needs assessment. *Health Educ Behav.* 1997;24(3):369–387. doi:10.1177/109019819702400309
6. Wang CC. Photovoice: a participatory action research strategy applied to women's health. *J Womens Health.* 1999;8(2):185–192. doi:10.1089/jwh.1999.8.185
7. Centers for Disease Control and Prevention. *Behavioral Risk Factor Surveillance System.* 2019. https://www.cdc.gov/brfss
8. Lytle LA, Nichaman MZ, Obarzanek E, et al. Validation of 24-hour recalls assisted by food records in third-grade children. The CATCH Collaborative Group. *J Am Diet Assoc.* 1993;93(12):1431–1436. doi:10.1016/0002-8223(93)92247-U
9. Ball SC, Benjamin SE, Ward DS. Development and reliability of an observation method to assess food intake of young children in child care. *J Am Diet Assoc.* 2007;107(4):656–661. doi:10.1016/j.jada.2007.01.003
10. Adams MA, Pelletier RL, Zive MM, Sallis JF. Salad bars and fruit and vegetable consumption in elementary schools: a plate waste study. *J Am Diet Assoc.* 2005;105(11):1789–1792. doi:10.1016/j.jada.2005.08.013
11. Cohen JFW, Smit LA, Parker E, et al. Long-term impact of a chef on school lunch consumption: findings from a 2-year pilot study in Boston middle schools. *J Acad Nutr Diet.* 2012;112(6):927–933. doi:10.1016/j.jand.2012.01.015
12. Glasgow RE, Vogt TM, Boles SM. Evaluating the public health impact of health promotion interventions: the RE-AIM framework. *Am J Public Health.* 1999;89(9):1322–1327. doi:10.2105/ajph.89.9.1322
13. Lobb R, Colditz GA. Implementation science and its application to population health. *Annu Rev Public Health.* 2013;34:235–251. doi:10.1146/annurev-publhealth-031912-114444
14. Glasgow RE, Emmons KM. How can we increase translation of research into practice? Types of evidence needed. *Annu Rev Public Health.* 2007;28:413–433. doi:10.1146/annurev.publhealth.28.021406.144145
15. RE-AIM. 2019. http://www.re-aim.org
16. *Center for Training and Research Translation. Healthy Food Environments Pricing Initiative.* 2019. http://www.centertrt.org/?p=intervention&id=1099
17. Leeman J, Myers AE, Ribisl KM, Ammerman AS. Disseminating policy and environmental change interventions: insights from obesity prevention and tobacco control. *Int J Behav Med.* 2015;22(3):301–311. doi:10.1007/s12529-014-9427-1
18. Leeman J, Sommers J, Leung MM, Ammerman A. Disseminating evidence from research and practice: a model for selecting evidence to guide obesity prevention. *J Public Health Manag Pract.* 2011;17(2):133–140. doi:10.1097/PHH.0b013e3181e39eaa
19. Leeman J, Sommers J, Vu M, et al. An evaluation framework for obesity prevention policy interventions. *Prev Chronic Dis.* 2012;9:E120. doi:10.5888/pcd9.110322

20. Damschroder LJ, Aron DC, Keith RE, et al. Fostering implementation of health services research findings into practice: a consolidated framework for advancing implementation science. *Implement Sci.* 2009;4:50. doi:10.1186/1748-5908-4-50

21. National Cancer Institute. *Making Health Communication Programs Work: A Planner's Guide.* Washington, DC: National Cancer Institute; 2004.

22. Lapka C, Jupka K, Wray RJ, Jacobsen H. Applying cognitive response testing in message development and pre-testing. *Health Educ Res.* 2008;23(3):467–476. doi:10.1093/her/cym089

23. *The Conclave Complete Social Media Measurement Standards June 2013.* 2019. https://docs.wixstatic.com/ugd/0b15ae_c4b5f3e188e143cca1ca263376fbb132.pdf

24. Agboola S, Hale TM, Masters C, et al. "Real-world" practical evaluation strategies: a review of telehealth evaluation. *JMIR Res Protoc.* 2014;3(4):e75. doi:10.2196/resprot.3459

25. Lau F, Kuziemsky C, eds. *Handbook of EHealth Evaluation: An Evidence-Based Approach.* Victoria, BC, Canada: University of Victoria; 2017.

26. World Health Organization. *Mhealth: New Horizons for Health Through Mobile Technologies (Global Observatory for Ehealth).* Geneva, Switzerland: World Health Organization; 2011:126.

27. Pew Research Center. *Demographics of Mobile Device Ownership and Adoption in the United States.* Washington, DC: Pew Research Center; 2019. https://www.pewinternet.org/fact-sheet/mobile

28. Davis TL, DiClemente R, Prietula M. Taking mHealth forward: examining the core characteristics. *JMIR Mhealth Uhealth.* 2016;4(3):e97. doi:10.2196/mhealth.5659

29. Tonkin E, Brimblecombe J, Wycherley TP. Characteristics of smartphone applications for nutrition improvement in community settings: a scoping review. *Adv Nutr.* 2017;8(2):308–322. doi:10.3945/an.116.013748

30. Marcolino MS, Oliveira JAQ, D'Agostino M, et al. The impact of mHealth interventions: systematic review of systematic reviews. *JMIR Mhealth Uhealth.* 2018;6(1):e23. doi:10.2196/mhealth.8873

31. Weber SJ, Dawson D, Greene H, Hull PC. Mobile phone apps for low-income participants in a public health nutrition program for Women, Infants, and Children (WIC): review and analysis of features. *JMIR Mhealth Uhealth.* 2018;6(11):e12261. doi:10.2196/12261

32. Firchow P, MacGinty R. Including Hard-to-Access Populations Using Mobile Phone Surveys and Participatory Indicators. *Sociol Methods Res.* 2017:1–28. doi:10.1177/0049124117729702

33. Ferrara G, Kim J, Lin S, et al. A focused review of smartphone diet-tracking apps: usability, functionality, coherence with behavior change theory, and comparative validity of nutrient intake and energy estimates. *JMIR Mhealth Uhealth.* 2019;7(5):e9232. doi:10.2196/mhealth.9232

34. McCallum C, Rooksby J, Gray CM. Evaluating the impact of physical activity apps and wearables: interdisciplinary review. *JMIR Mhealth Uhealth.* 2018;6(3):e58. doi:10.2196/mhealth.9054

IV

CURRENT AND FUTURE CHALLENGES IN PUBLIC HEALTH NUTRITION AND SUSTAINABILITY

CURRENT NUTRITION-RELATED HEALTH ISSUES AND CHALLENGES

AMANDA S. HEGE, KENDRA OO, AND JOANNA CUMMINGS

You do not solve the hunger problem by feeding people. . . . The problems of hunger and malnutrition can be solved only by ensuring that people can live in dignity by having decent opportunities to provide for themselves.

—George Kent, Freedom from Want

LEARNING OBJECTIVES

After reading and studying this chapter and its contents, you should be able to:

1. Identify nutrition-related health challenges worldwide.
2. Define food and nutrient needs for optimal health across the life span.
3. Describe the double burden of malnutrition.
4. Explain the four pillars of food security, which can be used to assess population nutritional status.
5. Describe the relationship among malnutrition, food security, hunger, and the overall health and wellness of a community.

INTRODUCTION

Food and nutrition have significant implications for the health and well-being of a population. The benefits of high consumption of fruits and vegetables are well known. There is strong evidence that links a healthy diet with optimal growth and development, high educational attainment, immune response, and longevity, in addition to decreasing the risk of developing obesity, diabetes, osteoporosis, cognitive decline, and certain types of cancer. This chapter identifies how food and nutrition can promote health, quality of life, and economic prosperity. Nutrition-related health issues and challenges, across the globe, from infancy through adulthood, are explored. The relationship among malnutrition, food security, hunger, and health, incorporating the four pillars of food availability, access, utilization, and stability, will be used in assessing and developing strategies that accelerate progress toward optimal health.

NUTRITION AND HEALTH-RELATED DISEASE TRENDS

Global Burden of Malnutrition

Malnutrition, the lack of proper nutrients to meet daily needs, is the largest single contributor to disease and poor health outcomes in the world. Referring to both the presence of **undernutrition** (insufficient intake of energy and nutrients to meet an individual's needs) and **overnutrition** (overconsumption of certain nutrients, such as protein, carbohydrates, and fat), the *2014 Second International Congress on Nutrition* framed this issue as "malnutrition in all forms." Undernutrition results from not getting enough energy from **macronutrients** (carbohydrates, protein, and fat) and **micronutrients**, thereby leading to low weight-for-height (wasting), low height-for-age (stunting), and low weight-for-age (underweight). Overnutrition results from an overconsumption of macronutrients and energy, and leads to overweight, obesity, and diet-related chronic diseases.

Globally, 795 million individuals are malnourished, including one in every four children.[1] The world's undernourished population is unevenly distributed with the majority living in Asia (more than 500 million). While the United States is considered the land of plenty, too many men, women, and children still struggle to put food on the table. According to Feeding America, the largest anti-hunger agency in the United States, approximately 41 million Americans and one in five U.S. children experience **food insecurity**—the lack of consistent access to enough food for an active, healthy life—putting them at a greater risk of various forms of malnutrition and poor health.[2] In mostly middle-income nations, where the economy has slowed or contracted, we see an increase in hunger, the extreme physical feeling of discomfort or weakness caused by a lack of food. If the current trends continue, the 2030 Sustainable Development Goals (to halve the number of stunted children) and the 2025 World Health Assembly target (to reduce the prevalence of low birth weight) will not be met.

It is possible to be overweight or obese from excessive calorie consumption but still not get enough vitamins and minerals to promote good health. The American Medical Association (AMA) designated obesity as a disease that contributes to 4 million deaths annually worldwide.[3] By 2050, 60% of males and 50% of females will have obesity.[4,5]

Food and Nutrition Needs for Optimal Health

The most widely recognized definition of healthful eating is a high intake of fruits and vegetables.[6] Proper nutrition includes the consumption of essential macronutrients (protein, carbohydrates, and fats) and micronutrients (vitamin A, iodine, iron, and zinc). Essential nutrients play a critical role in humoral immunity responses, cellular signaling and function, learning and cognitive function, work capacity, reproductive health, and the evolution of microbial virulence (Table 14.1).[7]

Dietary Recommendations

The basics of obtaining good nutrition incorporates a variety of foods across all five food groups (vegetables, fruits, grains, protein, and dairy; Figure 14.1).

Undernutrition and Disease

Recent estimates indicate that more than 2 billion people globally are at risk for vitamin A, iodine, and/or iron deficiency. The prevalence is especially high in Southeast Asia and sub-Saharan Africa. In many settings, more than one micronutrient deficiency exists, suggesting the need for simple approaches that evaluate and address multiple micronutrient malnutrition.[8]

TABLE 14.1 ESSENTIAL NUTRIENTS AND THEIR PRIMARY FUNCTIONS AND DIETARY SOURCES

NUTRIENT	FUNCTION	SOURCE
Macronutrient		
Protein (Nine essential amino acids in foods)	Repairs body tissues and cells; healthy functioning of immune system; manufacturing hormones	Beans and legumes, seeds, nuts, quinoa, beets, raw greens (kale, spinach), avocado, meat, fish, eggs, and dairy
Carbohydrate	Primary energy source; comprises 45% to 65% of diet	Apples, bananas, cauliflower, carrots, oats, brown rice, quinoa, chickpeas, kidney beans
Fat (Focus on healthy*)	Improves brain development, cell functioning, protects the body's organs, helps absorb vitamins and minerals	Almonds, walnuts, seeds, olives, avocados*
Micronutrient		
Vitamin A	Promotes good eyesight; as an antioxidant, maintains healthy teeth and skin; supports healthy pregnancy and breastfeeding; fat-soluble	Salmon, eggs, cooked sweet potato, winter squash, kale, collards, turnip greens, carrots, Swiss chard, spinach
Iodine	Regulates thyroid hormones; promotes proper bone and brain development during pregnancy and infancy	Cod, seaweed, yogurt, iodized salt, milk, enriched bread, shrimp
Iron	Functions of hemoglobin, protein needed to transport oxygen in the blood; promotes healthy pregnancy, increased energy, and improved athletic performance	Fortified grains, white beans, canned clams, lean ground beef, dark chocolate, beans, nuts, baked potato cooked spinach[†]
Zinc	Supports healthy immune system, heal wounds, and proper senses of taste and smell; promotes healthy pregnancy	Oysters, lean meat, poultry, seafood (crab and lobsters), fortified grains

*Sources of healthy, monounsaturated/polyunsaturated fats.
[†]Consuming vitamin C–rich foods alongside plant-based (non-heme) iron sources will increase absorption.
Source: Data from Kapil U, Bhavna A. Adverse effects of poor micronutrient status during childhood and adolescence. *Nutr Rev.* 2002;60(suppl 5):S84–S90. doi:10.1301/00296640260130803

Nutrient Deficiencies

Anemia, one of the major global nutrition concerns, is caused by a deficiency in iron and is associated with other nutrient deficiencies including vitamins A, B6, and B12; riboflavin; and folic acid.[9] General infections, chronic diseases, malaria, and helminth infestation can also contribute to developing anemia.

Iodine deficiency disorder (IDD) is a public health problem in 130 countries and affects about 13% of the world's population.[10] Globally, about 740 million people are affected by goiter and over 2 billion are considered at risk for IDD. The major consequence of IDD is impaired development of the fetal brain. Iodization of salt in the 1940s has been one of the most successful food fortification initiatives, but many countries lack access to this resource.

Zinc is a vital micronutrient for body function. Deficiency of zinc, which is essential for DNA and protein synthesis, can lead to growth failure in children. Subclinical zinc deficiency has been

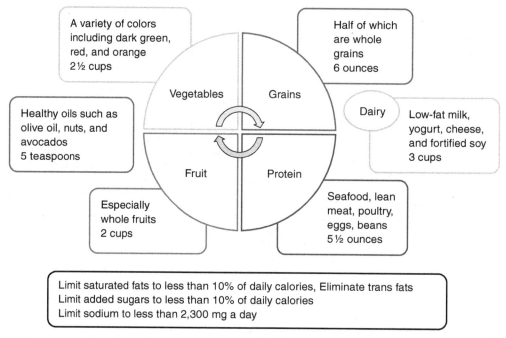

FIGURE 14.1 A healthy eating pattern for an average U.S. adult, 2,000 calories a day.

recognized as a significant limiting factor for growth among children in both developing and developed countries.[11]

Clinical vitamin A deficiency (VAD) affects over 2 million preschool children in over 60 countries and subclinical VAD is considered a problem for at least 250 million school-aged children and pregnant women. VAD has been shown to increase morbidity and mortality rates and to contribute to delayed growth and is the leading cause of blindness in children.

Infectious and Communicable Disease

The burden of infectious diseases coincides with malnutrition, recognized as "the primary cause of immunodeficiency worldwide."[12] Undernutrition is immunosuppressive and contributes to spread of **communicable diseases**, infectious diseases that are contagious. Protein deficiency (kwashiorkor) was historically believed to be the predominant basis of malnutrition. Severe protein deficiency bears a definite relationship to antibody formation and development of the immune system in infants and children. The immunosuppressive effect of undernutrition starts during intrauterine life, as maternal nutrition impacts immune function of the offspring. The top infectious diseases include:

Tuberculosis (TB) is caused by the bacterium *Mycobacterium tuberculosis,* which affects the lungs. Globally, it is estimated that 10 million people developed TB in 2018, a number that has remained relatively stable. The highest burden of disease is in adult men, accounting for 57% of all TB cases in 2018. Adult women accounted for 32% and children 11% of cases worldwide in 2018. Drug-resistant TB is a public health crisis and it is estimated that 500,000 people who developed TB in 2018 were resistant to rifampicin and 78% of them had multi-drug-resistant TB. Nearly 1.7 billion people, 23% of the world population, have latent TB infection and are at risk of developing active TB in their lifetime.[13]

HIV infection impairs the immune system, increasing susceptibility to opportunistic infections, weight loss, fever, and diarrhea. HIV-positive patients are 26 to 31 times more likely to develop active TB. Prevalence of HIV-TB infection is greatest in Africa. According to the Global Tuberculosis 2019 report, TB caused an estimated 1.2 million deaths among HIV-negative people and an additional 251,000 deaths among HIV-positive people.[13] HIV-positive individuals also have reduced appetite and an impaired ability to absorb food. One of the most concerning nutritional impacts of HIV infection is the emergence of severe weight loss and muscle wasting. Severe malnutrition is seen in advanced stages of HIV infection.

Neglected tropical diseases are a diverse group of diseases that thrive mainly among the poorest populations in tropical and subtropical conditions, often seen in populations without adequate sanitation and in close contact with infectious vectors, domestic animals, and livestock. WHO has publicized 17 neglected tropical diseases, which are endemic in 149 countries and affect more than 1 billion people with infested water. Soil-transmitted helminthiases are the most common parasitic infection, caused by nematode infections transmitted through oral–fecal transmission. Nematodes (e.g., hookworm, whipworm, roundworm) can cause anemia, vitamin A deficiency, stunted growth, malnutrition, intestinal obstruction, and impaired development. The parasitic burden in a person can cause undernutrition due to lack of appetite, poor intake due to food contamination, and an increased metabolic rate. Nutrient losses occur from vomiting, intestinal bleeding, diarrhea, and reduced absorption of nutrients. Secondary outcomes, such as reducing anemia and zinc and iodine deficiency have been observed. Key prevention strategies include proper hygiene, sanitation, and vaccination.

Acute respiratory infections are the leading cause of death in children under 5 years of age, with nearly 1 million documented deaths in 2018. Pneumonia is the most frequent infection and is caused by bacteria, viruses, and fungi.[126]

Diarrheal diseases are generally caused by poor hygiene, inadequate sanitation, and contaminated water. The most common bacterial infections are due to *Escherichia coli* (*E. coli*), *Vibrio*, *Salmonella*, *Shigella*, and *Clostridioides difficile* (*C. diff*); viral infections include rotavirus and protozoa like *Cryptosporidium* and *Giardia*. WHO estimates that diarrheal diseases affect 1.7 billion people annually and they constitute one of the leading causes of malnutrition in children.[126]

Measles causes over 135,000 deaths each year, despite being completely preventable by vaccine. The most vulnerable populations are pregnant women and children under 5 years of age, those with suppressed immune systems, and those with vitamin A deficiency.[127] Some of the most severe consequences of measles include dehydration, diarrhea, blindness, and respiratory infections.

Malaria occurs in two forms, caused by *Plasmodium falciparum* and *P. vivax*. There are over 2 million cases of malaria each year. From 2010 to 2016, malaria deaths were cut by 25% across the globe. However, in 2018, an estimated 228 million cases were reported and an estimated 405,000 people died, specifically impacting young children in sub-Saharan Africa.[128]

Between 1990 and 2017, early death from diarrhea, typhoid fevers, intestinal infections, respiratory infections, and tuberculosis, and maternal and neonatal disorders decreased globally, with the greatest declines in the least developed countries. According to the 2011–2020 WHO action plan, a global push to improve vaccine coverage resulted in a 79% reduction in deaths. As of 2015, global coverage of vaccines was 37% (129 countries) and 23% (84 countries) for pneumococcal and rotavirus. By 2025, WHO and UNICEF aim to reduce child mortality rates from pneumonia to 3/1,000 and from diarrhea to 1/1,000 of all live births.[129]

Overnutrition and Disease

Progress in reducing global mortality rates from disease has stalled or reversed primarily owing to an increase in **noncommunicable diseases (NCDs)**. Overweight and obesity are modifiable risk factors for NCDs including type 2 diabetes mellitus, cardiovascular disease, chronic respiratory disease, and cancers. Obesity is the top risk factor that contributes to disability-adjusted life years globally, even among high-income countries.[14] In 2016, NCDs accounted for 72.3% of all deaths globally and almost half (42%) of NCD deaths are premature (occurring before the age of 70).[15,16]

Factors Influencing Overnutrition

Poor diets are driving overnutrition and are a significant cause of death and disability worldwide. Although the importance of fruits and vegetables is recognized, 87% of the population consume too few vegetables and 75% do not meet the goal for recommended fruit intake.[17] On average, too many processed foods that contain high fructose corn syrup and added fats are consumed, characterizing the Western pattern diet (WPD) or standard American diet (SAD) that includes high intake of red and processed meats, packaged foods, butter, fried foods, high-fat dairy, corn, refined grains, and potatoes (Figure 14.2).[18]

Dietary consumption is influenced by the food system in which food is grown, harvested, processed, distributed, prepared, marketed, and disposed of in addition to nutritional, social, environmental,

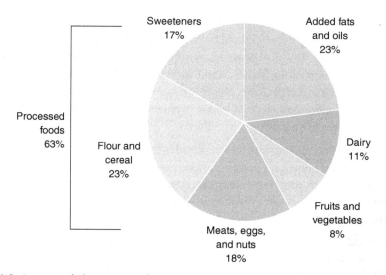

FIGURE 14.2 Average daily percent of calories in the standard American diet.

Source: From Hiza H, Casavale K, Guenther P, Davis C. Diet quality of Americans differs by age, sex, race/ethnicity, income, and education level. *J Acad Nutr Diet.* 2012;113(2):297–306. doi:10.1016/j.jand.2012.08.011

and economic drivers. Access to healthy, nutrient-dense food is identified as a leading challenge to sufficient intake.[19] Obesogenic food environments include "the sum of influences that the surroundings, opportunities, or conditions of life have on promoting obesity in individuals or populations," offering easy access to fast food restaurants and processed foods.[20] Consumers also report price as a primary challenge to adequate consumption.[21] Studies conducted in India show that income inequality had the same effect on the risk of being overweight as it did on being underweight.[22]

Assessing Overnutrition

Overweight and obesity are defined differently for each age group. Children under 5 years of age are not typically defined as being overweight or obese, as they are still growing and the child should maintain growth along the percentile trajectory. For school-age children and adolescents (ages 5 to 19 years), being overweight indicates having a **body mass index (BMI)** for age >1 standard deviation above the WHO growth reference standard median, whereas obesity is defined as having a BMI for age more than 2 standard deviations above. In the case of adults, overweight is a BMI ≥25 (except for Asian ethnicities); and obesity is a BMI ≥30.

Cultural competency is an important consideration when assessing and diagnosing NCDs. For example, there is a high prevalence of diabetes and cardiovascular disease in parts of Asia, where the average BMI is below 25, the typical threshold for overweight. South Asians tend to have less muscle and more abdominal fat compared to white Europeans, so the same BMI may represent a higher percentage of body fat in Asians. This highlights the limitations of BMI for assessing adiposity and cardio-metabolic risk. As diabetes may occur at lower BMIs in Asian populations, WHO has suggested a lower BMI cut-off point.[23] The traditional overweight range is 25.0 to 29.9 kg/m², whereas for Asian populations, there is an increased risk of cardiovascular disease when BMI is between 23.0 and 27.4 kg/m². For obesity, the traditional range is >30 kg/m² but for Asian populations it is >27.5 kg/m². Ethnic cut-off points have also been suggested for waist circumference.[24] Incorporating BMI and waist circumference cut-off points that are culturally sensitive into screening programs may help reduce the diabetes burden on these populations.

Overweight and Obesity

The **obesogenic culture** has spread worldwide, leading to adult BMI rising steadily by 2 percentage points per decade. Although undernutrition is still more prevalent than overnutrition among children, the opposite will be true by 2022 if increasing trends continue at their current rate.[25]

While Asia and Africa have the lowest overweight prevalence, together they accounted for nearly three-fourths of all overweight children under the age of 5. Oceania is an example of a region where the population is affected by the double burden of malnutrition, with high prevalence of both acute malnutrition (wasting) and overweight. China has more than 10,000 American-based fast-food restaurants (such as McDonald's) and increasing obesity rates that surpass 20% in some cities. An estimated 160 million Americans are either obese or overweight, accounting for nearly 30% of boys and girls under the age of 20 (Figure 14.3).[26] In 2016, nearly 40% of U.S. adults were obese, costing an estimated US\$147 billion annually. The medical cost for those with obesity is nearly US\$1,500 higher a year than for those of normal weight.[27]

Type 2 Diabetes

The International Diabetes Federation's projection of increases in worldwide adult type 2 diabetes showed the greatest rise between 2017 and 2045 to be in Southeast Asia (84% increase), the

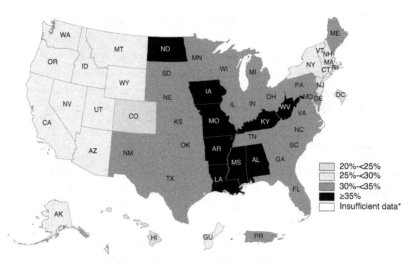

FIGURE 14.3 Prevalence* of self-reported obesity among U.S. adults by state and territory, Behavioral Risk Factor Surveillance System (BRFSS), 2017.

*Prevalence estimates reflect BRFSS methodological changes started in 2011. These estimates should not be compared to prevalence estimates before 2011.

Note: Sample size <50 or the relative standard error (dividing the standard error by the prevalence) ≥30%.

Source: Centers for Disease Control and Prevention. *Data & Statistics: Adult Obesity Facts.* 2018. https://www.cdc.gov/obesity/data/prevalence-maps.html

Middle East and North Africa (110% increase), and Africa (156% increase).[28] Type 2 diabetes occurs when the body does not produce enough insulin (a hormone that regulates blood sugar levels) or resists the effects of insulin, lacking the ability to maintain normal blood sugar levels. Primary risk factors include overweight and obesity, fat distribution in the abdomen, inactivity, family history, race (black, Hispanic, Asian), and age. It is managed with medication and typically can be cured through lifestyle changes including a healthy diet and physical activity.

Cardiovascular Disease

Referring to conditions that involve narrowed or blocked blood vessels, cardiovascular disease includes heart attack, chest pain (angina), and stroke. Heart damage or atherosclerosis, buildup of fatty plaque in the arteries, contributes to artery stiffening and inhibits the flow of blood to organs and tissues. Common causes are an unhealthy diet, overweight and obesity, smoking, stress, and lack of physical activity. It is the leading cause of death for both men and women and one in four Americans die of cardiovascular disease annually.[29]

Respiratory Disease

Nutrition plays a critical role in both preventing and managing certain respiratory diseases, including chronic obstructive pulmonary disease (COPD) and asthma. Maintaining a healthy weight is important.[30] For many, breathing is unconscious and effortless; however, for those with respiratory diseases, breathing requires a conscious effort and an increase in energy requirements. Unintentional weight loss can also be due to difficulty swallowing or chewing, mouth breathing that can alter the taste of food, coughing, fatigue, chronic mucus production, depression, or medication side effects.[31]

Cancer

According to WHO, between 30% and 50% of cancers can be prevented by proper nutrition. Cancer treatments, such as chemotherapy, radiation therapy, and surgery can contribute to side effects that impact appetite, leading to unintentional weight loss. Focusing on protein to support muscle strengthening and resisting infections, carbohydrates to sustain energy, and healthy fats to promote heart health, in combination with treatments, is helpful. Water consumption is vital to replenish healthy cell growth.[32]

Malnutrition in all forms can lead to serious negative health consequences. The development of vaccines and decreasing undernutrition have led to significant improvements such as declining trends in communicable diseases, such as infections and neonatal disorders; however, there has been a rapid increase in NCDs such as obesity, diabetes, cardiovascular disease, and cancers worldwide. Children who are overweight are at a higher risk of obesity, related diseases, and early death. Obtaining proper nutrition through a high intake of fruits, vegetables, and whole grains is essential in accelerating progress toward good health.

MATERNAL, INFANT, AND CHILD HEALTH

Maternal and Child Health Trends

Despite numerous advances and improvements in maternal and child health, malnutrition remains a significant challenge. Nearly half of all deaths in children under the age of 5 is attributed to poor nutrition.[4] Improving nutrition during the critical first 1,000 days, from conception to the child's second birthday, has the potential to save lives and allow millions of children to develop fully and thrive.

Micronutrient deficiency is a major contributor to malnutrition and the impact is more devastating in children, especially young infants. The condition of maternal and childhood undernutrition includes a wide array of consequences:

- Poor fetal growth, intrauterine growth restriction (IUGR) resulting in low birth weight;
- Stunting, a chronic restriction of growth in height indicated by short stature;
- Wasting, characterized by acute weight loss indicated by low weight-for-height; and
- Less visible micronutrient deficiencies.[122]

Stunting and wasting cause irreparable harm by impeding physical growth, significantly increasing the risk of chronic disease. Children who are stunted or born with IUGR have been shown to complete fewer years of schooling and earn less income as adults, hindering their cognitive growth and economic potential. Lower income, poor health, and reduced access to proper nutrition continue to impact the health of children born into future generations, establishing a repetitive cycle. The most prevalent diseases due to childhood micronutrient deficiencies are:

> *Anemia.* According to a systematic review of 23 nationally representative surveys, 37% of nonpregnant women and 24% of school children worldwide have anemia caused by a deficiency of iron.[33] In young children, the peak prevalence occurs around 18 months of age and then falls as iron requirements decline and iron intake is increased through complementary foods. Women of child-bearing age are at high risk for negative iron balance because of blood loss during menstruation and the substantial needs for iron during pregnancy.

Iodine deficiency disorder impairs motor and mental development of the fetus and increases risk of miscarriage and fetal growth restriction. Maternal supplementation with iodine improves pregnancy outcomes, and neurological and cognitive development of the infant.[34] Breast milk iodine content is very low in areas of endemic iodine deficiency, exacerbating depletion in infants. A meta-analysis showed that populations with chronic iodine deficiency have a 13.5-point reduction in IQ scores.[35]

Zinc deficiency disorder. Zinc is a vital micronutrient for body function and growth and is essential for DNA, protein synthesis, and several metalloenzymes. It is estimated that one third of the world population lives in countries with a high prevalence of zinc deficiency, resulting in increased risk of diarrhea, pneumonia, and malaria in children.[36,37]

Neural tube defects. Folic acid protects unborn babies against serious birth defects and can prevent against early pregnancy loss. Sources include leafy green vegetables, oranges, and beans and in fortified breads, pastas, and cereals. A prenatal vitamin is recommended for all women of childbearing age.[38]

Rickets. Vitamin D deficiency in utero can cause poor fetal growth and skeletal mineralization, and is followed by lower concentrations of vitamin D in breast milk. An estimated 35% to 80% of children in countries such as Turkey, India, Egypt, China, Libya, and Lebanon are vitamin D deficient owing to the practice of shrouding, avoidance of skin exposure to sunlight, and foods not being fortified with vitamin D.[39] A combination of vitamin D and calcium deficiency is recognized as the main cause of rickets.

Additional micronutrient deficiencies. Clinical VAD affects at least 2.8 million preschool children in more than 60 countries.[40] Children with shigellosis can lose a significant amount of vitamin A in the urine, thus further contributing to VAD. In women with malnutrition, the content of vitamin B12 in breast milk can be so low that symptoms of deficiency appear in their breast-fed infants, including failure to thrive, stunting, poor neurocognitive function, and global developmental delays. A supplement containing vitamins B, C, and E can decrease the prevalence of IUGR.

Factors Influencing Nutritional Status

Major contributing factors for undernutrition are prolonged and recurrent diarrhea, poor dietary intake, suboptimal breastfeeding, and low socioeconomic status. In recent years, the association of increased micronutrient losses, such as zinc and copper, with severe diarrhea has been well recognized. The risk of micronutrient deficiency in infancy and early childhood can also be compounded by the presence of low body stores from birth and poor complementary feeding practices. Thus, poor intake of complementary foods, as well as selection of unhealthy foods, may lead to iron and zinc deficiencies.

Poverty and socioeconomic inequity remain important factors in the presence of micronutrient deficiency. Among children 4 years of age and younger, food insecurity is associated with fair or poor health and puts children at risk for developmental delays.[41] Low-resource households are shown to have lower intakes of meat and dairy products and higher intake of cereal-based diets with poor iron and zinc bioavailability.

Drug Addiction and Substance Abuse

Addictive disorders have severe nutritional deficiencies and are linked with blood-borne diseases, including HIV infection and hepatitis C, that can exacerbate malnutrition. Although the United

States has only 5% of the world population, Americans consume nearly 80% of the world's opioid supply, with the highest rates seen among young adults (18–25 years old).[42] The prevalence of misuse is also higher in Europe, as well as Southwest and Central Asia (Iran, Pakistan, and Afghanistan), than the global average. Research shows an overlap between opioid misuse, opioid use disorder (OUD), and heroin use, contributing to malnutrition and death.[43]

One of the most vulnerable populations for OUD are pregnant women and neonates. The proportion of U.S. babies born with neonatal abstinence syndrome (NAS) increased fivefold from 2000 to 2012, disproportionately impacting rural and low-resource communities.[44] More than 86% of pregnancies conceived by women with OUD are unintended, compared with 31% of pregnancies in the general population.[45] NAS is characterized by excessive crying, increased muscle tone, tremors, and sleep disturbances in addition to significant gastrointestinal dysfunction including poor feeding, poor sucking and swallowing, vomiting, diarrhea, and weight loss.

A comprehensive treatment for OUD in pregnant women that includes medication-assisted therapy and proper nutrition is critical for limiting the effects of NAS on unborn children. Breastfeeding is protective against illicit drug use and increases maternal confidence; thus, breastfed infants are less likely to need pharmacologic treatment for NAS. During treatment and detoxification programs, unintentional weight loss, vitamin D deficiency, and protein deprivation are commonly observed in women. Increasing dietary intake of protein and reducing simple carbohydrates can help with treatment. Malabsorption of vitamins and minerals can also occur and a multivitamin that includes zinc, iron, calcium, vitamin D, chromium, potassium, magnesium, and other essential nutrients should be prescribed. Zinc helps with improving immune system and proper brain function; calcium and magnesium will reduce the incidence of nervous and muscular disorders that are common among this population.[46]

Child Nutrition

All newborns should be breastfed within 1 hour after birth ("kangaroo care"), exclusively breastfed for the first 6 months of life, and continue breastfeeding up to the second year of life. Recent reviews have shown that a lack of breastfeeding has led to a 47% to 157% increase in mortality rate in 6- to 11-month-old and 12- to 23-month-old children, respectively.[47] In Africa, Asia, Latin America, and the Caribbean, only 47% to 57% of infants younger than 2 months are breastfed.

Even with optimal breastfeeding, children will become stunted and malnourished if they do not receive an adequate quantity and quality of complementary foods after 6 months of age. Most stunting and wasting happens in the first 2 years of life when children have a high demand for nutrients and there are limitations in the diet. Children under the age of 2 also have a high rate of infectious diseases, which can adversely affect growth and nutritional status.

Prenatal nutritional environments are associated with the child's risk of developing cardiovascular disease, type 2 diabetes, and obesity in adulthood.[48] Studies show that offspring of pregnant women during famine had a lower birth weight and were predisposed to NCDs. Famine in early gestation increases the risk of cardiovascular disease, dyslipidemia, and obesity. Famine during midgestation increased microalbuminuria and renal function disorders. Famine in late gestation enhances the risk of type 2 diabetes. Malnourished conditions in fetal life with poor growth in utero (IUGR) lead to impaired glucose and energy metabolism, including enhanced production of hepatic glucose, decreased insulin sensitivity for muscle protein synthesis, and impaired pancreatic development.

Adolescent Nutrition

Adolescent nutrition is relevant to maternal nutrition, as pregnancies in adolescents have a higher risk of complications and higher mortality rate in mothers and poorer birth outcomes than pregnancies in older women.[49] Pregnancy in adolescence can also slow and stunt a girl's growth. There are 1.2 billion adolescents (10–19 years old) in the world, 90% of whom live in low- and middle-income countries where fertility rates are significantly higher. Additionally, adolescent fertility is three times higher in low- and middle-income countries.

Maternal Nutrition

Maternal obesity can lead to adverse maternal and fetal complications during pregnancy, delivery, and the postpartum period.[50] Obese pregnant women (prepregnant BMI >30 kg/m^2) are four times more likely to develop gestational diabetes mellitus and two times more likely to develop preeclampsia compared with women of a normal BMI (BMI 18.5–24.9 kg/m^2). During labor and delivery, maternal obesity is associated with maternal death, hemorrhage, cesarean delivery, or infection and a higher risk of neonatal and infant death, birth trauma, and infant macrosomia.[51]

Maternal undernutrition, including chronic energy and micronutrient deficiencies, is prevalent around the world. In some countries, more than 10% of women have BMI ranges from 10% to 19%. With a prevalence of low BMI in about 40% of women, the situation is considered critical in India, Bangladesh, and Eritrea. Maternal short stature is a risk factor for cesarean delivery, largely related to cephalopelvic disproportion. A meta-analysis of epidemiological studies found a 60% (95% CI [confidence interval] 50–70) increased need for assisted delivery among women in the lowest quartile of stature (146 cm–157 cm) compared to women in the highest quartile. Maternal undernutrition has little effect on the volume of composition of breast milk unless malnutrition is severe. The concentration of some micronutrients (vitamin A, iodine, thiamin, riboflavin, pyridoxine, and cobalamin) in breast milk is dependent on maternal status and intake, so the risk of infant depletion is increased by maternal deficiency. Maternal supplementation of these micronutrients increases the amount secreted in breast milk and can improve infant status.

Intervention Coverage Trends

There is a direct need to scale-up interventions that directly impact the nutritional status of women and children. Many of the highest impact interventions are found within the first 1,000 days and several contribute to achieving multiple targets (Table 14.2).

The double burden of undernutrition and overnutrition is increasingly a challenge for women of childbearing age. Undernutrition undermines the survival and growth of children, while obesity doubles the risk for complications including preeclampsia, gestational diabetes, and chronic disease for both mom and baby later in life. Appropriate nutrition assessment, intervention, and management are necessary for all women of childbearing age, specifically adolescent girls. Investments in nutrition interventions alone are not enough to reach the goals of healthy development; improvements in water and sanitation, agriculture, women's health, and education are also necessary to accelerate progress.

HEALTH PROMOTION FOR YOUNG ADULTS, SPECIFICALLY COLLEGE AND UNIVERSITY STUDENTS

Undergraduate college years are considered a critical transitional period for most traditional college students, especially in relation to health behaviors and consequences, as individuals begin to

TABLE 14.2 GLOBAL MATERNAL AND CHILD HEALTH INTERVENTIONS

INTERVENTION AND TARGET ADDRESSED	DESCRIPTION AND ASSUMPTIONS
For pregnant women and mothers of infants	
Micronutrient supplementation for pregnant women (stunting, anemia)	Includes iron and folic acid supplementation, and at least one additional micronutrient for approximately 180 days of pregnancy. Delivered as part of antenatal care.
Promotion of good infant and young child nutrition and hygiene practices (stunting, exclusive breastfeeding)	Individual or group-based counseling sessions to promote exclusive breastfeeding (0–5 months of age) and continued breastfeeding, and timely introduction and appropriate quality and quantity of complementary foods for children (6–24 months of age).
Balanced protein-energy supplementation (stunting)	Nutritional supplementation during pregnancy for pregnant women living under the poverty line (US$1.25/day). Delivered through existing community, health facility, or social safety net programs.
Intermittent preventive treatment for malaria in pregnancy (stunting, anemia)	Two doses of sulfadoxine-pyrimethamine for pregnant women (in malaria endemic areas only) delivered as part of antenatal care.
For infants and young children	
Vitamin A supplementation for children (stunting)	Two doses per year for children 6–59 months old delivered through mass campaigns.
Prophylactic zinc supplementation (stunting)	120 packets of zinc (10 mg/day) per child per year for children 6–59 months old. Delivered through community mechanisms similar to multiple micronutrient supplementation.
Public provision of complementary foods (stunting, wasting)	Supplemental foods for children 6 to 23 months of age, living under the poverty line delivered through community-based nutrition programs or existing social safety net programs.
Treatment of severe acute malnutrition (SAM; severe wasting)	Treatment of SAM with ready-to-use therapeutic foods (RUTF) in children 6 to 59 months of age with weight-for-height below 3 SD or MUAC <115 mm. Outpatient treatment for uncomplicated cases and inpatient treatment (in the stabilization phase) for patients with complications.
For women of reproductive age	
Iron and folic acid supplementation for nonpregnant women (anemia)	Weekly supplementation of 60 mg iron + 0.4 g folic acid delivered through public provision via schools, community health workers, hospitals, and private distribution for women above the poverty line.
For the general population	
Staple food fortification (anemia)	Fortification of wheat and maize flour as well as rice with iron and folic acid, and distributed through the marketplace.
Pro-breastfeeding social policies (exclusive breastfeeding)	Policies, legislation, and monitoring, and enforcement of policies related to the International Code of Marketing of Breast Milk Substitutes and subsequent resolutions, WHO Ten Steps integration into hospital accreditation, and maternity protection/leave.
National breastfeeding promotion campaign (exclusive breastfeeding)	Large scale efforts and use of mass media to promote breastfeeding.

MUAC, mid-upper arm circumference; SD, standard deviation.
Source: Adapted from Shekar M, Kakietek J, D'Alimonte M, et al. *Investing in Nutrition from the Foundation of Development.* The World Bank Group. http://documents.worldbank.org/curated/en/963161467989517289/pdf/104865-REVISED-Investing-in-Nutrition-FINAL.pdf

gain autonomy in lifestyle choices with less parental influence. Students transitioning into college life often undergo major lifestyle changes, including dietary behaviors, that can positively or negatively affect their physical and mental health. As this transitional stage is unique to young adults in college settings, it is important to discuss this population's health trends and influential factors on their health and nutritional statuses, independent of the broader adult population.

College and University Health Trends

According to the American College Health Association National College Health Assessment (ACHA-NCHA), 37% of college students ($n = 54,497$) were *overweight or obese* in 2019.[52] The obesity epidemic comes with an increased risk for developing chronic diseases, including type 2 diabetes and heart disease.[53] Proper nutrition is vital to achieving good physical, mental, and emotional development during young adulthood (18–25 years of age); however, nearly all college students report overnutrition, consuming the standard American diet, which includes less than five servings of fruits and vegetables per day.

In addressing overweight and obesity in young adults, it is important to be mindful of *disordered eating*. Nearly 20% of college students, both male and female, report an eating disorder. Increase in workload, less structure, and more focus on peers collide with anxiety, learning challenges, and poor self-esteem to create a "perfect storm" for eating disorders in this population. The most common disorders are *anorexia*, an emotional disorder characterized by an obsessive desire to lose weight by refusing to eat; *binge eating disorder*, characterized by recurrent binge-eating without any behaviors to counter the effects of overeating; and *bulimia*, a distortion of body image in which bouts of extreme overeating are followed by self-induced vomiting, purging, or fasting. Initiatives that promote healthy body image are becoming popular on campuses, such as *The Body Project,* a national group-based intervention that provides a forum for individuals to confront unrealistic beauty ideals.

College counseling centers recognize psychological problems, such as *stress, anxiety,* and *depression,* as a significant and growing concern on their campuses, leading to poor health among this population. Nearly all students report having some level of stress (98%) and 88% felt overwhelmed, 14% had seriously considered suicide, and 10% self-harmed themselves in the past 12 months.[52] Stress-related problems impact student well-being and academic performance, as numerous research studies show a link between poor mental health and overnutrition. Additionally, *sleep deprivation* (averaging under 6 hours a night) is associated with mental health problems and malnutrition in young adults.

Barriers to Achieving Good Health

Lifestyle Factors

Modifiable lifestyle factors contribute to malnutrition and poor health among college students, including unhealthy eating habits, excessive alcohol consumption or binge drinking, and physical inactivity.[54] Maintaining healthy eating habits as part of the daily routine is a common challenge for all age groups, but it is shown to be particularly challenging for young adults and college students. College students experience unhealthy lifestyle choices as they transition from adolescence to young adulthood, learning to manage social life, basic needs, finances, and coursework with less influence from parents or guardians. According to the American Heart Association and College of Sports Medicine, 150 minutes of moderate-intensity or 75 minutes of vigorous-intensity physical activity per week is recommended for young adults. However, only 46% of students met those recommendations, while 27% consumed five or more alcoholic beverages in one sitting at least once in the past 2 weeks.[52] Excessive calorie intake from binge drinking with the lack of physical activity can result in an unhealthy weight gain that exacerbates the overall health and well-being of college students.

Financial Hardship

The U.S. Government Accountability Office (GAO) estimates a nearly twofold increase in an average in-state net price (tuition, room, and board) for a full-time undergraduate student at public 4-year institutions over the past 30 years; while there was also an increase in the number of students from households with an income at or below 130% of the **poverty level**.[55] With the increase in cost of attendance, student loans are heavily relied upon to pay tuition and the critical expenses of basic needs, such as food, housing, medical care, and transportation.[56] Moreover, the least expensive campus dining plans in many universities are more expensive than the official USDA Thrifty Food Plan (US$1.79 per meal), recognized as the most affordable food plan by the USDA. These economic conditions, along with failures in built environment, such as transportation difficulties, place a significant financial burden on college students' ability to maintain good health.

Food and Nutrition Insecurity

A 2016 comprehensive survey of college students at 34 community colleges and 4-year colleges in 12 states found that 48% qualified as food insecure. Of those surveyed, 22% were identified as hungry, meaning they experienced very low food security.[57] Additionally, a recent study of 33,000 college students in seven states (Louisiana, Pennsylvania, New York, California, New Jersey, Wisconsin, and Wyoming) found that 9% of students experienced homelessness in the past year.[58] Food insecurity is linked with both age and ethnicity. Additionally, students who received need-based financial assistance were more likely to experience food insecurity, and childhood food insecurity was the most significant risk factor for college food insecurity.[59]

Food insecure students often experience difficulty concentrating, both in and out of class, and college food insecurity can undermine the educational success of many students, often leading to poor academic performance, increased rates of attrition, and delayed graduation.[56,59,60] Research at the University of Massachusetts, Boston, found that 80% of respondents indicated that food insecurity impacted their class performance and 25% reported dropping a class because of finances.[61]

As a means of coping with the overwhelming burden from various financial demands, students who are food insecure consume inexpensive, processed, energy-dense foods with significantly reduced amount of fruits, vegetables, legumes, dairy, and calcium compared to their counterparts.[62] Many food insecure college students downsize and/or skip meals to stretch their meal budget, resulting in unmet nutritional needs for individuals to sustain a healthy, active life.[59] As a result of these nutritional shortfalls, students commonly experience physical health problems, such as reduced energy levels, headaches, and fatigue along with mental health problems including irritability, anger, stress, and depression (see Box 14.1).

Limited knowledge in nutrition and meal planning along with lack of confidence in food preparation may also present a challenge to many college students.[63] Based on the ACHA-NCHA II survey, 48% of students did not receive any nutrition-related information and 67.3% desired such information from their universities. Knowledge and confidence in healthy nutrition practices,

BOX 14.1

EXAMPLE FROM THE FIELD: TIGHT BUDGET AND LACK OF HEALTHY FOOD LEADS TO POOR HEALTH FOR COLLEGE STUDENTS

As a first-generation college student, Kaira never knows if she is going to be able to afford the basic necessities of college—books, housing, and food. She received a scholarship that covers the full cost of tuition but quickly learned that this amount would not be enough.

Kaira is trying to figure out how to make ends meet and budget for the first time. Her family is "middle-class" and when applying for the FAFSA (the Federal Student Aid Form that qualifies students for federal grants, loans, or work-study programs based on need), she learned that her parents make too much money to receive financial assistance. On top of tuition, Kaira still had to pay more than US$4,000 per semester to live in the residence hall and US$1,500 for a meal plan, amounting to an additional US$11,000 per year. Additionally, she needed to pay for books, additional course fees, laundry, professional clothing, conferences, printer paper, and a number of other unanticipated charges. Her parents were able to cover half of those costs, leaving her with no choice but to work part-time. Sometimes, it was not enough to pay all the necessary expenses and she had to borrow short-term loans from Cash Advance. Kaira was glad she did not to have a car on campus as the price of the parking pass and gas would have made things even tighter. However, having no car and using unreliable public transportation made it harder for her to buy groceries, including healthy foods that are not accessible on campus. Furthermore, she did not have a lot of time in between classes, extracurricular activities, and her part-time job.

Cooking in the residence hall kitchen facility and planning meals was also new to her. As her first year progressed, she found herself skipping dinner, breakfast, and sometimes both, based on what she could afford with her meal plan. Sometimes, she chose to eat cheap, processed foods because it was convenient for her schedule, especially with limited hours of campus dining facilities. Kaira began to feel overwhelmed, irritated, and stressed, making it very difficult for her to concentrate on her studies. She had frequent headaches whenever she skipped meals and drank water to suppress hunger. During her first year, she started performing poorly in all her classes and the security of her scholarship was then threatened because of her low GPA. Kaira felt that, "I was letting my family down. I had worked so hard to earn scholarships so that the stress of finances was not an issue, but it still was." The stress of not being able to afford books and food, constant headaches from skipping meals, and depression led her to consider leaving the university after her first year.

such as meal planning and preparation, can improve students' ability to maintain healthy lifestyle practices including healthy eating habits and meal preparation.

Though nutrition plays an essential role in physical and mental health due to our body's needs for essential nutrients to maintain daily functions, it is often overlooked among college students. Young adults attending colleges and universities have an increased risk for malnutrition as they are navigating new responsibilities and many are paying bills, obtaining credit, and/or budgeting for the first time. Food and nutrition security at colleges and universities is interconnected with promoting psychological and physical well-being and academic development of all students. Integrating financial well-being, nutrition education, and mental health resources across campus will foster student well-being and success.

NUTRITIONAL NEEDS AND HEALTH CONDITIONS WHILE AGING

By the year 2050, the number of older adults, aged 65 and over, will exceed 1.2 billion and reach 22% of the world's population, outnumbering younger people worldwide.[64] Increased longevity in adults can largely be attributed to advances in healthcare and public health. In the first half of the 20th century, there were large improvements in infant and childhood health, contributing to an increase in average life expectancy from 65 to 72 years.[65] Maintaining good nutritional status is essential for sustaining health, functional independence, and obtaining a good quality of life.

Older Adult Nutrition Needs

Older adults experience changes in dietary needs as metabolism begins to slow and energy requirements decrease. A **nutrient-dense diet** is essential for achieving optimal health:

Water. The guidelines for water recommendations include the national standard of eight 8-ounce glasses per day. The less older adults drink, the less thirsty they become. A focus on encouraging fluid consumption will help ensure older adults have adequate water to maintain an appropriate body temperature, protect body organs and tissues, prevent constipation, lessen the burden on the kidneys, and absorb water-soluble vitamins and minerals. Adequate fluid can be achieved by offering water during the day by placing cups of water easily within reach.

Protein. Adults over the age of 65 have higher protein needs in order to maintain strong muscles, balance, and mobility. Protein naturally provides essential amino acids that the body needs, such as leucine, that preserves and rebuilds muscle. Excellent protein sources are beans and legumes, wild salmon, eggs, Greek yogurt, nuts, and seeds. Protein intake should be closely monitored by a healthcare team for those with impaired renal function.[66]

Carbohydrate. Foods containing carbohydrates supply energy to the body and fuel the brain and nervous system. Because many older adults can be impacted by constipation, fiber is essential for maintaining gut health and promoting regularity. It also helps lower the risk of heart disease and type 2 diabetes. Foods rich in fiber include whole grain breads and cereals, beans, lentils, sweet potatoes, prunes, and peas. Sugars naturally occur in many foods (fruit) and are added to processed foods and sweetened beverages. Older adults should focus on eating foods with naturally occurring sugars while avoiding added sugar.

Fat. Eating the right kind of fat is critical for maintaining a healthy heart. Attention should be placed on foods that are high in healthy fats while limiting foods with saturated and trans fats. Healthy, polyunsaturated, and monounsaturated fats can help to lower blood cholesterol levels and improve heart health. Saturated fats that should be limited occur naturally in many animal sources including fatty beef, pork, cream, butter, cheese, and other dairy products made from whole-fat milk.

Micronutrients. Older adults are at greater risk of micronutrient deficiencies, disproportionately impacting non-Hispanic, black, and low-income older adults (Table 14.3).[67]

Factors Influencing Nutritional Status

Physical Factors

As the body ages, physiological changes occur that can result in a decrease in nutrient and water intake, often referred to as the *anorexia of aging*. Taste and smell begin to decline, and many

TABLE 14.3 MICRONUTRIENT NEEDS OF OLDER ADULTS AND THEIR DIETARY SOURCES

MICRONUTRIENT	ROLE IN THE BODY	DIETARY SOURCES
Calcium and vitamin D	Maintain bone health	Three servings of calcium-rich foods or beverages a day, from fortified cereals, dark green leafy vegetables (that is, kale, spinach), milk, fortified plant beverages, calcium supplement or multivitamin with vitamin D
Vitamin B12	Maintains brain function and red blood cells	Lean meat, fish and seafood, fortified cereal, B12 supplement or multivitamin
Potassium	Maintains a healthy blood pressure (with low sodium intake)	Fruits (bananas, oranges, cantaloupes, apricots), vegetables (spinach, broccoli, potatoes, peas, mushrooms, cucumbers), beans, prepared foods with little or no added salt (add flavor with herbs and spices)

Source: Data from Weimer JR. Many elderly at nutritional risk. *USDA Food Rev.* 1997;20(1):42–48.

individuals experience a suppressed appetite due to delayed gastric emptying. Poor dentition may limit food choices to soft foods, and dry mouth (xerostomia) can make swallowing difficult.[68] Sensory decline decreases the enjoyment of food, leading to decreased variety and an increase in the use of salt and sugar to compensate for flavor.

Body water content decreases with age and many report a loss of sense of thirst.[69] Dehydration is associated with more hospital visits and contributes to impaired cognition, falling, and constipation.[70] In the United States the avoidable cost of hospitalizations due to dehydration is estimated at approximately US$1 billion annually.[71]

Individuals also become less physically active and many experience mobility constraints as they age. Physical inactivity can worsen quality of life, leading to poor mental health and premature death. Limited mobility can make it difficult to complete **activities of daily living (ADLs)**, such as walking and feeding oneself, and **instrumental activities of daily living (IADLs)**, such as driving, grocery shopping, and preparing meals.

Adults over the age of 70 experience changes in body composition, leading to an increase in fat mass and decrease in lean muscle mass.[72] Osteopenia is a normal loss of bone density that occurs with aging. The aging body becomes less efficient in utilizing and absorbing nutrients, contributing to higher levels of nutrient requirements in order to maintain adequate nutrition levels. Some medications may also inhibit the absorption of nutrients due to drug-nutrient interactions, most commonly impacting fluid and vitamin B12 levels.

Social Factors

Addressing **social determinants of health** (SDOH) is a critical component of promoting healthy aging. Encompassing the social, economic, and environmental factors that can affect health and quality of life, SDOH-related factors have significant implications for the ability of older adults to age in place and live independently. These factors include a stable income, affordable housing, safe neighborhoods, reliable transportation, social connectedness, adequate food and nutrition, and access to medical services.

Financial health is vital for the well-being of older adults. Many are nearing retirement or are already on a fixed income. Of adults surveyed by AARP aged 60 and above, 39% reported living in low-income households and 20% found it somewhat or very difficult to pay their monthly living expenses. Nearly 40% expressed concern about being able to stay in their home as they age.[73] Minority older adults, such as those with an African-American or Hispanic ethnicity, have higher rates of health problems, such as hypertension, diseases of the circulatory system, and diabetes, than do Whites.[74]

Those with *lower socioeconomic status* have reportedly poorer diets. As of 2017, 7.7% of older adults, or 5.5 million individuals, reported food insecurity and 22% report making trade-offs between food and other basic needs. While food may be available, older adults experience significant challenges in accessing affordable, healthy food. High medical expenses and the cost of housing can compete with available resources for food. Food purchased may not provide the nutrients necessary to maintain a good quality of life, and this population reports skipping meals often. Loss of mobility may affect their ability to utilize food in order to prepare balanced meals.

Social isolation is very common in the aging population and worsens the risk for developing other health conditions. More than one in five older adults report feeling lonely frequently or often. Those with lower incomes are at greater risk of being socially isolated and are almost twice as likely to report relationship dissatisfaction. This could be the result of living alone, lack of interactions with others during mealtime, and insufficient transportation.

Chronic Conditions and Disease Trends in Older Adults

The prevalence of chronic conditions among adults over 65 years of age is increasing due to high rates of obesity and diabetes. It is estimated that 91% of older adults have at least one chronic health condition and 77% have multiple chronic diseases.[75,76] The most common causes of death among older adults are *cancer* and *cardiovascular disease*. Over one third of all deaths are the result of heart disease, and hypertension is a major contributor that involves abnormally high blood pressure and is the most common chronic disease among adults over 65 years of age.[77]

The second most common chronic condition is *osteoarthritis*, associated with high levels of chronic pain and disability. More than half of the adults over the age of 85 have osteoarthritis, with women affected more commonly than men. Owing to high rates of obesity, the rate of severe hip and knee arthritis continues to increase as the overweight population ages. Treatments include pain management and joint replacement surgery, both with considerable risks. Osteoporosis, a severe weakening of bone density, is also common in adults 85 years of age and older, and bone density screening is recommended for women over age 65.

As the overweight population ages, the prevalence of *diabetes* among American older adults may increase more than 400% by 2050.[78] Diabetes is associated with cardiovascular disease, peripheral arterial disease, and peripheral neuropathy, contributing to diabetic foot ulcers and amputations. Regular examinations of the legs and feet are important to prevent amputations and manage ulcers. Managing diabetes should be individualized, as older adults are particularly at risk for hypoglycemia (low drops in blood sugar).

Older adults are at high risk for a stroke, marked by the lack of blood flow to the brain, and the fourth leading cause of death in the United States.[79] The most common type of stroke is ischemic and is caused by a blood clot or the narrowing of a blood vessel leading to the brain. A transient ischemic attack (TIA) is a "mini-stroke" and occurs when the symptoms only last a few minutes and then disappear. Older adults can lower their risk of stroke by controlling blood pressure, stopping smoking, effectively managing diabetes, getting regular exercise, and maintaining good cholesterol levels by eating healthy foods.

Approximately one in seven adults over the age of 50 suffer from *respiratory diseases* that restrict the flow of air out of the lungs. Common respiratory diseases are asthma and COPD, including emphysema and chronic bronchitis. Smoking is the leading cause of COPD; other factors include indoor and outdoor air pollution, low educational level, occupational hazards, and infections. There is a common misconception that shortness of breath is a normal part of aging and COPD often goes untreated. Early diagnosis and treatment can significantly improve the quality of life for aging adults. The best ways to avoid COPD are to lose weight and stop smoking.[80]

The rates of *dementia* may rise from 47 million in 2015 to 131 million in 2050, exceeding estimated costs of US$2 trillion worldwide.[81] Dementia is a decline in memory and commonly occurs in conjunction with other problems in language, mood, mental health, behavior, and decision-making, and can lead to an increased irritability, depression, and anxiety. The two most common types of dementia are Alzheimer's disease and vascular dementia, due to blockages in the brain's blood vessels. Dementia caused by infections, vitamin deficiencies, and medications can be improved and treatment should be started immediately. In addition, vitamin B12 intake and adequate hydration are protective factors against dementia.

Isolation, coupled with the change and loss experienced in older age, may lead to *depression*, a well-known cause of anorexia and weight loss. Later life can be a time of multiple losses through retirement, disability, and death of friends and family as well as changes in financial, social, and physical health. Approximately one in four older adults experience issues related to mental health, including both depression and anxiety.

Addressing Malnutrition to Achieve Optimal Nutritional Status

The National Health and Nutrition Examination Survey (NHANES) estimates that 16% of community-dwelling Americans older than 65 years consume fewer than 1,000 calories per day, placing them at high risk for undernutrition.[82] Undernutrition and unintentional weight loss can lead to a weakened immune system, infections, poor wound healing, higher risk of hospitalization, and increased risk of death. The loss of muscle mass, or sarcopenia, is attributed to inadequate protein intake and can lead to falls and fractures.

Individual Approaches

Improving nutritional status for aging individuals begins with assessing weight and functional status, dietary intake, medical history, and the current living situation (see Box 14.2). A *multidisciplinary health care team* is the most effective approach, including family members or caregivers. Obtaining an accurate assessment includes:

- Weight status including weight gain or loss, percent of change, and time period
- Learning if the individual is living independently, alone, with family or friends, or in an assisted living or skilled nursing facility
- Physical examination including dentition and ability to swallow, gastrointestinal and respiratory symptoms
- Mobility status including ability to complete ADLs and IADLS
- Cognitive and neurological conditions, such as depression, anxiety, or dementia
- Intake of food and fluids over a typical 24-hour period (24-hour dietary recall), meal preparation methods, and support for shopping for and preparing meals
- Medical history, including the presence of any chronic diseases
- Current use of medications, multivitamins, or supplements

BOX 14.2

EXAMPLE FROM THE FIELD: SIMPLE SOLUTIONS TO ADDRESSING MALNUTRITION IN OLDER ADULTS

An 85-year-old woman lives independently in a mobile home park. She has a 3-month history of intermittent abdominal pain, nausea, diarrhea, and gradual weight loss. Her daughter lives nearby and would prepare meals for her to warm in the microwave oven. The initial medical examination showed no underlying cause for the weight loss and abdominal symptoms. The patient was given medication for abdominal discomfort and was encouraged to add over-the-counter nutritional supplements to her daily diet. The patient's condition continued to decline. A referral led to a home visit by a case manager who discovered that the elderly woman's refrigerator was noisy and had been disturbing her sleep. The woman had attempted to address this problem by unplugging the refrigerator each evening at 8 pm when she prepared for bed. When informed of this situation, the family replaced the refrigerator, and the abdominal symptoms and weight loss subsided.[83]

Interventions for reversing malnutrition need to occur early. It can be effective to remove dietary restrictions, encourage the use of flavor enhancers, incorporate frequent small meals throughout the day, and offer liquid supplements between meals. While medications should not be considered as a primary treatment for malnutrition, adjusting to ones that do not have anorexia-producing side effects and using antidepressants that are appetite stimulating can be helpful. Social services assessments for the living situation can be essential.[84]

Community-Based Approaches

The United States offers a variety of health promotion programs and organizations for adults over the age of 60. The *National Council on Aging (NCOA)* "improve[s] the lives of millions of older adults, especially those who are struggling"[124] by providing services that promote well-being and maintain independence. The NCOA offers different programs across (a) social, (b) economic, (c) legal, and (d) nutrition services.

Meals on Wheels is an example of a well-known program that delivers fresh, healthy meals daily to home-bound adults and group feeding sites. Nearly 80% of low-income older adults are not receiving the home-delivered meals that they need. Operating in nearly every community in America, it addresses the challenges of malnutrition, hunger, and social isolation.

Health promotion services for older adults should be responsive to ethnic and socioeconomic diversity. Engaging the community in developing solutions is an effective strategy for developing approaches that are perceived as being accessible and acceptable by the aging population.[85] Participatory approaches that build trustful relationships include involving community health workers and members within marginalized groups. Services in disadvantaged areas can be more resource-demanding because of the time-consuming nature of both recruitment and delivery.

Older adults are exceptionally vulnerable to malnutrition and dehydration, and their negative effects on health. It is a common misconception that nutritional deficiencies are an inevitable consequence of aging. Consideration for nutrition status of older adults should be a routine part of caring for this population. Mealtime should be an enjoyable experience focused on social

BOX 14.3

EXAMPLE FROM THE FIELD: *INTERGENERATIONAL MENTORING PROGRAM* DECREASES ISOLATION AND ENCOURAGES HEALTHY EATING IN OLDER ADULTS

An *Intergenerational Mentoring Program* was established to promote healthy eating, community engagement, and environmental sustainability while focusing on improving social cohesion and food security in a community in Kentucky. One evening a week, a group of college students and older adults gather at a community center that is walking distance to the older adults' homes where they cook meals from recovered food. The older adults take a bag of groceries home that include fresh fruits and vegetables and dairy products. Of the older adults served, 92% expressed a decrease in isolation and 60% ate/drank more fruits, vegetables, whole grains, and water as a result of this program. Meal recipients shared, "I now eat better and made new friends." As a result of the program, the same group of older adults began weekly walks together and shared rides to the doctor and grocery store. The manager at the housing authority shared, "Most of the individuals that attend the program lived in the same building or next door to each other but they had never met one another. The relationships that the individuals built with one another is irreplaceable. They feel confident knowing that they have someone to turn to." The *Intergenerational Mentoring Program* effectively leveraged the power of the university to improve food security and health for older adults.

interaction and incorporating whole grains, fruits, vegetables, fish, nuts, lean proteins, and low-fat dairy while being mindful of the physical changes that occur with age. Identifying and treating nutrition issues early by listening to the challenges faced by older adults and understanding barriers to achieving optimal nutrition can increase longevity, promote good health, and foster independence (see Box 14.3).

MALNUTRITION, FOOD INSECURITY, AND HUNGER AND IMPLICATIONS FOR HEALTH

Health challenges and consequences associated with the double burden of malnutrition, food insecurity, and hunger are intrinsically linked and can be largely attributed to a failure of the **food system** in supplying affordable, accessible, and reliable *healthful food* for all. The 1945 Universal Declaration of Human Rights recognized the **Right to Food,** defined as the right to feed oneself with dignity, as a legal obligation under international law, thus recognizing that adequate food for health is not merely a promise to be met through charity but a right to be fulfilled through appropriate actions by governments and nonstate agencies.[86] The United Nations (UN) recognizes that, "[t]he right to adequate food is realized when every man, woman and child, alone or in community with others, have physical and economic access at all times to adequate food or means for its procurement."[125] This section connects the dots between malnutrition, food insecurity, and hunger and describes a framework for measuring and achieving food and nutrition security.

Food Security Framework

Food and nutrition security is multi-dimensional and comprises four essential components of (a) food *availability*, (b) food *access*, (c) food *utilization*, and (d) *stability*.[87]

Availability is an essential precursor for access, affordability, and utilization. As defined by the World Food Programme, "Food availability is the amount of food that is present in a country or area through all forms of domestic production, imports, food stocks and food aid."[88] Availability is dependent upon food and agricultural production in a region. Among the countries where adverse impacts of economic downturns on food security have been the strongest, the majority rely heavily on commodity exports and/or imports to supply food.

Access includes the physical, economic, and social means of obtaining food. Lack of physical access is illustrated by a scenario in which food is being produced, but not distributed appropriately, owing to inefficiency or lack of infrastructure. Market systems and community buying power are a vital component in considering the economics of food access as described, "Even in rural areas, most people, and especially the poor, rely on market systems to provide food and essential goods and services but also for selling their produce."[89] Specifically, urban, peri-urban, or rural low-resource communities have limited physical access to food because of a lack of full-service supermarkets or grocery stores. Finally, food may not be accessible to a particular social group or gender. For example, predominantly black or Hispanic neighborhoods are shown to have fewer full-service supermarkets than their White counterparts.[90]

Utilization is both the way in which the body makes use of the nutrients in the food and the household's food safety and preparation practices. Based on the World Food Summit, utilization includes having "safe, nutritious foods that meet dietary needs of all individuals."[91] Understanding healthy food selection, preparation, storage, and sanitation are needed to ensure adequate utilization. For example, food may be available or present in a country, as well as physically, socially, and economically accessible; however, if the household does not know how to cook healthy food, then food and nutrition insecurity may still exist.

Finally, *stability* of food availability, access, and utilization at all times is necessary to achieve nutrition security. Scenarios that can disrupt stability include poverty, unemployment, increased food costs, adverse changes in climate, public safety situations, and political conditions.

Connecting Food Security and Health

An integral component of the multi-dimensional nature of food security is its implications for nutritional status. As previously mentioned, food insecurity can lead to malnutrition and poor health through decreased eating of healthful food, increased risk of diet-related chronic diseases, poor mental health, depression, stress, anxiety, social exclusion, academic barriers, and increased healthcare costs.[92]

A number of research studies show a positive association between food insecurity and diet-related chronic diseases.[93] Fifty-eight percent of low or very low food secure households contain at least one member with high blood pressure and 33% have at least one member with diabetes.[94] Obesity and hunger may exist side by side within the same household or community, commonly known as the **hunger-obesity paradox**. Owing to limited financial resources, households that are food insecure use coping strategies that compromise health:

- Choosing cheaper food even though they know it is not the healthiest
- Forgoing the foods needed for special medical diets (e.g., diabetic diets)
- Making trade-offs between food and other basic necessities (e.g., housing)
- Engaging in cost-related medication underuse
- Postponing preventive or needed medical care

Causes associated with the hunger-obesity paradox are the result of low-income households facing unique challenges to adopting and maintaining healthful behaviors. The cycle of food insecurity and chronic disease begins when an individual or household has a lack of availability or physical access to healthy, affordable foods. Owing to the absence of full-service grocery stores and farmers' markets, residents may be forced to access food at convenience stores or gas stations, where fresh food and healthful options are limited or not present.

Low-resource households are less likely to have and use their own vehicle for regular food shopping;[95] thereby limiting purchases because of how much can be carried when walking or when using public transit or the length of time between shopping trips. For example, household shoppers without stable transportation may only go to a full-scale supermarket once a month and will purchase fewer perishable foods, such as fresh produce.[96]

When these households have the physical means of accessing healthy food, the more healthful options, like fresh produce, are perceived to be more expensive and possess a higher potential for waste.[97] Energy-dense, convenience foods that are filled with added sugars, fats, and refined grains are more popular with lower resource households because of lower cost. These foods are also lower in nutritional quality, contributing to an overconsumption of calories and resulting in weight gain and obesity.[98]

In addition to the decrease in the availability of affordable healthful foods, low-resource communities have a higher density of fast-food restaurants.[99] These restaurants predominantly offer a variety of energy-dense, nutrient-poor foods at relatively low prices. Research shows a diet rich in these foods is associated with weight gain and diet-related diseases.[100,101]

The financial and emotional pressures of food insecurity, coupled with low wage work, limited healthcare, inadequate transportation, poor housing, and neighborhood violence, contribute to extremely high levels of stress and poor mental health for these households. Research has linked stress and poor mental health to weight gain and obesity through stress-induced hormonal and metabolic changes.[102]

Environmental barriers to physical activity present significant challenges for low-resource communities. There are fewer parks, green spaces, and recreational facilities in lower income neighborhoods compared to their higher income counterparts.[103] When physical activity resources are available, they often have fewer natural features (e.g., trees) in addition to more trash and signs of damage.[104] Safety concerns are common barriers to being physically active. Because of neighborhood crime, children and adults are more likely to stay inside and engage in sedentary activities (e.g., television, video games).

Marketing and advertising for obesity-promoting products that encourage the consumption of energy-dense, unhealthful foods disproportionately impacts low-resource communities.[105,106] This type of marketing is shown to have an influence on the diet and contribute to obesity in youth and young adults.

Measurements of Food Security Status

The U.S. Department of Agriculture (USDA) utilizes a tiered approach to measure food security status of American households:

Food Secure

- High food security: No problems or anxiety about consistently accessing adequate food

- Marginal food security: Problems or anxiety at times about accessing adequate food, but the quality, variety, and quantity of food were not substantially reduced

Food Insecure
- Low food security: Reduced quality, variety, and desirability of diets, but the quantity of food intake and normal eating patterns were not substantially disrupted

Hungry
- Very low food security: At times during the year, eating patterns of one or more household members were disrupted and food intake reduced because the household lacked money or other resources for food

Food security status is determined by a household's economic ability to afford food. The U.S. Food Security Survey Module developed by the USDA Economic Research Service (ERS) asks if, in the last 12 months, the household cut the size of meals, skipped meals, ate less than they should, or went hungry because there was not enough money for food.[107] The risk for food insecurity increases when money to buy food is limited or not available. The most prevalent risk factor for food insecurity is poverty (Figure 14.4).[108]

Applying the Social-Ecological Model to the Food Insecurity Multidimensional Index (FIMI) to Promote Health Across the Life span

The Food and Agriculture Organization (FAO)'s Food Insecurity Multidimensional Index (FIMI) can be applied to all levels of the social-ecological model, including the macro (large national and legal systems), meso (organizations, communities, and ethnic groups), and micro (families, relationships, and individuals) levels (Figure 14.5).

Availability

Food and nutrition cannot be considered without also thinking about farming and agriculture. Enough nutrient-dense food is produced and there is sufficient capacity in the world to feed the world's population, now and in the future. Resilient small-scale farms that yield nutrient-dense crops (fruits and vegetables) are integral to a nation's food supply. The share of small-scale food producers compared to all producers ranges from 40% to 85% in Africa, Asia, and Latin America, 10% in Europe, and 2% in Germany, Denmark, France, and the Netherlands. The United States has experienced a rapid decline in small-scale farms and the production of labor-intensive crops on domestic soil; thus, foreign-grown produce consumed in the United States has increased nearly

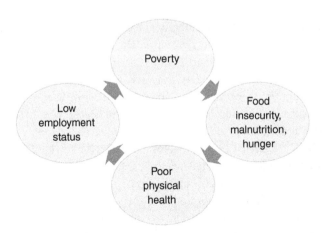

FIGURE 14.4 Poverty, food insecurity, malnutrition, and hunger are interrelated.

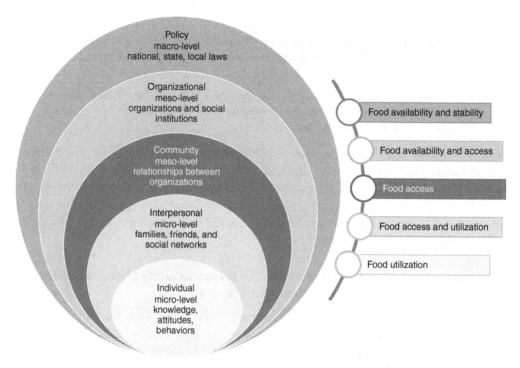

FIGURE 14.5 The social-ecological model (left) and corresponding food insecurity multidimensional index (right).

80%. During this time, if domestic farms maintained their market share of vegetable production, farm communities would have experienced an economic boost of US$4.9 billion, resulting in 89,000 jobs and raising the U.S. gross domestic product by US$12.4 billion in 1 year.[109]

Assessed at the macro (policy) and meso (community) levels, global government spending on agriculture and food production impact food availability. Spending typically prioritizes staple crops, such as corn, soybeans, rice, wheat, maize, and sugar cane, offering little to no nutritional value.[110] One of the largest portions of the U.S. Agriculture Adjustment Act (commonly known as the Farm Bill, the primary agricultural and food policy tool of the federal government) includes subsidies that artificially decrease the cost of commodities—wheat, corn, soybeans, tobacco, livestock and dairy—accounting for US$23 billion per year. The majority of subsidies support commercial farmers who have an average income of nearly US$200,000 and net worth just under US$2 million. While corn accounts for more than a quarter of the subsidy payments,[111] more than one-third of the U.S. corn crop is used to feed livestock, 13% is exported, 40% is used to produce ethanol, 9% is for plastics, 3% is for inputs including high-fructose corn syrup and corn oil, and less than 0.5% of the corn crop is used as food in the form of "sweet corn."[112] Some argue that sustainable, regenerative agriculture practices that support small-scale farms, diversify production, and strengthen resiliency (climate variability, natural disasters, or economic shocks) will contribute to improving dietary quality and overall health.[113]

Mitigating **food waste** is another contributing factor, as up to 40% of food in the United States goes uneaten. This preventable loss has profound effects on food security, the environment, and economy. Food waste is estimated to cost US$218 billion annually, approximately US$1,800 for a four-person American household. Interventions that reduce *pre-consumer waste*, on farms, in distribution and preparation, involve recovering and repurposing food. The *Bill Emerson Good Samaritan Act* protects food donors, including restaurants, institutions, and individuals, from liability when food is donated in all 50 states. *Post-consumer waste*, commonly known as "plate waste," is discarded by consumers at the time of consumption and can be mitigated by decreasing portion sizes, removing trays from "all-you-can-eat" buffets, and increasing awareness through demonstrations. Waste management practices in food service establishments should follow the *Food Waste Hierarchy* of (a) source reduction, (b) reuse to feed people, (c) reuse to feed animals, (d) reuse for industrial uses, (e) compost, and finally (f) contribute to a landfill.[114]

Access

Increasing access points to purchase fruits and vegetables is a method to promote healthful food consumption for all age groups. Typically assessed at the meso-level (community or organizational), research indicates that farmers' markets are associated with higher consumption of fruit and vegetables.[115] According to the USDA's Agricultural Marketing Service, consumer demand for locally sourced food continues to grow, contributing to an increase in the number of farmers' markets by 78% in one decade. Community-supported agriculture (CSA) is another method that increases consumption of healthy food while connecting consumers directly with farmers and involves purchasing a share from the farm in advance of the growing season. Financial incentives to join a CSA through "produce prescriptions" have been shown to effectively mitigate the consumer upfront cost and improve short- and long-term health outcomes.[116]

Various research studies sought to identify the barriers to intake and found that consumers reported price as a primary challenge to adequate consumption.[21] Governmental agencies offer safety-net programs that ensure adequate access to food for low-resource populations (Table 14.4).

According to the USDA, the majority of SNAP (Supplemental Nutrition Assistance Program) households and those receiving free or reduced-price school lunches, experienced food security while enrolled.[117] *Rewards-based incentive programs* for fruit and vegetable purchases, such as farmers' market incentive programs for WIC (Special Supplemental Nutrition Program for Women, Infants, and Children) or SNAP participants, are shown to address the dual challenge of food insecurity and malnutrition.[118] The USDA offers funding opportunities that support projects dedicated to increasing fruit and vegetable access among low-income consumers, including:

- Engaging public-private efforts to incentivize fruit and vegetable purchases with "point-of-sale double dollars" at food access points, including the Kentucky Double Dollars program that doubles the purchasing power of participants of SNAP, WIC, and the Seniors Farmers' Market Nutrition Program

- Making fresh fruits and vegetables more accessible to low-income families through grants to help farmers' markets install and operate electronic benefit transfer (EBT) card readers

- Gathering stakeholder input on stricter "depth of stock" requirements for SNAP retailers to better determine how to improve program integrity and expand the availability of more healthful foods to SNAP recipients, without compromising access to food for SNAP participants or unnecessarily burdening retailers that redeem SNAP benefits.

- The Healthy Incentives Pilot, designed to test the impact of incentivizing fruit and vegetable purchases among SNAP recipients that showed relatively small ongoing investment result in a 25% increase in fruit and vegetable consumption among adults.[123]

TABLE 14.4 FEDERAL FOOD ASSISTANCE PROGRAMS IN THE UNITED STATES

ACRONYM	FULL NAME	DESCRIPTION	POPULATION SERVED
SNAP	Supplemental Nutrition Assistance Program	Provides temporary benefits to low-income Americans to buy groceries	All age groups from infancy through older adults
TEFAP	The Emergency Food Assistance Program	Provides U.S. Department of Agriculture (USDA) commodities to families in need of short-term hunger relief through emergency food providers like food banks	All ages including those supplied through the national food bank network
CSFP	The Commodity Supplemental Food Program	Provides food assistance for low-income seniors through a monthly package of USDA commodities	All ages including supplying through the national food bank network
CACFP	The Child and Adult Care Food Program	Provides prepared nutritious meals and snacks to children and adults in designated child and adult care centers	Predominately for children (<5 years) and older adults
NSLP	The National School Lunch Program	Provides prepared nutritious lunch to qualified children during the school year	Predominately for school-age children (5–18 years)
SBP	The School Breakfast Program	Provides prepared nutritious breakfast to qualified children during the school year	Predominately for school-age children (5–18 years)
SFSP	The Summer Food Service Program	Provides prepared nutritious meals and snacks to qualified children during the summer	Predominately for school-age children (5–18 years)
WIC	Special Supplemental Nutrition Program for Women, Infants, and Children	A prescriptive, nonentitlement program that supplies nutritious foods for proper growth and development	Pregnant and lactating women, infants, and children

Utilization

Food utilization is assessed at the individual level and focuses on nutritional quality of food, in addition to personal food safety, storage, and preparation practices. The current food system offers an increased risk for food contamination owing to the distance between producers and consumers continuing to grow. The Centers for Disease Control and Prevention (CDC) reports that one in six Americans get sick, 128,000 are hospitalized, and 3,000 die from foodborne diseases each year.[119] There are often conflicts between food safety regulation and the cost of compliance for smallholder farmers, as stringent standards make it prohibitive for small-scale producers to enter markets and safe food that is inevitably monitored becomes less accessible to low-income consumers.

Nutrition education programs rooted in *behavior change theory* and *human-centered design* (a process that begins with the people in order to develop solutions that are tailored to their needs) are shown to be effective in addressing household food practices. For example, *Cooking Matters*®, a nutrition education program of *Share Our Strength,* empowers parents, caregivers, families, and children with the skills, knowledge, and confidence to shop for and cook healthy, affordable meals. The USDA continues to explore programs that effectively encourage the consumption of healthy foods, such as *SNAP-Ed* that offers strong nutrition education to change food behavior and improve health, specifically improving fruit and vegetable consumption for children and older adults, and providing shopping strategies and meal planning advice to help families serve more nutritious meals affordably through its *10-Tips Nutrition Series* and the *Thrifty Food Plan*.

Stability

Ensuring that food is available, accessible, and utilized "at all times," while addressing the interconnectedness of malnutrition, food insecurity, and hunger, involves policies that tackle systemic problems within the overall food system.[120] According to the UN, nations not supplying adequate food and nutrition services are violating international law. The second Sustainable Development Goal highlights the need for integration of global policy priorities in order to end hunger, achieve food security, improve nutrition, and promote sustainable agriculture.[121]

CONCLUSION

Malnutrition, food insecurity, and hunger all too often occur within the same communities and households. Largely because of a lack of financial resources, food insecure communities experience economic and environmental challenges to living a healthy life. Achieving optimal nutritional status is possible through food (a) availability, (b) accessibility, (c) utilization, and (d) stability. Ensuring the presence of these four components will lead to a *food and nutrition secure community* in which all residents can obtain a safe, culturally acceptable, nutritionally adequate diet through a sustainable food system that maximizes community self-reliance, social justice, and democratic decision-making.[130]

Encompassing both overnutrition and undernutrition, malnutrition is a global problem with such consequences as chronic diseases, poor child development, early mortality, and lack of economic productivity. All people must have sufficient physical, economic, and social access to healthful food at all times. The right to feed oneself with dignity is a legal obligation under international law. Adequate food for health is not merely a promise to be met through charity; it is one to be fulfilled through appropriate actions by governments and nonstate agencies. Social, economic, and environmental factors have a profound impact on nutrition-related health outcomes across the life span and call for integrated, system-based approaches.

KEY CONCEPTS

- The double burden of malnutrition, both undernutrition and overnutrition, is the largest single contributor to disease in the world and is an increasing challenge for women of childbearing age.

- Progress in reducing global mortality from disease has stalled or reversed primarily because of the increasing prevalence of NCDs, such as overweight and obesity, type 2 diabetes, cardiovascular disease, chronic respiratory disease, and certain types of cancers.

- Anorexia of aging is a common physical factor that contributes to malnutrition in older adults; however, it is preventable by addressing the social, economic, and environmental factors that promote quality of life and self-sufficiency.

- While investments in nutrition interventions and education are important, they should be integrated across the social-ecological model to accelerate progress toward good health.

- Food waste is a preventable loss that impacts the environment, economic viability, and food and nutrition security. Recovering and repurposing food play a critical role in mitigating food waste and improving population nutritional status.

- Sustainable, regenerative agriculture practices that support small-scale farms, diversify production, and strengthen resiliency (climate variability, natural disasters, or economic shocks) can contribute to food and nutrition security.

CASE STUDY: CHALLENGES FACED BY SINGLE MOTHER OF THREE

Jack, a 3-year-old boy, lives with his mother and two older siblings (4 and 7 years old). It is a 25-minute bus ride from their apartment to the WIC office or grocery store. Mom is single and makes about US$2,000 per month. Jack and his 4-year-old sibling are receiving WIC benefits. The oldest sibling, a 7-year-old girl, was on WIC until she aged out of the program at 5 years. She has always plotted in the 90th to 95th percentile in weight-for-age and BMI consistent at the 75th percentile, whereas Jack plots below the 3rd percentile and has triggered in the WIC system as "high risk" for malnutrition.

Seattle has been growing its technology industry, which has put pressure on the housing market, and the family had to relocate last year because of the rise in rent for their two-bedroom apartment. The new apartment has one bedroom; the older children share the bedroom. Mom and Jack sleep on a pull-out couch in the living room. The apartment has an efficiency kitchen. Mom has complained to the landlord about mold around the windows and is concerned with the frequency of ear infections for the older children and her persistent cough, but there are no other housing options.

Mom reports consistently using the WIC money to purchase food for the children and admits she gives the food to all the children as it is "too hard to tell one of them not to eat this food or that food when everyone is hungry." Her SNAP benefits change with her work schedule and unpredictable child-support payments and they rely on the nearest food pantry during the last week of the month. Last summer, the family received US$35 in WIC farmers' market vouchers, of which she was able to spend US$20. In June, she hopes to find an eligible farmer's market closer to their apartment.

She states mealtimes are the hardest time of day for her because her oldest daughter finishes her plate and will also eat any food left on the plates of her younger siblings. Mom says she is very happy to see her older daughter eating and praises her for eating so well at each meal. Mom struggles to get Jack to eat anything at mealtime and she has force-fed him many times to make sure he ate something that day. Mom has become so frustrated lately that she now makes three evening meals, one for each child, in an attempt to appease them all and get Jack to eat. She has tried to get a "routine" down, but struggles because of changes in her work schedule, children getting sick, commute from day care and school to home, and exhaustion.

Mom gets up at 3:00 am each day to go to her first minimum wage job. She wakes the children by 3:30 am and they are in day care near the school from 4:00 am until 6:00 pm at night when she gets off her second job. Day care has set mealtimes, schedules, and foods and the oldest daughter receives free breakfast and lunch at school. Mom reports that Jack does not eat well at day care either.

Access and time to shop for foods is a challenge for mom. The closest grocery store, food pantry, and WIC office to their neighborhood is a 30-minute bus ride. The WIC office is open from 8 am to 4 pm, Monday to Wednesday and Friday, and from 8:00 am to 5:45 pm on Thursdays. She is worried about using the coupons at the market as her first and only experience at the market proved stressful and overwhelming. She was not familiar with how to shop at the market, did not bring her own bags, heard some customers make side comments about her WIC coins, and when she arrived home, she did not know how to cook or prepare some of the vegetables. Mom understands the importance of having the children eat a more diverse variety of vegetables but struggles with overcoming the barriers.

Over the past few weeks, Jack has begun to drink more milk, so mom has offered this to him any time she can throughout the day and encouraged day care to "continually offer him milk" as she sees this as some type of nutrition he is getting if he will not eat. Mom is happy that Jack is drinking milk. She used to feel guilty wasting it because the family receives so much of it through WIC; it had been a challenge to consume it before it spoiled.

At the most recent WIC appointment, Jack's hemoglobin was <10 mg/dL and he was diagnosed with anemia in addition to being at high risk for malnutrition. Mom is encouraged to feed him more red meat each day to help bring up his iron stores and to reduce the amount of milk he is drinking as the milk may be a substitute for food.

Case Study Questions

1. Each of us has an individual perspective of the world and this impacts our awareness of different situations and relationships. Reflecting on your worldview, what are some ways your perspective impacts your understanding of the family situation, challenges, and barriers in this case study?

2. Thinking about the WIC Farmers' Market Program, what are some food availability (agricultural) impacts? What are social/cultural food access impacts?

3. Thinking about the recommendation by the WIC clinician for Jack's mom to increase his red meat consumption to improve his anemia, what are the barriers, challenges, and impacts of this recommendation? In what ways does food utilization play a role?

SUGGESTED LEARNING ACTIVITIES

Activity #1: Film Showing and Reflection

The film *A Place at the Table* introduces the notion that food is a right, not only a need. Watch the film and write a reflection paper discussing:

- What does the film say about food being a basic human right? Provide some clear examples.
- What does the film say about the role of agricultural subsidies and their impact on U.S. food security?
- How can we end hunger? Describe two examples from the film.
- Reflect on how this information relates to your future career goals.

Activity #2: Applying Chapter 14 Key Concepts to a Community-Based Case Study

1. Review the following *Activity #2 Case Example.*

2. Discuss the following questions (in a group/class discussion or an individual/reflection paper):

   - In what ways does *Fresh Stop* address nutrition-related health issues and challenges across the lifespan?

   - Does this model strengthen the resiliency and capacity of small-scale vegetable farms?

   - How do *Fresh Stop Markets* address the three-pillars of food access (social, physical, and economic)?

   - Agency is an important factor in considering food availability, access, and utilization. Does this model support food choice and democratic decision-making?

   - Food cooperatives, such as *Fresh Stop,* are not a new approach to ensuring food access. While the model is piloted in the United States, how could it be replicated across the globe?

   - Is this a sustainable approach? What are ways that government and nongovernment agencies can use this model to promote community food and nutrition security?

Activity #2 Case Example

Anna, a 65-year-old woman, is responsible for the care of her two grandchildren (4 and 7 years old). Her daughter, the children's mother, has opioid use disorder. Anna recently gained custody of the grandchildren and they are now living in Anna's one-bedroom apartment. Recently retired, Anna has a fixed income of about US$1,900 per month and receives US$16 per month in SNAP benefits.

Since she was 18 years old, Anna worked as a cook at a nearby restaurant and she prides herself on her cooking ability. Recently, her knees have started "giving me trouble" and she cannot stand for long periods of time. She has type 2 diabetes and the medical cost of doctor's visits and medications have put a strain on her finances. Her doctor is constantly telling her to lose weight.

There is a store on the corner where she can buy some food; however, despite her numerous requests, bananas are the only fresh food option. About once a month, she takes the bus to the nearest full-scale supermarket that is 40 minutes away, round-trip. Even with Anna's cooking knowledge, she struggles to make meals that she knows are good for their health and that both kids will eat.

While attending a children's event at the community center, she heard about a group trying to bring more fresh food options into their neighborhood. She was hesitant to attend the meeting the following evening because she was feeling drained and exhausted. The meeting offered dinner and childcare, so she decided to attend and felt that she had "nothing to lose." At the meeting, she learned about *Fresh Stop,* which pulls the community resources together to buy fresh produce from fruit and vegetable farms around the area. Anna also met another single grandparent caring for her grandchildren and, for the first time, did not feel so alone.

Anna walked with the kids to the first market and was surprised to see all the beautiful fruits and vegetables displayed. The market included activities for the kids and a chef was demonstrating how to make a stir-fry from some of that day's vegetables. With her SNAP benefits, Anna bought one fresh produce share and got a voucher for another free share, providing an entire month's supply of fresh fruits and vegetables for only US$10.

Over the course of the summer, Anna shared, "My knees no longer bother me and I am able to walk with my friends. The only change I made was eating the food from here." Anna lost 45 pounds that summer and eliminated her diabetic medication, essentially curing her diabetes.

Fresh Stop Markets offers opportunities to provide affordable access to fresh, local fruits and vegetables for low-income citizens, while supporting the economics of small farmers and fostering relationships within neighborhoods. Customers can pay a discounted price with subsidized Double Dollars vouchers with WIC and SNAP, ranging from US$0 to US$25 (for a two-week produce share). Produce is provided from a cooperative group of farmers at prices above wholesale, providing farmers with a guaranteed market without the stress of supplying an entire CSA share. In one year, *Fresh Stop* connects 1,400 unique families (4,200 individuals) with farm-fresh produce grown by 50 local farmers. Community food projects like the *Fresh Stop Market* bridge the gap between food insecure eaters and resource stressed local farmers—addressing food, farm, and nutrition issues.

REFLECTION QUESTIONS

1. What are the essential nutrients for all age groups?

2. How does the double burden of malnutrition impact the economic viability of a nation?

3. Is food and nutrition security a national security issue? Please describe.

4. What are the primary nutrition considerations for pregnant women?

5. Thinking beyond food access, what role does food security play in educational attainment? Alleviating the cycle of poverty?

6. How do social determinants of health impact disease progression through the life span?

7. Who holds the primary responsibility of ensuring food for all? Should this be addressed at the local, state, national, international level? By government or private agencies?

CONTINUE YOUR LEARNING RESOURCES

RESOURCE	DESCRIPTION	WEBSITE LINK
USDA ChooseMyPlate	Provides practical information to individuals, health professionals, nutrition educators, and the food industry to help individuals find their healthy eating style and build it throughout their lifetime.	www.choosemyplate.gov
USDA Lifecycle Nutrition	Information about proper nutrition from preconception through older adults.	www.nal.usda.gov/fnic/ lifecycle-nutrition-0

RESOURCE	DESCRIPTION	WEBSITE LINK
Sustainable Development Goals	A call for action by all UN countries—poor, rich and middle-income—to promote prosperity while protecting the environment.	sustainabledevelopment.un.org
First Thousand Days	The leading nonprofit organization working in the United States and around the world to ensure women and children have the healthiest first 1,000 days.	thousanddays.org/why-1000-days
The Hope Center	Home to an action research team using rigorous research to drive innovative practice, evidence-based policy-making, and effective communications to support #RealCollege students.	hope4college.com
The Body Project	A group-based intervention that provides a forum for women and girls to confront unrealistic beauty ideals and engages them in the development of healthy body image through verbal, written, and behavioral exercises.	www.nationaleatingdisorders.org/get-involved/the-body-project
Healthy Campus	"Sister document" to Healthy People, and much of the development process for Healthy Campus 2020 was guided by the Healthy People framework.	www.acha.org/healthycampus
Food and Agriculture Organization (FAO), High Level Panel of Experts	The High Level Panel of Experts (HLPE) on food security and nutrition has been created as part of the reform of the international governance of food security to advise the Committee on World Food Security (CFS).	www.fao.org/cfs/cfs-hlpe/reports/en Nutrition and Food Systems: www.fao.org/3/a-i7846e.pdf
Feeding America, Hunger + Health	Educate, connect, and engage cross-sector professionals at the intersection of food insecurity, nutrition, and health.	hungerandhealth.feedingamerica.org
Academy of Nutrition and Dietetics, Future of Food Initiative	Positioning the Academy and its members to address the issues of global food security, hunger, and malnutrition.	eatrightfoundation.org/why-it-matters/public-education/future-of-food

GLOSSARY

Activities of daily living (ADLs): Basic self-care tasks, such as walking and feeding oneself, that one encounters on a daily basis.

Body mass index (BMI): A measurement that can be used to screen for weight categories that may contribute to health problems. BMI is not a direct diagnostic of the body fatness or health of an individual and is calculated as Weight (kg)/height (m)^2.

Communicable diseases: Also known as infectious diseases; illnesses that result from infection, presence and growth of pathogenic biological agents.

Food insecurity: Lack of consistent access to enough food for an active, healthy life.

Food system: The path that food travels from field to fork that includes the growing, harvesting, processing, packaging, transporting, marketing, consuming, and disposing of food.

Hunger-obesity paradox: Occurrence of high rates of obesity among individuals with low resources due to a lack of access to healthy food.

Instrumental activities of daily living (IADLs): Activities, such as driving, grocery shopping, and preparing meals, that require complex thinking and organizational skills.

Macro- and micronutrients: Macronutrients refer to the carbohydrates, fats, and protein necessary for the basic components of a healthy diet. Micronutrients include the essential nutrients, such as vitamin A, iodine, iron, and zinc. Essential macro- and micronutrients play a critical role in humoral immunity responses, cellular signaling and function, learning and cognitive function, work capacity, reproductive health, and the evolution of microbial virulence.

Malnutrition: The lack of proper nutrients to meet daily needs and the largest single contributor to disease and poor health outcomes worldwide.

Noncommunicable diseases: Illnesses that are not transmissible directly from one person to another. NCDs include heart diseases, cancers, diabetes, chronic kidney disease, and Alzheimer's disease, among others.

Nutrient-dense diet: Consumption of foods that are high in essential nutrients and lower in "empty calories" and follow the dietary recommendations.

Obesogenic culture: The sum of influences that the surroundings, opportunities, or conditions of life have on promoting obesity in individuals or populations.

Overnutrition and undernutrition: Malnutrition in all forms refers to both overnutrition (an overconsumption of food that leads to overweight, obesity, and diet-related chronic diseases) and undernutrition (not getting enough energy from nutrients).

Poverty: The state of not having enough resources to provide for a person's basic needs of food, shelter, clothing, clean air, and clean water. A multifaceted concept that includes social, economic, and political elements.

Right to food: Defined by the UN as the right to feed oneself with dignity.

Social determinants of health: Encompass the social, economic, and environmental factors that can affect the health and quality of life of a population.

REFERENCES

1. World Health Organization. *Malnutrition.* 2018. https://www.who.int/news-room/fact-sheets/detail/malnutrition
2. Coleman-Jensen A, Rabbitt M, Gregory C, Singh A. *Household Food Security in the United States in 2016.* Washington, DC: U.S. Department of Agriculture, Economic Research Service; 2017. https://www.ers.usda.gov/webdocs/publications/84973/err-237.pdf?v=0
3. Institute for Health Metrics and Evaluation. *Global Burden of Disease (GBD) Compare/Viz Hub.* Seattle, WA: Institute for Health Metrics and Evaluation; 2019. https://vizhub.healthdata.org/gbd-compare
4. Food and Agriculture Organization. *The State of Food Security and Nutrition in the World 2019. Safeguarding Against Economic Slowdowns and Downturns.* Rome, Italy: Food and Agriculture Organization; 2019. http://www.fao.org/state-of-food-security-nutrition/en
5. Agha M, Agha R. The rising prevalence of obesity: part A: impact on public health. *Int J Surg Oncol.* 2017;2(7):e17. doi:10.1097/IJ9.0000000000000017

6. Falk LW, Sobal J, Bisogni CA, et al. Managing healthy eating: definitions, classifications, and strategies. *Health Educ Behav.* 2001;28(4):425–439.

7. Kapil U, Bhavna A. Adverse effects of poor micronutrient status during childhood and adolescence. *Nutr Rev.* 2002;60(suppl_5):S84–S90. doi:10.1301/00296640260130803

8. Ramakrishnan U. Prevalence of micronutrient malnutrition worldwide. *Nutr Rev.* 2002;60(5 Pt 2):S46–S52. doi:10.1301/00296640260130731

9. Kejo D, Petrucka PM, Martin H, et al. Prevalence and predictors of anemia among children under 5 years of age in Arusha District, Tanzania. *Pediatr Health Med Ther.* 2018;9:9–15. doi:10.2147/PHMT.S148515

10. Vir S. Current status of iodine deficiency disorders and strategy for its control in India. *Indian J Pediatr.* 2002;69:589. doi:10.1007/BF02722687

11. Ploysangam A, Falciglia G, Brehm B. Effect of marginal zinc deficiency on human growth and development. *J Trop Pediatr.* 1997;43(4):192–198. doi:10.1093/tropej/43.4.192

12. Katona P, Katona-Apte J. The interaction between nutrition and infection. *Clin Infect Dis.* 2008;46(10):1582–1588. doi:10.1086/587658

13. World Health Organization. *Global Tuberculosis Report, 2019.* Geneva, Switzerland: World Health Organization; 2019.

14. NCD Risk Factor Collaboration. Worldwide trends in body-mass index, underweight, overweight, and obesity from 1975 to 2016: a pooled analysis of 2416 population-based measurement studies in 128.9 million children, adolescents, and adults. *Lancet.* 2017;390(10113):2627–2642. doi:10.1016/S0140-6736(17)32129-3

15. GBD 2016 Causes of Death Collaborators. Global, regional, and national age-sex specific mortality for 264 causes of death, 1980-2016: a systematic analysis for the Global Burden of Disease Study 2016. *Lancet.* 2017;390:1151–1210. doi:10.1016/S0140-6736(17)32152-9

16. Institute for Health Metrics and Evaluation. *Findings from the Global Burden of Disease Study 2017.* Seattle, WA: Institute for Health Metrics and Evaluation; 2018.

17. U.S. Department of Agriculture. *Current Eating Patterns in the United States.* 2015. https://health.gov/our-work/food-nutrition/2015-2020-dietary-guidelines/guidelines/chapter-2/current-eating-patterns-in-the-unitedstates/

18. Hiza H, Casavale K, Guenther P, Davis C. Diet quality of Americans differs by age, sex, race/ethnicity, income, and education level. *J Acad Nutr Diet.* 2012;113(2):297–306. doi:10.1016/j.jand.2012.08.011

19. Troesch B, Biesalski HK, Bos R, et al. Increased intake of foods with high nutrient density can help to break the intergenerational cycle of malnutrition and obesity. *Nutrients.* 2015;7(7):6016–6037. doi:10.3390/nu7075266

20. Lake A, Townshend T. Obesogenic environments: exploring the built and food environments. *J R Soc Promot Health.* 2006;126(6):262–267. doi:10.1177/1466424006070487

21. Reicks MM, Randall JL, Haynes BJ. Factors affecting consumption of fruits and vegetables by low-income families. *J Am Diet Assoc.* 1994;94(11):1309–1311. doi:10.1016/0002-8223(94)92467-8

22. Subramanian SV, Kawachi I, Smith GD. Income inequality and the double burden of under- and overnutrition in India. *J Epidemiol Community Health.* 2007;61:802–809. doi:10.1136/jech.2006.053801

23. WHO Expert Consultation. Appropriate body-mass index for Asian populations and its implications for policy and intervention strategies. *Lancet.* 2004;363(9403):157–163. doi:10.1016/S0140-6736(03)15268-3

24. World Health Organization. *Waist Circumference and Waist-Hip Ratio. Report of a WHO Expert Consultation.* Geneva, Switzerland: World Health Organization; 2011.

25. Jaacks L, Slining M, Popkin B. Recent trends in the prevalence of under- and overweight among adolescent girls in low- and middle-income countries. *Pediatr Obes.* 2015;10(6):428–435. doi:10.1111/ijpo.12000

26. Centers for Disease Control and Prevention. *Data & Statistics: Adult Obesity Facts.* 2018. https://www.cdc.gov/obesity/data/prevalence-maps.html

27. Finekelstein E, Trogdon J, Cohen J, Dietz W. Annual medical spending attributed to obesity: payer-and service-specific estimates. *Health Aff.* 2009;28(1):w822–w831. doi:10.1377/hlthaff.28.5.w822

28. International Diabetes Federation. *Facts and Figures.* 2019. https://idf.org/52-about-diabetes.html

29. Centers for Disease Control and Prevention. *Heart Disease in the United States.* 2017. https://www.cdc.gov/heartdisease/facts.htm

30. Berthon BS, Wood LG. Nutrition and respiratory health—feature review. *Nutrients*. 2015;7(3):1618–1643. doi:10.3390/nu7031618

31. Ferreira I, Brooks D, Lacasse T, Goldstein R. Nutritional support for individuals with COPD: a meta-analysis. *Chest*. 2000;117(3):672–678. doi:10.1378/chest.117.3.672

32. McCullough ML, Patel AV, Kushi LH, et al. Following cancer prevention guidelines reduces risk of cancer, cardiovascular disease, and all-cause mortality. *Cancer Epidemiol Biomarkers Prev*. 2011;20(6):1089–1097. doi:10.1158/1055-9965.EPI-10-1173

33. Petry N, Olofin I, Boy E, et al. The effect of low dose iron and zinc intake on child micronutrient status and development during the first 1000 days of life: a systematic review and meta-analysis. *Nutrients*. 2016;8(12):773. doi:10.3390/nu8120773

34. Glinoer D, Delange F. The potential repercussions of maternal, fetal, and neonatal hypothyroxinemia on the progeny. *Thyroid*. 2000;10(10):871–887. doi:10.1089/thy.2000.10.871

35. Bleichrodt N, Born MP. A metaanalysis of research on iodine and its relationship to cognitive development. In Stanbury JB, ed. *The Damaged Brain of Iodine Deficiency*. New York, NY: Cognizant Communication Corporation; 1996:195–200.

36. Aggarwal A, Monsivais P, Drewnowski A. Nutrient intakes linked to better health outcomes are associated with higher diet costs in the US. *PLoS One*. 2012;7(5):e37533. doi:10.1371/journal.pone.0037533

37. Sazawal S, Dhingra U, Dhingra P, et al. Effects of fortified milk on morbidity in young children in north India: community based, randomised, double masked placebo controlled trial. *BMJ*. 2007;334:140.

38. Dean SV, Lassi ZS, Imam AM, Bhutta ZA. Preconception care: nutritional risks and interventions. *Reprod Health*. 2014;11(3):S3. doi:10.1186/1742-4755-11-S3-S3

39. Holick MF. High prevalence of vitamin D inadequacy and implications for health. *Mayo Clin Proc*. 2006;81(3):353–373. doi:10.4065/81.3.353

40. World Health Organization. *Global prevalence of vitamin A deficiency in populations at risk 1995–2005. WHO Global Database on Vitamin A Deficiency*. Geneva, Author; 2009.

41. Drennen C, Coleman S, Ettinger de Cuba S, et al. Food insecurity, health, and development in children under age four years. *Pediatrics*. 2019;144:e20190824. doi:10.1542/peds.2019-0824

42. Rudd R, Seth P, David F, Scholl L. Increases in drug and opioid-involved overdose deaths—United States, 2010–2015. *MMWR Morb Mortal Wkly Rep*. 2016;65:1445–1452. doi:10.15585/mmwr.mm655051e1

43. National Academies of Sciences, Engineering, and Medicine. Trends in opioid use, harms, and treatment. In: Phillips J, Ford M, Bonnie R, eds. *Pain Management and the Opioid Epidemic: Balancing Societal and Individual Benefits and Risks of Prescription Opioid Use*. Washington, DC: National Academies Press; 2017. https://www.ncbi.nlm.nih.gov/books/NBK458661

44. Villapiano N, Winkelman T, Kozhimannil K, et al. Rural and urban differences in neonatal abstinence syndrome and maternal opioid use, 2004–2013. *JAMA Pediatr*. 2017;171(2):194–196. doi:10.1001/jamapediatrics.2016.3750

45. Heil S, Jones H, Arria A, et al. Unintended pregnancy in opioid-abusing women. *J Subst Abuse Treat*. 2011;40(2):199–202. doi:10.1016/j.jsat.2010.08.011

46. Nabipour S, Ayu Said M, Hussain Habil M. Burden and nutritional deficiencies in opiate addiction—systematic review article. *Iran J Public Health*. 2014;43(8):1022–1032.

47. Imdad A, Bhutta ZA. Effect of preventive zinc supplementation on linear growth in children under 5 years of age in developing countries: a meta-analysis of studies for input to the lives saved tool. *BMC Public Health*. 2011;11 Suppl 3:S22. doi:10.1186/1471-2458-11-S3-S22

48. Piernas C, Miles DR, Deming DM, et al. Estimating usual intakes mainly affects the micronutrient distribution among infants, toddlers and pre-schoolers from the 2012 Mexican National Health and Nutrition Survey. *Public Health Nutr*. 2016;19(6):1017–1026. doi:10.1017/S1368980015002311

49. Yu SH, Mason J, Crum J, et al. Differential effects of young maternal age on child growth. *Glob Health Action*. 2016;9:31171. doi:10.3402/gha.v9.31171

50. Van Lieshout RJ, Taylor VH, Boyle MH. Pre-pregnancy and pregnancy obesity and neurodevelopmental outcomes in offspring: a systematic review. *Obes Rev*. 2011;12(5):e548–e559. doi:10.1111/j.1467-789X.2010.00850.x

51. Aviram A, Hod M, Yogev Y. Maternal obesity: implications for pregnancy outcome and long-term risks—a link to maternal nutrition. *Int J Gynaecol Obstet*. 2011;115 Suppl 1:S6–S10. doi:10.1016/S0020-7292(11)60004-0

52. American College Health Association. *American College Health Association-National College Health Assessment II: Undergraduate Student Executive Summary Spring 2019*. Silver Spring, MD: American College Health Association; 2019.

53. Stephens J, Althouse A, Tan A, Melnyk B. The role of race and gender in nutrition habits and self-efficacy: results from the Young Adult Weight Loss Study. *J Obes*. 2017;2017:1–6. doi:10.1155/2017/5980698

54. Yahia N, Wang D, Rapley M, Dey R. Assessment of weight status, dietary habits and beliefs, physical activity, and nutritional knowledge among university students. *Perspect Public Health*. 2016;136(4):231–244. doi:10.1177/1757913915609945

55. U.S. Government Accountability Office. *Food Insecurity: Better Information Could Help Eligible College Students Access Federal Food Assistance Benefits*. Report to Congressional Requesters GAO-19-95. Washington, DC: Government Accountability Office; 2018. https://www.gao.gov/assets/700/696254.pdf

56. Broton KM, Goldrick-Rab S. Going without: an exploration of food and housing insecurity among undergraduates. *Educ Res*. 2018;47(2):121–133. doi:10.3102/0013189X17741303

57. Dubick J, Mathews B, Cady C. *Hunger on Campus*. The Challenge of Food Insecurity for College Students. 2016. https://studentsagainsthunger.org/wp-content/uploads/2016/10/Hunger_On_Campus.pdf

58. Goldrick-Rab S, Richardson J, Hernandez A. *Hungry and Homeless in College: Results from a National Study of Basic Needs Insecurity in Higher Education*. 2017. https://www.higheredtoday.org/2017/03/17/hungry-homeless-college-results-national-study-basic-needs-insecurity-higher-education

59. Martinez S, Glik D, Malan H, Watson T. College students identify university support for basic needs and life skills as key ingredient in addressing food insecurity on campus. *Calif Agric*. 2017;71(3):130–138. doi:10.3733/ca.2017a0023

60. Morris L, Smith S, Davis J, Null D. The prevalence of food security and insecurity among Illinois University Students. *J Nutr Educ Behav*. 2016;48(6):376–382.e371. doi:10.1016/j.jneb.2016.03.013

61. Silva M, Kleinert W, Sheppard A, et al. The relationship between food security, housing stability, and school performance among college students in an urban university. *J Coll Stud Ret*. 2017;19(3):284–299. doi:10.1177/1521025115621918

62. Hanbazaza M, Ball G, Farmer A, et al. A comparison of characteristics and food insecurity coping strategies between international and domestic postsecondary students using a food bank located on a university campus. *Can J Diet Pract Res*. 2017;78(4):208–211. doi:10.3148/cjdpr-2017-012

63. Knol L, Robb C, McKinley E, Wood M. Very low food security status is related to lower cooking self-efficacy and less frequent food preparation behaviors among college students. *J Nutr Educ Behav*. 2018;51(3):357–363. doi:10.1016/j.jneb.2018.10.009

64. United Nations, Department of Economic and Social Affairs, Population Division. *World Population Ageing 2013*. ST/ESA/SER.A/348; 2013.

65. World Health Organization. *Global Health Observatory Data: Life Expectancy*. 2016. https://www.who.int/gho/mortality_burden_disease/life_tables/situation_trends_text/en

66. Houston DK, Nicklas BJ, Ding J, et al. Dietary protein intake is associated with lean mass change in older, community-dwelling adults: the Health, Aging, and Body Composition (Health ABC) Study. *Am J Clin Nutr*. 2008;87(1):150–155. doi:10.1093/ajcn/87.1.150

67. Weimer JR. Many elderly at nutritional risk. *USDA Food Rev*. 1997;20(1):42–48.

68. Watson L, Leslie W, Hankey C. Under-nutrition in old age: diagnosis and management. *Rev Clin Gerontol*. 2006;15:1–12.

69. Kenney WL, Chiu P. Influence of age on thirst and fluid intake. *Med Sci Sports Exerc*. 2001;33:1524–1532. doi:10.1097/00005768-200109000-00016

70. Mentes J. Oral hydration in older adults: greater awareness is needed in preventing, recognizing, and treating dehydration. *Am J Nurs*. 2006;106:40–49. doi:10.1097/00000446-200606000-00023

71. Xiao H, Barber J, Campbell E. Economic burden of dehydration among hospitalized elderly patients. *Am J Health Syst Pharm*. 2004;61:2534–2540. doi:10.1093/ajhp/61.23.2534

72. Kyle UG, Genton L, Hans D, et al. Age-related differences in fat-free mass, skeletal muscle, body cell mass and fat mass between 18 and 94 years. *Eur J Clin Nutr*. 2001;55:663–672. doi:10.1038/sj.ejcn.1601198

73. Pooler J, Srinivasan M. *Issue Brief: Social Determinants of Health and the Aging Population*. AARP Foundation and IMPAQ International; 2018. https://www.impaqint.com/sites/default/files/issue-briefs/Issue%20Brief_SDOHandAgingPopulation_0.pdf

74. Agency for Healthcare Research and Quality. *National Healthcare Disparities Report 2013.* Rockville, MD: Agency for Healthcare Research and Quality; 2014.

75. Anderson G. *Chronic Care: Making the Case for Ongoing Care.* Princeton, NJ: Robert Wood Johnson Foundation; 2010.

76. Rabin B, Brownson R, Haire-Joshu D, et al. A glossary for dissemination and implementation research in health. *J Public Health Manag Pract.* 2008;14(2):117–123. doi:10.1097/01.PHH.0000311888.06252.bb

77. Federal Interagency Forum on Aging-Related Statistics. *Older Americans 2016: Key Indicators of Well-Being.* 2016. https://agingstats.gov/docs/LatestReport/Older-Americans-2016-Key-Indicators-of -WellBeing.pdf

78. Kirkman MS, Briscoe VJ, Clark N, et al. Diabetes in older adults. *Diabetes Care.* 2012;35(12):2650–2664. doi:10.2337/dc12-1801

79. National Institute on Aging. *Stroke.* 2017. https://www.nia.nih.gov/health/stroke

80. Mannimo D, Buist A. Global burden of COPD: risk factors, prevalence, and future trends. *Lancet.* 2007;370:9589. doi:10.1016/S0140-6736(07)61380-4

81. Alzheimer's Disease International. *World Alzheimer Report 2015: The Global Impact of Dementia.* London: Alzheimer's Disease International; 2015.

82. Endoy MP. Anorexia among older adults. *Am J Nurse Pract.* 2005;9(5):31–38.

83. Evans C. Malnutrition in the elderly: a multifactorial failure to thrive. *Perm J.* 2005;9(3):38–41. doi:10.7812/TPP/05-056

84. Huffman G. Evaluating and treating unintentional weight loss in the elderly. *Am Fam Phys.* 2002;65(4):640–650.

85. Srivarathan A, Jensen AN, Kristiansen M. Community-based interventions to enhance healthy aging in disadvantaged areas: perceptions of older adults and health care professionals. *BMC Health Serv Res.* 2019;19(1):7. doi:10.1186/s12913-018-3855-6

86. Food and Agriculture Organization. *Voluntary Guidelines to Support the Progressive Realization of the Right to Adequate Food in the Context of National Food Security.* Rome, Italy: Food and Agriculture Organization of the United Nations; 2005. http://www.fao.org/3/a-y7937e.pdf

87. Napoli M, De Muro P, Mazziotta M, et al. *Towards a Food Insecurity Multidimensional Index (FIMI).* Rome, Italy: Food and Agriculture Organization of the United Nations; 2011.

88. World Food Programme. *Emergency Food Security Assessment Handbook.* 2nd ed. Rome, Italy: World Food Programme; 2009:170. https://documents.wfp.org/stellent/groups/public/documents/manual_ guide_proced/wfp203244.pdf

89. Albu M, Murphy E. *Market Analysis Tool in Rapid-Onset Emergencies.* Practical Action Consulting, Warwickshire, CV23; 2007. http://www.cashlearning.org/downloads/marketanalysisinemergencies -phaseonereportfinal.pdf

90. Galvez M, Morland K, Raines C, et al. Race and food store availability in an inner city neighborhood. *Public Health Nutr.* 2007;11:624–631. doi:10.1017/S1368980007001097

91. Food and Agriculture Organization. *World Food Summit: Rome Declaration on World Food Security and World Food Summit Plan of Action.* Rome, Italy: Food and Agriculture Organization; 1996.

92. Food Research & Action Center. *The Impact of Poverty, Food Insecurity, and Poor Nutrition on Health and Well-Being.* 2017. https://frac.org/wp-content/uploads/hunger-health-impact-poverty-food-insecurity -health-well-being.pdf

93. Holben DH, Taylor CA. Food insecurity and its association with central obesity and other markers of metabolic syndrome among persons aged 12 to 18 years in the United States. *J Am Osteopath Assoc.* 2015;115(9):536–543. doi:10.7556/jaoa.2015.111

94. Weinfield NS, Mills G, Borger C, et al. *Hunger in America 2014.* Chicago, IL: Feeding America; 2014.

95. Ver Ploeg M, Mancino L, Todd JE, et al. *Where Do Americans Usually Shop for Food and How Do They Travel To Get There? Initial Findings from the National Household Food Acquisition and Purchase Survey.* Washington, DC: U.S. Department of Agriculture, Economic Research Service; 2015.

96. Wiig K, Smith C. The art of grocery shopping on a food stamp budget: factors influencing the food choices of low-income women as they try to make ends meet. *Public Health Nutr.* 2009;12(10):1726–1734. doi:10.1017/S1368980008004102

97. Darmon N, Drewnowski A. Contribution of food prices and diet cost to socioeconomic disparities in diet quality and health: a systematic review and analysis. *Nutr Rev.* 2015;73(10):643–660. doi:10.1093/ nutrit/nuv027

98. Kant AK, Graubard BI. Energy density of diets reported by American adults: association with food group intake, nutrient intake, and body weight. *Int J Obes*. 2005;29:950–956. doi:10.1038/sj.ijo.0802980

99. Fleischhacker SE, Evenson KR, Rodriguez DA, Ammerman AS. A systematic review of fast food access studies. *Obes Rev*. 2011;12(5):e460–e471. doi:10.1111/j.1467-789X.2010.00715.x

100. Pereira MA, Kartashov AI, Ebbeling CB, et al. Fast-food habits, weight gain, and insulin resistance (the CARDIA study): 15-year prospective analysis. *Lancet*. 2005;365(9453), 36–42. doi:10.1016/S0140-6736(04)17663-0

101. Powell LM, Nguyen BT. Fast-food and full-service restaurant consumption among children and adolescents: effect on energy, beverage, and nutrient intake. *JAMA Pediatr*. 2013;167(1):14–20. doi:10.1001/jamapediatrics.2013.417

102. Leung CW, Epel ES, Willett WC, et al. Household food insecurity is positively associated with depression among low-income Supplemental Nutrition Assistance Program participants and income-eligible nonparticipants. *J Nutr*. 2015;145(3):622–627. doi:10.3945/jn.114.199414

103. Mowen AJ. *Parks, Playgrounds, and Active Living*. San Diego, CA: Active Living Research, San Diego State University; 2010.

104. Neckerman KM, Lovasi GS, Davies S, et al. Disparities in urban neighborhood conditions: evidence from GIS measures and field observation in New York City. *J Public Health Policy*. 2009;30(suppl 1):S264–S285. doi:10.1057/jphp.2008.47

105. Powell LM, Wada R, Kumanyika SK. Racial/ethnic and income disparities in child and adolescent exposure to food and beverage television ads across the U.S. media markets. *Health Place*. 2014;29:124–131. doi:10.1016/j.healthplace.2014.06.006

106. Yancey AK, Cole BL, Brown R, et al. A cross-sectional prevalence study of ethnically targeted and general audience outdoor obesity-related advertising. *Milbank Q*. 2009;87(1):155–184. doi:10.1111/j.1468-0009.2009.00551.x

107. U.S. Department of Agriculture. *U.S. Household Food Security Survey Module*. Washington, DC: U.S. Department of Agriculture, Economic Research Service; 2012. https://www.ers.usda.gov/media/8271/hh2012.pdf

108. RTI International Center for Health and Environmental Modeling. *Current and Prospective Scope of Hunger and Food Security in America: A Review of Current Research*. Research Triangle Park, NC: RTI International; 2014. https://www.rti.org/sites/default/files/resources/full_hunger_report_final_07-24-14.pdf

109. Census of Agriculture. *Farm Demographics*. 2014. https://www.agcensus.usda.gov/Publications/2012/Online_Resources/Highlights/Farm_Demographics.

110. HLPE. *Nutrition and food systems*. A report by the High Level Panel of Experts on Food Security and Nutrition of the Committee on World Food Security, Rome; 2017.

111. Farm Subsidy Database. *Environmental Working Group*. 2014. http://farm.ewg.org

112. Foley J. It's time to rethink America's corn system. Scientific American. March 5, 2013. https://www.scientificamerican.com/article/time-to-rethink-corn

113. Food and Agriculture Organization. The Future of Food and Agriculture: Alternative Pathways to 2050. Rome, Italy: Food and Agriculture Organization; 2018:224. Licence: CC BY-NC-SA 3.0 IGO. http://www.fao.org/3/I8429EN/i8429en.pdf

114. Hall KD, Guo J, Dore M, Chow CC. The progressive increase of food waste in America and its environmental impact. *PLoS One*. 2009;4(11):9–14. doi:10.1371/journal.pone.0007940

115. Jilcott Pitts SB, Gustafson A, Wu Q, et al. Farmers' market use is associated with fruit and vegetable consumption in diverse southern rural communities. *Nutr J*. 2014;13:1. doi:10.1186/1475-2891-13-1

116. Rossi JJ, Woods TA, Allen JE. Impacts of a Community Supported Agriculture (CSA) voucher program on food lifestyle behaviors: evidence from an employer-sponsored pilot program. *Sustainability, MDPI, Open Access Journal*. 2017;9(9):1–21.

117. Coleman-Jensen A, Rabbitt M, Gregory C, Singh A. *Household Food Security in the United States in 2018, ERR-270*. Washington, DC: U.S. Department of Agriculture, Economic Research Service; 2019.

118. Owens N, Donley A. The impact of the Farmers' Market Nutrition Program on participating Florida farmers: a research note. *J Rural Soc Sci*. 2015;30(1):Article 6. https://egrove.olemiss.edu/jrss/vol30/iss1/6

119. Centers for Disease Control and Prevention. *Estimates of Foodborne Illness in the United States*. 2011. https://www.cdc.gov/foodborneburden

120. Friel S, Ford L. Systems, food security, and human health. *Food Secur*. 2015;7:437. doi:10.1007/s12571-015-0433-1

121. United Nations. *Sustainable Development Goal 2: Targets and Indicators. Sustainable Development Goals*. 2019. https://sustainabledevelopment.un.org/sdg2

122. Bhutta ZA, Salam RA. Global nutrition epidemiology and trends. *Ann Nutr Metab*. 2012;61(suppl 1):19–27. doi:10.1159/000345167

123. U.S. Department of Agriculture. *Study Shows Strong Nutrition Education Can Lead to Healthier Food Choices by Supplemental Nutrition Assistance Program Recipients*. https://www.fns.usda.gov/pressrelease/2013/fns-001313. Published December 5, 2013.

124. National Council on Aging. About NCOA. https://www.ncoa.org/about-ncoa

125. Office of the High Commissioner for Human Rights. CESCR General Comment No. 12: The Right to Adquate Food (Art. 11). https://www.refworld.org/pdfid/4538838c11.pdf. Published May 12, 1999.

126. World Health Organization. *Household air pollution and health*. 2020. https://www.who.int/news-room/fact-sheets/detail/household-air-pollution-and-health

127. World Health Organization. *Measles*. 2020. https://www.who.int/news-room/fact-sheets/detail/measles

128. World Health Organization. *Malaria*. 2020. https://www.who.int/news-room/fact-sheets/detail/malaria

129. World Health Organization. *UNICEF-WHO-The World Bank Group, Joint child malnutrition estimates-Levels and trends*. 2019. https://www.who.int/nutgrowthdb/estimates2018/en/

130. Bellows A, Hamm M. U.S.-based community food security: influences, practice, debate. *J Study Food Soc*. 2002;6(1):31–44. doi:10.2752/152897902786732725

PROFESSIONAL DEVELOPMENT NEEDS AND STRATEGIES IN PUBLIC HEALTH NUTRITION

KYLE L. THOMPSON AND OLIVIA ANDERSON

LEARNING OBJECTIVES

1. Articulate the necessity and importance of continuous **professional** development throughout the career course of each public health nutrition (PHN) professional.

2. Describe strategies and methods for professional **self-assessment** and development.

3. List and identify professional organizations to support professional growth and networks in PHN.

4. Describe the importance of the **grantsmanship** process for PHN professionals.

5. Describe the steps in the grantsmanship process.

6. Develop a plan for **lifelong learning** and growth as a professional.

INTRODUCTION

Who is a professional? What is **professionalism?**

As PHN continues to assume increasing prominence within the broader field of public health, the importance of defining professional attributes for PHN practitioners grows. The word *professional* is derived from the Middle English word *profession*, which described the act of professing one's vows to a religious community; the Middle English word sprang from the Latin word *profiteri*, "to declare publicly."[1] Thus, a professional is someone who publicly declares—or vows—skill in a certain area of service or knowledge. Today, professionals can be defined as persons who move into a paid occupation that includes extensive training toward the development of formal qualifications and expertise.

Professionalism has been referred to in terms of specific **competencies**, expertise, and skills expected for the profession. While professionalism can also be defined subjectively, with different individuals holding different views on which characteristics constitute professional behavior, several traits are commonly associated with professionalism. Professional traits in healthcare careers include but are not limited to **competence** in the discipline practiced, reliability, calmness under pressure, flexibility, problem-solving capabilities, an empathetic and compassionate demeanor, excellent communication skills, a neat appearance, confidence without arrogance, a strong work ethic, good self-management and organizational abilities, accountability for one's own actions, understanding and accepting one's own limits, and acceptance of responsibility for continuing education and improvement of skills.[2,3] Professionalism may also be indicated by **certification** and/or **credentialing** by professional boards, such as the National Board of Public Health Examiners or, for dietetics professionals, the Commission on Dietetic Registration.[4,5]

Even though the term *profession* does not have one standard definition, several features are commonly associated with the word.[6] A profession encompasses a specific body of knowledge and field of practice, establishes a required course of training and credentialing for practitioners, develops ethical standards for practice and holds members of the profession accountable to those standards, and practices for the public good.[6] For the benefit and protection of the public, professions—and professionals—are expected to regulate themselves.

Because the field of PHN is still emerging, the formulation of professional standards for practitioners is in its initial stages.[7] This situation presents challenges for those who wish to confirm their PHN skills with appropriate credentialing, and for those seeking to educate future practitioners. However, along with challenges come great opportunities to define the profession, to delineate its scope of practice, and to develop educational and training opportunities that result in the confirmation of specific professional skills and competencies, all focused on the public good. Organizations such as the Association of State Public Health Nutritionists (ASPHN), the World Public Health Nutrition Association (WPHNA), and the Association of Graduate Programs in Public Health Nutrition (AGPPHN) have identified the training and equipping of future PHN leaders and practitioners as a priority action initiative.

This chapter discusses the importance of professional development throughout the span of one's career. In addition, this chapter discusses the development of guidelines for professional performance in PHN, suggests strategies for continuing professional development, provides a summary of professional organizations to support ongoing professional growth, leadership development, and emphasizes the development of grantsmanship skills as a key area of professional development.

THE IMPORTANCE OF CONTINUOUS PROFESSIONAL DEVELOPMENT

In a seminal article published in 1999 in the *Journal of the American Dietetic Association* (now the *Journal of the Academy of Nutrition and Dietetics*), Roberta L. Duyff, MS, RD, stated, "With our first breath we start a journey of learning. It is an adventure – for life and for our development as nutrition professionals."[8] Once one completes a program of study and enters the professional world, the process of learning has, in many ways, only begun.

The field of PHN, which incorporates subsets of both public health and nutrition knowledge, shares the broad spectrum of practice and the burgeoning body of knowledge common to both disciplines. Because the field of PHN is rapidly developing and changing, practitioners must be accountable for maintaining and improving knowledge, skills, and professional attributes. The importance of professional development may be highlighted by a question: Would you, as a patient, want to be treated by a physician who graduated from medical school and completed his or her residency 20 years ago, but has made no effort to update his or her skills or engage in **continuing professional education (CPE)** since that date? Such a practitioner would have failed to align his or her practice with one of the key characteristics of both a professional and a profession: self-accountability and self-regulation.

Public health nutritionists, who work with groups and populations to promote health, disease prevention, and quality of life through nutrition, have a responsibility to stay current with knowledge and skills in order to effectively deliver evidence-based, high-quality nutrition interventions to their populations served. Professional development as public health nutritionists is a career- and lifelong endeavor. PHN training programs should teach the process and skills of continuing professional development as part of the standard curriculum.

STRATEGIES AND METHODS OF PROFESSIONAL DEVELOPMENT

Levels of Professional Development

The **Dreyfus Model of Skill Acquisition (DMSA)** is frequently used to conceptualize levels of skill development in health professions education.[9–12] The DMSA has defined the following levels of competence for adult learners: novice, advanced beginner, competent, proficient, and expert.[9] The DMSA describes a progression in which a novice begins by carefully following rules while under supervision. Over time, the novice develops proficiency and expertise that facilitate independent, creative, ethical practice at multiple levels of influence, along with the ability to supervise and mentor others.[9,10,13–15]

New practitioners should adopt a realistic view of the process of professional development. While a newly graduated PHN practitioner may have a great deal of knowledge gained from study and the completion of experience-based projects, seasoned professionals point out that true proficiency in practice comes only with time.[10,13] Time is required to interact with a wide variety of people and situations; to internalize the learning that occurs at the intersections of knowledge, experience, and practice; and to develop the confidence that enables one to progress toward higher levels of practice. Realistic attitudes include the understanding that career progression is seldom smooth. Significant professional growth may occur in the process of accepting and dealing with obstacles, challenges, and failures that inevitably transpire during the course of one's career. Personal and professional preferences may indicate a desire to remain at a competent or proficient level throughout one's career, rather than seeking to practice as an expert. And professionals may operate at a high level in one area of competence, while performing as a beginner in another, more recently pursued area. Accurate perceptions of the stages of professional development will assist PHN professionals in understanding what to expect of themselves at various locations on the professional development continuum.

Several nutrition- and health-related professions have named and defined levels of professional development, working within the context of the DMSA. The Academy of Nutrition and Dietetics (AND) provides minimum standards of practice for core functions of the nutrition and dietetics technician and the registered dietitian nutritionist (RDN).[16] Practitioners of focus areas of dietetics—examples include clinical nutrition management, oncology nutrition, education of nutrition and dietetics practitioners, and others—are described as "competent," "proficient," or "expert."[17] In a seminal book published in 1984, Patricia Benner defined five levels of practice in the nursing profession: novice, advanced beginner, competent, proficient, and expert, aligning with the DMSA.[9,13,18] It is important to remember that practitioners of various health disciplines may simultaneously function as experts in some focus areas and as competent in others.[11] Important, too, is the recognition that not every proficient professional desires to reach the expert level of practice, which typically involves managerial/executive responsibilities.[10] While the exact terminology may vary among disciplines, health professions in general recognize that there are levels of practice and that there is a progression of development that occurs as novice practitioners gain experience over time. Table 15.1 provides a chart aligning the DMSA with levels of PHN practice.

Standards for Professional Development

Specific content areas for professional development for PHN practitioners are in formation. *Competencies* have been described by the Accreditation Council for Education in Nutrition and Dietetics (ACEND) as the "the described knowledge, skills, and judgment needed to perform as a professional."[19] Like other health professions, the ACEND has developed competencies, which are currently used to guide the education of dietetics professionals, including dietetic technicians, registered (DTRs), and RDNs.[19] The ACEND competencies, like competencies designed for other health professions, are used for purposes beyond novice practitioner training: (a) as a framework for CPE; (b) assessment of practitioner competency; (c) benchmarking for practitioner credentialing; (d) career planning; and (e) formulation of job descriptions.[7,19]

In 2011, the WPHNA published a background paper on the process of establishing competency areas for global PHN workers.[7] The WPHNA authors provide a rationale for the development of specific competencies for PHN practitioners. They explain that professional skills for public health nutritionists differ from those required for clinical nutrition practice and state that their model:

> recognises that population-based and promotional-preventative actions are required to address malnutrition in both forms *[under- and overnutrition]*. This requires different work that *compliments* clinical practice and consequently requires additional competencies, the knowledge, skills, and attitudes to perform this work.[7]

The background paper identifies 10 **core competency** areas for global PHN professionals. The 10 competencies, or functions, are encompassed within three broad areas of practice and may be summarized as follows:

1. Research and analysis: Primary competencies include monitoring, assessing, and communicating population nutrition data and nutrition needs.

2. Build capacity: Primary competencies include developing community, organizational, and workforce capacity.

3. Intervention management: Primary competencies include planning, implementing, managing, and evaluating interventions; enhancing community knowledge of healthful nutrition; advocating for healthful nutrition policy, nutrition equity, and the meeting of nutrition needs for all throughout the life span.

Table 15.2 provides a chart of the 10 core competencies described by the WPHNA. In the competency document provided in Table 15.2, the WPHNA has identified three categories of workforce personnel that can be roughly aligned with levels of practice for global public health nutritionists.[7] Competencies are determined to be **core** or **complementary** for each of the three practitioner types described: frontline, manager, and specialist.[7]

The AGPPHN in 2013 published competencies for training PHN professionals. PHN practitioners from a variety of educational and government agencies in the United States assisted in the preparation of this document. The competency document is available on the AGPPHN website.

TABLE 15.1 ALIGNMENT OF THE DMSA WITH LEVELS OF PHN PRACTICE

DMSA LEVEL	PRACTITIONER EXAMPLE	TYPICAL CHARACTERISTICS
Novice	PHN student in final phases of initial educational program Example: Student completing a field experience or capstone project	• Lacks experience that would otherwise provide context to inform applications of rules and guidelines to experiences • Carefully follows rules, policies, and guidelines • Requires ongoing supervision and mentoring • Collaborative and team skills are emerging • Professionalism is emerging
Advanced beginner	Newly graduated PHN employee in first employment setting Example: New WIC nutritionist working in a county health department	• Begins to gain a variety of experiences, which provide context for applications of rules and guidelines to situations • Carefully follows rules, policies, and guidelines • Requires supervision and mentoring; begins to work independently and assume responsibility for specific tasks • Competence is emerging • Demonstrates collaborative and team skills • Displays professionalism by practicing in an ethical and responsible manner • Engages in ongoing professional development; process is guided by mentors
Competent	PHN practitioner (2 or more years' work experience) Example: Food and nutrition educator for a multicounty group of food pantries served by a regional food bank	• Synthesizes lessons learned from experiences and situations; has developed a context to inform applications of rules, policies, and guidelines; innate sense of "what to do" has emerged and continues to develop • Works independently; takes responsibility for specific tasks and own performance • Competence is consistent and well established • Demonstrates good collaborative and team skills • Displays professionalism by practicing in an ethical and responsible manner • Engages in ongoing professional development; process is guided by self and mentors

(continued)

TABLE 15.1 ALIGNMENT OF THE DMSA WITH LEVELS OF PHN PRACTICE *(continued)*

DMSA LEVEL	PRACTITIONER EXAMPLE	TYPICAL CHARACTERISTICS
Proficient	Experienced PHN practitioner with a track record of excellence (8 or more years' work experience) Example: SNS for a county school district	• Has developed an innate sense of "what to do"; rules, policies, and guidelines have become internalized and provide the context for practice • Works independently; takes responsibility for own performance; may supervise/manage the work of others • Track record of excellence in performance is well established • Demonstrates excellent collaborative and team skills; may engage in collaboration and team-building • Consistently displays professionalism by practicing in an ethical and responsible manner • Engages in ongoing professional development; process is guided by self and informed by mentors
Expert	Seasoned PHN practitioner with broad experience, a track record of excellence and accomplishment, and evident leadership abilities Example: Regional director of the USDA FNS	• Highly developed, innate sense of "what to do"; rules, policies, and guidelines have become internalized and provide the context for practice • Establishes organizational vision, goals, and initiatives; applies and manages resources; directs and manages staff in accomplishing goals • Mentors emerging leaders • Track record of excellence and accomplishments is well established • Leads collaboration and team-building efforts • Consistently displays professionalism by practicing in an ethical and responsible manner • Engages in ongoing professional development; process is guided by self and informed by mentors

DMSA, Dreyfus Model of Skill Acquisition; FNS, food and nutrition service; PHN, public health nutrition, SNS, school nutrition specialist; USDA, U.S. Department of Agriculture; WIC, Special Supplemental Nutrition Program for Women, Infants, and Children.

Source: Data from Brody RA, Byham-Gray L, Touger-Decker R, et al. Identifying components of advanced-level clinical nutrition practice: a Delphi study. *J Acad Nutr Diet.* 2012;112(6):859–869; Dreyfus SE, Dreyfus HL. *Mind Over Machine.* New York, NY: Free Press; 1998; Martin K. *The Improvement Professional's Evolving Role: From Practitioner to Coach.* 2011. https://www.slideshare.net/KarenMartinGroup/the-improvement-professionals-evolving-role-from-practitioner-to-facilitator-oto-coac/13-Dreyfus_Model_ofSkill_AcquisitionStuart_Hubert

TABLE 15.2 WPHNA'S 10 CORE FUNCTIONS FOR GLOBAL PUBLIC HEALTH NUTRITIONISTS, WITH FUNCTIONS OF KEY WORKFORCE ACTORS AT THE FRONTLINE, MANAGER, AND SPECIALIST LEVELS

CATEGORY	CORE PHN FUNCTION	FRONT LINE	MANAGER	SPECIALIST
Research and analysis	1. Monitor, assess, and communicate population nutritional health needs and issues 2. Develop and communicate intelligence about determinants of nutrition problems, policy impacts, intervention effectiveness, and prioritization through research and evaluation	Core Core	Core Core	Core Core
Build capacity	3. Develop the various tiers of the PHN workforce and its collaborators through education, disseminating intelligence, and ensuring organizational support 4. Build community capacity and social capital to engage in, identify, and build solutions to nutrition problems and issues 5. Build organizational capacity and systems to facilitate and coordinate effective PHN action	Complementary Core Core	Core Complementary Core	Core Core Core
Intervention management	6. Plan, develop, implement, and evaluate interventions that address the determinants of priority PHN issues and problems and promote equity 7. Enhance and sustain population (community) knowledge and awareness of healthful eating so that dietary choices are informed choices 8. Advocate for food- and nutrition-related policy and government support to protect and promote health 9. Promote, develop, and support healthy growth and development throughout all life stages 10. Promote equitable access to safe and healthy food so that healthy choices are easy choices	Core Complementary Core Core	Complementary Complementary Complementary Complementary	Core Core Core Core

Core function, those functions that are regarded as absolutely necessary, without which would imply gaps in public health capacity; **complementary functions,** may be core in some contexts, often complementary to the work of the PHN specialist; PHN, public health nutrition; WPHNA, World Public Health Nutrition Association.
Source: From Hughes R, Shrimpton R, Recine E, Margetts B. *A Competency Framework for Global Public Health Nutrition Workforce Development: A Background Paper.* London, UK: World Public Health Nutrition Association; 2011. http://www .wphna.org/htdocs/downloadsapr2012/12-03%20WPHNA%20Draft%20competency%20standards%20report.pdf

Strategies for Professional Development

In her article on lifelong learning, Roberta Duyff outlined a process that has been adapted and utilized as a framework for professional development by the AND, as well as other professional organizations.[8] Since Duyff's article was published in 1999, various iterations of the professional development process have been implemented by health professions. However, the basic principles of repeated cycling through a process of self-assessment, **goal setting**, **strategic planning**, plan implementation, and further self-assessment and evaluation remain key components of professional development.[8] The goal of professional development is continuous growth in professional competency throughout the career span. Table 15.3 lists steps in the professional development process.

Step One: Self-Assessment

Self-assessment is a core component of professional development, and a vital element of lifelong learning.[20-22] Self-assessment has been defined as the ability to compare and judge one's own performance against a standard of practice.[23] Ideally, professionals should be able to review their practice, identify areas for improvement, and plan activities to fill the knowledge and skill gaps identified.

Self-assessment consists of three important and complementary tasks. First, the professional chooses a standard of performance and performs a comparison of actual performance with that standard. PHN professionals may choose to use the WPHNA competencies as a comparative standard. Second, the professional seeks constructive feedback and further education, experiences, or remediation as needed.[23] Third, the professional defines current and desired future professional roles, and thinks ahead to establish a timeline for growth.[24] Several professional organizations

TABLE 15.3 STEPS IN THE PROFESSIONAL DEVELOPMENT PROCESS

STEP	DESCRIPTION	THE CYCLE REPEATS
1. Self-assessment	Comparison of one's own performance to a selected standard	
2. Goal setting	Based on the results of self-assessment, development of specific goals for professional development and performance improvement	
3. Strategic planning	The process of planning experiences and activities designed to achieve desired goals	
4. Implementation	The process of implementing planned experiences and activities	
5. Repeat the professional development process	The process of periodically and regularly reviewing the results of professional development and repeating the cycle, beginning with self-assessment	

Source: Data from Duyff RL. The value of lifelong learning: key element in professional career development. *J Acad Nutr Diet.* 1999;99(5):538–543; Commission on Dietetic Registration. *Professional Development Portfolio Guide with Essential Practice Competencies.* 2019. https://www.cdrnet.org/vault/2459/web/files/PDP%20Guide%E2%80%942020.pdf; Doran GT. There's a S.M.A.R.T. way to write management's goals and objectives. *Manag Rev.* 1981;70:35–36.

encourage practitioners to ask themselves questions like, "Where do I want to be in 3 years? In 5 years?"[21]

Professionals engage in self-assessment continually, as daily tasks and events, and perhaps weekly and monthly performance indicators, indicate opportunities for improvement. Planning for comprehensive self-assessment at regular intervals—perhaps annually or semiannually—is important to ensure that this important process is not overlooked. Governing bodies of health professions nearly always mandate participation in a regular process of professional development, including self-assessment, as a requirement for maintaining credentialing.

Researchers have found that accurate self-assessment is notoriously difficult.[25,26] Human nature impacts self-evaluation. A natural tendency is to overlook areas to improve because identification of deficiencies is uncomfortable and the effort required to correct them may be substantial and inconvenient.[26] Any number of contextual factors may affect one's ability to self-assess, including one's general life situation, practice environment, and a myriad of other influences.[23] Individuals are prone to rate themselves too high or too low compared to the chosen standard.[25] Professionals may lack a systematic method for self-evaluation, not understand which performance criteria should be self-assessed, or simply not understand the importance of self-assessment. For this reason, it is important to remember that self-assessment also includes seeking external feedback. Thus, an accurate self-assessment would include consideration of such evidence as performance reviews, comments, and input from colleagues and clients, customer satisfaction surveys, and other objective evidence.

Systematic self-assessment provides meaningful comparisons that are helpful in planning professional development activities. Based on the results of a comprehensive self-assessment that includes personal reflection and objective evidence, the professional is ready to construct and implement a strategic plan for development.

Step Two: Goal Setting

Based on the results of self-assessment, the PHN professional should set professional development goals. The concept of **SMART goals** has been popular since 1981, when George T. Doran wrote an article proposing the concept.[27] The acronym defines a process for creating goals that are specific, measurable, achievable, realistic, and timely.[27] Timely goals may include both short-term (1 year or less) and long-term (usually considered 3–5 years) goals. Goals should be prioritized in order of importance.

For example, a PHN practitioner may decide that improvement of grantsmanship skills is a professional priority. Examples of SMART goals directed at this priority include:

- "I will request a mentor in grantsmanship from my supervisor, and will make the request within 2 weeks of implementing this strategic plan" (S—request a mentor in grantsmanship; M—the task is either done or not; A—the goal is achievable within the current employment situation; R—the goal is realistic and feasible to accomplish; T—the goal is timely).

- "I will register for and attend a webinar on grant writing within 3 months of implementing this strategic plan" (S—register for and attend a webinar on grantsmanship; M—the task is either done or not; A—the goal is achievable within the current employment situation; R—the goal is realistic and feasible to accomplish; T—the goal is timely).

■ "I will complete and submit a community foundation grant application for a new commercial refrigerator for our local food pantry within 6 months of implementing this strategic plan" (S—complete and submit a community foundation grant application; M—the task is either done or not; A—the goal is achievable within the current employment situation; R—the goal is realistic and feasible to accomplish; T—the goal is timely).

SMART goals are more likely to be achieved than poorly defined, general statements such as, "I want to be a better public health nutrition professional."

When setting goals, professionals should consider profession-specific requirements for the maintenance of credentialing. Such requirements may involve earning a specific number of CPE hours or credits, or participating in certain activities, over a specified period of time.[21] The strategic plan should include activities directed toward meeting the profession's credentialing standards. Table 15.4 provides a description of SMART goals. Table 15.4 provides a description of SMART goals, based on a PHN practitioner's work assignment to plan community-focused grocery store tours.[40]

TABLE 15.4 SMART GOALS: EXPLANATION AND EXAMPLES

SMART GOAL CRITERION	EXPLANATION	"DO THIS" EXAMPLE	"DON'T DO THIS" EXAMPLE
1. **S**pecific	The goal is clearly defined and described	"I will plan and deliver a 45-minute grocery store tour focused on packing a healthful lunch box for school or work."	"I will get better at doing grocery store tours."
2. Measurable	It is clear whether or not the goal has been reached.	"The delivery date for the tour is May 6, 20__. I've communicated and collaborated with the store manager on all details of the tour. The lesson plan for the tour will be delivered to my supervisor by April 21, 20__, for review and revision. I will market the tour for 4 weeks preceding the tour, with a goal of attaining 8–10 participants."	"I'll try to deliver the tour sometime soon."
3. Achievable	A reasonable person would conclude that the goal is achievable, given current circumstances.	"Given my current practice environment, I am very sure that I can be successful with the tour."	Does not consider
4. Realistic	Given the resources, time, and facilities available, a reasonable person would conclude that this goal is feasible.	"Given the resources, time, and facilities available to me, this tour is realistic and feasible to accomplish."	Does not consider
5. Timely	A time limit is set for achievement of the goal.	"I'll deliver the tour on May 6, 20__, will evaluate the event with my supervisor within 2 weeks following the tour, and will develop next steps within 3 weeks following the tour."	"Hopefully I'll get this done sometime this year."

Source: From Doran GT. There's a S.M.A.R.T. Way to write management's goals and objectives. *Manage Rev.* 1981;70:35–36.

Steps Three and Four: Strategic Planning and Implementation

Strategic planning for professionals occurs after (a) self-assessment reveals directions and desires for career development, areas of interest to be explored or strengthened, and/or performance indicators to be improved and (b) goals for professional development are established. Professional development possibilities encompass an expansive range of topics and include both profession-specific skills and general professional skills. Professionals may choose to plan strategically for development in four areas that have been defined by Duke University Human Resources: "technical skills, social skills, aptitudes (natural talents), attitudes (ways of looking at things."[28] Another way of looking at areas for development is to categorize skills as "hard," or technical and profession-specific, and "soft," or people- and attitude-oriented.[41] Both types of skills are important targets for professional development.

Strategic planning sets the direction for professional development, but the most carefully formulated strategic plan is useless unless it is implemented. Thus, steps three and four—strategic planning and implementation—are inseparable. The strategic plan includes participation in activities and personal growth initiatives that are aligned with the attainment of desired goals. The professional must consider barriers to achieving components of the strategic plan and take action to address those barriers.[24] The practitioner should be aware that professional development plans created for employment or credentialing purposes usually require approval from designated parties, often a job supervisor or professional credentialing board.

Professionals should document their development activities, including reflections on self-assessment, goals based on the results of self-assessment, the strategic plan for attaining desired goals, and the activities and initiatives directed toward professional growth.[24] A simple Internet search will reveal a number of professional development planning tools, and many professional organizations provide their own templates, along with online recording of professional activities and continuing education credits. **Documentation** should include copies of continuing education credits awarded, certifications earned, and competencies demonstrated, along with any other records that indicate professional growth. Records of professional development should "tell the story" of one's career growth and development over time.

Step Five: Repeat the Professional Development Process

Professional development is an ongoing process throughout the career span. When the timeline for one professional development plan expires, the practitioner should repeat the process, beginning with self-assessment and an evaluation of the results of the previous plan. As the professional development process is repeated in cyclic fashion, growth in professional competence, and progression through the various levels of competence, should result.

ENGAGEMENT IN PROFESSIONAL ORGANIZATIONS TO PROMOTE PROFESSIONAL DEVELOPMENT

Profession-specific organizations serve practitioners in a myriad of ways, and are key resources supporting professional development. Examples of such organizations include but are not limited to the ASPHN, the American Public Health Association (APHA), and the AND. Involvement in professional organizations can be a fulfilling and rewarding component of one's career throughout the career span, and is *highly* recommended for PHN professionals.

Participation in professional organizations offers a number of benefits, including but not limited to:

- *Alignment with a professional group* that offers an established code of ethics and a variety of other practice resources

- **Networking** *opportunities* on a variety of levels: local, state, regional, national, and international

- *Leadership opportunities,* including committee/task force/practice initiative participation; leadership of practice groups focused on areas of interest; writing and editing newsletters and other organizational publications; program planning for state/regional/national meetings; consulting on issues of importance to the profession—perhaps providing input for government initiatives at the request of local, state, or national policy makers; running for and holding an elected office in the organization

- *Services* such as professional liability insurance, job postings, **mentorship,** profession-related news updates, and a variety of others

- *Involvement* in profession-wide initiatives (examples include the AND *Evidence Analysis Library* and the *National Fruit and Vegetable Nutrition Council* of the ASPHN)

- *Publications,* including scholarly journals (examples include *American Journal of Public Health, Journal of Nutrition Education and Behavior*), trade magazines, and newsletters

- *Continuing education events and opportunities,* both face to face and online

- *Staying up to date* with new developments in the profession, along with opportunities to influence the profession's future

Perusal of organizational websites will provide a wealth of information regarding opportunities for involvement in professional development activities. These may include meetings, current concerns and initiatives, and networking opportunities. Table 15.5 provides examples of professional organizations and selected benefits of membership.

Leadership Development

Chapter 1 emphasizes that leadership development and other professional development training is a critical focus for PHN professionals as they work to meet the nutrition-related needs of the public and often involved in the leadership of multidisciplinary, stakeholder groups to promote population health through nutrition services, interventions, initiatives and policy, systems, and environmental change.[42] In addition, the vital importance of building capacity in the area of leadership skills of public health nutrition professionals is emphasized across the professional associations referred to in this chapter. For example, WPHNA's website affirms the significance of leadership and scholarship to strengthen the evidence base for effective action as vital to the field. ASPHN states that developing skilled leaders in public health nutrition is a critical component of all their work and provide examples of effective leadership training programs offered in the U.S. such as Johns Hopkins Maternal and Child Health Leadership Skills Development Series; The Academy of Nutrition and Dietetics Leadership Certificate of Training; and The National WIC Association Leadership Academy.

SKILLS FOR EFFECTIVE GRANTSMANSHIP IN PHN

Collaboration and Innovation

As an expert in the field of PHN, one must constantly remain innovative. **Innovation,** in other words, is at the forefront of research ideas that are funded. To a novice or even a seasoned

TABLE 15.5 SELECTED EXAMPLES OF PROFESSIONAL ORGANIZATIONS OF POTENTIAL BENEFIT TO PHN PROFESSIONALS

ORGANIZATION	CONTACT INFORMATION	MISSION	EXAMPLES OF SERVICES PROVIDED TO MEMBERS (THESE ASSOCIATIONS PROVIDE MANY OTHER MEMBER BENEFITS IN ADDITION TO THOSE MENTIONED IN THE FOLLOWING)
Academy of Nutrition and Dietetics (AND)	Academy of Nutrition and Dietetics 120 South Riverside Plaza, Suite 2190 Chicago, Illinois 60606-6995 Phone: 800/877-1600 Phone: 312/899-0040 www.eatright.org	To impact health internationally through nutrition and foods	• EatRight Careers and job postings • *Journal of the Academy of Nutrition and Dietetics* • *Food and Nutrition* magazine • Continuing professional education opportunities • Online certificates of training, including a certificate in PHN • National conference (FNCE)
American Public Health Association (APHA)	APHA 800 I Street, NW Washington, DC 20001 202-777-2742 www.apha.org	Improve the health of the public and achieve equity in health status (APHA, 2019)	• Sections/Special Primary Interest Groups • *The Nation's Health/American Journal of Public Health* • Professional development webinars • APHA Annual Meeting and Expo • Networking opportunities • Public health CareerMart
American Association of Family and Consumer Sciences (AAFCS)	AAFCS 400 N. Columbus St., Ste. 202 Alexandria, VA 22314 703-706-4600 www.aafcs.org/home	To provide leadership and support for professionals whose work assists individuals, families, and communities in making informed decisions about their well-being, relationships, and resources to achieve optimal quality of life	• Archived and live webinars • *Journal of Family and Consumer Science* • Affiliate membership in state AAFCS • Annual conference • Professional assessments and certifications • Job and career center
Association of Graduate Programs in Public Health Nutrition (AGPPHN)	agpphn.org	To promote the public's health through assessment, policy development, assurance of and accessibility to food and nutrition programs and services through the promotion of excellence in the graduate education of qualified professionals	• Curriculum guide for PHN programs (available to members) • Networking opportunities

(continued)

TABLE 15.5 SELECTED EXAMPLES OF PROFESSIONAL ORGANIZATIONS OF POTENTIAL BENEFIT TO PHN PROFESSIONALS (continued)

ORGANIZATION	CONTACT INFORMATION	MISSION	EXAMPLES OF SERVICES PROVIDED TO MEMBERS (THESE ASSOCIATIONS PROVIDE MANY OTHER MEMBER BENEFITS IN ADDITION TO THOSE MENTIONED IN THE FOLLOWING)
Association of State Public Health Nutritionists (ASPHN)	ASPHN P.O. Box 37094 Tucson, AZ 85740-7094 814-255-2829 asphn.org	To strengthen nutrition policy, programs, and environments for all people through development of PHN leaders and collective action of members nationwide	• Educational training, workshops, and meetings • The Development Digest: A Professional Growth Blog for Public Health Nutritionists • Health Equity Internship • Annual meeting • Publications and resources • Job postings
International Society of Behavioral Nutrition and Physical Activity (ISBNPA)	www.isbnpa.org/index.php?r=site/contact www.isbnpa.org	To stimulate, promote, and advocate innovative research and policyin the area of behavioral nutrition and physical activity toward the betterment of human health worldwide	• Networking opportunities • International Journal of Behavioral Nutrition and Physical Activity • Leadership opportunities • Membership and job directory • Special interest groups • Mentoring • Annual meeting
National Rural Health Association (NRHA)	NRHA 4501 College Blvd.; Suite 225 Leawood, KS 66211-1921 Phone: 816-756-3140 www.ruralhealthweb.org	To provide leadership on rural health issues through advocacy, communications, education, and research	• Annual Rural Health Conference • Rural Horizons/Journal of Rural Health • NRHA Connect (rural health social networking site) • Career Center • Government Affairs Action Alerts • Participation in committees, councils, and other groups
School Nutrition Association (SNA)	SNA 2900 S. Quincy Street, Suite 700 Arlington, VA 22206 Tel (703) 824-3000 schoolnutrition.org	Core purpose: Well-nourished students, prepared to succeed We empower and support school nutrition professionals in advancing the accessibility, quality, and integrity of school nutrition programs	• Certificates and credentialing (Certificate in School Nutrition, School Nutrition Specialist [SNS] Credential) • School Nutrition Magazine/The Journal of Child Nutrition and Management Learning Center (training, webinars, resources) • CEUs • Annual School Nutrition Industry Conference • Member awards and scholarships

(continued)

TABLE 15.5 SELECTED EXAMPLES OF PROFESSIONAL ORGANIZATIONS OF POTENTIAL BENEFIT TO PHN PROFESSIONALS *(continued)*

ORGANIZATION	CONTACT INFORMATION	MISSION	EXAMPLES OF SERVICES PROVIDED TO MEMBERS (THESE ASSOCIATIONS PROVIDE MANY OTHER MEMBER BENEFITS IN ADDITION TO THOSE MENTIONED IN THE FOLLOWING)
Society for Nutrition Education and Behavior (SNEB)	SNEB 3502 Woodview Trace Suite 300 Indianapolis, IN 46268 317-328-4627 or 1-800-235-6690 www.sneb.org	To promote effective nutrition education and healthy behavior through research, policy, and practice	• Webinars, including recorded webinars for continuing education • *Journal of Nutrition Education and Behavior* • Job postings • Annual conference • Opportunities to influence nutrition-related public policy • Journal club
Society for Public Health Education (SOPHE)	SOPHE 10 G Street N.E. Suite 605 Washington, DC 20002 202-408-9804 www.sophe.org	To provide global leadership to the profession of health education and health promotion and to promote the health of society	• SOPHE Annual Conference • *Health Education and Behavior/Health Promotion Practice/Pedagogy in Health Promotion* • Member awards and scholarships • Networking • Journal self-studies and online courses for professional development • Live webinars
World Public Health Nutrition Association (WPHNA)	WPHNA Charles Darwin House 12 Roger Street London WC1N 2JU UK	To promote and strengthen public health nutrition, as a profession and discipline with responsibility to understand, protect, and improve nutrition-related population health and well-being	• World Nutrition Conferences • *World Nutrition Journal* • Opportunity to report member news on the WPHNA website • Certification as a Global Public Health Nutritionist (eGPHN) • Opportunities to participate in advocacy and other WPHNA activities • Free membership for graduate and undergraduate students

CEUs, continuing education units; FNCE, Food and Nutrition Conference and Expo; PHN, public health nutrition.

Sources: From Academy of Nutrition and Dietetics. *Academy Mission, Vision and Principles.* 2019. https://www.eatrightpro.org/about-us/academy-vision-and-mission/mission-and-vision-statements; American Public Health Association. *Our Mission.* 2019. https://www.apha.org/about-apha/our-mission; American Association of Family and Consumer Sciences. *About Us.* 2019. https://www.aafcs.org/about/about-us; Association of Graduate Programs in Public Health Nutrition. *About.* https://agpphn.org; Association of State Public Health Nutritionists. *About ASPHN.* https://asphn.org/about; International Society for Behavioral Nutrition and Physical Activity. *About Us.* 2019. https://www.isbnpa.org/index.php?r=about/index; Slabach B, National Rural Health Association. *About the National Rural Health Association.* 2019. https://www.ruralhealthweb.org/about-nrha; School Nutrition Association. *Vision & Mission.* 2019. https://schoolnutrition.org/AboutSNA/VisionMission; Society for Nutrition Education and Behavior. *SNEB Mission.* 2019. https://www.sneb.org/about; Society for Public Health Education. *Our Mission.* 2019. https://www.sophe.org/about/mission; World Public Health Nutrition Association. *World Nutrition.* 2012. http://www.wphna.org/htdocs/2012_jan_wn2_editorial.htm

professional, the generation of new, impactful ideas can be daunting. New ideas stem from the identification of gaps in one's respective discipline. An individual may identify a gap, but developing the solution to address those gaps is most often created through collaborations.

Collaboration is an approach so common in research that it is now expected that an appropriate team of experts will be identified when generating a proposal.[29] The basis of collaborative research is that everyone involved provides creative solutions to work toward the same goal, a broad aim intended to foster a public health impact.[30] With a common goal in mind, the diverse perspectives and specific areas of expertise that make up a collaborative research team result in the generation of **process-oriented objectives**. Each team member is assigned specific and measurable tasks that contribute to reaching the goal. Collaboration that supports innovation works best when each individual has intrinsic motivation for the success of the work and confidence in their abilities to contribute to the research project being proposed.[29,31] To create the process-oriented objectives, it is vital that researchers first establish the end goal and/or aims of the project. Only then can meaningful tasks be developed that contribute to accomplishing the project's end goal.[32] This approach is referred to as backward design and is used frequently as the best practice in curriculum development but can be effectively applied to research proposals.

The Writing Process

Once the framework of the research project is established, the details can be fleshed out. Before writing the full proposal, there are a few key steps that fuel the writing process.

- *Thoroughly read through the **request for proposal (RFP)** guidelines and discuss your proposal idea with a program officer.* A program officer is a contact person who is listed on the RFP who can advise whether your project fits within the scope of the RFP or agency. If so, the program officer can then be your advocate through the writing process.[29] These steps provide affirmation that the agency/organization is the best fit for the work. Federal databases are available to see which types of projects particular programs fund and to learn who is funding particular researchers (an example is found at federalreporter.nih.gov). Foundations typically provide a database of funded projects and their principal investigators within their website.

- *Understand the written components required for the proposal.* For example, the National Institutes of Health (NIH) format includes the following components: (a) Background, (b) Specific Aims, (c) Research Strategy, (d) Significance, (e) Innovation, and (f) Approach. Each component will have a description as to what is expected including content, formatting, and length.[33] The NIH, for example, provides sample applications along with step-by-step guidance for preparing and submitting a proposal (an example is found at www.niaid.nih.gov/grants-contracts/sample-applications). Similar resources are available from other agencies and will give the researcher an opportunity to read a sample proposal before writing.

- *Write a generic outline.* When an understanding of the required components of a proposal is established, an outline initiates the actual writing process by thinking through each component and ensuring that the proposed research will meet the expectations of reviewers. Table 15.6 includes some key questions to answer when generating the outline.

- *Understand expectations of reviewers.* The review process for each agency differs, but what is common among reviewers is that they will determine whether or not the investigator has followed the written proposal guidelines. Because the review process

TABLE 15.6 REFLECTIVE QUESTIONS THAT ELICIT RESPONSES CRUCIAL TO COMMON GRANT APPLICATION COMPONENTS

QUESTION	TYPE OF APPLICATION COMPONENT THE ANSWER COULD ADDRESS
What are you proposing?	Cover Letter; Abstract
Why is this work important to the field of public health nutrition?	Background; Significance; Innovation; Letters of Support
What exactly do you plan to accomplish?	Specific Aims; Objectives
How are you going to accomplish these objectives?	Approach; Methodology; Research Strategy; Preliminary Work
How are you equipped?	Resources; Personnel
How much will it cost? How can institutional resources help?	Budget; Budget Justification
Additional information	Appendix

Source: Data from Bonetta L. Project Management. In: Bonetta L, ed. *Making the Right Moves: A Practical Guide to Scientific Management for Postdocs and New Faculty.* Research Triangle Park, NC: Burroughs Welcome Fund & Chevy Chase, MD: Howard Hughes Medical Institute; 2006.

is different for every agency, it may be hard to know exactly what the reviewers are looking for. Volunteering to be a reviewer will give a researcher the most insight into the process for a specific agency, if the agency is a potential key funding source. However, sitting as a reviewer may not always be feasible. Agencies have developed resources such as webinars, in-person seminars, and even mock review panels available online (an example is found at www.youtube.com/watch?v=lzBhKeR6VIE). Taking advantage of these resources will help a researcher to comprehend what reviewers are looking for and will help the researcher to carefully craft and target the proposal.

■ *Have someone read the proposal before submitting.* To the **principal investigator** and the rest of the research team, the research proposal may seem to flow logically from beginning to end; this is to be expected because the research team is familiar with both the topic and the proposal. However, a critical reading of the proposal by an individual external to the project will ensure that others perceive the significance and methodology as having intellectual merit, yet can be understood by a person or persons outside the collaborative research team. The best circumstances are to have someone with funding from the same agency or who has served as a reviewer to evaluate the proposal.

Grant Management Strategies

Writing the proposal and submitting it is one feat, but once the proposal is funded, then the real work begins. Managing a research project is a skill in itself and varies dramatically across research groups. Management of a project entails tracking work, communicating with collaborators, overseeing research assistants, and making sure the resources identified in the proposal are still available.[34] The following tasks may jump-start a management plan for any principal investigator:

- Identify specific tasks.
- Determine the duration of every task.
- Determine the person(s) needed to complete each task.
- Identify potential constraints.
- Decide on order of tasks.
- Develop a detailed schedule (see Exhibit 15.1 as an example).
- Revise schedule as necessary.

Fortunately, many tools and strategies are available to utilize that provide guidance to manage a project. Google Suite (G Suite) and Microsoft Office, for example, have online capabilities to share documents and other tools in real time, so an investigator could share a working agenda with multiple people or share a folder filled with relevant literature to the project. There are also messenger systems such as Slack, which can be used to communicate with all or selected team members. Slack has the capability to share files, conduct online meetings, and even sync with G Suite apps. Providing an overview of the project timeline and schedule of activities will help the team to plan, remain organized, and stay on track.[34] Certain types of graphics such as a **Gantt chart** and **Program Evaluation and Review Technique (PERT) chart** can be used and easily revised as the project progresses (Exhibit 15.1). These graphics can also be useful to help identify potential constraints within the project timeline.

Developing Writing Skills

Writing does not come naturally to most individuals, but like any professional skill, it is something that can be developed over time. **Writing skills** start in graduate school through courses that require research papers. The formatting of research papers is similar to that of a grant, especially in regard to identifying a problem or gap that has sufficient background associated with it.[35] The understanding of the framework of a research project and the mechanics of formatting, such as sections, headers, and citations are learned through writing assignments. Low-stake opportunities such as internal grants or volunteering to write the first draft of a grant for a PhD or postdoc advisor is a way to practice grant writing. These grants are often shorter in length, yet require the same components as larger federally funded or foundational grant proposals. Such grants give the researcher an opportunity to practice grant writing and following instructions. Additionally, mentors or colleagues may be more receptive to providing constructive feedback when they are asked to evaluate a proposal shorter in length. Many institutions have some form of writing centers that provide support such as writing workshops for both graduate students and faculty. And finally, there is a handful of literature to help guide professional development in writing.[35-38]

Grantsmanship Summary

PHN researchers spend their career tackling important public health issues, yet this process is much more efficient and effective if a researcher has funding to support his or her goals. Developing an innovative, intellectually sound proposal takes skill but is something that does not have to be done alone. Finding collaborators who share the same public health goals can enrich the proposal and prove to reviewers that the work proposed is feasible. There are important steps to take before writing the proposal that will increase the likelihood of it being funded. Once funded, there is

EXHIBIT 15.1

SAMPLE GANTT CHART FOR A SIMULATION PILOT STUDY

PROJECT ACTIVITIES AND PHASE	RESPONSIBLE PERSONS	JUL	AUG	SEP	OCT	NOV	DEC	JAN	FEB	MAR	APR	MAY	JUN
Simulation Pilot Study	All												
IRB Submission Draft	Anne, Stan												
IRB Submission Feedback	Deb, Joe												
Zoom to Discuss Submission	All												
Send Qualtrics Access to Anne	Deb, Joe												
Final IRB Submission	All												
Training Plan for Stan	All												
Simulation Models Shipped to Practice Site	Stan												
Practice Simulation	Deb, Joe, Stan												
Dress Rehearsal	Deb, Joe, Stan												
Pilot Study Date	All												
Data Analysis	Anne												
Manuscript Draft	Anne, Stan												
Manuscript Submission	Anne												

IRB, Institutional Review Board.

a plethora of project management tools to help organize the research team. Finally, developing writing skills is often not prioritized in the busy life of a researcher, yet one can actively seek out professional development opportunities to strengthen writing skills.

CONCLUSION

Professionals who serve the public—including PHN professionals—have an ethical obligation to practice with competence and compassion. For this reason, professionals have a responsibility to maintain and improve technical and people skills, to stay current with developments in their fields, and to practice in full alignment with their profession's code of ethics. Because grant funding is vital to many PHN initiatives, development of grant writing skills is an important area of professional development for PHN practitioners.

Professional development can be a lifelong adventure of learning and growth. Regular attention to self-assessment, strategic planning, implementation of professional development activities, and cyclic reassessment is likely to reveal new career directions, new opportunities, and ultimately, greater fulfillment in one's professional service throughout the career span.

KEY CONCEPTS

1. Concepts of *professions* and *professionalism* inform the behaviors and attitudes of *professionals*. Essentially, a professional is one who is capable in a specific area of skill or knowledge, practices that skill or applies that knowledge within an ethical framework, and self-regulates one's own performance and behavior, for the public good.

2. The DMSA suggests that levels of professional development may encompass novice, advanced beginner, competent, proficient, and expert practitioners.

3. Professional competencies and credentialing in the field of PHN are still in development, but professional organizations are working toward this goal.

4. Research and data analysis, capacity-building, and intervention management have been proposed as key competency areas for PHN professionals.

5. PHN practitioners must be accountable for maintaining and improving knowledge, skills, and professional attributes.

6. SMART goals are specific, measurable, achievable, realistic, and timely. Time-related goals may include both short-term (1 year or less) and long-term (usually considered 3–5 years) goals. Goals should be prioritized in order of importance.

7. Professional development is a repeating cycle, which includes self-assessment, goal setting, strategic planning, plan implementation, and further self-assessment and evaluation. The goal of professional development is continuous growth in professional competency throughout the career span.

8. Membership and active participation in professional organizations form a key strategy for professional development.

9. Grantsmanship skills include collaboration with other professionals, understanding how to read RFPs and write a grant that meets RFP requirements, and managing awarded grants.

10. Grant writers should strive to continuously improve their writing skills.

CASE STUDY 1: PROFESSIONAL DEVELOPMENT: SETTING GOALS FOR A COMMUNITY NUTRITION AND WELLNESS EDUCATOR SEEKING TO MOVE INTO MANAGEMENT AND DIRECTORSHIP

JT is employed in a county health department as a community nutrition and wellness educator. His responsibilities include countywide initiatives for nutrition education, as well as social marketing for the nutrition education initiatives. JT holds a bachelor's degree in nutrition and wellness from an accredited university. He is just entering his third year in community nutrition practice.

JT's self-assessment included a review of his annual evaluations, which have overall been excellent. His supervisor identified a need for JT to further develop his skills in food and nutrition education, suggesting that he pursue an advanced degree. JT identified interests in the area of social media marketing, further nutrition education training, and grantsmanship. He would also like to follow a career path that eventually leads him to management and directorship opportunities in PHN.

Case Study Questions

Based on this description, answer the following questions:

1. Write two short-term (3-year) and two long-term (5-year) SMART goals for JT.

2. For each SMART goal, create a hypothetical timetable for achieving the goal.

3. For each SMART goal, describe two specific activities that JT could engage in that would promote progress toward achieving the goal.

4. Contextualize your goals, timeline, and activities by creating an overall strategic plan for JT's achievement of his professional development objectives. You may wish to develop a table to present your strategic plan.

5. Assume that 5 years have passed. What steps would JT take to review his strategic plan, assess his progress, and begin another cycle of professional development?

CASE STUDY 2: GRANTSMANSHIP: NUTRITION EDUCATOR APPLYING FOR A GRANT TO TEACH COOKING SKILLS CLASSES IN THE COMMUNITY

CJ works as a nutrition educator for a nationally affiliated food bank that serves 189 constituent food pantries in a 22-county region of a state. She has learned of a grant that will provide up to $35,000 to conduct cooking skills classes in food pantry settings. CJ decides to apply for the grant.

Case Study Questions

Based on this description, answer the following questions:

1. CJ decides to assemble a team of colleagues to collaborate in the grant writing effort. List five individuals who could make valuable contributions to the team. For each individual, list two contributions they could make to the project.

2. Create two specific objectives for the project.

3. In regard to the RFP, what should CJ be careful to do?

4. How might the grantor's program officer be helpful to CJ?

5. How can CJ learn more about the expectations of the reviewers who will be considering the grant application?

6. Once the grant application is completely drafted, what is an important step for CJ to complete before final submission?

7. If you were mentoring CJ in grantsmanship, what are two suggestions you could provide to her in regard to developing and improving her writing skills?

SUGGESTED LEARNING ACTIVITIES

1. Choose three health professions, and use the Internet to locate their standards for professional practice, as well as their professional development requirements. Review the standards and requirements you have located. How are these similar and how do they differ among the professions? What overarching principles for professional development do you see among the professions?

2. Write and reference a 750-word (about three double-spaced pages) position paper describing your views on *professionalism* and its meaning for PHN professionals.

3. Perform a professional self-assessment using the WPHNA core competencies found in Table 15.2. Compare your current development to the standards, using both self-identified data and feedback gathered from objective sources. Reflect on your own goals, interests, and plans for the future, and include these reflections in your self-assessment. Based on your self-assessment, what do you see as areas for future professional development and growth? Prepare a written document describing the results of your self-assessment.

4. Create at least three SMART goals related to your own professional development. Ask a classmate or colleague to review your goals to ensure that they are specific, measurable, achievable, realistic, and timely.

5. Select one of your own professional development goals and then create a strategic plan to attain that goal. Include specific activities and experiences that you will engage in as you work toward your goal. How will you document your progress toward the goal and demonstrate your professional growth?

6. Create a list of at least 10 resources to promote professional development in PHN practice. You may include professional development organizations in your list. Justify your choice of each resource.

7. Use the Internet to locate three RFPs from three different funding entities. Create a table comparing and contrasting the three RFPs, including the required written components for the completed grant proposal. Comment on similarities, differences, and overarching principles that you have identified as a result of this experience.

8. Interview a PHN professional who has been successful in attaining grant funding. Ask that person for tips, hints, and suggestions on the grantsmanship process. How did the person get started with grant writing? What advice would he or she provide regarding selecting appropriate funding opportunities, writing the grant, and managing the grant once funded?

9. Participate in a writing workshop or webinar. After the experience, write a brief reflection on your learning.

10. Create a list of 10 writing resources available on the Internet. At least five of these resources should provide instruction for academic and/or technical writing. Justify your choice of each resource.

REFLECTION QUESTIONS

1. When you hear the word *professional,* what characteristics come to your mind? Which of these characteristics do you see as most important? Provide a rationale for your answer.

2. Provide a rationale for this statement: "It is imperative that professionals engage in continuous professional development throughout the career span."

3. What is the relationship of time to professional development? You may wish to locate and read the paper written by Brody, Byham-Gray, and Touger-Decker[13] for more information on this topic.

4. The WPHNA has identified three broad areas of PHN practice, along with 10 core competencies categorized within the three areas (see Table 15.2). Which of the three broad areas might you consider most important? Are there specific core competencies that you would prioritize for your own professional development? Justify your answers.

5. What are methods for performing self-assessment? What are challenges to self-assessment, and how may these be addressed?

6. What are the components of SMART goals? Describe each component.

7. Describe the process of strategic planning and plan implementation. How might you follow up on the implementation of your own strategic plan for professional development? How would you document your activities, experiences, and accomplishments during execution of your plan?

8. What are some reasons that grantsmanship is a key area for professional development for public health nutritionists?

9. Develop your own definition of *collaboration.* List at least three reasons collaboration is vital to the grantsmanship process.

10. According to this chapter, what are the five basic steps to writing a grant? Describe each step.

11. What are at least three practical methods for improving writing skills throughout the course of one's career?

12. What is the basic goal of professional development throughout the career span? Ultimately, who do you think is the beneficiary of each professional's development?

CONTINUE YOUR LEARNING RESOURCES

The Academy of Nutrition and Dietetics. https://www.eatright.org.
The American Public Health Association. https://www.apha.org.
The American Association of Family and Consumer Sciences. https://www.aafcs.org/home.

Association of Graduate Programs in Public Health Nutrition. https://agpphn.org.
Association of State Public Health Nutritionists. https://asphn.org.
International Society for Behavioral Nutrition and Physical Activity. https://www.isbnpa.org.
National Rural Health Association. https://www.ruralhealthweb.org.
School Nutrition Association. https://schoolnutrition.org.
Society for Nutrition Education and Behavior. https://www.sneb.org.
Society for Public Health Education. https://www.sophe.org.
World Public Health Nutrition Association. https://www.wphna.org.

GLOSSARY

Certification: The process of providing official verification of an accomplishment or degree of attainment.[6]

Collaboration: The act of working with others to accomplish a desired common goal.

Competence: The ability to perform professional tasks in a satisfactory manner. Appropriate knowledge, skills, and judgment are considered prerequisites to competence.[4]

Competencies: Specific skills that a professional is expected to be able to perform in a satisfactory manner.

Complementary competency: According to the WPHNA, functions that may be helpful to a PHN professional, but would not, if lacking, represent a gap in the ability to carry out key public health functions. In some practice environments, competencies normally considered complementary may actually be core.[9]

Continuing professional education (CPE): The means by which professionals stay current with their professions' standards and maintain and improve competency throughout the career span. In order to retain certification/credentialing, professionals are often required to meet CPE requirements as established by their professional organizations. CPE terminology may vary; for example, some professions use continuing professional education units (CPEUs) or other variants of the term.

Core competency: According to the WPHNA, core competencies represent functions that, if lacking, would represent gaps in the ability to carry out key public health functions.[9]

Credentialing: The process of granting credentials as an indicator of title, achievement, and/or other aspects of someone's background, usually to indicate that the credentialed person is qualified to do something.[8]

Documentation (in regard to professional development): Artifacts saved by a professional as proof of engagement in professional development activities and CPE; these may include certificates, diplomas, calendars, products of learning, hour and experience logs, and a variety of other indicators. Documentation of professional development is required by most professional organizations and employers.

Dreyfus Model of Skill Acquisition (DMSA): A model of levels of professional practice, frequently used in professional development processes including self- and employer/professional organization assessment of performance. DMSA levels include novice, advanced beginner, competent, proficient, and expert.[12,13]

Gantt chart: A project management tool that may be useful during the grant writing process; a Gantt chart uses a visual presentation of horizontal lines to compare actual performance to expected performance per time period.[37]

Goal setting: The process of identifying and articulating specific desired outcomes to be achieved by efforts exerted.

Grantsmanship: The overall process of obtaining and managing funding provided by grantors for research and projects. The grantsmanship process includes identifying appropriate funding opportunities, assembling collaborative teams to address identified opportunities, writing funding requests, and managing funded projects.

Innovation: The process of bringing forth new ideas, products, methods, and/or ways of doing tasks.

Lifelong learning: The process and attitude underlying continuing professional development; that is, the process of continuously learning throughout the career and life span.[11]

Mentorship: The process by which a more experienced person helps to guide the professional growth of a less experienced person.

Networking: The process by which a professional builds relationships and connections with other individuals and organizations for the purpose of furthering professional and personal growth, optimizing professional efforts, and developing effective initiatives and collaborations for the benefit of the public.

Program Evaluation and Review Technique (PERT) chart: PERT is a project management tool that may be useful during the grant writing process. PERT identifies *what* tasks are necessary; *who* will complete each task; and *when* each task will be completed. Before subsequent tasks can be started, previous tasks must be completed.[38]

Principal investigator: The lead researcher; also considered the researcher who initiates and spearheads a particular research project; usually the first author on any publications resulting from the research.

Process-oriented objectives: Project objectives that are focused on the process of carrying out the project rather than directly on the project outcomes. For example, a process-oriented objective for a grant project might include scheduling a call or visit with the granting organization's program officer in order to obtain direction for writing the grant proposal.

Profession: A group comprising those who perform a specific activity for payment, such as medicine or nursing; encompasses a specific body of knowledge and field of practice, establishes a required course of training and credentialing for practitioners, develops ethical standards for practice and holds members of the profession accountable to those standards, and practices for the public good.[9]

Professional: A person who is paid to utilize a skill; the process of becoming and maintaining professional status often requires extensive education and experience, formal credentialing, and completion of ongoing continuing education requirements throughout the career span.[1]

Professionalism: The skills, behaviors, and attitudes expected of a professional. Professionalism may include displaying competence in the discipline practiced, reliability, calmness under pressure, flexibility, problem-solving capabilities, an empathetic and compassionate demeanor, excellent communication skills, a neat appearance, confidence without arrogance, a strong work ethic, good self-management and organizational abilities, accountability for one's own actions, understanding and accepting one's own limits, and acceptance of responsibility for continuing education and improvement of skills.[2–4,39]

Request for proposal (RFP): A document issued by a grant funding individual or organization; describes the nature and purpose of a specific grant opportunity, eligibility requirements and specific instructions for preparing the grant application, instructions for submitting the application, and other materials such as the contact information for the organization's program officer.

Self-assessment: The process of comparing and judging one's own performance against a standard of practice; consists of reviewing one's practice, identifying areas for improvement, and planning activities to fill the knowledge and skill gaps identified.[24,25]

SMART goals: Goals that are specific, measurable, achievable, realistic, and timely. SMART goals are more likely to be achieved than goals that are general and poorly defined.[29]

Strategic planning (in regard to professional development): The overall process of setting goals, determining time frames, planning activities, monitoring progress, and evaluating results of professional development.

Writing skills: A key component of grantsmanship; encompasses the ability to write clearly and succinctly, to correctly use expected conventions of written expression, to follow instructions for written work such as grant applications, and to review and edit preliminary work by oneself and with feedback from collaborators and reviewers.

REFERENCES

1. Oxford University Press. Profession. In: Oxford University Press, ed. *Lexico*. Oxford, UK; Oxford University Press; 2019.
2. MPH Programs List: Advocates for Public Health Education. *10 Qualities and Skills Public Health Employers Want From You*. 2019. https://mphprogramslist.com/10-qualities-and-skills-public-health-employers-want-from-you
3. Hamilton J. *6 Qualities of Truly Great Health and Community Care Professionals*. 2019. https://www.opencolleges.edu.au/blog/2017/11/06/ca-6-qualities-truly-great-health-professionals
4. National Board of Public Health Examiners. *CPH: Certified in Public Health*. 2019. https://www.nbphe.org
5. Commission on Dietetic Registration. *Commission on Dietetic Registration: The Credentialing Agency for the Academy of Nutrition and Dietetics*. 2019. https://www.cdrnet.org
6. Wurm-Schaar M. Professionalism: an exemplar for the sciences. *Biochem Pharmacol*. 2015;98(2):313–317. doi:10.1016/j.bcp.2015.06.026
7. Hughes R, Shrimpton R, Recine E, Margetts B. *A Competency Framework for Global Public Health Nutrition Workforce Development: A Background Paper*. London, UK: World Public Health Nutrition Association; 2011. http://www.wphna.org/htdocs/downloadsapr2012/12-03%20WPHNA%20Draft%20competency%20standards%20report.pdf
8. Duyff RL. The value of lifelong learning: key element in professional career development. *J Acad Nutr Diet*. 1999;99(5):538–543. doi:10.1016/S0002-8223(99)00135-2
9. Dreyfus SE. The Five-Stage Model of Adult Skill Acquisition. *Bull Sci Technol Soc*. 2004;24(3):177–181. doi:10.1177/0270467604264992
10. Benner P. Using the Dreyfus Model of Skill Acquisition to describe and interpret skill acquisition and clinical judgment in nursing practice and education. *Bull Sci Technol Soc*. 2004;24:188–199. doi:10.1177/0270467604265061
11. Academy of Nutrition and Dietetics. *Academy Standards Learning Module, Part 1: Guiding RDN and NDTR Practitioner Competence and Advancement*. Chicago, IL: Academy of Nutrition and Dietetics; 2019.
12. Kirkpatrick K, Mackinnon R. Technology-enhanced learning in anaesthesia and educational theory. *Contin Educ Anaesth Crit Care Pain*. 2012;12:263–267. doi:10.1093/bjaceaccp/mks027

13. Brody RA, Byham-Gray L, Touger-Decker R, et al. Identifying components of advanced-level clinical nutrition practice: a delphi study. *J Acad Nutr Diet.* 2012;112(6):859–869. doi:10.1016/j.jand.2012.02.022

14. Dreyfus SE, Dreyfus HL. *Mind Over Machine.* New York, NY: Free Press; 1998.

15. Martin K. *The Improvement Professional's Evolving Role: From Practitioner to Facilitator to Coach.* 2011. https://www.slideshare.net/KarenMartinGroup/the-improvement-professionals-evolving-role-from -practitioner-to-facilitator-oto-coac/13-Dreyfus_Model_ofSkill_AcquisitionStuart_Hubert

16. The Academy Quality Management Committee. Academy of Nutrition and Dietetics: Revised 2017 Standards of Practice in Nutrition Care and Standards of Professional Performance for Registered Dietitian Nutritionists. *J Acad Nutr Diet.* 2018;118(1):132–140. doi:10.1016/j.jand.2018.01.012

17. Journal of the Academy of Nutrition and Dietetics. *Focus Area Standards for RDNs Collection.* 2019. https://jandonline.org/content/focus

18. Benner P. *From Novice to Expert: Excellence and Power in Clinical Nursing Practice.* Menlo Park, CA: Addison-Wesley; 1984.

19. Accreditation Council for Education in Nutrition and Dietetics. *ACEND Standards Update: Competency Based Education.* February 2018. https://www.eatrightpro.org/-/media/eatrightpro-files/acend/ standardsupdatefebruary2018.pdf?la=en&hash=F1B92E526A20087889681CD29E3626E790F25BA8

20. McGinnis PQ, Guenther LA, Wainwright SF. Development and integration of professional core values among practicing clinicians. *Phys Ther.* 2016;96(9):1417–1429. doi:10.2522/ptj.20150189

21. Commission on Dietetic Registration. *Professional Development Portfolio Guide With Essential Practice Competencies.* 2019. https://www.cdrnet.org/vault/2459/web/files/PDP%20Guide%E2%80%942020.pdf

22. Boud D. *Enhancing Learning Through Self-Assessment.* London, UK: Kogan Page; 1995.

23. Al-Kadri H, Al-Moamary MS, Al-Takroni H, et al. Self-assessment and students' study strategies in a community of clinical practice: a qualitative study. *Med Educ Online.* 2012;17(1):11204. doi:10.3402/ meo.v17i0.11204

24. University of Nebraska-Lincoln Office of Graduate Studies. *The Individual Professional Development Plan (IPDP): A Career Management Tool.* 2019. https://www.unl.edu/gradstudies/connections/ individual-professional-development-plan-ipdp-career-management-tool

25. Forsman H, Jansson I, Leksell J, et al. Clusters of competence: relationship between self-reported professional competence and achievement on a national examination among graduating nursing students. *J Adv Nurs.* 2010;76(1):199–208. doi:10.1111/jan.14222

26. Regehr G, Eva K. Self-assessment, self-direction, and the self-regulating professional. *Clin Orthop Relat Res.* 2006;449:34–38. doi:10.1097/01.blo.0000224027.85732.b2

27. Doran GT. There's a S.M.A.R.T. way to write management's goals and objectives. *Manag Rev.* 1981;70: 35–36.

28. Duke Human Resources. *Professional Development Plan.* n.d. https://hr.duke.edu/managers/ performance-management/professional-development-plan

29. Jividen J. *Writing a competitive research grant proposal.* Paper presented at: School of Public Health Grant Writing Workshop; June 1, 2017; Ann Arbor, MI.

30. Paulus P. Groups, teams, and creativity: the creative potential of idea-generating groups. *Appl Psychol.* 2000;49(2):237–262. doi:10.1111/1464-0597.00013

31. Ryan RM, Deci EL. Self-determination theory and the facilitation of intrinsic motivation, social development, and well-being. *Am Psychol.* 2000;55:68–78. doi:10.1037/0003-066X.55.1.68

32. Wiggins G, McTighe J. Backward design. In: McTighe GWJ, ed. *Understanding by Design.* Upper Saddle River, NJ: Pearson Education; 2005:13–28.

33. Gemayel R, Martin SJ. Writing a successful fellowship or grant application. *FEBS J.* 2017;284:3771–3777. doi:10.1111/febs.14318

34. Bonetta L. Project management. In: Bonetta L, ed. *Making the Right Moves: A Practical Guide to Scientific Management for Postdocs and New Faculty.* Research Triangle Park, NC: Burroughs Wellcome Fund & Chevy Chase, MD: Howard Hughes Medical Institute; 2006.

35. Ibrahim AM, Dimick JB. Writing for impact: how to prepare a journal article. In: Markovac J, Kleinman M, Englesbe M, eds. *Medical and Scientific Publishing.* Cambridge, MA: Academic Press; 2018.

36. Fuller LM. A field guide to medical writing training. *Med Writing.* 2013;22(1):17–22. doi:10.1179/2047 48012X13560931063636

37. Gopen GD, Swan JA. The science of scientific writing. *Am Sci.* 1990;78(6):550–558.

38. Mensh B, Kording K. Ten simple rules for structuring papers. *PLoS Comput Biol.* 2017;13(9):e1005619. doi:10.1371/journal.pcbi.1005619

39. Oxford University Press. Professionalism. In: Oxford University Press, ed. *Lexico.* Oxford, UK: Oxford University Press; 2019.

40. Thompson K, Silver C, Pivonka E, Gutschall M, McAnulty L. Fruit- and vegetable-focused grocery store tour training kit and grant to promote peer-on-peer nutrition education utilizing nutrition and dietetics students. *J Nutr Educ Behav.* 2015;47(5):472–476.

41. Walsh S, Arnold B, Pickwell-Smith B, Summers B. What kind of doctor would you like me to be? *Clin Teach.* 2016;13:98–101. doi:10.1111/tct.12389

42. Shrimpton R, Hughes R, Recine E, et al. Nutrition capacity development: a practice framework. *Public Health Nutr.* 2013;7(3):682–688. doi:10.1017/S1368980013001213

SUMMARY STATEMENTS ON SUSTAINABILITY AND PUBLIC HEALTH NUTRITION

SONYA JONES AND DENNIS LANIGAN

LEARNING OBJECTIVES

1. Become familiar with the four interrelated crises of environmental destabilization, energy depletion, economic hegemony of neoliberal capitalism, and social inequities that threaten ecosystem **sustainability** and **resilience**.

2. Consider economic, agroecological, and rights-based approaches to creating more sustainable food and nutrition systems.

3. Evaluate the extent to which current summary statements on nutrition and sustainability use available approaches to build sustainable and resilient food systems.

INTRODUCTION

In 2014, a group of prominent nutrition scientists and professionals charged with revising the Dietary Guidelines for Americans were directed by the U.S. Congress to not consider any evidence related to the environment in making recommendations. Congress had heard that the committee was interested in gathering information about how agricultural practices and environmental impacts of the food system might also be relevant to nutrition recommendations. Why would the people concerned about the Dietary Guidelines for Americans be considering "the environment" in their recommendations? In this chapter, we put human nutrition in a broad context of sustainability with hopes of elucidating many of the connections between how food is produced and human health. We first describe the interrelated crises of environment, energy, economics, and equity that threaten the sustainability of the human food supply. We then explore the agroecological, economic, and rights-based approaches that form the basis of a systems response to these crises. Last, this chapter examines summary statements, including the Sustainable Development Goals, Healthy People 2020 and 2030, and the EAT-Lancet recommendations against the approaches described. We provide recommendations for how nutrition professionals can become allies with the many movements for a more sustainable food system and provide case studies of communities seeking sustainability reform.

DEFINING SUSTAINABILITY FOR PUBLIC HEALTH AND NUTRITION

Sustainability is a buzzword in nutrition and public health, and like most buzzwords, it has many meanings defined by many different stakeholders. From an environmental perspective, sustainability is a way of interacting with our natural environment that maintains ecological system balance and conserves resources for future use. From an economic perspective, sustainability is the wise investments of finances in activities that will generate their own future finances. From a social perspective, sustainability is the maintenance of relationships among humans that ensure security and stability. All three of these realms—environmental, economic, and social—are important for nutrition and public health. In each of these domains, numerous scientific disciplines are pointing to challenges that threaten human security, stability, and healthful roles in the ecosystems. Ensuring socially, economically, and environmentally sustainable food systems therefore is a critical focus for future public health nutrition policy and programs.

The Interrelated Sustainability Crises

While the United Nations Sustainable Development guidelines and most public health nutrition literature focuses on a so-called "triple bottom line" (i.e., people, planet, and profit), here we use the Post Carbon Institute's framing of four-part crises (E4) of environment, energy, economics, and equity.[1] We briefly describe the specific aspects of these challenges related to human food systems.

Environment

The natural environments in which human food systems are located are the sources of the energy, nutrients, water, and resilience needed to sustain human life. Ecologists describe the state in which ecosystems are tending toward stability, beauty, and resilience as "right relationships."[2] Human food systems "right relationships" would be those in which solar energy is converted into sugars that plant consumers can use as energy and, in turn, other companions can use to ensure water and nutrients are available to plants. Note that right relationship in a human food system, therefore, is not human-centric but includes humans as participants in the system. Humans and other participants in right relationship share the risks and benefits. For example, a person might grow greens to eat in his or her yard using only sunshine and the soil available. If the soil lacks nutrients, then the greens will suffer and the person might not be able to eat those greens. Likewise, if a human applies compost to the soil, both the human and greens benefit. Humans have found ways to reduce the short-term risks of participating in the food system by replacing ecosystem relationships with human technological alternatives. We briefly describe some of the human–environment relationships that require urgent attention for sustainability.

TOPSOIL LOSS

Topsoil is the living skin of Earth's landmasses. It includes microorganisms, minerals, and nutrients for plants. The Food and Agriculture Organization reported in 2015 that only 60 years of topsoil are left for farming if soil degradation continues at the current rate.[3] The latest assessment of land degradation released in 2016 estimated that topsoil losses are leading to decreases in productivity of crops, forests, grasslands, and rangelands.[4] Wetland areas, such as rain forests, have been the hardest hit, with 87% lost globally in the past 300 years. Areas that lose topsoil become degraded land or deserts. The causes of soil degradation include agricultural practices of tilling and pesticide and fertilizer application, overgrazing animals, deforestation, and industrialization.

BOX 16.1

HIGHLIGHT ON POLYFACE FARMS

Joel Salatin of Polyface Farms is widely recognized as a "soil health guru." Polyface Farms operates on six principles, which together lead to great soil health. Polyface Farms is **grass-based**, meaning that live-stock and poultry move frequently to different fields of grass to graze and offer landscape healing through their manures, scratching, and hooves. The farm also focuses on the **individuality** of plants and animals by providing habitats that allow them to express their distinctiveness. Also, the farm seeks to build **community** by selling only in their own bioregion. Soil building is accomplished through following **Nature's Template** by mimicking the natural patterns of ecosystems. **Earthworms** are central to the biological tillage of soils at Polyface Farms. Last, the farm believes in **transparency**. Anyone is welcome to visit, learn from, and see the farm. Polyface Farms sells to 5,000 consumers and 50 restaurants in Virginia.

The soils wash away in the water, creating water pollution, blow away in the wind, become acidi-fied through application of chemicals, or are compacted and crusted.

Some farming and forestry practices actually build soil rather than causing erosion (Box 16.1).[5] These practices include biological tillage, cover crops, composting, using organic matter mulches, crop rotations, managed grazing, maintenance of bacterial and fungal communities, and planting nitrogen-fixing and deep-rooted companion plants to provide natural fertilization.

FRESHWATER DEPLETION

If soil is the living skin of land, water might be thought of as the circulatory system of Earth. Freshwater is essential for all aspects of human food systems. Nineteen hot spots around the world, including California, north-west China, northern and eastern India, and the Middle East are all rapidly depleting their freshwater.[6] From 2011 to 2016, California suffered a severe drought, in which aquifers receded by 16 million acre-feet per year and 1,900 wells dried up.[7] Heavy rains in 2017 dropped 228% more rain than usual in California, creating flooding, but not replenish-ing underground aquifers (which would require about 4 years to replace that amount of water). Treating waste and stormwaters and desalinizing ocean waters are only partial solutions, as each requires a lot of energy.

Some countries, such as Australia, have instituted policies that allow the country to limit the impact of droughts through water conservation policies and allowing people to trade water, which halved the amount of water used in businesses and residences.[8] Other countries, such as Israel, treat and recycle a large majority of water used, even sewage water.[9] Last, many initiatives capture and conserve rainwater. Most expert panels agree that conservation and frugal manage-ment of existing water infrastructure (e.g., fixing leaky pipes), drip irrigation, and drought-re-sistant crop selections that require less water are all required to maintain the availability of freshwater. Agroecologists work to maintain freshwater through supporting local water cycles. For instance, the role of trees in all aspects of the water cycle is now widely understood.[10] Forests are the most efficient sources of precipitation after oceans according to forestry studies because trees pull water from the ground, release it during photosynthesis and normal exhalation, and capture and slow water as it falls.[11] Agroecologists often include trees in agricultural designs to manage water.

NITROGEN FIXATION

Nitrogen is a nutrient required by plants and animals to make proteins, including the proteins that plants require to make chlorophyll. Plants use nitrates that have been "fixed" by *Rhizobium* bacteria that live in the root nodules of nitrogen-fixing plants, such as legumes, and in healthy soil. Other symbiotic and associative relationships between bacteria and plants also exist to fix nitrogen for plants, and scientists describe these relationships as intricate and specific (e.g., only certain strains of bacteria will fix nitrogen for particular types of plants).

In 1913, humans discovered a way to "fix" nitrogen using natural gas, creating chemical fertilizers. The industrial generation of nitrogen fertilizer consumes approximately 30% of all the energy used in agricultural production.[12] Excess nitrates run off farms, impacting rivers and streams, affecting the biodiversity and productivity of aquatic and land ecosystems. A common effect is for the excess nitrogen to fertilize algae in coastal areas, which in turn depletes oxygen from the water systems and creates dead zones. This process is called eutrophication. Likewise, industrially fixed nitrate is present in drinking water.

In the bacterially driven nitrogen cycle, soil bacteria would transform these nitrates back into nitrogen forms that are released as gases into the air. These gases are part of the greenhouse gas effect of agriculture, and greater amounts are released when either industrial nitrogen fertilizers or manures are applied to crops.[13] These greenhouse gas emissions can be reduced by not tilling soil and using cover crops over the winter.

PHOSPHORUS DEPLETION

All living things require phosphorus as a key building block of DNA and RNA. Plants require phosphorus, therefore, for every aspect of growth including photosynthesis, respiration, reproduction, and making sugars. Unlike the other cycles that support life, such as water and nitrogen, phosphorus does not circulate as a gas in the air as part of its normal cycle. The largest stores of phosphorus are found in sedimentary rocks. As these rocks weather in the rain, phosphates leach into the soil. Plants absorb and use the phosphates and animals absorb phosphates through consuming these plants. Plants that are left to decay in place, such as cover crops, leave phosphorus to be reabsorbed into the soil.

The first manufactured phosphorus for use in fertilizers came from animal bones, but mining operations began soon after. About 90% of all phosphorus mined is used for food production, primarily to create fertilizers. Mined phosphorus will eventually become unavailable, and some researchers estimate that this will happen in about 70 years.[14] Because phosphate circulates locally rather than atmospherically, global trade in food also affects the global distribution of phosphorus. For instance, when the United States imports fruits and vegetables grown in other countries, all of the nutrients drawn out of the exporting country's soil are also imported. The phosphorus then becomes part of U.S. waste management systems as the food is consumed or wasted. Thus, phosphorus depletion is more likely to happen earliest in countries that export agricultural products and do not have a local supply of phosphorus.

Phosphorus can be locally conserved through agriculture practices that focus on local consumption of agricultural products and efficient waste management programs that recycle nutrients back into local soil.[15] Ecological sanitation, for instance, focuses on both the public health goals of safely managing sewage and recycling nutrients back into agricultural systems. Sweden, for example, has developed a system for removing nutrients from urine water. Advocates call for a plan for phosphorus security to manage the global and political processes needed to make these low-tech, low-cost solutions possible.

MONOCULTURE, MONOCROPPING, AND BIODIVERSITY LOSS

The Intergovernmental Science-Policy Platform on Biodiversity and Ecosystem Services (IPBES) concluded that land-based species have fallen by 20% since 1990, 40% of amphibian species have been lost, and 33% of corals and marine mammals are threatened. Some 9% of domesticated animal breeds are now extinct, and 1,000 more are threatened.[16] One third of marine stocks are being overharvested, and 60% are being maximally sustainably fished. Likewise, the genetic diversity of livestock animals has also declined precipitously.

Insect populations are experiencing mass extinctions.[17] In agriculture, particular attention has been given to the decline in pollinating insects, such as monarch butterflies, which have experienced a 90% population loss in the 20 years between 1999 and 2019,[18] and honeybees, which have lost 87% of their population in the same period.[19] While some insects negatively affect the human food system, many others are beneficial. Beneficial insects not only pollinate plants, allowing them to produce fruits, nuts, and seeds, but also keep negative insect populations in check.

Edible plant species are also in decline. Since the 1990s, about 75% of plant diversity has been lost as farmers select high-yielding, genetically uniform varieties over local variations of plants. About 75% of the world food supply is produced currently from 12 plant species.[20] Diseases can have a much wider impact without genetic diversity. For instance, the most common form of banana sold globally, the Cavendish, accounts for 99% of all banana exports in 2019. The Cavendish is suffering from two fungal diseases which is likely to affect banana production in 130 countries. In addition, the lack of agrobiodiversity leads to a less varied and healthful human diet.

Monocropping is planting the same plants in the same land year after year. Diseases and pests that affect a particular plant also continue to grow in those soils, so monocropped plants are less productive and more disease-prone. For instance, tomatoes are affected by a variety of fungal diseases and bacterial diseases. Growing tomatoes in the same field where plants were previously affected by a fungus will lead to a reinfection of the next year's crop.

Numerous strategies are available to support plant and animal diversity and include growing local, heirloom plant varieties, saving seeds from local varieties, rotating crops, and intercropping plants with beneficial companions. Likewise, converting land to animal, insect, and wild edible habitats can support existing populations. Maintaining existing forest ecosystems with large and diverse populations is also critical.

CARBON REGULATION

Carbon, particularly the carbon released through methane and carbon dioxide, plays an important role in climate regulation. Agricultural activities, including animal manures, transportation, and soil disturbance all release carbon into the atmosphere and contribute to warming. Other agricultural activities, such as food forests, agroecology, and no-till farming, sequester carbon in plants and ground and contribute to a well-regulated climate cycle. Forests through both trees and soil can release methane into the atmosphere but also sink carbon dioxide into trees and soil.

Energy

FROM SOLAR TO FOSSIL FUELS

In a functioning ecosystem, the primary source of energy is sunshine. Simply put, plants convert sunlight into sugars that fuel their own growth and health, feed a host of microorganisms in the soil, feed sugar-preferring mammals, birds, and insects, and allow plants to breath in carbon dioxide and release water into the air. Thus, the sun energizes water, mineral, food, reproduction, communications, and eco-communities. Across the food system, these complex energy-exchange systems have been replaced by fossil fuels in industrial agriculture. Take, for example, pollination. In the solar-powered ecosystem, birds and insects adapted to local plants will consume sugar, pick up pollen, and carry it to other plants, transferring the solar energy created by the plants. In industrial agriculture, honeybees are driven in trucks from farm to farm across thousands of miles using fossil fuels to aid the process of pollinating plants. Across the entire food system—from production, transportation, processing, packaging, retail, food services, to household storage and preparation—the energy inputs are about 14.2 quads (1×10^{15} BTU), which generates about 1.75 quads of food energy for people to eat.[21]

Fossil fuels are used in many agricultural processes, including creating nitrogen and phosphorus fertilizers, irrigation, fuels, machinery, drying harvests, seed productions, and herbicide production. Between 1910 and 1983, energy inputs into corn production alone in the United States increased by 810%.[22] Livestock production also requires fossil fuel inputs to maintain animal confinements, transportation, and feed production.

RENEWABLE ENERGY CANNOT POWER INDUSTRIAL AGRICULTURE ALONE

Heinberg and Fridley[23] argue that renewable energy sources, such as windmills, solar panels, and biomass, while important, cannot alone fuel agricultural needs for several reasons: (a) the intermittent availability of energy generated from wind and solar; (b) liquid fuels that fuel machines and transportation cannot be replaced entirely by electric power or biofuels because of the horsepower needs of large machinery; (c) the other uses of fossil fuels to create agricultural inputs from cement, rubber, and glass to feed and fertilizer; (d) the spatial distribution and location of renewable energy resources will be tied to places where it is more sunny, windier, rivers flow, and biomass can be grown; and (e) renewable energy sources are unlikely to generate the quantities of energy needed to support large population centers.

Economics

THE FOCUS ON GROWTH

The current global hegemony of neoliberal capitalism focuses on a model of constant economic activity, measured as gross domestic product (GDP), and an expectation that GDP will increase, also known as economic growth. Growth in an economy can come from extracting more natural resources from Earth and selling them. For example, phosphorus and water are extracted and sold in human food systems. Growth might also come from hiring more people, paying them better wages, or selling more food at higher prices. In short, globally, the generally accepted economic model currently focuses on "more" economic activity rather than healthy, sustainable, just, or "better" economic activity.

Several alternatives for measuring progress in a country have been developed that consider greener and socially desirable alternatives to GDP. The United Nations tracks the Human Development Index as a measure of the possibility to "do and be" and includes life expectancy, school enrollment, adult literacy, and other well-being data. Ecological footprints measure how much of a productive field is needed to maintain humans and process their wastes. Last, the Happy Planet Index combines information from the ecological footprint with expected lifetime and life satisfaction to create an index for each country. Rich countries, such as the United States and European countries, tend to have high ecological footprints and high Human Development

Indices while countries in Latin America, such as Costa Rica and Panama, have high Happy Planet Indices.[24]

TRADE LIBERALIZATION

As country-level economies become more and more globally engaged in international trade (**globalization**) as a growth strategy, export-driven commodity agriculture creates numerous challenges. Otero and colleagues[25] have found that **trade liberalization** policies effectively create relationships of dependency in which economically dominant countries, such as the United States, import "luxury foods," such as fruits and vegetables, while protecting grain and meat markets. Trade partners, such as Mexico, Turkey, and Brazil, on the other hand, have shifted their diet toward more imported grains and meats and produce less of the food that their citizens eat. Trade relationships are not stable, however, and global political differences often create trade challenges. An embargo against a country that is dependent on importing basic foodstuffs can quickly create a humanitarian crisis. Some countries are responding to the challenge of trade dependency by creating national policies of **food sovereignty**. Fair trade agreements developed between private entities, such as small farmers and retailers who agree to a minimum price for a product and a better distribution of profits.

EXTERNALIZED COSTS

Because of the increasing distances and isolation between fields, processing centers, and consumers, many of the costs of agricultural production and processing are externalized. Examples of **externalized costs** in the food system range from the costs of water pollution from excess fertilizer and animal manure washing into our rivers and eventually oceans to the costs of diabetes treatment and management from excess simple sugar and carbohydrate consumption. The Environmental Protection Agency (EPA) explained that the costs of water pollution with excess nutrients (e.g., fertilizers) would include the impacts to commercial fishing, real estate, tourism and recreation, healthcare, and drinking water treatment.[26] Summarizing the available studies on these different areas, the EPA found that millions of dollars of economic activity were lost daily in affected communities in each category. For example, in one study, communities along the coast of Maine lost $2.45 million because of reduction in shellfish and clam harvests related to bed closures in polluted waters. In another, the state of Ohio paid $13 million to treat water from Grand Lake for drinking water due to a blue-green algae outbreak.*

ECOLOGICAL ECONOMICS

The field of ecological economics brings into alignment the understanding that Earth has finite resources, or planetary boundaries, and no system on Earth, including the economy, can exceed Earth's boundaries. In the "safe operating zone," economies can distribute goods and resources that support human life in ways that do not exceed the planet's ecological ceilings.[27]

Likewise, ecological economics emphasizes that wealth should be measured as the material, spiritual, artistic value of things needed to maintain high-value relationships (e.g., fertile land and happy families). The modern money system of wealth is based on a social agreement that banks can create money through fractional reserve–based lending. This system could be transformed into a living economy through transparent rules that favor communities and have strict controls on speculative trading of debt. Numerous groups from the National Association

---

*Blue-green algae grows quickly in nutrient-rich waters, such as those polluted by manure or fertilizers.

for the Advancement of Colored People to presidential candidates have called for debt reform. Some communities have responding by developing local currencies, such as "BerkShares" in the Berkshire, Massachusetts region that started to support local food businesses and grew to be a regional lender that supports local businesses, organizations, and people.[28]

Equality

CRISIS OF COMMUNITY GOVERNANCE

Elinor Ostrom's Nobel Prize–winning work on the resilience of social systems demonstrates that under certain conditions, the so-called "tragedy of the commons" will develop while in other conditions, communities and nations will reliably protect ecosystems. Through a series of studies on communities that were able to engage collectively with ecosystem resources without depleting them, she developed the following principles of governance: (a) define clear group boundaries; (b) match rules governing use of common goods to local needs and conditions; (c) ensure that those affected by the rules can participate in modifying the rules; (d) make sure the rulemaking rights of community members are respected by outside authorities; (e) develop a system, carried out by community members, for monitoring members' behavior; (f) use graduated sanctions for rule violators; (g) provide accessible, low-cost means for dispute resolution; and (h) build responsibility for governing the common resource in nested tiers from the lowest level up to the entire interconnected system (Case Study 1).[29]

As the *Community Resilience Reader*[1] notes, the ability of institutions to ensure an equitable, transparent, and democratic model of sharing resources such as the one described by Elinor Ostrom is reaching a crisis. Community decision-making authority in the United States, for instance, is affected by four interrelated challenges. First, state legislatures use the doctrine of "state preemption"[30] to remove decision-making authority from local communities and define the relationship between the state and local government as a "parent–child" relationship. Next, the doctrine of corporate personhood allows corporations to claim rights to the protections of free speech, search and seizure, and equal protection.[31] This doctrine allows corporations' "rights" to supersede community decision-making. The third challenge is treating nature as property without rights. An individual or corporation who owns a part of a river, forest, wetland, or soil has the legal right to harm it. Last, the regulatory process in the United States often involves a citizen input period in which communities are supposed to have a voice in the permits that regulatory agencies grant.[32] However, the permitting process is superseded by property rights and corporate personhood so that regulatory agencies are constrained in their ability to respond to community desires.

UNEQUAL DISTRIBUTION OF FOOD

Globally, several widely varying estimates suggest that increases in production are needed to support global population growth. Other studies find that poverty, or the inability to purchase food commodities on the global marketplace, is the root cause of food insecurity. In the United States, a country that exports $140 billion worth of food and wastes an estimated 40% of food along the supply chain, about 12% of the population is food-insecure or has inadequate income to ensure an adequate food supply. Addressing access to food in the United States and globally therefore has to focus on poverty alleviation and increasing agricultural production. The United Nations and International Food Policy Research Institute say that increases in production have to be on small-scale farms, using low-input, high-yielding approaches, such as agroecology, to realize the greatest increases in food security globally.[33,34]

AUSTERITY

While the post–world wars period was a time of social development in many countries in which a social safety net was institutionalized, several factors have led to the systematic dismantling of programs that ensured living wages, affordable childcare, food, housing, healthcare, and retirement security. These so-called **austerity** measures are instituted primarily to address debt in a country economy. For instance, Greece cut social security, public worker wages, and social welfare programs after renegotiating debt payments with the Eurozone.[35,36] In the United States, public welfare programs were reformed in 1997, leading to a redistributing of spending away from direct cash assistance to individual poor families and toward organizations that provide services, such as job training. Austerity measures are widely understood to reduce human food security and cause civil unrest.[37,38] Alternatives to austerity include progressive tax reforms that redistribute wealth across populations, debt forgiveness to individuals and countries, and cooperatively and democratically managed corporations (e.g., **stakeholder corporations**).

HOW WE RESPOND TO THE INTERRELATED CRISES

While the interrelated challenges of environment, energy, economics, and equity are daunting, ecological thought leaders suggest that we are at a critical turning point in human evolution.[39] In short, we have an incredible opportunity to reimagine humans as part of thriving ecosystems with agriculture integrated into that ecosystem. We have numerous tools at our disposal to undergo such a transition, including market-based economic approaches, agroecological approaches, and rights-based approaches. A brief overview of the different approaches is provided in this section.

Correcting Market Failures

When a business is thriving even though the cost of creating its product is higher than the price it charges, economics theory considers this a market failure. Market failures in which prices are lower than costs happen when the costs are being externalized. Correcting the market failure of externalized costs can happen through public policy or changes in corporation practice and governance. Some of the costs that are externalized along the food supply chain include the costs of water, air, and soil pollution; the difference between wages paid and living wages; the costs of healthcare for uninsured workers; the costs of greenhouse gas emissions; and the costs of poor animal care and management. Public policy corrections for externalized costs are often thought of as fiscal policies that collect taxes and subsidies. For instance, collecting taxes on sugar-sweetened beverages to pay for the health consequences of excess sugar consumption is a market correction of the externalized health costs of sugar.

Correcting market failures for pollution have been proposed, including charging discharge fees and taxing for emissions (i.e., polluter pays).[40] Each of these requires a regulatory framework that describes what polluting activities are, how much pollution costs society and therefore should be paid by polluters, and who all the responsible parties are. For instance, releasing chicken manure into a river through farm runoff might be the responsibility of the individual chicken farmer, the corporation that contracts the farmer to raise chickens, or the community with poor stormwater management. Given the complications of developing regulations for these systems, polluter pays policies have not gained traction in many places. Some countries in the European Union do charge "green taxes" for undesirable agricultural practices.[41]

Market incentives, such as subsidizing conservation activities (e.g., crop rotations or forest management) or tying the receipt of production subsidies to particular conservation practices, are also used to internalize the costs of ecosystem services by redirecting agriculture practices toward environmentally friendly approaches. Likewise, market incentives can and are used to encourage agricultural practices that support fair wages and conservative energy use. The challenge of using market incentives to increase the sustainability of human food systems is similar to using taxes and fees. Each of these approaches requires that policy-makers can agree on and estimate the cost of the negative impacts of a food system practice and that they have the political will to pay incentives or charge taxes to make the market correction. Agriculture, however, is a "frontier economic" activity that encourages that the location of production is removed from the externalized costs. In short, farmers prefer that wastes are downwind, downstream, and off the farm and therefore do not perceive their impact in the same way as people living where the wastes are located. This distance between people affected by market failures and those externalizing the costs of production creates contention in the process of assigning responsibility and costs.[40]

Ensuring the Rights of Nature, Humans, and Communities

Public policy can also be used to develop a legal framework for nature, human, and community rights. **Rights of Nature** are laws that recognize that ecosystems, such as oceans, rivers, and forests, have as much a right to live as humans. The traditional framework for these systems has been to treat them as private property, and Rights of Nature laws instead focus on the right of an ecosystem to exist, persist, and regenerate. Bolivia wrote the Universal Declaration of the Rights of Mother Earth in 2010 and ratified it into Bolivian law.[42] Following this lead, other communities have passed laws recognizing the rights of particular ecosystems, including the Colombian Amazon Rainforest, the Te Urewera forest and Whanganui River of New Zealand, and the Ganges and Yamuna rivers in India.[43] In 2019, Toledo, Ohio residents passed a law recognizing the rights of Lake Erie. The law recognizes the right of the lake to exist, flourish, and naturally evolve, and gives residents of Toledo the ability to sue polluters on behalf of the lake. Rights of Nature laws are new, and as they develop, they are likely to be challenged based on the laws that create a crisis of community governance.

Numerous human rights, as elaborated first in the 1948 Universal Declaration of Human Rights, are supportive of the right to food. For brevity's sake, we focus here only on the right to food. The right to food as defined by the Food and Agriculture Organization is the right to feed oneself adequately. In 1976, the General Assembly of the United Nations developed the International Covenant on Economic, Social, and Cultural Rights (ICESCR). It recognizes the right of everyone to an adequate standard of living including adequate food. In 2016, 164 state parties have adopted the covenant. The United States is not a state party. Twenty-three countries have explicit laws that protect the right to food of some or all of the population. For instance, Bolivia, Ecuador, Brazil, Haiti, Kenya, South Africa, Nepal, and Nicaragua all explicitly recognize the rights of all their citizens to food. Costa Rica recognizes the rights to food for indigenous populations, and Colombia, Cuba, Honduras, Mexico, Panama, and Paraguay recognize children's right to food. Another 31 countries have implicit laws that recognize the right to food within a broader human rights framework.

Rights to food laws create state obligations to monitor food security, implement changes across the food system, and create transparent and participatory processes for enforcing rights. In Brazil, the Fome Zero movement created 7,000 local capacity-building projects that distributed food, generated income, established urban vegetable gardens, and supported agrarian reforms. This movement supported rights to food legislation in Brazil. A National Council for Food and

Nutritional Security (CONSEA) was developed of civil and governmental stakeholders to consider food rights, and a working group reviews all Brazilian policies for their compliance with the right to food.

Some communities and countries have recognized the right to food sovereignty. In 2018, the state of Maine passed An Act to Recognize Local Control Regarding Food Systems. After the state law, cities and towns passed local ordinances in support of the state law. The Maine policy encourages food self-sufficiency for citizens through (a) local control, which preserves the ability of communities to produce, process, sell, purchase, and consume local foods; (b) small-scale farming and food production to preserve family farms and local foodways; (c) improved health and well-being by reducing hunger and improved access to wholesome, nutritious, and sustainable farms and fish; (d) self-reliance and personal responsibility promotion by allowing individuals to prepare, process, advertise, and sell food directly to consumers; and (e) rural economic development that supports the environmental and social wealth of rural communities. Communities that participate by developing a local ordinance are freed from state regulations and some federal rules as well, such as requiring kitchen licensing for selling processed foods directly to consumers. Such food sovereignty laws may have unintended consequences of decreased food safety, although communities with such laws have not had increases in food-borne illnesses.

Agroecological Systems

Agroecological systems are designed agricultural systems that integrate social and ecological principles and that seek to optimize interactions among plants, animals, humans, and the environment. Agroecological projects operate on 10 principles described by the Food and Agricultural Organization (Box 16.2). Agroecology is not a new practice, as most traditional and indigenous communities produce human food based on these principles, but several projects around the world have sustainably intensified food production using these projects (Case Study 2).

BOX 16.2

AGROECOLOGICAL SYSTEM PRINCIPLES (FAO)

1. **Diversity.** Agroecological systems maximize diversity of species and genetic resources in a variety of ways. Agroforestry systems organize plants and trees of different heights to mimic forest stories and allow for complementary intercropping. Likewise, people and other species eating in an agroecological system are eating a more diverse diet, and diverse animal and plant crops enhance the diversity of insect and supporting microbiomes, increasing soil health and resilience.

2. **Cocreation** and sharing of knowledge. Agroecology is local and therefore requires local adaptations to environmental, social, economic, and political contexts. Thus, agroecology requires participatory knowledge creation where traditional and indigenous knowledge and scientific knowledge are all used to develop a local agroecological system.

(continued)

BOX 16.2

AGROECOLOGICAL SYSTEM PRINCIPLES (*CONTINUED*)

3. **Synergy.** Agroecology seeks to create synergies across key functions in the food system. Biological synergies might include planting nitrogen-fixing alongside sugar-producing plants. Rice paddies might integrate fish and ducks. At the landscape level, agroecology uses trees and terracing to control soil erosion and manage water.

4. **Efficiency.** Agroecological systems are designed to use abundant and free natural resources, such as solar energy and atmospheric carbon and nitrogen, to produce food. Agroecological systems often have higher yield ratios than other systems.

5. **Recycling.** Natural ecosystems do not create "waste" and therefore agroecological systems imitate this by recycling nutrients, biomass, and water in the system. For instance, deep-rooted trees capture nutrients that shallow-rooted annual crops cannot, and leaf mulch from those trees can nourish annual crops.

6. **Resilience.** Agroecological systems have a greater capacity to recover from shocks, such as drought, floods, hurricanes, or pest attacks. For instance, the water management practices of agroforestry and cover cropping retain more topsoil in floods than other systems.

7. **Human and social values.** Agroecological systems value human dignity, equity, and inclusion by putting the people who produce, distribute, and consume in the system at the center of all decision-making.

8. **Culture and food traditions.** Agroecological systems seek to reintegrate humans with their local ecology and therefore the cultural skills, traditions, and adaptations that fit locally are honored and integrated. For instance, culinary traditions around locally adapted food varieties are core knowledge for agroecological systems. Appalachian Americans' tradition of gathering and cooking ramps in the springtime is a culinary tradition that integrates humans with their local environment.

9. **Responsible governance.** Agroecological systems need transparent, accountable, and inclusive mechanisms of governance to make agroecology possible and sustainable. For example, land governance would ensure the rights of the rural poor to access ecosystem services for agroecology.

10. **Circular and solidarity economy.** Agroecological systems support local producers and consumers through virtuous circles of economic development that increase incomes of food producers and maintain fair prices for consumers.

Perhaps the most dramatic of these projects is the Loess Plateau in China.[44] The region was named for dry powdery soil that blew in the wind after centuries of land degradation through agriculture. An agroecology project worked with local farmers to institute several changes, including farmers retaining rights to lands they worked, contouring and terracing hills for soil retention, planting trees to manage soil erosion, and managing animal grazing. The results were that 2.5 million people in four poor provinces were lifted out of poverty as farmer incomes more than doubled from $70 per person to $200 per person. The natural vegetation cover increased from 17% to 24%. Soil erosion into the Yellow River decreased by more than 100 million tons per year. Food security increased as not only grain production increased in the region, but also a wide range of high-quality and high-value products were grown.

SUMMARY STATEMENTS ON FOOD AND SUSTAINABILITY

Given the urgency of the E4 crisis and the potential of economic, rights-based, and agroecological approaches to quickly address unsustainable human food system practices, numerous consensus statements of nutrition and sustainability have been released. Here we summarize and evaluate the statement from the Sustainable Development Goals, Healthy People 2020 and 2030 goals and objectives, and the EAT-Lancet Commission report on human diet in the Anthropocene. We provide Tables 16.1 and 16.2 to summarize the extent to which these statements address challenges identified in this chapter and use approaches described here.

Sustainable Development Goals

In 2015, the United Nations adopted the 2030 Agenda for Sustainable Development. This high-level commitment includes 17 goals with accompanying strategies focused first and foremost on eliminating poverty in all its forms and second on healing and securing the planet. The 17 Sustainable Development Goals incorporate principles of agroecology, call for market corrections, and focus on human rights assurances. In particular, the Sustainable Development Goal to eliminate hunger by 2030 focuses on the dangerous role of trade liberalization policies in threatening the sustainable livelihoods of people all over the world, stating that to eliminate hunger we need to "prevent distortions in world agricultural markets, including the elimination of all forms of agricultural export subsidies. Those subsidies mask market signals, reduce competitiveness and can lead to environmental damage and the inequitable distribution of benefits."[45] Likewise, in the same goal, a strong emphasis is placed on agroecological sustainable intensification of agriculture, in particular, agrobiodiversity.

Healthy People 2020 and 2030

Healthy People 2020 does not have an explicit goal related to the health or sustainability of human food systems. It does include objectives related to environmental health, nutrition, and social determinants of health that are directly related to the E4 crisis of sustainability. Environmental health objectives include a focus on water conservation and eutrophication (e.g., clean beaches) as well as a reduction in pesticide exposures. Likewise, the social determinants of health framework used to develop 2020 goals employs rights-based approaches to ensuring health, such as ending poverty and child hunger and reducing food insecurity. The 2030 framework similarly employs environmental, social, and nutritional objectives that could address human food system sustainability through public health.

EAT-Lancet Commission on Food in the Anthropocene

In 2019, a Lancet Commission released a report that outlined five key strategies for a healthy and sustainable diet using an ecological economics framework.[46] The strategies included:

1. Seeking international and national commitments to shift toward healthy diets. Healthy diets, as defined by the commission, are those that focused on plant-based foods and substantially reducing consumption of animal foods and sugar.

(*text continues on page 434*)

TABLE 16.1 SUMMARY STATEMENT GOALS, OBJECTIVES, OR RECOMMENDATIONS THAT RELATE TO AREAS OF THE HUMAN FOOD SYSTEM CRISES IN ENVIRONMENT, ENERGY, ECONOMICS, AND EQUALITY

	ENVIRONMENT						ENERGY		ECONOMICS			INEQUALITY		
	SOIL	WATER	PHOSPHORUS	NITROGEN	BIODIVERSITY	CARBON	FOSSIL FUELS	RENEWABLE ENERGY	FOCUS ON GROWTH	EXTERNALIZED COSTS	TRADE LIBERALIZATION	COMMUNITY GOVERNANCE	DISTRIBUTION OF FOOD	AUSTERITY
Sustainable Development Goals														
1. No poverty														X
2. Zero hunger					X						X	X	X	X
3. Good health and well-being														X
4. Quality education														X
5. Gender equality														X
6. Clean water and sanitation		X												
7. Affordable, clean energy							X	X						
8. Decent work and economic growth									X					
9. Industry, infrastructure, innovation									X					
10. Reduce inequality														X

TABLE 16.1 SUMMARY STATEMENT GOALS, OBJECTIVES, OR RECOMMENDATIONS THAT RELATE TO AREAS OF THE HUMAN FOOD SYSTEM CRISES IN ENVIRONMENT, ENERGY, ECONOMICS, AND EQUALITY (continued)

	ENVIRONMENT						ENERGY		ECONOMICS			INEQUALITY		
	SOIL	WATER	PHOSPHORUS	NITROGEN	BIODIVERSITY	CARBON	FOSSIL FUELS	RENEWABLE ENERGY	FOCUS ON GROWTH	EXTERNALIZED COSTS	TRADE LIBERALIZATION	COMMUNITY GOVERNANCE	DISTRIBUTION OF FOOD	AUSTERITY
11. Sustainable cities and communities												X		
12. Responsible consumption and production										X	X			
13. Climate action						X								
14. Life below water					X									
15. Life on land					X									
16. Peace, justice, and strong institutions												X	X	X
17. Partnerships for goals												X		
Healthy People 2020 and 2030														
Environmental Heath Objectives														
6. Reduce per capita water withdrawals and consumption		X												
7. Increase the numbers of days that beaches are open for swimming		X												
10. Reduce pesticide exposures that result in visits to ED					X									

(continued)

TABLE 16.1 SUMMARY STATEMENT GOALS, OBJECTIVES, OR RECOMMENDATIONS THAT RELATE TO AREAS OF THE HUMAN FOOD SYSTEM CRISES IN ENVIRONMENT, ENERGY, ECONOMICS, AND EQUALITY (continued)

	ENVIRONMENT						ENERGY		ECONOMICS			INEQUALITY		
	SOIL	WATER	PHOSPHORUS	NITROGEN	BIODIVERSITY	CARBON	FOSSIL FUELS	RENEWABLE ENERGY	FOCUS ON GROWTH	EXTERNALIZED COSTS	TRADE LIBERALIZATION	COMMUNITY GOVERNANCE	DISTRIBUTION OF FOOD	AUSTERITY
11. Reduce the amount of toxic pollutants released into the environment					X									
20.7 Reduce exposure to DDT (DDE) in the population					X									
Nutrition and Weight Status Objectives														
4. Increase the proportion of Americans who have access to a retail outlet that sells a variety of foods that are encouraged by the Dietary Guidelines for Americans													X	
13. Reduce household food insecurity and in doing so reduce hunger														X
Social Determinants of Health Objectives														
2. Proportion of persons living in poverty														X
6. Proportion of persons eligible to participate in elections who are registered to vote												X		

(continued)

TABLE 16.1 SUMMARY STATEMENT GOALS, OBJECTIVES, OR RECOMMENDATIONS THAT RELATE TO AREAS OF THE HUMAN FOOD SYSTEM CRISES IN ENVIRONMENT, ENERGY, ECONOMICS, AND EQUALITY *(continued)*

	ENVIRONMENT						ENERGY		ECONOMICS			INEQUALITY		
---	SOIL	WATER	PHOSPHORUS	NITROGEN	BIODIVERSITY	CARBON	FOSSIL FUELS	RENEWABLE ENERGY	FOCUS ON GROWTH	EXTERNALIZED COSTS	TRADE LIBERALIZATION	COMMUNITY GOVERNANCE	DISTRIBUTION OF FOOD	AUSTERITY
EAT-Lancet Commission														
1. Shift to healthy diet										X				
2. Reorient agriculture to produce healthy food					X					X				
3. Sustainably intensify production	X	X	X	X										
4. Strong coordinated governance of land and oceans		X			X									
5. Halve food losses through waste									X					

DDE, dichlorodiphenyldichloroethylene; DDT, dichlorodiphenyltrichloroethane.

TABLE 16.2 SUMMARY STATEMENTS ON SUSTAINABILITY AND NUTRITION CALL FOR AGROECOLOGICAL, ECONOMICS, AND RIGHTS-BASED APPROACHES TO IMPROVING HUMAN FOOD SYSTEMS SUSTAINABILITY

	AGROECOLOGICAL APPROACHES										MARKET CORRECTIONS					RIGHTS-BASED APPROACHES		
	DIVERSITY	COCREATION OF KNOWLEDGE	SYNERGY	EFFICIENCY	RECYCLING	RESILIENCE	HUMAN AND SOCIAL VALUES	CULTURAL TRADITIONS	RESPONSIBLE GOVERNANCE	CIRCULAR SOLIDARITY ECONOMY	POLLUTER PAYS PRINCIPLE	FAIR COMPENSATION	FAIR TRADE	STAKEHOLDER CORPORATIONS	MARKET INCENTIVES	RIGHTS OF NATURE	HUMAN RIGHTS	FOOD SOVEREIGNTY
Sustainable Development Goals																		
1. No poverty	X																X	
2. Zero hunger			X	X	X	X	X		X				X	X			X	
3. Good health and well-being																	X	
4. Quality education																	X	
5. Gender equality																	X	
6. Clean water and sanitation			X		X	X			X									
7. Affordable, clean energy				X		X												
8. Decent work and economic growth				X								X					X	
9. Industry, infrastructure, innovation											X							
10. Reduce inequality																	X	
11. Sustainable cities and communities				X		X											X	

TABLE 16.2 SUMMARY STATEMENTS ON SUSTAINABILITY AND NUTRITION CALL FOR AGROECOLOGICAL, ECONOMICS, AND RIGHTS-BASED APPROACHES TO IMPROVING HUMAN FOOD SYSTEMS SUSTAINABILITY (continued)

	AGROECOLOGICAL APPROACHES										MARKET CORRECTIONS					RIGHTS-BASED APPROACHES		
	DIVERSITY	COCREATION OF KNOWLEDGE	SYNERGY	EFFICIENCY	RECYCLING	RESILIENCE	HUMAN AND SOCIAL VALUES	CULTURAL TRADITIONS	RESPONSIBLE GOVERNANCE	CIRCULAR SOLIDARITY ECONOMY	POLLUTER PAYS PRINCIPLE	FAIR COMPENSATION	FAIR TRADE	STAKEHOLDER CORPORATIONS	MARKET INCENTIVES	RIGHTS OF NATURE	HUMAN RIGHTS	FOOD SOVEREIGNTY
12. Responsible consumption and production												×						
13. Climate action	×					×	×	×	×	×								
14. Life below water	×		×	×	×	×			×									
15. Life on land																		
16. Peace, justice and strong Institutions																×		
17. Partnerships for goals		×							×									
Healthy People 2020 and 2030																		
Environmental Heath Objectives																		
6. Reduce per capita water withdrawals and consumption				×	×													
7. Increase the numbers of days that beaches are open for swimming																		

(continued)

TABLE 16.2 SUMMARY STATEMENTS ON SUSTAINABILITY AND NUTRITION CALL FOR AGROECOLOGICAL, ECONOMICS, AND RIGHTS-BASED APPROACHES TO IMPROVING HUMAN FOOD SYSTEMS SUSTAINABILITY (continued)

	AGROECOLOGICAL APPROACHES										MARKET CORRECTIONS					RIGHTS-BASED APPROACHES		
	DIVERSITY	COCREATION OF KNOWLEDGE	SYNERGY	EFFICIENCY	RECYCLING	RESILIENCE	HUMAN AND SOCIAL VALUES	CULTURAL TRADITIONS	RESPONSIBLE GOVERNANCE	CIRCULAR SOLIDARITY ECONOMY	POLLUTER PAYS PRINCIPLE	FAIR COMPENSATION	FAIR TRADE	STAKEHOLDER CORPORATIONS	MARKET INCENTIVES	RIGHTS OF NATURE	HUMAN RIGHTS	FOOD SOVEREIGNTY
10. Reduce pesticide exposures that result in visits to ED																		
11. Reduce the amount of toxic pollutants released into the environment																		
20.7 Reduce exposure to DDT (DDE) in the population																		
Nutrition and Weight Status Objectives																		
4. Increase the proportion of Americans who have access to a retail outlet that sells a variety of foods that are encouraged by the Dietary Guidelines for Americans																	X	
13. Reduce household food insecurity and in so doing reduce hunger																	X	

(continued)

TABLE 16.2 SUMMARY STATEMENTS ON SUSTAINABILITY AND NUTRITION CALL FOR AGROECOLOGICAL, ECONOMICS, AND RIGHTS-BASED APPROACHES TO IMPROVING HUMAN FOOD SYSTEMS SUSTAINABILITY *(continued)*

	AGROECOLOGICAL APPROACHES										MARKET CORRECTIONS					RIGHTS-BASED APPROACHES		
	DIVERSITY	COCREATION OF KNOWLEDGE	SYNERGY	EFFICIENCY	RECYCLING	RESILIENCE	HUMAN AND SOCIAL VALUES	CULTURAL TRADITIONS	RESPONSIBLE GOVERNANCE	CIRCULAR SOLIDARITY ECONOMY	POLLUTER PAYS PRINCIPLE	FAIR COMPENSATION	FAIR TRADE	STAKEHOLDER CORPORATIONS	MARKET INCENTIVES	RIGHTS OF NATURE	HUMAN RIGHTS	FOOD SOVEREIGNTY
Social Determinants of Health Objectives																		
2. Proportion of persons living in poverty																	X	
6. Proportion of persons eligible to participate in elections who are registered to vote																	X	
EAT-Lancet Commission																		
1. Shift to healthy diet	X								X								X	
2. Reorient agriculture to produce healthy food			X	X														
3. Sustainably intensify production			X	X	X	X												
4. Strong coordinated governance of land and oceans									X									
5. Halve food losses through waste																		

DDE, dichlorodiphenyldichloroethylene; DDT, dichlorodiphenyltrichloroethane.

2.   Reorientation of agricultural priorities from producing high quantities of food to producing healthy food.

3.   Sustainably intensifying food production to increase high-quality output through efficient uses of fertilizer and water, recycling phosphorus, enhancing biodiversity within agricultural systems, and implementing climate mitigation strategies.

4.   Strong and coordinated governance of land and oceans, including no new agricultural lands, restoration of degraded land, and ensuring that fisheries are managed to support healthy oceans.

5.   At least, halve food losses and waste throughout the supply chain using technological solutions.

These strategies advance our understanding of human nutrition's relationship to the planet in many important ways. The commission did not integrate a complete systems perspective of the impacts of human nutrition on Earth, and future commissions should more directly consider that plant-based agriculture, as cited in the report, is a widely variable activity. Some types of plant-based agriculture, particularly the types focused on high output and efficiency, will continue to have negative environmental impacts whether the crops are spinach for humans or corn for livestock. Other types of plant-based agriculture can actually have multiple systems-level environmental benefits, such as agroecological approaches that integrate forests, rivers, and animal grazing into the agricultural system.

FUTURE DIRECTIONS

While each of these summary statements provides critical agenda setting for policy-makers to improve the sustainability of human food systems, future leadership is needed to fully integrate agroecological, market-based economics and rights-based approaches into our policies. Of particular note is that none of these documents explicitly articulates mechanisms to increase community governance of food systems, change corporate behavior through market incentives, taxes, or changes in incorporation, or using Rights of Nature laws to protect critical ecosystems. These frontiers in sustainability will need to be integrated into future recommendations to fully transition toward a sustainable human food system. Another consideration for future recommendations is a reframing of the role of agriculture in ecosystems. Archeological evidence suggests that humans have a long history of using agriculture to enhance the biodiversity, local water cycle, and nutrient cycling in ecosystems.[47] Thus, land and ocean governance approaches not only need to rein in the excesses of **extractivism** but also empower indigenous and traditional communities to lead the way in managing their local ecosystems. Also notably lacking from these summary statements are explicit actions to develop or maintain cultural traditions and values that reintegrate humans into local ecosystems, such as local food culinary traditions.

Developing Novel Partnerships for Food Sustainability, Security, and Sovereignty

Public health nutritionists will need to become effective partners with several different types of stakeholders to increase the sustainability of the human food system. As agroecological principles emphasize, resolving the interrelated E4 crises will involve cocreating knowledge with indigenous and traditional communities that have wisdom about how to live in local ecosystems. Public health nutritionists can develop such partnerships by developing their capacity to speak multiple languages, approach groups with cultural humility, and address unequal privileges. Interprofessional collaborations are also essential, and novel partnerships could include environmental health advocates; legal advocates versed in community, Rights of Nature, and human rights; and economists familiar with the variety of market-based strategies that can reform food system impacts on humans and ecosystems.

CONCLUSION

Sustainability is a multidimensional concept that integrates our hopes for an ecological, economic, and social future. The sustainability of human food systems is threatened by interrelated crises in energy, environmental, economic, and social systems. Urgent needs to reduce human demands for nonrenewable energy, to build soil, to protect biodiversity, and to close the phosphorus and nitrogen loops locally are balanced against the need to develop systems of governance that allow communities to manage and control agroecological systems, locally and more equitably across social groups. The global economic shift toward **neoliberalism** can be appropriately governed through a variety of market-based mechanisms if systems of governance support better financial and political regulation of large corporations. The United Nations Sustainable Development Guidelines, Healthy People 2020 and 2030, and the recent EAT-Lancet report all make recommendations that support a more sustainable food supply using a variety of approaches. Public health nutritionists can support efforts to create an ecologically, economically, and socially sustainable human food system by forming alliances with communities that are using agroecological approaches to sustainably intensify food production, seeking community rights to govern the food system, and demanding market corrections for externalized costs of food production and processing.

KEY CONCEPTS

- Sustainability is a multidimensional idea that encompass ecological, economic, and social domains. Both equity within human groups and a rebalancing of human relationships with their ecosystem are required for sustained human life on Earth.

- The human food system is facing four interrelated crises: environment, economic, energy, and equity.

- Agroecology is the system of approaches that integrates human food systems and humans into local ecology.

- Rights-based approaches include developing a framework to ensure every human has the right to a nutritious food supply throughout life, protecting the Rights of Nature to exist and flourish, and the rights of communities to govern their local food system and supporting ecosystem services.

- In the current global economy, many of the negative consequences of the food system are external to the cost of the foods we purchase in retail settings. Numerous approaches, from "polluter pays" fees to incentives for sustainable farming practices, can correct market failures such as externalized costs.

- Public health nutritionists can be allies to communities seeking to sustainably intensify food production through agroecological and rights-based approaches by focusing on cultural humility, relinquishing privilege, and study of ecocentrism.

CASE STUDY 1: A CRISIS OF COMMUNITY GOVERNANCE IN THE FOOD SYSTEM IN SOUTH CAROLINA

Farmers along the Edisto River in South Carolina disagreed with a decision by the South Carolina Department of Health and Environmental Control to allow a regulatory permit to Walther Farms of Michigan, which grows potatoes for potato chips, allowing unlimited withdrawals of water from the Edisto River. They were concerned about the amount of water that would be available on their farms if this large farm were allowed to withdraw the 800 million gallons per month needed for irrigation. The Environmental Law Project sued the state on behalf of farmers, community members, and citizens concerned with the environment. The South Carolina Supreme Court ruled that farmers are free to take as much water from the river as they can. Continued pressure from community groups forced the regulatory agencies to set some upper limits on the amount of water that can be withdrawn from the river, but the local community has no authority to limit the size, type, or environmental harms of local megafarms.

Related news articles are listed as follows:

- Potato farm water fight heading back to South Carolina Supreme Court: www.postand-courier.com/news/potato-farm-water-fight-heading-back-to-south-carolina-supreme/article_9733ec4a-a77c-11e7-a417-cfd683b52b33.html.

- Thirsty mega-farms face crackdown after DHEC vote Thursday: www.greenvilleonline.com/story/news/2018/11/09/thirsty-mega-farms-face-crackdown-after-dhec-vote-thursday/1942948002.

Case Study Questions

1. What are the human health consequences of growing potatoes for potato chips?

2. What are the environmental health consequences of growing only one variety of potato over a large area?

3. What are the alternatives that community groups have to protect rivers from excessive extraction?

4. How might a community resist megafarms from locating in their community?

5. Reflection question 1: In what watershed do you live? Check out these tools to learn more about your watershed and how it is impacted: water.usgs.gov/wsc/watersheds.html#Tools.

6. Reflection question 2: What agricultural practices could reduce the amount of water needed? Check out the National Resource Conservation Center for ideas: www.nrcs.usda.gov/wps/portal/nrcs/main/national/nwmc.

CASE STUDY 2: RWANDA'S AGRICULTURAL AND ENVIRONMENTAL STRATEGIES

The country of Rwanda recognizes the effects of climate change and poverty on the country and has developed a cross-sector strategy of green growth that includes the Crop Improvement Program, the Girinka program, and an animal nutrition program. The Crop Improvement Program provides mineral fertilizers and improved seeds to farmers. The Girinka program provides a cow to poor farmers. The animal nutrition program provides an on-farm mix of forage legumes and grasses to raise animals without grazing. Each of these programs is designed to reduce the environmental impact of farming while improving the livelihood of farmers. A study estimated how much food was available in calories and how much emissions were created by each program in different ecological zones in Rwanda. The study assumed that 2,500 calories per day per person was an adequate food availability. The study showed the following results: Girinka reached the lowest number of households, but improved food availability the most among poor households. Thus, Girinka was able to reduce the number of households with less than 2,500 calories per day available by 11%. However, the highest greenhouse gas emissions were also from Girinka households due to manure and methane emissions. The animal nutrition program reached more middle and high food availability households and therefore only reduced the percentage of households with less than 2,500 calories per day per person by 3%. Improving animal nutrition did not increase greenhouse gas emissions as improved feeding tends to lead to less methane emissions from animals. The Crop Improvement Program reached 94% of households and therefore people with all levels of food availability, and it increased the percentage of households with adequate food availability by 6%. It also had the least impact on greenhouse gas emissions.

Case Study Questions

1. Should the Rwandan government consider total calories available as the best indicator of nutrition for people in Rwanda? What else should be considered?

2. Should the Rwandan government consider other factors besides greenhouse gas emissions in evaluating the environmental impact of these programs? What else should they consider?

3. Based on the study finding, how should the Rwandan government implement its policy for green development?

4. Who should be involved in deciding which strategies are selected for green development?

5. Reflection question 1: Check out your carbon footprint at www3.epa.gov/carbon-footprint-calculator. What factors were considered in calculating your impact on emissions?

6. Reflection question 2: What if Rwanda instead took an approach like Bolivia did and ensured human and natural rights? What programs would they consider instead of these three? Check out unfccc.int/files/cooperation_and_support/financial_mechanism/standing_committee/application/pdf/annex_2._implementation_joint_mitigation.pdf.

SUGGESTED LEARNING ACTIVITIES

1. Start a worm bin (vermicompost) to see, up close, how organic matter is created.

2. Research how long it takes to create 1 inch of topsoil.

3. Investigate indigenous foodways in your area.

4. Volunteer at a local farm, river cleanup, or community garden.

5. Grow some of the foods that you recommend that others consume, such as leafy greens.

6. Plant a native food tree in your community. Many communities have tree planting programs.

REFLECTION QUESTIONS

1. Agroecological principles rely on trees with their deep roots, tall canopies, and many leaf surfaces to create and sustain local water cycles. Look around the place where you live. Are trees helping to soak up rainwater? Does your local stream flood often? Where would you place trees in your local landscape to help support better water retention and flood management?

2. EAT-Lancet suggests that certain dietary principles, such as not eating red meat, should be adopted universally across all cultures to support a healthy planet. What are the ecological, economic, and social considerations of creating a universal set of dietary recommendations?

3. Community rights advocates emphasize local governance of the food supply. Look for your community's emergency preparedness plan. Is there a food section? How many days of food are available in your community? How might you sustainably intensify food production and storage?

4. Many people concerned with the sustainability of the food supply get involved with campaigns to "vote with your fork" in which they try to affect system behavior through consumer choice. Consider the example of meat consumption. How would refusing to purchase meat in grocery stores and in restaurants change the role of animals in the agroecology of communities?

CONTINUE YOUR LEARNING RESOURCES

Read more about the planetary boundaries concept from the Stockholm Resilience Centre: https://www.stockholmresilience.org/research/planetary-boundaries/planetary-boundaries/about-the-research/the-nine-planetary-boundaries.html.

Paul BK, Frelat R, Birnholz C, et al. Agricultural intensification scenarios, household food availability and greenhouse gas emissions in Rwanda: ex-ante impacts and trade-offs. *Agric Syst.* 2018;163:16–26. https://www.sciencedirect.com/science/article/pii/S0308521X17301749.

GLOSSARY

Austerity: The policies and practices of cutting government spending on social safety nets.

Externalized costs: Costs of creating an item for sale that are not included in the price. In food systems, some externalized costs include the costs of air, water, and soil that are not paid for by food producers but rather by people living in the communities affected by dirty water, poor air quality, or contaminated soil.

Extractivism: "Those activities which remove large quantities of natural resources that are not processed (or processed only to a limited degree), especially for export. Extractivism is not limited to minerals or oil. Extractivism is also present in farming, forestry and even fishing."[48] Extractivism often involves extracting resources from a resource rich area for sale and use in another area. Countries in the equatorial region are sometimes referred to as subject to the "resource paradox" of being resource rich but cash poor.[49] Products such as bananas, coconuts, and chocolate are agricultural examples of global extractivist economies, where large quantities of bananas, for instance, are grown in Central America and the Caribbean for consumption in the United States.

Fair trade agreement: "[P]artnership, based on dialogue, transparency and respect, that seeks greater equity in international trade. It contributes to sustainable development by offering better trading conditions to, and securing the rights of, marginalized producers and workers – especially in the [global] South."[50]

Food sovereignty: The "right of each nation or region to maintain and develop their capacity to produce basic food crops with the corresponding productive and cultural diversity. The emerging concept of food sovereignty emphasizes farmers' access to land, seeds, and water while focusing on local autonomy, local markets, local production-consumption cycles, energy and technological sovereignty, and farmer-to-farmer networks."[51]

Globalization: The "integration of markets, transportation systems, and communication systems to a degree never witnessed before - in a way that is enabling corporations, countries, and individuals to reach around the world farther, faster, deeper, and cheaper than ever before, and in a way that is enabling the world to reach into corporations, countries, and individuals farther, faster, deeper, and cheaper than ever before."[52] While globalization has been a part of human social and economic development for centuries, with a great increase in the period of European colonization of the Americas, Africa, and Asia, globalization as we describe in this section is a process that really began in the post–World War II period.

Neoliberalism: A political economy that focuses on free market capitalism with policies that focus on trade liberalization, austerity, deregulation, and privatization. Neoliberalism seeks to reduce the role of the public sector to create more of a role for the private sector.

Resilience: "The ability of a system—like a family, a country, or Earth's biosphere—to cope with short-term disruptions and adapt to long-term changes without losing its essential character." While sustainability focuses on outcomes, resilience focuses on process. "Building resilience means intentionally guiding a system's process of adaptation so as to preserve some qualities and allow others to fade away, all while retaining the essence—or *identity*—of the system. In a human community, identity is essentially determined by what people value about where they live; therefore, the *people* who inhabit a community must be at the heart of the resilience-building process."[53]

Rights of Nature: The rights of ecosystems to exist, persist, and flourish. Rights of Nature are part of indigenous and traditional understandings of human food systems and have been written into laws in countries, such as Bolivia, Ecuador, and New Zealand. When the rights of a natural ecosystem, such as a forest or river, are recognized, then human advocates have legal recourse to protect the ecosystem against extractivism.[54]

Stakeholder corporation: A corporation that is legally bound to seek the best interests of all stakeholders, including workers, customers, and neighbors rather than the financial interests of shareholders (i.e., shareholder corporations). Stakeholder corporations are a way of reforming corporate behavior by engaging a wider set of voting members in the corporation's decisions and changing the primary focus from profit to social good.

Sustainability: "Development that meets the needs of the present without compromising the ability of future generations to meet their own needs."[55] Many organizations focus on three Ps to define sustainability—people, planet, and profit.[45] Sustainability requires intergenerational equity (people), maintenance of Earth's ecosystems (planet), and the ability of people to exchange goods and services fairly (profit). Others focus on the sustainability crisis in the four Es—environment, energy, equity, and economy.[1] In this view, extractivist capitalism (economy) depletes natural resources (environment), using nonrenewable energy sources (energy), and creating and perpetuating poverty and institutional racism (equity).

Trade liberalization: The removal of barriers to the free movement of goods between countries, including tariffs, licensing, and quotas. Trade liberalization often is accomplished through free trade agreements. Agricultural products and environmental protections are subject to free trade agreements and limit local groups' abilities to implement environmental conservation and social justice initiatives.

REFERENCES

1. Lerch D. *The Community Resilience Reader: Essential Resources for an Era of Upheaval.* Washington, DC: Island Press; 2017.
2. Leopold A. The land ethic. In: Ndubisi FO, ed. *The Ecological Design and Planning Reader.* New York, NY: Springer Publishing Company; 2014:108–121.
3. Food and Agriculture Organization. *Status of the World's Soil Resources (SWSR)–Main Report.* Rome, Italy: Food and Agriculture Organization of the United Nations and Intergovernmental Technical Panel on Soils; 2015;650.
4. Intergovernmental Science-Policy Platform on Biodiversity and Ecosystem Services. *The IPBES Assessment Report on Land Degradation and Restoration.* Bonn, Germany: Secretariat of the Intergovernmental Science-Policy Platform on Biodiversity and Ecosystem Services; 2018.
5. Magdoff F, Van Es H. *Building Soils for Better Crops.* Beltsville, MA: Sustainable Agriculture Network; 2000.
6. Famiglietti JS. The global groundwater crisis. *Nat Clim Chang.* 2014;4(11):945. doi:10.1038/nclimate2425
7. Richey AS, Thomas BF, Lo MH, et al. Quantifying renewable groundwater stress with GRACE. *Water Resour Res.* 2015;51(7):5217–5238. doi:10.1002/2015WR017349
8. Murray–Darling Basin Authority. *Guide to the Proposed Basin Plan.* Canberra, Australia: Murray–Darling Basin Authority; 2010.
9. Anderson J. The environmental benefits of water recycling and reuse. *Water Sci Technol Water Supply.* 2003;3(4):1–10. doi:10.2166/ws.2003.0041
10. Locatelli B, Vignola R. Managing watershed services of tropical forests and plantations: can meta-analyses help? *For Ecol Manag.* 2009;258(9):1864–1870. doi:10.1016/j.foreco.2009.01.015
11. Wright JS, Fu R, Worden JR, et al. Rain forest-initiated wet season onset over the southern Amazon. *Proc Natl Acad Sci U S A.* 2017;114(32):8481–8486. doi:10.1073/pnas.1621516114
12. Pimentel D, Pimentel M, Karpenstein-Machan M. Energy use in agriculture: an overview. *Agricultural Engineering International: CIGR Journal.* 1999. www.cigrjournal.org/index.php/Ejournal/article/view/1044
13. Munch J, Velthof GL. Denitrification and agriculture. In: Bothe H, Ferguson SJ, Newton WE, eds. *Biology of the Nitrogen Cycle.* St. Louis, MO: Elsevier Science; 2007:331–341.
14. Cordell D, Drangert J-O, White S. The story of phosphorus: global food security and food for thought. *Glob Environ Chang.* 2009;19(2):292–305. doi:10.1016/j.gloenvcha.2008.10.009
15. Ashley K, Cordell D, Mavinic D. A brief history of phosphorus: from the philosopher's stone to nutrient recovery and reuse. *Chemosphere.* 2011;84(6):737–746. doi:10.1016/j.chemosphere.2011.03.001
16. Potts SG, Imperatriz-Fonseca V, Ngo H, et al. *Summary for Policymakers of the Assessment Report of the Intergovernmental Science-Policy Platform on Biodiversity and Ecosystem Services (IPBES) on Pollinators, Pollination and Food Production.* Bonn, Germany: Intergovernmental Science-Policy Platform on Biodiversity and Ecosystem Services; 2016.
17. Ceballos G, Ehrlich PR, Dirzo R. Biological annihilation via the ongoing sixth mass extinction signaled by vertebrate population losses and declines. *Proc Natl Acad Sci U S A.* 2017;114(30):E6089–E6096. doi:10.1073/pnas.1704949114
18. Thogmartin WE, Wiederholt R, Oberhauser K, et al. Monarch butterfly population decline in North America: identifying the threatening processes. *R Soc Open Sci.* 2017;4(9):170760–170760. doi:10.1098/rsos.170760

19. Juers E. Management plan for the rusty patched bumble bee (Bombus affinis) in Indiana (2017-2027). *Reproduction.* 2017;6:7.
20. Dumaresq D, Carpenter D, Lockie S. The human ecology of agrobiodiversity. In: Lockie S, Carpenter D, eds. *Agriculture, Biodiversity and Markets: Livelihoods and Agroecology in Comparative Perspective.* London, UK: Earthscan Publications; 2010.
21. Center for Sustainable Systems. *U.S. Food System Factsheet.* Ann Arbor, MI: Center for Sustainable Systems; 2017.
22. Pimentel D, Williamson S, Alexander CE, et al. Reducing energy inputs in the US food system. *Hum Ecol.* 2008;36(4):459–471. doi:10.1007/s10745-008-9184-3
23. Heinberg R, Fridley D. Other uses of fossil fuels: the substitution challenge continues. In: Heinberg R, Fridley D. *Our Renewable Future.* New York, NY: Springer Publishing Company; 2016:95–113.
24. Szigeti C, Tóth G, Borzán A, Farkas S. GDP alternatives and their correlations. *J Environ Sustain.* 2013;3(3):3. doi:10.14448/jes.03.0002
25. Otero G, Pechlaner G, Gürcan EC. The political economy of "food security" and trade: uneven and combined dependency. *Rural Sociol.* 2013;78(3):263–289. doi:10.1111/ruso.12011
26. United States Environmental Protection Agency. *A Compilation of Cost Data Associated With the Impacts and Control of Nutrient Pollution.* Washington, DC: U.S. Environmental Protection Agency; 2015.
27. Raworth K. A doughnut for the anthropocene: humanity's compass in the 21st century. *Lancet Planet Health.* 2017;1(2):e48–e49. doi:10.1016/S2542-5196(17)30028-1
28. Shubik M. *Simecs, Ithaca Hours, Berkshares, Bitcoins and Walmarts.* Cowles Foundation Discussion Paper No. 1947. 2014. https://ssrn.com/abstract=2435902
29. Ostrom E. *Design principles of robust property-rights institutions: what have we learned.* 2008.
30. Weiland PS. Federal and state preemption of environmental law: a critical analysis. *Harv Environ Law Rev.* 2000;24:237.
31. Ripken SK. Corporations are people too: a multi-dimensional approach to the corporate personhood puzzle. *Fordham J Corp Financ Law.* 2009;15:97.
32. Godschalk DR, Brody S, Burby R. Public participation in natural hazard mitigation policy formation: challenges for comprehensive planning. *J Environ Plann Manag.* 2003;46(5):733–754.
33. Delgado CL, Narrod CA, Tiongco MM, de Camargo Barros GSA. *Determinants and Implications of the Growing Scale of Livestock Farms in Four Fast-Growing Developing Countries.* Vol. 157. Washington, DC: International Food Policy Research Institute; 2008.
34. United Nations Conference on Trade and Development. *Trade and Environment Review 2013: Wake Up Before It's Too Late.* Geneva, Switzerland: United Nations Conference on Trade and Development; 2013.
35. Ifanti AA, Argyriou AA, Kalofonou FH, Kalofonos HP. Financial crisis and austerity measures in Greece: their impact on health promotion policies and public health care. *Health Policy.* 2013;113(1–2):8–12. doi:10.1016/j.healthpol.2013.05.017
36. Pappas TS, O'Malley E. Civil compliance and "political Luddism" explaining variance in social unrest during crisis in Ireland and Greece. *Am Behav Sci.* 2014;58(12):1592–1613. doi:10.1177/0002764214534663
37. Dowler E, Lambie-Mumford H. Introduction: hunger, food and social policy in austerity. *Soc Policy Soc.* 2015;14(3):411–415. doi:10.1017/S1474746415000159
38. Stuckler D, Basu S. How austerity kills. *The New York Times.* May 12, 2013.
39. Macy J, Johnstone C. *Active Hope: How to Face the Mess We're in Without Going Crazy.* Novato, CA: New World Library; 2012.
40. Buttel FH. Internalizing the societal costs of agricultural production. *Plant Physiol.* 2003;133(4):1656–1665. doi:10.1104/pp.103.030312
41. Albrecht J. The use of consumption taxes to re-launch green tax reforms. *Int Rev Law Econ.* 2006;26(1):88–103. doi:10.1016/j.irle.2006.05.007
42. Vidal J. Bolivia enshrines natural world's rights with equal status for Mother Earth. *The Guardian.* April 10, 2011.
43. Community Environmental Legal Defense Fund. *Rights of Lake Erie Recognized in Historic Vote.* 2019. https://celdf.org/2019/02/rights-of-lake-erie-recognized-in-historic-vote
44. Zhao G, Mu X, Wen Z, et al. Soil erosion, conservation, and eco-environment changes in the Loess Plateau of China. *Land Degrad Dev.* 2013;24(5):499–510. doi:10.1002/ldr.2246

45. United Nations General Assembly. Sustainable development goals. *Transforming Our World: The 2030 Agenda for Sustainable Development*. 2015. https://www.unfpa.org/resources/transforming-our-world-2030-agenda-sustainable-development

46. Willett W, Rockström J, Loken B, et al. Food in the Anthropocene: the EAT–Lancet Commission on healthy diets from sustainable food systems. *The Lancet*. 2019;393(10170):447–492.

47. Denevan WM. *Cultivated Landscapes of Native Amazonia and the Andes*. Oxford, UK: Oxford University Press on Demand; 2003.

48. Acosta A. Extractivism and neoextractivism: two sides of the same curse. In: Lang M, Mokrani D, eds. *Beyond Development: Alternative Visions From Latin America*. Amsterdam, The Netherlands: Transnational Institute; 2013:61–86.

49. McKay BM. Agrarian extractivism in Bolivia. *World Dev.* 2017;97:199–211. doi:10.1016/j.worlddev.2017.04.007

50. World Trade Organization. *Who We Are: Definition of Fair Trade*. wfto.com/who-we-are

51. Altieri MA. Agroecology, small farms, and food sovereignty. *Mon Rev.* 2009;61(3):102–113. doi:10.14452/MR-061-03-2009-07_8

52. Friedman TL. *The Lexus and the Olive Tree: Understanding Globalization*. New York, NY: Farrar, Straus and Giroux; 2000.

53. Lerch D. Six foundations for building community resilience. In: Lerch D, ed. *The Community Resilience Reader*. New York, NY: Springer Publishing Company; 2017:9–42.

54. Andrade PA. The government of nature: post-neoliberal environmental governance in Bolivia and Ecuador. In: de Castro F, Hogenboom B, Baud M, eds. *Environmental Governance in Latin America*. London, UK: Palgrave Macmillan; 2016:113–136.

55. Brundtland GH, Khalid M, Agnelli S, Al-Athel S. *Our Common Future*. New York, NY: United Nations; 1987.

FUTURE CHALLENGES, TRENDS, AND OPPORTUNITIES

GIZEM TEMPLETON, NIHAL DESTAN AYTEKIN HATIK, AND
HILARY A. CAMPBELL

LEARNING OBJECTIVES

1. Understand and explain future trends in population growth, urbanization, and climate change.

2. Describe specific challenges that will need to be addressed in the global food system.

3. List several new approaches or agricultural technologies that have been proposed to address these challenges.

INTRODUCTION

Humans evolved while hunting and gathering what was available in their surrounding environment. The beginnings of agriculture—planting, tending, and harvesting foods—changed hunting/gathering **lifeways** and allowed larger groups of people to live in one place. As a result, the food supply became more stable and manageable. More recently, food industrialization had changed food lifeways in ways that are just as significant. Today, more people on the planet have access to food that is grown elsewhere through trade and/or food aid than ever before. This globalization and commodification of food makes understanding the global food system more complex, and more difficult to predict and forecast.

Of particular concern is that the global food system does not feed people equitably or sustainably. According to the 2019 Revision of World Population Prospects, the world population is estimated to reach 9.7 billion in 2050 and 10.9 billion by the end of the century.[1] The estimated population growth adds further pressure to the global food system. In this final chapter, we describe the challenges and opportunities in growing enough food for all people to live a healthy life. We also address the sustainability of agriculture, the equitable distribution and access to food by all humans, and the reciprocal relationship between climate change and farming practices.

GLOBAL HEALTH TRENDS

Set against the backdrop of feeding an ever-increasing world population, supplying food for all people, with diversified diets, is an issue of global concern. After succeeding in reducing the number of people living with chronic hunger over the past several decades, we have reached a stumbling point. Beginning in 2015,[2] the trend of success in eliminating hunger has reversed and each year the number of people going hungry increases. As we are writing this chapter, over 820 million people are chronically hungry, and this number is rising globally.[3] Ongoing hunger has severe consequences, especially on vulnerable populations such as infants and young children. Forty-five percent of the deaths in children under 5 years of age are attributed to maternal and child malnutrition. Globally, almost 50 million children are wasted and 149 million children are stunted.[2]

Hidden hunger, also known as micronutrient deficiencies, affects an estimated 2 billion people worldwide.[4] The most common micronutrient deficiencies are iron, zinc, iodine, folate, and vitamin A. Such micronutrient deficiencies may lead to cognitive and physical disability; preventable blindness; diseases and conditions such as diarrhea, anemia, stunting, and even death.[4]

One in three women of reproductive age suffers from iron deficiency anemia.[2] Iron deficiency leads to impaired cognitive abilities that cannot be reversed. Anemia affects 800 million women and children globally, and iron deficiency causes the vast majority of anemia. Zinc deficiency increases the rate of stunting, puts 1 billion people at risk, and causes 116,000 deaths of children under 5 years of age per year.[5] Vitamin A deficiency causes night blindness for almost 10 million pregnant women and 5.2 million children and 105,700 childhood deaths annually.[6]

At the same time, overweight and obesity are also rising. About 2 billion adults, 40 million children under 5 years of age, and 338 million children aged 5 to 18 are overweight.[2] The overweight and obesity problem is no longer just a high-income county problem. Low-income countries are also facing these challenges, particularly as industrialized and commodity foods spread across the globe. Chronic hunger and obesity are often concurrent problems.

The combination of these three forms of malnutrition (hunger, micronutrient deficiency, and overnutrition), which can be observed in the same country's context or even at the household or the individual level, is called the **triple burden of malnutrition**. The **global nutrition index** is a useful tool for understanding the triple burden of malnutrition as a single statistic at the national, regional, and global levels. The global nutrition index uses three metrics of (a) protein–energy malnutrition, (b) micronutrient deficiency, and (c) obesity (% female obesity). The global nutrition index analysis for 1990–2015 (calculated for 186 countries) shows a decreasing trend in undernutrition but increased overnutrition.[7] The triple burden of malnutrition is considered to be a global emergency. The Food and Agriculture Organization (FAO) estimates the cost of malnutrition as US$3.5 trillion per year, translating into US$500 per individual.[8]

The prevalence of hunger and overnutrition differs depending on the region, country, city, and even postal zip codes. Figure 17.1 shows how variable hunger and obesity are dependent on the region.[9] To generalize, it appears that once a region starts curbing the hunger problem, the obesity problem picks up. This is largely due to a concept called **nutrition transition**, defined by Popkin[10] as the shift toward a Western-style diet higher in fat, sugar, and refined carbohydrates and lower levels of physical activity, which comes as a result of economic, epidemiological, and demographic transition. Although overweight and obesity were once a developed country issue, rising incomes and changing consumption patterns are now resulting in increasing obesity in developing countries as well.

Rapid urbanization and discrepancies in purchasing power are some of the main drivers in the nutrition transition. As a result, populations begin to exhibit an upward trend toward overweight and obesity as well as diet-related **noncommunicable diseases** (NCDs) in urban areas. Healthy diets in urban areas can be expensive and hard to access.[11]

As cities continue to grow, low-income segments of the urban population in particular can find it difficult to afford healthy diets. More than half of the world population today lives in urban

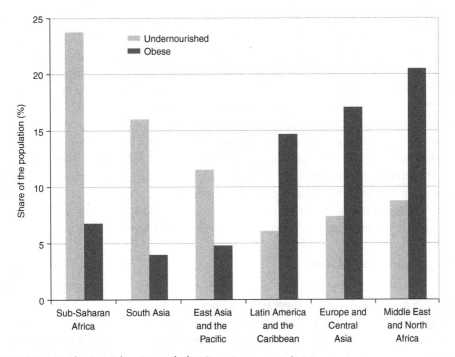

FIGURE 17.1 Undernourishment and obesity rates per region.

Source: From World Bank Group. *Ending Poverty and Hunger by 2030: An Agenda for the Global Food System.* Washington, DC: World Bank Group; 2015. https://openknowledge.worldbank.org/handle/10986/21771 License: CC BY 3.0 IGO.

areas, compared to only one in three people as recently as 1950. By 2050, the urban population is forecasted to be 68% globally. And, as urbanization continues to rise, land and labor dedicated for agriculture will also be reduced. This adds a further dimension of complexity to the challenge of global nutrition.[12]

According to the **Lancet Global Burden of Disease report**, NCDs cause 11 million deaths a year as a consequence of inadequate diets.[13] The Lancet team selected 15 dietary risk factors and looked at the impact of such variables on mortality across 195 nations. The Lancet team found that diets low in whole grains, low in fruits, and high in sodium may be the cause of more than 50% of mortality rates due to NCDs. The team estimated that improving dietary intake of populations could prevent one in five deaths globally.[13] **The EAT-Lancet commission report** presented a framework to reach optimal dietary intake while also focusing on sustainability of food production worldwide.[14] Neither sustainable agriculture nor optimal diets are possible without taking a holistic food-system approach, engaging multiple stakeholders, and a strong commitment.

By 2050, we need to have solutions and systems in place that can feed an estimated 10 billion people. We know that healthy diets play an important role not only for the sustained health of individuals but also for the overall well-being and prosperity of human society.[15] The lack of sustainable and scalable solutions to global hunger has serious consequences.

FOOD SYSTEMS AND ENVIRONMENTAL HEALTH

As explained in detail in Chapter 4, Behavioral Aspects of Public Health Nutrition, a food system consists of everything that happens in the food chain: growing, harvesting, processing, packaging, distributing, consuming, and disposal of food. The global food system encompasses multiple other systems, such as the agricultural system, water system, energy system, and financial system. Multiple food systems—from local to regional to global—coexist, interact, and impact each other. Socioeconomic, political, and economic factors all drive food systems and affect human health and well-being. With the advancements in the industrialization of food, a **"conventional" food system** has emerged. A conventional food system mainly focuses on increasing the yield and production of agricultural and horticultural crops while reducing the cost of food.[16]

Recently, a desire toward alternative food systems has also emerged. The complexity and interconnectedness of the food system calls for a holistic approach to achieve a more sustainable food system, that is, supply safe, affordable, and adequately nutritious food for all. We also need food systems that preserve the environment and are resilient in the face of unforeseen challenges. In this section, we describe the challenges created by the conventional food system, from food waste to climate change to loss of biodiversity, and an alternative model called **agroecology**. We also present different scenarios of the future proposed by the **World Economic Forum**.

Food Loss and Food Waste

As a result of food loss or food waste, we currently fail to use an estimated one third of our food produced globally. Food loss occurs during the initial parts of the food chain (e.g., growth, harvesting, processing) whereas food waste happens at the retail and consumption levels.[17] In either scenario, the overall food system is damaged, whether in the form of missed opportunity to increase access to nutritious food, unnecessary contribution to greenhouse gas emissions, or depleted soil resources. Food loss is more common in low-income countries, whereas food waste happens more in middle-income to higher income countries. Since there are multiple potential reasons for food loss, different approaches should be used to combat this problem.

Food loss, mainly occurring in the developing world, may be minimized by focusing on producer needs. Food producers need public or private investment in infrastructure, storage, and processing facilities, connecting growers with markets to sell their products, as well as increasing knowledge and capacity of food chain workers to handle food safely.[17]

Food waste, on the other hand, could be minimized by focusing on retailer and consumer attitudes. In high-income countries, there are more food/calories produced than the population needs. This results in food waste down the food chain.[17] This may occur by stocking shelves of supermarkets with more food than what can be sold by "sell-by" dates, discarding food products due to minor cosmetic deviations, or the processing facilities or consumers being able to "afford" to waste foods due to their income level or through processing inefficiencies. Increasing public awareness may curb the majority of these problems and could significantly reduce food waste. For example, although more food is being produced relative to population needs in more affluent countries, not all citizens can afford the foods. More attention is being paid to this challenge by transporting foods to people who could otherwise not afford it, donations to soup kitchens and food pantries, or selling so-called **ugly produce** at a bargain price next to the standard-looking produce in the aisle.[18]

Effect of Agrochemicals

To keep pace with the demand for food in the 20th century, rapid increases in agricultural production were driven largely by advances in agrochemicals such as pesticides and fertilizers. However, these chemicals are now known to be associated with negative health effects on exposed agricultural workers, negative effects on aquatic life exposed to agricultural runoff, as well as beneficial pollinators such as bees and animals upstream in the food chain such as birds and small mammals.[19] The global need for fresh water already strains the system, and the need to safeguard water quality and reduce contamination and runoff will deepen.[19]

Increased Urban Farming

Urban farming may also become more common as population density increases, putting pressure on agricultural land availability.[20] Increasing urbanization alongside increasing population growth is likely to infringe on agricultural land adjacent to current urban areas. Researchers have estimated 1.8% to 2.4% of global croplands, particularly in Asia and Africa, could be lost to urban expansion by 2030.[21] Urban food production could result in lowering the energy burden of agriculture by reducing the need for long-distance transportation and large-scale storage, among other mechanisms. However, care would have to be taken to avoid unintended consequences, such as increased energy demand for water treatment and distribution in urban environments as compared to traditional croplands.[22]

Climate Change

Climate change is now recognized as one of the world's most significant public health challenges. Our collective future and global food security are threatened by climate change because it adversely affects biodiversity and rising carbon dioxide levels are projected to cause plants/crops to lose nutrition levels by 17% when compared with current conditions.[23]

In addition, the temperature of the Earth is rising, caused in part by increased carbon dioxide levels in the atmosphere.[24] The **Intergovernmental Panel on Climate Change (IPCC)**[25] estimates global warming will reach 1.5°C above preindustrial levels between 2030 and 2052 if warming continues at the current rate. This could cause increased average temperatures both on land and in the ocean, heavy precipitation in some places, and droughts in other places.[25] Continued rising temperatures will lead to higher sea levels, changes in rainfall patterns, and potentially an increase in extreme weather events.[24] Without substantial efforts to limit global warming, rising global temperatures will cause increasingly catastrophic results.[26]

Crop Yield

An early simulation predicted that crop yield may increase due to higher levels of carbon dioxide available for use in photosynthesis. However, more recent simulations indicate crop yield will likely decrease, especially across tropical areas that overlap with regions that are already struggling with food insecurity such as South Asia and Central Africa.[24] A systematic review suggests that staple crop yields of wheat, maize, sorghum, and millet would be more adversely impacted than rice, cassava, and sugarcane. Rural areas will be disproportionately affected in terms of water availability, food security, and agriculture due in part to shifting locations of food production.[25]

Changes in Nutritional Value

Increased carbon dioxide will affect the nutritional value of some crops, including wheat, rice, potatoes, soy, and peas These staple crops provide much of the protein and micronutrients in the diets of people in low-income countries.[27] Changes in the nutritional value of just these crops are predicted to result in an additional 175 million people to become zinc-deficient. Further, an estimated 4 billion women of childbearing age and children under 5 years of age in countries already struggling with the prevalence of more than 20% anemia would lose more than 4% of dietary iron intake.[13]

Livestock Production and Meat Reliance in Diets

The IPCC predicts that livestock production will be adversely affected as a result of global warming effects on feed quality, spread of diseases, and reduced water resource availability. Fisheries and agroforestry will also be affected.[27] In high- and middle-income countries and in urban areas, among populations, meat consumption generally has been increasing. The FAO data also show a rapid increase in meat consumption whereas a slower increase is shown for fruits and vegetables.[28]

The EAT-Lancet Commission suggests limiting production/consumption of red meat as production causes significant greenhouse gas emission.[14] Another reason for this recommendation is that a portion of the cattle feed could be converted into edible foods for humans. Lastly, the production of feed grain creates its own environmental impact. To date, studies on crop yield changes due to climate change have not rigorously addressed grassland productivity and livestock feed needs. Neither have researchers quantified the potential impact of increased extreme weather events on livestock production.[24] Some researchers advocate for decreased livestock production and decreased consumption of animal protein. They argue that livestock are a difficult-to-mitigate source of increased greenhouse gases that stimulate global warming and climate change.[25] This group advocates increased uptake of plant-based diets and vegetable protein consumption. Insects have also been proposed as a sustainable alternative protein source.[20]

Alternative Systems: Agroecology

Another significant concern for the food and nutrition security agenda is the **global syndemic** of obesity, undernutrition, and climate change. Food systems are significant contributors to this syndemic. Healthy diets tend to be expensive and more challenging for people to access.[11] Our global engagement with both climate change and food security/nutrition needs to be reshaped, bringing in specific attention to equity issues, sustainability, and environmental impact. It is crucial to understand the interlinkage of climate change and the food system so that systematic and holistic solutions can be developed. Agroecology as an alternative to industrial food systems promises to deliver these ambitious goals.[29]

Though agroecology has multiple definitions, it can be broadly defined as a holistic agricultural system that encompasses ecological, social, political, and economical dimensions to result in a sustainable and resilient food system. Agroecology is a circular system, keeping an ecological approach at its heart to mimic natural cycles, such as water and nitrogen cycles. At the same time, agroecology supporters believe that a sustainable food system cannot be achieved in the absence of food sovereignty. Agroecology prioritizes diversity over uniformity and equity over the accumulation of wealth in the hands of a small number of corporations.[29]

Future Food-System Scenarios

The World Economic Forum, with multiple partners, created a scenario analysis report for the future of global food systems.[30] Taking into consideration predictable trends and critical uncertainties, this report highlights the issue that the global food system change can follow many different trajectories. Though it is not possible to predict with certainty, a scenario analysis of these different directions may guide planning and decision-making processes moving forward. The World Economic Forum lays out the four scenarios based on demands (resource-intensive consumption vs. resource-efficient consumption) and markets (high connectivity and low connectivity; see "Shaping the Future of Global Food Systems: A Scenarios Analysis" at www3.weforum.org/docs/IP/2016/NVA/WEF_FSA_FutureofGlobalFoodSystems.pdf). The first scenario is "Unchecked Consumption" in which the demand toward Western-style diets (high in sugar, fat, salt, and animal-based foods) keeps increasing everywhere around the world. Business, government, and society keep making decisions in a "business-as-usual" manner. This is defined as deferring mitigating solutions to environmental degradation to the future, even though most of the environmental issues are irreversible by then.

The second scenario is **"Open-Source Sustainability,"** which is arguably the scenario that places the most number of people in relative advantage. Governments and businesses integrate the Sustainable Development Goals into their strategies. Food value chains become more transparent, and consumers shift toward a more resource-efficient food supply and demand.

The third scenario, "Survival of the Richest," would be caused by public and private sectors acting on immediate concerns as opposed to long-term environment-friendly approaches and governments deciding to protect their countries. This scenario would result in increased malnutrition in all forms.

The last scenario discussed in the report is **"Local Is the New Global."** Governments and businesses focus on sourcing locally and shift toward meeting resource-efficient food supply and demand. Though this scenario would create positive impact for some geographies, others may suffer due to lack of arable land, resources, and technology.

As these possible example scenarios demonstrate, multiple stakeholders (public and private sectors, consumers, and growers) need to work toward a balance in which we can achieve a future global food system that is efficient, sustainable, inclusive, and nutritious.[30]

INNOVATIVE TECHNOLOGIES AND COMMUNICATION STRATEGIES

Biofortification to Address Micronutrient Deficiencies

Micronutrient deficiencies, discussed previously as hidden hunger, affect many people around the world. Low-income, rural families are particularly affected due to limited access to nutritious food. Low-income farming family diets may rely on staple crops that are accessible to them or that they grow, and these crops may not be nourishing enough, resulting in micronutrient deficiencies. There are several ways to address hidden hunger, such as fortification of the foods or supplementation. One complementary convention is **biofortification**, which is enriching staple crops commonly consumed by the rural poor with vitamins and minerals. The goal is to make sure that these populations will have sufficient micronutrient levels to support the healthy growth and development of children to meet their full potential. And also so that adults can live healthy lives and contribute to the productivity and economic development of their countries. The founder of the HarvestPlus program Howarth Bouis shared the World Food Prize in 2016 with other pioneers for advancements in biofortification technology. The **HarvestPlus** program is part of the Consultative Group for International Agricultural Research (CGIAR) Research Program on Agriculture for Nutrition and Health (A4NH). The CGIAR is a global agriculture research partnership with a vision for a food secure future. In partnership with multiple agricultural research centers and local partners, they provide global leadership on biofortification.[31]

Biofortification can be accomplished using three different methods: plant breeding, transgenic techniques, and agronomic practices, that includes examples such as adding vitamins and minerals to fertilizers.[31] To date, all the biofortified crops released through the efforts of HarvestPlus and its partners were developed using conventional plant breeding. By the end of 2018, more than 340 varieties of 11 biofortified crops were officially distributed in over 40 countries, with funding from HarvestPlus and its partners such as CGIAR's International Potato Center (CIP).

HarvestPlus focuses on three essential micronutrients that are often lacking in diets, iron, zinc, and vitamin A in multiple staple crops, such as maize, beans, rice, pearl millet, sweet potato, sorghum, and wheat.[32] There is evidence that biofortification does not compromise yields, are more climate-smart and disease-resistant, and when consumed, biofortified crops generate a significant impact on consumers' nutrition and health. Improved health outcomes such as improved cognitive skills have been documented. Studies show that farmers are willing to grow, and consumers are eager to consume biofortified products.[31]

Use of Big Data in Agriculture

Big data—the analysis of vast amounts of information from many sources—will continue to become an even more important part of agriculture. Common applications of big data in an agricultural context include remote monitoring of crops and field conditions, and precise planting and fertilization activities—also referred to as **precision agriculture**. Big data can also be used for monitoring and predicting weather phenomena that affect crops and informing farming and harvesting decisions. Big data application can also help track agricultural production and sustainability practices and communicate that information to consumers. This would make it possible to "trace a head of lettuce back to the row of the field from which it was harvested" and even "who was working on the crew that particular day." One potential use of this information is better automated data collection to track progress against sustainability goals of consumer-facing companies like Walmart and Unilever. Better and more detailed product tracking can also be used for food safety verification, and foodborne illness surveillance and response. A variety of scanning and screening technologies, alongside appropriately powerful analytic platforms, can be implemented toward this goal.[33]

Nanotechnology also has shown some potential in the form of nanoparticle-based biosensors to contribute to precision agriculture by detecting pollutants and pathogens, as well as monitoring growth and health of crops.[34] However, it is important to note that uneven access to advanced agricultural technology has the potential to exacerbate food system disparities.[30]

Genetically Modified Organisms (GMOs)

GMOs have been around for over 35 years. In agriculture, there have been many ambitions in embarking on this biotechnological journey of gene modification. Even though improving the nutritional content and creating climate change resistance is generally mentioned, the existing genetically modified crops confer three properties around insect damage, viral infections, and tolerance to herbicides. There has been considerable controversy around the public acceptance around the safety of the GMOs. Furthermore, the proprietary rights imposed by the seed companies on the farmers have created additional challenges.[35,36]

Caution is urged as GMOs and other technologies to increase agricultural production are implemented more widely. The agrochemical boom that fueled the "green revolution" doubled agricultural productivity in the 20th century, but also created substantial negative effects that linger long after they were discovered and mitigation was attempted.[19]

FOOD POLICY HURDLES AND BARRIERS

The food system is complex, and policy interventions have many downstream consequences. Today, it is common for concurrent contradictory policies to be in place. For example, this includes efforts in the European Union to increase localization of dairy production at the same time as relaxed quotas that incentivize global dairy competition, which inadvertently work against smaller local dairies.[37]

In the United States, the most significant piece of legislation for both agriculture and food security is the Farm Bill. This is an omnibus legislation that is reauthorized by Congress every five years—most recently in 2018—and that establishes spending of approximately $86 billion per year. The largest budget item is the Supplemental Nutrition Assistance Program (SNAP), formerly known as the food stamp program. More than 42 million low-income individuals receive SNAP benefits, which gives them a monthly budget to purchase food at stores and farmers' markets. The rest of the Farm Bill addresses agricultural topics such as crop insurance and environmental conservation. The legislation is the subject of contentious debate and requires compromise to pass. Some argue that SNAP should be turned into its own separate piece of legislation, and this has been unsuccessfully attempted. Others argue for more provisions that tie agricultural and SNAP provisions together, such as initiatives to increase SNAP enrollee intake of and demand for fresh fruits and vegetables, which would also benefit farmers.[38]

In recent years, in addition to helping people meet their caloric needs, as in the SNAP program, there have been policy initiatives to limit the caloric intake, especially in the form of liquid calories. With the increasing rates of obesity, public health officials and policy makers look for solutions to curb the problem, and decreasing sugar-sweetened beverage (SSB) consumption can be one of the solutions. There have been multiple SSB taxes, also known as soda taxes, passed in different localities and in different countries. There is more research to be done to optimize the amount of tax (e.g. how many cents, on what basis; ounce of soda vs. grams of sugar).[39] However, research has demonstrated that soda taxes prove to be effective in reducing soda consumption.[40] Despite this evidence, the progress to implement soda taxes throughout the countries suffering from the obesity epidemic has been slow. Obesity-related policies that target mainly the food industry have always been met with resistance, mainly due to the strong lobbying power of the global agricultural and food businesses.[41]

ACHIEVING FOOD EQUITY

The current global food system fails to distribute the food grown to malnourished people in equitable ways.[42] One third of the food being grown is wasted or lost.[17] We produce enough food to feed everyone in the world and yet one in nine people go hungry today. There are numerous inequities in the current system, most notably on the basis of income level, race/ethnicity, and gender. With the commodification of food, low-income people have lost their ability to afford food. Ironically, a majority of the people dealing with chronic hunger are employed in agriculture.[43]

In the context of **low- and middle-income countries (LMICs)**, about three out of four people in poverty live in rural areas, most of whom are working in agriculture. The majority of these farmers are undernourished as a result of their income level.[42] The reasons for this situation are not singular and thus achieving food equity in this area will not be simple either. Access to food by the poor is shaped by a multitude of factors, such as land ownership, hourly wages, agricultural vulnerability, access to water, sanitation, storage, and processing technology to name a few.

High-income countries, despite having more food than their population needs, fail to provide equitable access to nutritious food. For example, in the United States, the food system operates through historically established structural inequalities based on a person or community's race and ethnic background, and income.[44] The Farm Bill, as discussed in detail in Chapter 4, Behavioral Aspects of Public Health Nutrition, is a significant shaping mechanism for the food system in the United States. The Haas Institute for a Fair and Inclusive Society defines **structural racialization** as follows: "The set of practices, cultural norms, and institutional arrangements that are reflective of, and help to create and maintain, racialized outcomes in society—reinforcing group based advantages and disadvantages." The impact of racialized policies in the form of health and economic disparities is widely evident. For example, in every part of the food chain, from farm to fork, food laborers of color get paid less than their white counterparts. Neighborhoods with the least access to nutritious foods also house mostly racially marginalized populations.[44] Though there are a lot of charity models trying to address the food and economic insecurities, they result in upholding the status quo, which drives these inequities in the first place.[44]

Gender inequality is also a vital issue of concern in global food security and nutrition agenda. In developing countries, differential food allocation within a household is a key problem. Women or disabled members of vulnerable and low-income families do not get the most nutritious food available to the family.[45]

Women also tend to be disadvantaged in accessing/sharing resources, new technologies, and responsibilities within communities or households.[46] Policies are needed to improve nutrition by increasing women's assets, control over income and decision-making, and through empowerment to make decisions that will enhance family health and nutrition. It is vital to address gender (reducing gender disparities as a cross-cutting issue) in public health policies/strategies/programs.[47]

Investments in nutrition policies and programs also need to focus on adolescent girls, women of childbearing age, and pregnant and lactating women. Malnourished women give birth to malnourished babies. Healthy generations can only be ensured by improving the quality and access to nutritious diets for all. It is crucial to support breastfeeding, provide safe food with adequate water and sanitation as well as education and knowledge and capacity-building in communities.[48]

Similarly, an increased number of studies highlight a direct link between malnutrition and disability,[49,50] and there is a rising interest to understand the links between disability and malnutrition better. Disability-sensitive policies and programs can enhance nutrition and prevent or decrease disabilities and their impact.[49]

CONCLUSION

The current global food system does not ensure equitable access to nutritious food, and this creates a measurable and negative burden on individuals, communities, and society broadly. As a global society, we face multiple challenges such as increase in world population, loss of biodiversity, environmental degradation, and climate change. There are also many opportunities to move toward a thriving society by creating a sustainable food system that respects the environment and provides sovereignty to the communities around nutritious and culturally appropriate food. With the advancements of technology and communication around the globe, food-system stakeholders may choose to coordinate and collaborate toward a just food environment. Though the future by definition is unknown, we have the power to shape it.

KEY CONCEPTS

- Population growth, urbanization, and climate change will put increasing pressure on the food system.
- Future challenges include ensuring food security while also addressing disparities and equity issues.

- Technological advancements and policy levers offer tools to address challenges, but many are controversial, may not be evenly distributed, and can cause unintended consequences in the complex food system.

CASE STUDY 1: FOOD SOVEREIGNTY IN URBAN UNITED STATES: AN URBAN FARMING COMMUNITY IN SOUTH CENTRAL LOS ANGELES

After the Los Angeles riots in 1992, a community garden in South Central Los Angeles was created in a 14-acre vacant land as a Food Bank project to bring fresh fruits and vegetables into a food desert. This land was located in one of the most impoverished areas of Los Angeles, which was a neighborhood of majority people of color. Throughout the years, the community garden turned into an urban farm, which housed 350 families who grew between 100 and 150 different species of plants.[51] The community of mostly Latinx immigrant farmers and African American residents came together to create a microcosm of food sovereignty. It all came to a halt when the real-estate developer who originally owned most of this vacant land came back to reclaim it in 2003. The farming community did not want to leave the land they have been cultivating for all this time. This led to an epic battle, which involved the developer, farming families, local residents, and the city government. Ultimately, the developer won the lawsuit and evicted all the farmers in 2006 despite numerous grassroots movements to preserve it. Though the developer was planning to build a warehouse, the lot remains idle and empty many years after being demolished. You can watch a documentary based on the South Central Farm, *The Garden* by Impact Partners.

Case Study Questions

- When you get involved in an existing community garden or in planning a new one to increase fresh fruit and vegetable consumption, how can you best guide the community you are serving from their land being demolished later on?

- Is it possible to achieve food sovereignty, partially defined as people's right to have control over how the food is grown and the food system operates, in a capitalistic society?

- Have you come across any other examples of nonfood policies impacting people's access to land and nutritious food, for example, zoning?

CASE STUDY 2: VITAMIN A SWEET POTATO IN UGANDA: BIOFORTIFICATION ENHANCING NUTRITION FOR VULNERABLE POPULATIONS

Sweet potato biofortified with vitamin A is a prominent example of how the impact of biofortification has been catalyzed over the years. Its success in enhancing nutrition for vulnerable rural populations was recognized with the World Food Prize 2016. It has also been declared as one of the most innovative ways to feed the planet,[52] and it was among the 25 best inventions of 2016 by Time Magazine. By the end of 2018, 145 varieties of vitamin A sweet potato were released in Africa, Asia, Latin America, and the Caribbean, facilitated by HarvestPlus and the International Potato Center. Biofortification added varying farmer benefits to sweet potato. These are high-yielding, virus-resistant, and drought-tolerant. In addition, biofortified sweet potatoes provide up to 100% of daily vitamin A yields for the consumers. On the other hand, the global estimated prevalence of vitamin A deficiency in children under 5 years of age is 29%. The prevalence is almost 50% in sub-Saharan Africa.[6] Consumption of vitamin A sweet potatoes with high beta carotene content is an effective way of addressing vitamin A deficiency.

Ninety-five percent of the sweet potato is grown in developing countries. It is an important staple food, specifically in sub-Saharan Africa and in Uganda. At the very beginning, implementers were concerned about the adoption of the vitamin A sweet potato by the population in Uganda, due to its orange color. Rural farmers were concerned about the biased knowledge that these products were genetically modified, which was not the case. The reason behind this concern was the limited knowledge and awareness of traditional breeding technologies to produce biofortified crops. Another prominent adoption concern was the changed cooking trait. The vitamin A sweet potato was softer when cooked traditionally compared with the regular sweet potato. Providing nutrition education and access to the nutrition messages, communicating the behavior change in an efficient way, branding with the color "orange," and raising awareness toward the benefits of biofortification were key to attaining success in adoption and creating demand, as well as eliminating the potential bias.

HarvestPlus provided the necessary information and training to farmers on how to use the potato vines for the following seasons sustainably and on the nutritional benefits of the biofortified crop.[53] Women were easier to convince since the mothers were able to observe the positive impact on their children's health (such as reducing the incidence and duration of diarrhea).[54] Becoming aware of the biofortified crops' health impact was effective on several men, as well. However, men were also keen to have their sweet potato the way they were used to, with the same dry structure. At that point, it was important to focus on the cooking traits and let the consumers know that it takes less time to prepare the biofortified sweet potato, which is a benefit. Besides, if they steam it instead of boiling, which is more commonplace, they can still have the same preferred texture of the sweet potato meal.

It has also been crucial to have the ownership of national policy makers and other stakeholders such as the private sector to have vitamin A sweet potato highlighted in the national food system and scaling up the nutrition and health impact.[55] Product and market developments along the value chain were centralized among stakeholders' efforts, and private sector's ownership was crucial in scaling up. Besides, years of effort led to Uganda's inclusion of biofortification in its policies and programs, with the support of the National Biofortification Technical Working Group, established in 2019, consisting of public authorities, and other key stakeholders from the private sector, academia, multilateral institutions, and so on, to promote biofortification in national policies, strategies, and programs.

Case Study Questions

- What would be the best practices to drive the behavior change in a country with cultural barriers? How might adoption be facilitated/enhanced within the community?

- How should the government assess the impact of increased rates of adoption on public health?

- Should the government relate the impact assessment with other indicators besides the nutrition outcomes? If so, which ones?

- Who should be involved in deciding which scaling-up strategies should be in place and implement them?

- Reflection question: Imagine that a nutrition policy officer who works for an international organization wants to decide on an optimum way to make a right investment to overcome the iron deficiency in a target rural population, whose diets rely on staple crops they grow in Rwanda. This population has limited access to nutritious diets and iron supplements, or food fortified with iron is limited. What should be this nutritionist's strategy? Which significant impact would this nutritionist's investment bring?

SUGGESTED LEARNING ACTIVITIES

- Explore these maps (www.impactlab.org/map) and choose a couple of locations to see how the climate change might play out in that area.

- Learn about on-the-ground agroecology practices, saving seeds, and increasing biodiversity on the website www.navdanya.org/

- Trade agreements, transnational corporations, and U.S. agricultural policy are behind the scenes shaping the food environment that you live in. Discover these at the Shahidi Project of University of Berkeley (shahidi.berkeley.edu).

REFLECTION QUESTIONS

- Please read the four scenarios proposed by the World Economic Forum[30] and discuss which one is more likely. Play out the scenarios in a neighborhood/area/region of your choosing, for example, your hometown, a community you are working with, or where you go to school.

- We know that the food system is not racially just, but how would you go about measuring the inequities? Check out these suggested metrics and discuss which one you might be able to use in some of the issues that you are passionate about: www.canr.msu.edu/resources/measuring-racial-equity-in-the-food-system

CONTINUE YOUR LEARNING RESOURCES

USDA Farm Bill Implementation (www.usda.gov/media/press-releases/2019/04/12/usda-update-farm-bill-implementation-progress)
FAO Agriculture/ Nutrition update report websites (www.fao.org/publications/en/)
STAP (stapgef.org/publications)

GLOSSARY

Agroecology: There is no single definition of agroecology. The Food and Agriculture Organization (FAO) organized a database of different definitions. For this chapter's purposes, it is defined as "a more environmentally and socially sensitive approach to agriculture, one that focuses not only on production, but also on the ecological sustainability of the productive system. This definition implies a number of features about society and production that go well beyond the limits of the agricultural field."[56]

Biofortification: This "is the process by which the nutritional quality of food crops is improved through agronomic practices, conventional plant breeding, or modern biotechnology. Biofortification differs from conventional fortification in that biofortification aims to increase nutrient levels in crops during plant growth rather than through manual means during processing of the crops."[57]

Conventional food systems: These aim to maximize economies of scale, lowering overall consumer costs and maximizing production. Conventional food systems generally utilize vertical integration, economic specialization, and global trade. Conventional food systems are based on the low cost of fossil fuels, the manufacturing of chemical fertilizers (also dependent on low-cost petroleum), the processing of food, and the packaging of food. Although conventional food systems often produce more food than alternative systems, they often do so by compromising the ecosystem and the health of the consumer (Food System Wiki).

The EAT-Lancet commission report: 2019 summary report on the convening of 37 leading scientists from 16 countries across a variety of disciplines with the focus of developing global evidence-based objectives for the achievement of healthy diets and sustainable food production.

Global nutrition index: With the understanding that a single number would help rank countries based on the nutrition status, a global nutrition index was created modeled after the human development index. Three nutritional parameters are taken into account: nutritional deficit, obesity, and food security. Nutritional deficit is calculated through the data compiled by the Global Burden of Disease study. Obesity was measured via World Health Organization (WHO) country statistics. Food security was measured by the Food and Agriculture Organization (FAO) data on percentage undernourishment in a given country.[58]

Global syndemic: The Lancet Commission defines global syndemic as the coexistence of "three pandemics—obesity, undernutrition, and climate change. It affects most people in every country and region worldwide. They constitute a syndemic, or synergy of epidemics, because they co-occur in time and place, interact with each other to produce complex sequelae, and share common underlying societal drivers."[11]

HarvestPlus: Organization whose mission is the biofortification of agricultural crops to reduce malnutrition around the world.

Hidden hunger: This also known as "micronutrient deficiencies, occurs when the quality of food that people eat does not meet their nutrient requirements, so they are not getting the essential vitamins and minerals they need for their growth and development."[59] "A chronic lack of vitamins and minerals often has no visible warning signs so that people who suffer from it may not even be aware of it. Its consequences are nevertheless disastrous: hidden hunger can lead to mental impairment, poor health and productivity, or even death."[60]

Intergovernmental Panel on Climate Change (IPCC): The United Nations body for assessing the science related to climate change.

Lancet Global Burden of Disease report: 2017 report on one of the most comprehensive international observational epidemiological studies to date relative to mortality and morbidity due to chronic diseases, injuries, and other risk factors to health at local to global levels.

Lifeways: The customs and practices of a culture or society.

Local Is the New Global: Where governments and businesses focus on sourcing locally and shift toward meeting resource-efficient food supply and demand.

Low- and middle-income countries (LMICs): These encompass the countries categorized as low and middle income by the World Bank. According to this classification, low-income countries have gross national income (GNI) of $1,025 or less and middle-income countries have GNI between $1,026 and $3,995.[61]

Noncommunicable diseases: A disease that cannot be transmitted from one person to another.

Nutrition transition: When diets shift toward higher amounts of processes with lots of fat, salt, and sugar, bringing along related degenerative diseases, nutrition transition occurs. This term was coined by Barry Popkin in the 90s. Many factors, some of which are urbanization, increases in income, and roles both the food industry and the state play, concurrently result in nutrition transition.[10]

Open-Source Sustainability: Contemporary phrase to refer to a variety of questions related to the financial support, burnout, and diversity within the open source community.

Precision agriculture: It "is the application of technologies and principles to manage spatial and temporal variability associated with all aspects of agricultural production for the purpose of improving crop performance and environmental quality."[62]

Structural racialization: This is "the set of practices, cultural norms, and institutional arrangements that are reflective of, and help to create and maintain, racialized outcomes in society— reinforcing group-based advantages and disadvantages."[44]

Triple burden of malnutrition: There are three types of malnutrition: undernutrition, micronutrient deficiencies, and overnutrition. The fact that all three can exist within the same country, family, and even the same person throughout the life span is called triple burden of malnutrition.

Ugly produce: In the conventional food system, only the cosmetically appealing and standardized produce make it to the supermarket shelves. This means "ugly produce" that do not fit the cosmetic standards of retailers get wasted. Starting in Europe, there were food waste reduction campaigns, which sold so-called ugly produce at bargain prices.[18]

World Economic Forum: An international organization headquartered in Geneva, Switzerland that meets on a yearly basis to discuss major issues concerning the world political economy.

REFERENCES

1. United Nations. *World Population Prospects—Population Division—United Nations.* 2019. https://population.un.org/wpp/Publications
2. The State of Food Security and Nutrition in the World (SOFI). *SOFI 2019—The State of Food Security and Nutrition in the World.* 2019. http://www.fao.org/state-of-food-security-nutrition/en
3. World Health Organization. *Global Hunger Continues to Rise, New UN Report Says.* 2018. https://www.who.int/news-room/detail/11-09-2018-global-hunger-continues-to-rise---new-un-report-says
4. Bailey RL, West KP, Black RE. The epidemiology of global micronutrient deficiencies. *Ann Nutr Metab.* 2015;66(suppl 2):22–33. doi:10.1159/000371618
5. Black RE, Victora CG, Walker SP, et al. Maternal and child undernutrition and overweight in low-income and middle-income countries. *Lancet.* 2013;382(9890):427–451. doi:10.1016/S0140-6736(13)60937-X
6. Stevens GA, Bennett JE, Hennocq Q, et al. Trends and mortality effects of vitamin A deficiency in children in 138 low-income and middle-income countries between 1991 and 2013: a pooled analysis of population-based surveys. *Lancet Glob Health.* 2015;3(9):e528–e536. doi:10.1016/S2214-109X(15)00039-X
7. Peng W, Berry EM. Global nutrition 1990–2015: a shrinking hungry, and expanding fat world. *PLOS One.* 2018;13(3):e0194821. doi:10.1371/journal.pone.0194821
8. Food and Agriculture Organization. *The State of Food and Agriculture 2013.* Rome: Food and Agriculture Organization; 2013. http://www.fao.org/3/i3300e/i3300e00.htm
9. World Bank. *Ending Poverty and Hunger by 2030: An Agenda for the Global Food System.* Washington, DC: World Bank; 2015. https://openknowledge.worldbank.org/handle/10986/21771
10. Popkin BM. Nutritional patterns and transitions. *Popul Dev Rev.* 1993;19(1):138–157. doi:10.2307/2938388

11. Swinburn BA, Kraak VI, Allender S, et al. The global syndemic of obesity, undernutrition, and climate change: the Lancet Commission report. *Lancet.* 2019;393(10173):791–846. doi:10.1016/S0140-6736(18)32822-8

12. United Nations, Department of Economic and Social Affairs, Population Division. *World Urbanization Prospects: The 2018 Revision (ST/ESA/SER.A/420).* New York, NY: United Nations; 2019.

13. Afshin A, Sur PJ, Fay KA, et al. Health effects of dietary risks in 195 countries, 1990–2017: a systematic analysis for the Global Burden of Disease Study 2017. *Lancet.* 2019;393(10184):1958–1972. doi:10.1016/S0140-6736(19)30041-8

14. Willett W, Rockström J, Loken B, et al. Food in the Anthropocene: the EAT–Lancet Commission on healthy diets from sustainable food systems. *Lancet.* 2019;393(10170):447–492. doi:10.1016/S0140-6736(18)31788-4

15. Food and Agriculture Organization. *The future of food and agriculture – Alternative pathways to 2050.* Rome; 2018:224.

16. IPES-Food. *From Uniformity to Diversity: A Paradigm Shift from Industrial Agriculture to Diversified Agroecological Systems.* Report by the International Panel of Experts on Sustainable Food Systems (IPES-Food). 2016. http://www.ipes-food.org/images/Reports/UniformityToDiversity_FullReport.pdf

17. Food and Agriculture Organization. *Global Food Losses and Food Waste—Extent, Causes and Prevention.* Rome: Food and Agriculture Organization; 2011.

18. Muth MK, Birney C, Cuéllar A, et al. A systems approach to assessing environmental and economic effects of food loss and waste interventions in the United States. *Sci Total Environ.* 2019;685:1240–1254. doi:10.1016/j.scitotenv.2019.06.230

19. Carvalho FP. Pesticides, environment, and food safety. *Food Energy Secur.* 2017;6(2):48–60. doi:10.1002/fes3.108

20. Sims R, Bierbaum R, Leonard S, Whaley C. A Future Food System for Healthy Human Beings and a Healthy Planet. Washington, DC: Scientific and Technical Advisory Panel to the Global Environment Facility; 2018.

21. d'Amour CB, Reitsma F, Baiocchi G, et al. Future urban land expansion and implications for global croplands. *Proc Natl Acad Sci U S A.* 2017;114(34):8939–8944. doi:10.1073/pnas.1606036114

22. Mohareb E, Heller M, Novak P, et al. Considerations for reducing food system energy demand while scaling up urban agriculture. *Environ Res Lett.* 2017;12(12):125004. doi:10.1088/1748-9326/aa889b

23. Smith MR, Myers SS. Impact of anthropogenic CO_2 emissions on global human nutrition. *Nat Clim Change.* 2018;8(9):834–839. doi:10.1038/s41558-018-0253-3

24. Wheeler T, von Braun J. (2013). Climate change impacts on global food security. *Science.* 2013;341(6145):508–513. doi:10.1126/science.1239402

25. Intergovernmental Panel on Climate Change. Summary for policymakers. In: Masson-Delmotte V, Zhai P, Pörtner HO, et al, eds. *Global Warming of 1.5°C. An IPCC Special Report on the Impacts of Global Warming of 1.5°C Above Pre-Industrial Levels and Related Global Greenhouse Gas Emission Pathways, in the Context of Strengthening the Global Response to the Threat of Climate Change, Sustainable Development, and Efforts to Eradicate Poverty.* Geneva, Switzerland: World Meteorological Organization; 2018:32.

26. Intergovernmental Panel on Climate Change. (2014). *Climate Change 2014: Synthesis Report. Contribution of Working Groups I, II and III to the Fifth Assessment Report of the Intergovernmental Panel on Climate Change.* In: Pachauri RK, Meyer LA, eds. *Core Writing Team.* Geneva, Switzerland; Author; 2014:151.

27. Fanzo J, Davis C, McLaren R, Choufani J. The effect of climate change across food systems: implications for nutrition outcomes. *Glob Food Secur.* 2018;18:12–19. doi:10.1016/j.gfs.2018.06.001

28. Food and Agriculture Organization. *3. Global and Regional Food Consumption Patterns and Trends.* 2015. http://www.fao.org/3/ac911e/ac911e05.htm

29. Burlingame B, Dernini S, eds. Sustainable Diets: Linking Nutrition and Food Systems. Wallingford, UK: CABI; 2018.

30. Nayyar S, Dreier L. *Shaping the Future of Global Food Systems: A Scenarios Analysis.* A report by the World Economic Forum's System Initiative on Shaping the Future of Food Security and Agriculture Prepared in collaboration with Deloitte Consulting LLP. Geneva, Switzerland: World Economic Forum; 2017:28.

31. Bouis HE, Saltzman A. Improving nutrition through biofortification: a review of evidence from HarvestPlus, 2003 through 2016. *Glob Food Secur.* 2017;12:49–58. doi:10.1016/j.gfs.2017.01.009

32. HarvestPlus. *Catalyzing Biofortified Food Systems, 2018 Annual Report.* 2018. https://www.harvestplus.org/knowledge-market/in-the-news/catalyzing-biofortified-food-systems-2018-annual-report

33. Ahearn MC, Armbruster W, Young R. Big data's potential to improve food supply chain environmental sustainability and food safety. *Int Food Agribus Manag Rev.* 2016;19(A):155–171.

34. Ranjan S, Dasgupta N, Lichtfouse E, eds. *Nanoscience in Food and Agriculture.* Cham, Switzerland: Springer Publishing; 2016.

35. Jones HD. Future-proofing regulation for rapidly changing biotechnologies. *Transgenic Res.* 2019;28(2):107–110. doi:10.1007/s11248-019-00143-4

36. World Health Organization. *Frequently Asked Questions on Genetically Modified Foods.* 2014. http://www.who.int/foodsafety/areas_work/food-technology/faq-genetically-modifi ed-food/en

37. Smith J, Lang T, Vorley B, Barling D. Addressing policy challenges for more sustainable local–global food chains: policy frameworks and possible food "futures." *Sustainability.* 2016;8(4):299. doi:10.3390/su8040299

38. Mozaffarian D, Griffin T, Mande J. The 2018 Farm Bill—Implications and Opportunities for Public Health. *JAMA.* 2019;321(9):835–836. doi:10.1001/jama.2019.0317

39. Benjamin BL, Taubinsky D. Should we tax soda? An overview of theory and evidence. *J Econ Perspect.* 2019;33(3):202–227.

40. Park H, Yu S. Policy review: implication of tax on sugar-sweetened beverages for reducing obesity and improving heart health. *Health Policy Tech.* 2019;8(1):92–95. doi:10.1016/j.hlpt.2018.12.002

41. Nestle M. *Food Politics: How the Food Industry Influences Nutrition and Health.* Berkeley, CA; University of California Press; 2007.

42. Food and Agriculture Organization. *Contribution to the 2014 United Nations Economic and Social Council (ECOSOC) Integration Segment.* 2014. Retrieved from https://www.un.org/en/ecosoc/integration/pdf/foodandagricultureorganization.pdf

43. Sharma P, Dwivedi S, Singh D. Global poverty, hunger, and malnutrition: a situational analysis. In: Singh U, Praharaj CS, Singh SS, Singh NP, eds. Biofortifi cation of Food Crops. New York, NY: Springer Publishing; 2016:19–30. doi:10.1007/978-81-322-2716-8_2

44. Ayazi H, Esheikh E. *The US Farm Bill: Corporate Power and Structural Racialization in the United States Food System.* Haas Institute for a Fair and Inclusive Society at the University of California, Berkeley website; 2015. http://haasinstitute.berkeley.edu/farm-bill-report-corporate-power-and-structural-racialization-us-food-system

45. Belinda D, Asiyati C. *Gender and Food Insecurity in Southern African Cities.* Southern African Migration Programme; 2016.

46. Townsend RF, Ceccacci I, Cooke S, et al. *Implementing Agriculture for Development: World Bank Group Agriculture Action Plan (2013-2015).* Washington, DC: The World Bank; 2013; No. 77911:1–132. http://documents.worldbank.org/curated/en/331761468152719470/Implementing-agriculture-for-development-World-Bank-Group-agriculture-action-plan-2013-2015

47. Diiro GM, Seymour G, Kassie M, et al. Women's empowerment in agriculture and agricultural productivity: evidence from rural maize farmer households in western Kenya. PLoS ONE. 2018;13(5):e0197995. doi:10.1371/journal.pone.0197995

48. Branca F, Piwoz E, Schultink W, Sullivan LM. Nutrition and health in women, children, and adolescent girls. *BMJ.* 2015;351:h4173. doi:10.1136/bmj.h4173

49. Groce N, Challenger E, Berman-Bieler R, et al. Malnutrition and disability: unexplored opportunities for collaboration. *Paediatr Int Child Health.* 2014;34(4):308–314. doi:10.1179/2046905514Y.0000000156

50. Kerac M, Postels DG, Mallewa M, et al. The interaction of malnutrition and neurologic disability in Africa. *Semin Pediatr Neurol.* 2014;21:42–49. https://www.sciencedirect.com/science/article/pii/S1071909114000047

51. Peña D. Farmers Feeding Families: Agroecology in South Central Los Angeles, Keynote address presented to the National Association for Chicana and Chicano Studies, Washington State University, Pullman, WA March 4, 2006. Retrieved from https://ucdenver.instructure.com/courses/344129/files/4015468/download?wrap=1

52. HarvestPlus. *Orange Sweet Potato One of the Most Innovative Ways to Feed the Planet, Says USAID Administrator*. HarvestPlus. 2013. https://www.harvestplus.org/node/1818

53. International Potato Center. *Sweetpotato Facts and Figures*. https://cipotato.org/crops/sweetpotato/sweetpotato-facts-and-figures

54. Jones KM, de Brauw A. Using agriculture to improve child health: promoting orange sweet potatoes reduces diarrhea. *World Dev*. 2015;74:15–24. doi:10.1016/j.worlddev.2015.04.007

55. Tanumihardjo SA, Ball A-M, Kaliwile C, Pixley KV. The research and implementation continuum of biofortified sweet potato and maize in Africa. *Ann N Y Acad Sci*. 2017;1390(1):88–103. doi:10.1111/nyas.13315

56. U.S. Department of Agriculture. *Sustainable Agriculture: Definitions and Terms. Related Terms*. Alternative Farming Systems Information Center. https://www.nal.usda.gov/afsic/sustainable-agriculture-definitions-and-terms-related-terms#term1

57. World Health Organization. *Biofortification of Staple Crops*. http://www.who.int/elena/titles/biofortification/en

58. Rosenbloom JI, Kaluski DN, Berry EM. A global nutritional index. *Food Nutr Bull*. 2008;29(4):266–277. doi:10.1177/156482650802900403

59. Food and Agriculture Organization. *What is hidden hunger?* [Video] http://www.fao.org/about/meetings/icn2/news-archive/news-detail/en/c/265240

60. United Nations Regional Information Centre for Western Europe. *Hidden Hunger—Missing Minerals*. https://www.unric.org/en/latest-un-buzz/28946-hidden-hunger-hidden-problem

61. World Health Organization. *Definition of regional groupings*. https://www.who.int/healthinfo/global_burden_disease/definition_regions/en/

62. Pierce FJ, Nowak P. Aspects of precision agriculture. In: Sparks DL, ed. *Advances in Agronomy*. Vol. 67. New York, NY: Academic Press. 1999:1–85. doi:10.1016/S0065-2113(08)60513-1

APPENDIX: WEBSITES WITH EVIDENCE-INFORMED PROGRAMS TO IMPROVE DIET AND EXERCISE BEHAVIORS OF COMMUNITIES

KAREN L. PROBERT AND BECKY ADAMS

COMPREHENSIVE WEBSITES WITH EVIDENCE-BASED PROGRAMS PLUS ADVANCED SUPPORT RESOURCES

Title: CDC Community Health Improvement Navigator

Sponsor: U. S. Department of Health and Human Services, Centers for Disease Control and Prevention (CDC)

Description: The CDC Community Health Improvement Navigator (CHI Navigator) Database of Interventions is a tool that helps you identify *interventions that work* in four action areas—socioeconomic factors, physical environment, health behaviors, and clinical care. The CHI Navigator is a one-stop-shop of program planning resources including the database of evidence-informed programs. A key goal of the website is to support hospitals in improving community health as a hospital shifts from a focus on volume of services to an orientation toward improved health outcomes of communities served. (*Source:* Centers for Disease Control and Prevention. *CDC Community Health Improvement Navigator website.* 2019. www.cdc.gov/chinav)

Title: What Works for Health

Sponsor: Robert Wood Johnson Foundation

Description: "A menu of evidence-informed policies and programs that can make a difference locally." Another full-service website for evidence-informed program planning. The What Works for Health program database is one component of the County Health Rankings & Roadmaps website that also includes information and resources on assessment, prioritization, evaluation, and collaboration. (*Source:* Robert Wood Johnson Foundation. *What Works for Health website.* 2019. https://www.countyhealthrankings.org/take-action-to-improve-health/what-works-for-health)

WEBSITES GEARED TOWARD SPECIFIC FEDERAL FUNDING STREAMS

Title: DNPAO Proven Strategies

Sponsor: U.S. Department of Health and Human Services, Centers for Disease Control and Prevention, Division of Nutrition, Physical Activity, and Obesity

Description: On this website, CDC lists "proven strategies that support healthy eating, physical activity, and breastfeeding in child care, health care, school, worksite, and community-wide settings." (*Source:* Division of Nutrition, Physical Activity, and Obesity. *Division of Nutrition, Physical Activity, and Obesity, Proven Strategies website.* 2019. https://www.cdc.gov/nccdphp/dnpao/proven-strategies.html)

Title: MCH Evidence

Sponsor: National Center for Education in Maternal and Child Health with funding from U.S. Department of Health and Human Services, Health Resources and Services Administration

Description: The evidence-informed program database is one component of the website. The MCH Evidence website is a comprehensive approach to advance Title V, Maternal and Child Health (MCH) Block Grant state plans. The website incorporates the expertise of four MCH-focused organizations and includes an intervention database and innovative technical assistance. Interventions are pulled from Innovation Station, a searchable database of emerging, promising, and best practices in MCH developed by the Association of Maternal and Child Health Programs. (*Source:* National Center for Education in Maternal and Child Health. *MCH Evidence website.* 2019. https://www.mchevidence.org)

Title: Research-Tested Intervention Programs (RTIPs)

Sponsor: U.S. Department of Health and Human Services, National Cancer Institute

Description: "RTIPs is a searchable database of evidence-based cancer control interventions and program materials and is designed to provide program planners and public health practitioners easy and immediate access to research-tested materials." (*Source:* National Cancer Institute. *Research-Tested Interventions Programs website.* 2019. rtips.cancer.gov/rtips)

Title: SNAP-Ed Toolkit

Sponsor: Regional Nutrition Education Centers of Excellence, National Coordination Center at the University of Kentucky with funding from U.S. Department of Agriculture

Description: A collection of evidence-based* obesity prevention and policy, system, and environmental change interventions. The interventions in the toolkit are only a partial list of interventions that are used in SNAP-Ed. All the interventions are intended to achieve the goal of helping SNAP-eligible households make healthy eating and physical activity choices on a limited budget. (*Source:* U.S. Department of Agriculture. *SNAP-Ed Toolkit website.* 2019. https://wicworks.fns.usda.gov)

———————

*Term used on SNAP-Ed Toolkit website but not all interventions meet the strict definition of evidence-based as per the typology for classifying interventions by level of scientific evidence.

Title: WIC Works Resource System

Sponsor: U.S. Department of Agriculture, Food and Nutrition Service (FNS)

Description: "The WIC Works Resource System (WIC Works) is an online education, training and resource center for state, local and clinic staff administering the Special Supplemental Nutrition Program for Women, Infants, and Children (WIC)." WIC Works is "the primary means to share FNS resources as well as resources from a variety of program partners, including WIC state and local agencies, WIC clinics, other federal agencies, and non-government entities that offer WIC-relevant resources." (*Source:* U.S. Department of Agriculture. *WIC Works Resource System website.* 2019. https://wicworks.fns.usda.gov)

WEBSITES WITH EVIDENCE-BASED ONLY PROGRAMS

Title: Healthy People 2020 Evidence-Based Resources

Sponsor: U.S. Department of Health and Human Services, Office of Disease Prevention and Health Promotion

Description: Database with evidence-based resources selected by subject matter experts. Resources must have evidence of effectiveness, feasibility, reach, sustainability, and transferability. Each resource has been rated and classified according to specific criteria. (*Source:* Office of Disease Prevention and Health Promotion. *Healthy People 2020 Evidence-Based Resources.* 2019. https://www.healthypeople.gov/2020/tools-resources/Evidence-Based-Resources)

Title: The Community Guide

Sponsor: Community Preventive Services Task Force

Description: A resource to help practitioners select interventions that improve health and prevent disease. The guide to Community Preventive Services (The Community Guide) includes evidence-based programs that consider health outcomes and cost effectiveness. Findings are describes as recommended with strong evidence or sufficient evidence, recommended against or insufficient evidence. The findings are based on systematic reviews of peer-reviewed literature. (*Source:* Community Preventive Services Task Force. *The Community Guide.* https://www.thecommunityguide.org)

WEBSITES WITH PROGRAMS BUT FUNDING STOPPED

For the three resources listed in this section, a website exists but funding to support continued maintenance has stopped.

Title: AHRQ Innovations Exchange

Sponsor: U.S. Department of Health and Human Services, Agency for Healthcare Research and Quality (AHRQ)

Description: The Innovations Exchange includes clinical and nonclinical activities and tools that vary in their degree of novelty, effect on quality, and level of supporting evidence. Funding ended September 2016 and nothing has been added since. Other current websites pull information from the database on this website. (*Source:* Agency for Healthcare Research and Quality. *AHRQ Health Care Innovations Exchange website.* 2019. https://innovations.ahrq.gov)

Title: Center TRT

Sponsor: U.S. Department of Health and Human Services, Centers for Disease Control and Prevention, Division of Nutrition, Physical Activity, and Obesity

Description: "The Interventions section of the website provides resources designed to support the planning, implementation, and evaluation of evidence-supported nutrition, physical activity and obesity prevention interventions." (*Source:* UNC Center for Health Promotion and Disease Prevention. *Overview.* http://centertrt.org/?p=interventions_overview)

Title: Community Health Online Resource Center

Sponsor: U.S. Department of Health and Human Services, Centers for Disease Control and Prevention, National Center for Chronic Disease Prevention and Health Promotion

Description: A searchable database "populated with practice-based resources to help you implement changes to prevent disease and promote healthy living in your community. The resources include webinars, model policies, toolkits, guides, fact sheets, and other practical materials which are organized by content areas." Most recent entries in the database were in 2017. (*Source:* Centers for Disease Control and Prevention. *Community Health Online Resource Center.* 2019. https://www.cdc.gov/nccdphp/dch/online-resource/index.htm)

WEBSITES LISTING RESOURCES FROM MULTIPLE SOURCES

Title: Collection of Online Resources & Inventory Database: Organized and Readily Accessible (CORIDOR)

Sponsor: U.S. Department of Health and Human Services, Centers for Disease Control and Prevention, National Center for Chronic Disease Prevention and Health Promotion

Description: The resources included on this website "are primarily practice-based and represent science and practice promoted by CDC and CDC-funded partners to address chronic disease conditions and risk factors. Tools include model policies and programs, guides, case studies, toolkits, and other resources for a variety of audiences with a range of skills." (*Source:* Centers for Disease Control and Prevention. *CORIDOR.* 2019. https://nccd.cdc.gov/CORIDOR)

Title: Rural Health Information Hub

Sponsor: Federal Office of Rural Health Policy

Description: This website includes evidence-based toolkits for rural community health. "The step-by-step guides help practitioners build effective programs. Resources and examples are drawn from evidence-informed and promising programs." For some of the websites listed in this section, the Rural Health Information Hub includes the strengths and limitations from the rural perspective. *Source:* Rural Health Information Hub. *Rural Health Information Hub website.* 2019. https://www.ruralhealthinfo.org)

INDEX

CPSIA information can be obtained
at www.ICGtesting.com
Printed in the USA
BVHW051924240820
587197BV00008B/172